OXFORD MEDICAL PUBLICATIONS

# Oxford Handbook of
# Primary Care and
# Community Nursing

D0050582

## Published and forthcoming Oxford Handbooks in Nursing

Oxford Handbook of Adult Nursing
Oxford Handbook of Cancer Nursing
Oxford Handbook of Cardiac Nursing, 2e
Oxford Handbook of Children's and Young People's Nursing, 2e
Oxford Handbook of Clinical Skills for Children's and Young People's Nursing
Oxford Handbook of Clinical Skills in Adult Nursing
Oxford Handbook of Critical Care Nursing
Oxford Handbook of Dental Nursing
Oxford Handbook of Diabetes Nursing
Oxford Handbook of Emergency Nursing
Oxford Handbook of Gastrointestinal Nursing
Oxford Handbook of Learning and Intellectual Disability Nursing
Oxford Handbook of Mental Health Nursing
Oxford Handbook of Midwifery, 2e
Oxford Handbook of Musculoskeletal Nursing
Oxford Handbook of Neuroscience Nursing
Oxford Handbook of Nursing Older People
Oxford Handbook of Orthopaedic and Trauma Nursing
Oxford Handbook of Perioperative Practice
Oxford Handbook of Prescribing for Nurses and Allied Health Professionals
Oxford Handbook of Primary Care and Community Nursing, 2e
Oxford Handbook of Renal Nursing
Oxford Handbook of Respiratory Nursing
Oxford Handbook of Women's Health Nursing

# Oxford Handbook of
# Primary Care and Community Nursing

**Second edition**

Edited by

# Vari Drennan
Professor of Health Care & Policy Research,
Faculty of Health, Social Care & Education,
Kingston University & St. George's University of London, UK

# Claire Goodman
Professor of Health Care Research,
Centre for Research in Primary and Community Care,
University of Hertfordshire, UK

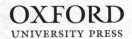

# OXFORD
UNIVERSITY PRESS

# OXFORD
UNIVERSITY PRESS

Great Clarendon Street, Oxford, OX2 6DP,
United Kingdom

Oxford University Press is a department of the University of Oxford.
It furthers the University's objective of excellence in research, scholarship,
and education by publishing worldwide. Oxford is a registered trade mark of
Oxford University Press in the UK and in certain other countries

Published in the United States of America by Oxford University Press
198 Madison Avenue, New York, NY 10016, United States of America

British Library Cataloguing in Publication Data
Data available

Library of Congress Control Number: 2013945066

ISBN 978–0–19–965372–0

Printed in Great Britain on acid-free paper by
Ashford Colour Press Ltd., Gosport, Hampshire.

# Acknowledgements

This second edition builds on the previous edition and the input from all of those who helped us then. Our thanks as ever go to all the nurses and health visitors who provided feedback on the first edition, read and commented on drafts of edition two, and likewise to the former members of the Primary Care Nursing Research Unit (2001–2007) in the Department of Primary Care, University College London. We thank too our anonymous reviewers for their helpful comments and our OUP editors who persevered with us.

As ever, we are indebted to our families who have supported us through a second edition.

# Preface

Primary care and community nurses work in a wide range of settings, their work involves addressing the multiple public health, prevention, treatment, and care needs of their patients and local communities. These nurses include practice nurses, nurse practitioners, district nurses, community staff nurses, health visitors, school nurses, walk-in centre nurses, sexual health and contraceptive service nurses, community paediatric nurses, and occupational health nurses. In an environment of constant change and reorganization, and increasing expectations for what nursing has to deliver for people and families living at home, it is important to have a resource that recognizes the complexity of their work and seeks to enable them to base practice on best evidence.

Primary care and community nurses are both generalists and specialists, working with individuals and their families and carers at different stages of their life. This book cuts across the traditional service divisions between primary care-based specialist nursing practitioners, nurses working in general practice, and those employed by community services. It responds to health policy and professional trends that require a flexible, patient-centred service increasingly provided outside of hospitals. It is a valuable resource for nurses involved in new types of services, nurses in public health, and those with widening responsibilities for health promotion, screening programmes, first contact triage, chronic disease management, care management, and child and adult protection.

This book addresses primary care and community nurses' need to readily access evidence-based information for a very broad range of conditions, and across an extensive range of preventive care and treatment techniques. It is intended as a quick reference source guide for nurses working in primary care and community health services that supports them in everyday clinical decision-making. As well as evidence-based clinical knowledge, the book also addresses the organizational knowledge that nurses need to be able to work in primary care and community, and across different organizations, and the interface of the statutory and voluntary sectors in health, education, and social care. It is written by primary care and community nurses who are directly engaged in current practice, research, education, and policy developments.

We welcome feedback and suggestions for new topics in future editions.

Vari M Drennan & Claire Goodman

# Contents

# Contents

# List of contributors

**Verity Abrahms**
Health visitor,
Suffolk County Council, UK

**Sue Beckwith**
Freelance Nursing Care
Consultant, UK

**Helen Bedford**
Senior Lecturer in Children's
Health, Centre for Epidemiology
and Biostatistics, UCL,
Institute of Child Health,
London, UK

**Jane Black**
Designated Nurse, Safeguarding
Children, NHS Norfolk, UK

**Jane Chiodini**
Independent travel nurse
consultant, www.janechiodini.
co.uk/home/

**Maggie Cooper**
Freelance Cervical Screening
Trainer, www.cscourses.co.uk

**Toity Deave**
Associate Professor for
Family & Child Health,
Centre for Child & Adolescent
Health, University of the West
of England, Bristol, UK

**Catherine Evans**
NIHR Clinical Lecturer in
Palliative Care, Honorary Clinical
Nurse Specialist Palliative
Care Sussex Community NHS
Trust, Cicely Saunders Institute,
Department of Palliative Care
Policy and Rehabiliation, King's
College London, London, UK

**David Elliman**
Consultant in Community Child
Health, Whittington Health,
London, UK

**Suzanne Everett**
Senior Nurse Practitioner,
Camberwell Sexual Health
Department, Kings College
Foundation Hospital &
Senior Lecturer, Middlesex
University, London, UK

**Madeleine Flanagan**
Principal Lecturer Skin Integrity/
Dermatology, School of Medical
& Life Sciences, University of
Hertfordshire, Hatfield, UK

**Penny Franklin**
Associate Professor in Health
Studies (Prescribing), Faculty of
Health, Education and Society,
University of Plymouth,
Plymouth, UK

**Penny Louch**
Clinical Lead/Lead Nurse
Practitioner, Health E1 Homeless
Medical Centre, London, UK

**Caroline McGraw**
Lecturer, School of Health
Sciences, City University, London;
UK & Lead District Nurse
for Education and Training,
Whittington Community
Health Services, London, UK

**Sandra McGregor-Read**
School Nurse Team Leader
School Nursing Service, CNWL,
Camden Provider Services,
London, UK

**Janet Medforth**
Lecturer in Midwifery, Sheffield University, Sheffield, UK

**Kevin Miles**
Manager Health Programmes, Oil Search Health Foundation, Port Moresby, Papua New Guinea

**Professor Christine Norton**
Burdett Professor of Gastro-intestinal Nursing, Florence Nightingale School of Nursing and Midwifery, King's College, London, and Nurse Consultant, St Mark's Hospital, London, UK

**Lynda Roderique**
Senior Lecturer (children's nursing), Faculty of Health, Social Care & Education, Kingston University & St George's University of London, London, UK

**Ann Skingley**
Senior Lecturer, Department of Health & Social Welfare, Canterbury Christ Church University, Canterbury, UK

**Ken Spearpoint**
Consultant Nurse, Resuscitation, Imperial College Health care & Principal Lecturer Medical Simulation, University of Hertfordshire, Hatfield, UK

**Val Thurtle**
Senior Lecturer (health visiting), University of Hertfordshire, Hatfield, UK

**Mandy Wells**
Nurse Consultant, Integrated Bladder and Bowel Care, Exeter PCT, East Devon PCT, Mid Devon PCT and the Royal Devon and Exeter Foundation NHS Trust, and Honorary Lecturer, Kings College, London and University of Plymouth, Plymouth, UK

**Jane Wright**
Senior Lecturer (primary care/school nursing), New Buckinghamshire University, High Wycombe, UK

# Symbols and abbreviations

| | |
|---|---|
| ↑ | increased |
| ↓ | decreased |
| → | leading to |
| > | greater than |
| < | less than |
| ≥ | equal to or greater than |
| ≤ | equal to or less than |
| ♂ | male |
| ♀ | female |
| ° | degrees |
| 1° | primary |
| 2° | secondary |
| ❶ | warning |
| 🕮 | topic cross reference |
| ℛ | website |
| AA | attendance allowance |
| AAA | abdominal aortic aneurysms |
| AABR | auditory brain responses |
| ABPM | ambulatory blood pressure monitoring |
| ACE | angiotensin-converting enzyme |
| ACP | advance care planning |
| ACTH | adrenocortitrophic hormone |
| ADH | antidiuretic hormone |
| ADHD | attention-deficit hyperactivity disorder |
| ADL | activities of daily living |
| ADR | adverse drug reaction |
| AED | automated external defibrillation |
| AF | atrial fibrillation |
| AFB | acid-fast bacilli |
| AIDS | acquired immune deficiency syndrome |
| ALL | acute lymphoblastic leukaemia |
| ALO | actinomycete-like organism |
| ALS | amyotrophic lateral sclerosis |
| ALT | alanine aminotransferase |
| AMD | age-related macular degeneration |
| AML | acute myeloid leukaemia |
| AMTS | Abbreviated Mental Test Score |

| ANP | advanced nurse practitioner |
| AO | accountable officer |
| AOB | any other business |
| APMS | alternative provider medical services |
| ARB | angiotensin II receptor blocker |
| ASAP | as soon as possible |
| ART | antiretroviral therapy |
| ASBO | anti-social behaviour order |
| ASD | atrioseptal defect |
| AUDIT | alcohol use disorders identification test |
| BBV | blood-borne virus |
| BCC | basal cell carcinoma |
| BCG | Bacille Calmette–Guérin vaccine |
| bd | twice a day |
| BED | binge eating disorder |
| BLS | basic life support |
| BMD | bone mineral density |
| BMI | body mass index |
| BNF | *British National Formulary* |
| BP | blood pressure |
| BPH | Benign prostatic hypertrophy |
| BPSD | behavioural and psychological symptoms of dementia |
| BSA | body surface area |
| BSL | British Sign Language |
| BST | British Summer Time |
| BV | bacterial vaginosis |
| CAA | Constant Attendance Allowance |
| CAB | Citizens Advice Bureau |
| CAF | Common Assessment Framework |
| CAMHS | Child and Adolescent Mental Health Services |
| CBA | controlled before-and-after |
| CBT | cognitive behavioural therapy |
| CCB | calcium channel blocker |
| CCG | clinical commissioning group |
| CD | controlled drug |
| CDD | conduct disorder |
| CDRs | controlled drug registers |
| CDS | community dental service |
| CE | Conformité European mark |
| CF | cystic fibrosis |

| CFA | craniofacial abnormality |
| CGIN | cervical glandular intraepithelial neoplasia |
| CHD | coronary heart disease |
| CHP | Community Health Partnerships |
| CIN | cervical intraepithelial neoplasia |
| CKD | chronic kidney disease |
| CLAPA | Cleft Lip and Palate Association |
| CLDT | community learning disabilities team |
| CLL | chronic lymphocytic leukaemia |
| CMHT | community mental health team |
| CMO | chief medical officer |
| CMP | clinical management plan |
| CMV | cytomegalovirus |
| CNO | chief nursing officer |
| CNS | clinical nurse specialist |
| C/O | complain of |
| COC | combined oral contraceptive |
| CONI | Care of Next Infant Scheme |
| COPD | chronic obstructive pulmonary disease |
| COSSH | Control of Substances Hazardous to Health |
| CP | cerebral palsy |
| CPA | care programme approach |
| CPD | continuing professional development |
| CPR | cardiopulmonary resusitation |
| CQC | Care Quality Commission |
| CRB | Criminal Records Bureau |
| CrD | Crohn's disease |
| CRF | chronic renal failure |
| CSCI | continuous subcutaneous infusion |
| CSF | cerebrospinal fluid |
| CSPQ | community specialist practice qualification |
| CSSD | Central Sterile Services Department |
| CT | computed tomography |
| CTC | Child Tax Credit |
| CVA | cerebrovascular accident |
| CVAD | central venous access device |
| CVD | cardiovascular disease |
| CVS | chorionic villus sampling |
| CXR | chest X-ray |
| DAFNE | dose adjustment for normal eating |

| DDH | developmental dysplasia of hips |
| DES | direct-enhanced services |
| DEXA | dual energy X-ray absorptiometry |
| DH | Department of Health |
| DHSSPS | Department of Health Social Services & Public Safety |
| DI | Donor insemination |
| DKA | diabetic ketoacidosis |
| DLA | Disability Living Allowance |
| DM | diabetes mellitus |
| DMPA | Depo-Provera |
| DN | district nurse |
| DNACPR | Do Not Attempt Cardiopulmonary Resuscitation |
| DOB | date of birth |
| DOT | directly observed therapy |
| DPA | Data Protection Act 1998 |
| DRE | digital rectal examination |
| DU | duodenal ulceration |
| DVT | deep vein thrombosis |
| DWP | Department of Works and Pensions |
| EAR | estimated average requirements |
| EC | emergency contraception |
| ECG | electrocardiogram |
| ECT | electro-convulsive therapy |
| ED | emergency department |
| EDD | expected date of delivery |
| EEG | electroencephalography |
| eGFR | estimated glomerular filtration rate |
| EHO | environmental health officer |
| ENT | ear, nose, and throat |
| EoLC | end-of-life care |
| EPA | enduring power of attorney |
| EPDS | Edinburgh Postnatal Depression Scale |
| EPP | expert patient programme |
| EqIA | Equality Impact Assessments |
| ESA | Employment and Support Allowance |
| ESL | English as a second language |
| ETF | enteral tube feeding |
| FB | foreign body |
| FBC | full blood count |
| FBOA | foreign body airway obstruction |

| FEV | forced expiratory volume |
| --- | --- |
| FH | family history |
| FI | faecal incontinence |
| FNP | Family Nurse Partnership Programme |
| FPG | fasting plasma glucose |
| FSH | follicle stimulating hormone |
| FSIDS | Foundation for Sudden Infant Death Syndrome (now the Lullaby Trust) |
| FVC | forced vital capacity |
| GA | general anaesthetic |
| GDS | geriatric depression scale |
| GI | gastrointestinal |
| GMS | general medical service |
| GORD | gastro-oesophageal reflux disease |
| GP | general practioner |
| GPES | General Practice Extraction Service |
| GPN | general practice nurse |
| GPwSI | GP with special interests |
| GRE | glycopeptide-resistant enterococci |
| GSF | Gold Standard Framework |
| GTN | glyceryl trinitrate |
| GU | gastric ulceration |
| GUM | genitourinary medicine |
| h | hour |
| hrs | hours |
| HAV | hepatitis A virus |
| Hb | haemoglobin |
| HBeAg | hepatitis B 'e' antigen |
| HBsAg | hepatitis B surface antigen |
| HBPM | home blood pressure monitoring |
| HBV | hepatitis B virus |
| HCA | health care assistant |
| HCP | Healthy Child Programme |
| HCV | hepatitis C virus |
| HDL | high-density lipoprotein |
| HEI | Higher Education Institution |
| HEV | hepatitis E virus |
| HFAC4 | *Health for all children*, 4th edition |
| HFPEF | heart failure with preserved ejection fraction |
| HIA | health impact assessment |

| HIV | human immunodeficiency virus |
| HME | heat and moisture exchanger |
| HNA | health needs assessment |
| HONK | hyperosmolar non-ketotic coma |
| HPA | Health Protection Agency |
| HPC | Health Professions Council |
| HPV | human papillomavirus |
| HRA | Human Rights Act |
| HRT | hormone replacement therapy |
| HSC | Health & Safety Commission |
| HSE | Health and Safety Executive |
| HV | health visitor |
| Hx | history |
| IAPT | Improving Access to Psychological Therapies |
| IBD | inflammatory bowel disease |
| IBS | irritable bowel syndrome |
| ICP | integrated care pathways |
| ICSI | intracytoplasmic sperm injection |
| IEP | individual education plan |
| IFCC | International Federation of Clinical Chemistry and Laboratory Medicine |
| IFG | impaired fasting glucose |
| IgE | immunoglobulin E |
| IHD | ischaemic heart disease |
| IM | intramuscular |
| IMCA | independent mental capacity advocate |
| IMD | indices of multiple deprivation |
| INR | international normalized ratio |
| IPSS | International Prostate Symptom Score |
| IRAS | Integrated Research Application System |
| IS | income support |
| ITS | interrupted time series |
| IUD | intrauterine device |
| IUS | intrauterine system |
| IV | intravenous/ly |
| IVF | *in vitro* fertilization |
| JSA | Job Seekers Allowance |
| KSF | knowledge and skills framework |
| LA | local authority |
| LABA | long-acting beta-2 agonists |

| LARC | long-acting reversible contraception |
|------|--------------------------------------|
| LBC | liquid-based cytology |
| LCG | local commissioning group |
| LD | learning disability |
| LDL | low-density lipoprotein |
| LDP | local delivery plan |
| LEA | local education authority |
| LES | locally-enhanced services |
| LFT | liver function test |
| LGV | lymphogranuloma venereum |
| LH | luteinizing hormone |
| LHB | local health board |
| LHRH | luteinizing hormone-releasing hormone |
| LLETZ | large loop excision of the transformation zone |
| LMP | last menstrual period |
| LPA | lasting power of attorney |
| LSCB | Local Safeguarding Children Board |
| LTC | long-term condition |
| LTOT | long-term oxygen therapy |
| LUNSERS | Liverpool University Neuroleptic Side Effect Rating Scale |
| LVF | left ventricular function |
| LVSD | left ventricular systolic dysfunction |
| MA | megestrol acetate |
| MAU | Medical Assessment Unit |
| MCADD | medium-chain acyl-CoA dehydrogenase deficiency |
| MC&S | microscopy, culture, and sensitivity |
| MCV | mean corpuscular volume |
| MDR | multi-drug resistant |
| MDRTB | multi-drug resistant tuberculosis |
| MDT | multi-disciplinary team |
| MHRA | Medicines and Health Care Products Regulatory Agency |
| MI | myocardial infarction |
| MLD | manual lymphatic drainage |
| MM | malignant melanoma |
| MMR | measles, mumps, and rubella vaccine |
| MMSE | Mini Mental State Examination |
| MND | motor neurone disease |
| MPA | medroxyprogesterone acetate |
| MRC | Medical Research Council |
| MRSA | methicillin-resistant *Staphylococcus aureus* |

| MS | multiple sclerosis |
|---|---|
| MSH | melanocyte-stimulating hormones |
| MSM | men who have sex with men |
| MSU | mid-stream specimen of urine |
| mths | months |
| MUST | Malnutrition Screening Tool |
| NAAT | nucleic acid amplification test |
| NAIR | National Arrangements for Incidents involving Radioactivity |
| NCT | National Childbirth Trust |
| NELH | National Electronic Library for Health |
| NET-EN | norethindrone enanthate |
| NG | nasogastric |
| NGT | nasogastric tube |
| NGU | non-gonococcal urethritis |
| NHL | non-Hodgkin's lymphoma |
| NHS | National Health Service |
| NHSBSA | NHS Business Services Authority |
| NICE | National Institute for Health and Care Excellence |
| NIHR | National Institute of Health Research |
| NIHR CPS | NIHR centralised system for NHS research permssions |
| NIPPV | non-invasive ventilation |
| NMC | Nursing and Midwifery Council |
| NMSC | non-melanoma skin cancer |
| NOFTT | non-organic failure to thrive |
| NP | nurse practitioner |
| NPC | National Prescribing Centre |
| NPSA | National Patient Safety Agency |
| NRES | National Research Ethics Service |
| NRL | natural rubber latex |
| NRLS | National Reporting and Learning System |
| NRT | nicotine replacement therapy |
| NSAID | non-steroidal anti-inflammatory drug |
| NSCSP | NIHR coordinated system for NHS research permission |
| NSF | National Service Framework |
| OA | osteoarthritis |
| OAE | oto-acoustic emissions |
| od | once a day |
| ODD | oppositional defiant disorder |
| OH | occupational health |
| OOH | out-of-hours |

| OGTT | oral glucose tolerance test |
|------|------|
| OPD | outpatient department |
| OT | occupational therapy/therapist |
| OTC | over-the-counter medicines |
| pa | per annum |
| PALS | Patient Advice and Liaison Service |
| PBP | progressive bulbar palsy |
| PCB | polychlorinated biphenyl |
| PCP | *Pneumocystis* pneumonia |
| PCO | primary care organization |
| PCV | pneumococcal conjugate vaccine |
| PD | Parkinson's disease |
| PDA | patent ductus arteriosus |
| PDP | personal development plan |
| PDSA | Plan-Do-Study-Act |
| PE | pulmonary embolism |
| PEFR | peak expiratory flow rate |
| PEG | percutaneous endoscopic gastrostomy |
| PEP | post-exposure prophylaxis |
| PET | positron emission tomography |
| PfPC | Preferred Priorities for Care |
| PGD | patient group directions |
| PHCHR | parent-held child health record |
| PHCT | primary health care team |
| PHMB | polyhexamethylene biguanide |
| PICC | peripherally inserted central catheter |
| PID | pelvic inflammatory disease |
| PIL | patient information leaflet |
| PIN | personal identification number |
| PIP | Personal Independence Payment |
| PKU | phenylketonuria |
| PLB | pursed lip breathing |
| PMA | progressive muscular atrophy |
| PMH | past medical history |
| PMS | personal medical service |
| PN | partner notification |
| PND | postnatal depression |
| po | *per os* (by mouth) |
| POM | prescription-only medicine |
| POP | progestogen-only pill |

| PPC | pre-payment certificate |
| PPDP | Practice Professional Development Plans |
| PPE | personal protective equipment |
| PPI | patient and public involvement |
| PPP | personal professional profile |
| PREP | Post-Registration Education and Practice Standards |
| prn | *pro re nata* (as required) |
| PROM | patient-reported outcome measures |
| PSA | prostate-specific antigen test |
| PSD | patient-specific direction |
| PSHE | personal, social, and health education |
| PTSD | post-traumatic stress disorder |
| PTT | prothrombin time |
| PUVA | psoralen and UVA |
| PVD | peripheral vascular disease |
| QMAS | Quality Management and Analysis System |
| QOF | quality and outcomes framework |
| QoL | quality of life |
| RA | rheumatoid arthritis |
| RCC | red cell count |
| RCN | Royal College of Nursing |
| RCT | randomized controlled trial |
| RIDDOR | Reporting of Injuries, Diseases and Dangerous Occurrence Regulations |
| RH | retrobulbar haemorrhage |
| RTA | road traffic accident |
| Rx | treatment |
| S | serum |
| SAP | single assessment process |
| SARC | sexual assault referral centre |
| SARS | severe acute respiratory syndrome |
| SATs | Standard Assessment Tests |
| SC | subcutaneous |
| SCC | squamous cell carcinoma |
| SCJ | squamocolumnar junction |
| SEN | special educational needs |
| SEHD | Scottish Executive Health Department |
| SENCO | special educational needs coordinator |
| SENDIST | Special Educational Needs and Disability Tribunal |
| SIGN | Scottish Intercollegiate Guidelines Network |

| SLD | simple lymphatic drainage |
| SLE | systemic lupus erythematosus |
| SLT | speech and language therapy/therapist |
| SMP | statutory maternity pay |
| SN | school nurse |
| SOB | shortness of breath |
| SOP | standard operating procedure |
| | |
| SRE | sex and relationship education |
| SS | sickle cell |
| SSP | statutory sick pay |
| SSRI | selective serotonin reuptake inhibitor |
| STI | sexually-transmitted infection |
| SIDS | sudden infant death syndrome |
| TB | tuberculosis |
| TC | total cholesterol |
| TCA | tricyclic antidepressants |
| tds | three times a day |
| TENS | transcutaneous electrical nerve stimulation |
| TFT | thyroid function tests |
| TG | triglycerides |
| TIA | transient ischaemic attack |
| TOIL | time off in lieu |
| TOP | termination of pregnancy |
| TSE | testicular self-examination |
| TSH | thyroid-stimulating hormone |
| TVT | tension-free vaginal tape |
| UC | ulcerative colitis |
| U&Es | urea and electrolytes |
| UPSI | unprotected sexual intercourse |
| URTI | upper respiratory tract infection |
| US | ultrasound |
| USS | ultrasound scan |
| UTI | urinary tract infection |
| UV | ultraviolet |
| UVA | ultra violet A (ray) |
| UVB | ultra violet B (ray) |
| VDRL | Venereal Disease Research Laboratory test |
| VF | ventricular fibrillation |
| VSD | ventriculoseptal defect |

| VRE | vancomycin-resistant enterococci |
|-----|----------------------------------|
| VTE | venous thrombolytic embolism |
| WCC | white cell count |
| WEN | Women's Environmental Network |
| WHO | World Health Organization |
| wks | weeks |
| WTC | Working Tax Credit |
| YOT | youth offending team |
| yrs | years |

# The context of health care

# UK health profile

The UK population was 62.3 million in 2012[1]. Key projected demographic changes include increased percentages of adults aged over 65yrs, particularly in the oldest group, i.e. aged over 80yrs.

Health is influenced by a number of factors as summarized in Fig. 1.1.

## Major causes of death

- Majority of deaths occur in those aged 65yrs and over.
- The three leading causes are:
  - Circulatory diseases (includes heart disease and stroke) nearly 2 ♂:1 ♀.
  - *Cancers*—four most common are breast, lung, colorectal, and prostate.
  - Respiratory diseases.
- Leading causes of death varies with age and sex:
  - *1–4yrs*—is congenital abnormalities.
  - *5–35yrs*—land transport accidents and suicide, with a mortality rate of 2♂:1♀.
  - *35–65yrs*—breast cancer in ♀, coronary heart disease (CHD) in ♂.
  - *65yrs and over*—CHD for both sexes.

## Health inequalities

People are likely to experience worse health than the rest of the population if they experience one or more of the following—material disadvantage, lower educational attainment, and/or insecure employment[2]. The indices of multiple deprivation (IMD) are used extensively to analyse patterns of deprivation (see *Atlas of Deprivation*[3]). There is also evidence that living in materially deprived neighbourhoods contributes to worse health for individuals and that inequalities are widening (see Marmot Review[4]).

### Average life expectancy

Life expectancy is 82.1yrs for ♀, 78.1 yrs for ♂ yrs. However, the average socio-economic and geographic gradients for males in some areas is <74yrs (see Public Health Observatories[5]).

### Infant mortality

Infant mortality was 4.3 per 1000 live births in England and Wales in 2010. However, there is considerable variation by area and socio-economic status of the parents, with higher rates in babies with fathers in manual occupations, and where only the mother registered the baby. Highest rates are found for teenage mothers and lowest where the mother was 30–34yrs.

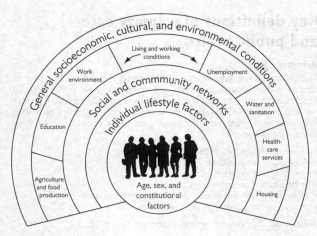

**Fig. 1.1** Influences on health.
Reproduced with kind permission of the authors. Dahlgren G, Whitehead M. (1993). *Tackling inequalities in health: what can we learn from what has been tried?* Working paper prepared for the King's Fund International Seminar on Tackling Inequalities in Health, Ditchley Park, Oxfordshire. London, King's Fund. Accessible in: Dahlgren G, Whitehead M. (2007) European strategies for tackling social inequities in health: Levelling up Part 2. Copenhagen: WHO Regional Office for Europe.

## References

[1]Office for National Statistics. New 2011 Census statistics. Available at: 🔗 www.ons.gov.uk/ons/index.html

[2]World Health Organization (2008). *Closing the gap in a generation: health equity through action on the social determinants of health.* Geneva: WHO. Available at: 🔗 www.who.int/social_determinants/thecommission/finalreport/en/index.html

[3]Atlas of Deprivation 2010 (2011). Available at: 🔗 http://www.ons.gov.uk/ons/rel/regional-trends/atlas-of-deprivation--england/2010/atlas-of-deprivation-2010.html

[4]Marmot M, et al. (2010) *Fairer Society Health Lives: The Strategic Review of Health Inequalities in England post 2010* (The Marmot Review). Available at: 🔗 http://www.instituteofhealthequity.org/projects/fair-society-healthy-lives-the-marmot-review

[5]Public Health England (2013). The Network of Public Health Observatories. Available at: 🔗 www.apho.org.uk/

## Further information

Northern Ireland Statistics and Research Agency (2013). Available at: 🔗 www.nisra.gov.uk/index.html

National Records of Scotland (2013). Information about Scotland's People. Available at: 🔗 www.gro-scotland.gov.uk/index.html

# Key definitions of primary care and public health

## Primary care

The Declaration of Alma Ata[1] stated that primary care is the first level of contact that individuals, the family, and community have with a national health system, bringing health care as close as possible to where people live and work. WHO re-affirmed the importance of primary care with the aim of better health care for all[2]. It is the first element of a continuing health care process.

The five principles that underpin primary care are:
• Accessibility to health services.
• Use of appropriate technology.
• Individual and community participation.
• Increased health promotion and disease prevention.
• Intersectoral cooperation and collaboration.

See also 📖 Overview of services in primary care, p. 12.

## Public health

The purpose of public health is to create conditions so that people can be healthy. It is the science and art of preventing disease, prolonging life, and promoting physical and mental health through the organized efforts of society. It has a collective, rather than an individual view of the health needs and health care of a population.

The aim of public health bodies is to achieve this purpose by:
• Promotion of a safe environment.
• Control of community infections.
• Health promotion.
• Organization of medical and nursing service for early identification and treatment of ill health and disease.
• Health protection.

*Underpinning values of public health*
• Equity and social inclusion.
• Participation, collaboration, and community empowerment.
• Social justice where health is a basic human right.

See also 📖 Health needs assessment, p. 11.

## References

[1]Declaration of Alma Ata (1978). International Conference on Primary Health Care, Alma-Ata, USSR, 6-12 September 1978. Available at: ℘ http://www.who.int/publications/almaata_declaration_en.pdf
[2]WHO (2008). *The World Health Report 2008—Primary Health care (Now More Than Ever)* Geneva: WHO. Available at: ℘ http://www.who.int/whr/2008/whr08_en.pdf

## Further information

Public Health England (2013). Health Protection Agency. Available at: ℘ http://www.hpa.org.uk/HPAwebHome/
Public Health Agency Northern Ireland. Available at: ℘ www.publichealth.hscni.net/
Public Health Wales. Available at: ℘ www.publichealthwales.wales.nhs.uk/
Scotland's Health Improvement Agency. Available at: ℘ www.healthscotland.com/

# Generic long-term conditions model

## Background

There are ~15 million people in England with at least one long-term condition (LTC), i.e. a condition that cannot be cured, but can be managed with medication and/or therapy. Prevalence of LTCs varies across geographical regions. Multiple factors influence variations such as age (most significant), socio-economic status, and lifestyle.

## Key points

- People with a LTC often intensive users of health- and social care services, including community services, urgent and emergency care, and acute services.
- Conditions rising most quickly are cancers, chronic kidney disease (CKD), and diabetes.
- Number of people with one LTC expected to be relatively stable, but those with multiple LTCs expected to ↑ to 2.9 million in 2018 from 1.9 million in 2008.

The generic LTC care model identifies three elements for service improvement:

- Risk profiling.
- Neighbourhood care teams.
- Self care/shared decision-making.

This is a structured approach that aims to match care to need, stratifying the local population into three levels of need (derived from a USA Kaiser Permanente LTC model):

- *Tier 1:* focuses on complex needs and accounts for around 5% of people. Nursing interventions could include case management dedicated one-to-one support for people (e.g. a community matron) with regular contact.
- *Tier 2:* a medium level of need (around 25%). Nursing interventions can include use of personalized care planning:
  - Placing the person at centre of decision-making about their care.
  - Agreeing plan of how that care will be delivered.
  - It can also support the use of assistive technology.
  - Telephone coaching arrangements to help people to remain independent and self-care for as long as possible.
- *Tier 3:* low-level needs. Conditions under control (around 70%). Nursing interventions focus on enabling patients and their carers to develop knowledge, skills, and confidence to care for themselves effectively. The Expert Patient Programme or equivalent can support this (📖 Expert patients, p. 303).

## Further information

Department of Health (2010). *Generic long term conditions model.* Available at: ℘ http://webarchive.nationalarchives.gov.uk/+/www.dh.gov.uk/en/Healthcare/Longtermconditions/DH_120915

DH (2012) *Long Term Conditions Compendium of Information: Third Edition.* Available at: ℘ https://www.gov.uk/government/publications/long-term-conditions-compendium-of-information-third-edition

Policies on LTC are available on each country's central health department website. See the NHS in Northern Ireland, Scotland, and Wales

# The National Health Service (NHS)

The UK NHS was established on 5 July 1948 to provide a comprehensive range of health services to all in need. It is free at the point of delivery and paid for through taxation. Some services also incur subsidized charges, e.g. NHS prescriptions in primary care (England only). The NHS UK budget was £106 billion 2011–12.

Decisions about health policy have been devolved to each of the four countries of the UK. Consequently, structures and policy priorities are different in each country. The Isle of Man and the Channel Islands have independent health service structures.

In each country, there is a senior government minister responsible for health and publicly funded health services. Within government agreed policies, the central NHS administration sets overall priorities and some specific targets. Local NHS bodies (e.g. Community Health Partnership in Scotland, and Primary Care Trust Clusters or Clinical Commissioning Groups in England) plan, commission, and sometimes also manage and monitor services for the residents of a defined area—usually co-terminus with a Local Authority (LA). Each country has its own arrangements for assessing the quality of health care ([] Quality and outcomes framework, p. 66). England has moved further than other countries in separating commissioning organizations from provision of services organizations. The NHS in all countries is subject to periodic re-organization and the latest information is on the country specific websites listed in [] References, p. 7.

In all countries, general practice (primary medical care) is part of the NHS, but provided through specific contracts, not directly managed by the administrative structures of the NHS ([] General practice, p. 13).

## The NHS in England

The Department of Health provides central direction to both commissioning bodies and service-providing organizations within the NHS. There is a published NHS Constitution[1] stating principles, rights, and responsibilities. NHS England provides the overall commissioning direction and at the local area level Clinical Commissioning Groups (CCGs). Public Health Departments are part of LAs. All NHS provided services are within organizations called NHS Trusts and Foundation Trusts (indicating they have greater financial autonomy). Some services are funded (or commissioned) from the NHS, but provided by the private for-profit sector or not-for-profit voluntary sector or social enterprises. Community health services are mainly provided by NHS Trusts. The patient and public involvement (PPI) voice is through Health Watch.

## NHS in Northern Ireland

The Department of Health, Social Services, and Public Safety (DHSSPS) provides the central direction for the NHS. The Health and Social Care Board arranges, or commissions, delivers, and monitors health and social care supported by five Local Commissioning Groups (LCGs). Five Health and Social Care Trusts provide services for the residents in their areas including primary care services. The Patient and Client Council provides the focus for PPI including social care.

## Scotland

The Scottish Government Health Directorate (SEHD) provides the central direction of the NHS, overseeing the work of 14 area NHS boards and Special Health Authorities, e.g. NHS 24 (provides a 24-hr telephone advice line). In each Board there are Community Health Partnerships (CHPs) responsible for health improvement, greater integration of primary, secondary, and social care services, as well as the planning and management of community health services. The Scottish Health Council provides the PPI focus.

## Wales

The Department of Health and Social Services provides the central direction to the NHS with three regional offices and three services in Wales (e.g. the Ambulance Trust). Seven local health boards (LHBs) plan, secure, and deliver health services in their area. These are matched by seven Community Health Councils providing the PPI perspective.

## Reference

[1]Department of Health (2012) *NHS Constitution*, DH-_132961. London: DH. Available at: http:// www.nhs.uk/choiceintheNHS/Rightsandpledges/NHSConstitution/Documents/2013/ the-nhs-constitution-for-england-2013.pdf

## Further information

Community Health Councils in Wales. Available at: www.wales.nhs.uk/sitesplus/899/home
Community Health Partnerships Available at: www.chp.scot.nhs.uk/
Department of Health. Available at: www.gov.uk/government/organisations/department-of-health
Department of Health, Social Services, and Public safety. Available at: www.dhsspsni.gov.uk/ index.asp
Healthwatch. Available at: www.healthwatch.co.uk/
NHS in England. Consultant treatment outcomes. Available at: www.england.nhs.uk/
NHS Scotland. Scottish Health on the Web. Available at: www.show.scot.nhs.uk
Health in Wales. Available at: www.wales.nhs.uk
The Patient and Client Council. Available at: www.patientclientcouncil.hscni.net/
Scottish Health Council. Available at: www.scottishhealthcouncil.org/home.aspx

# NHS entitlements

The NHS provides health care in the UK. It is paid for through taxation. People living or working in the UK are entitled to free or subsidized (e.g. charges for dentists, opticians, prescriptions unless low income) treatments at the point of care, as are people taken ill whilst in the UK for a short stay. Some countries have a reciprocal agreement, where UK residents can get free medical treatment, and residents of that country can get the same in the UK.

## People coming from overseas

Treatment is always free at the point of care for:
• Accidents and emergency treatment.
• Compulsory psychiatric treatment.
• Certain communicable diseases, e.g. TB, cholera, food poisoning, malaria, and meningitis, STIs, but testing only for HIV virus (not treatment).
• Family planning.

Entitlement to NHS treatment depends on the length (>6mths) and purpose of residence in the UK, not nationality. A person who is regarded as ordinarily resident, i.e. their stay in the UK has some permanence and stability, is eligible for free treatment by 1° medical services. Overseas visitors to the UK are not regarded as ordinarily resident and subject to charging regulations if they do not meet this description. Exceptions include:
• Asylum seekers and refugees given leave to remain in the UK, or awaiting results of an application to remain.
• EEA nationals with forms E112 or E128.
• Any person, whether ordinarily resident or not, requiring treatment that a GP regards as emergency or immediately necessary (for <14 days).

GPs may offer to accept patients on a private basis, and charge if their stay is <6mths. Regulations are periodically reviewed.

## Further information

For detailed policies on each UK country's central website, see ⬚ The National Health Service (NHS), p. 6.
Citizens Advice Bureau. Available at: ℬ www.citizensadvice.org.uk/

# Commissioning of services

Commissioning (or funding services) is a set of planned activities undertaken with the intended outcome of measurable improvement in the health and wellbeing of resident populations, involving the implementation of change to secure the most effective and efficient use of resources. It includes:
- The assessment of need (📖 Public Health in the NHS, p. 10 and 📖 Health Needs Assessment, p. 11) and strategy development.
- The identification of priorities and investment planning.
- Service specification (including quality and development).
- Service contracting, including financial flows.
- Service monitoring of activities under the contract for individuals and populations.

In England commissioning for 2° and tertiary care services now uses a system of payment by results so that commissioners specify:
- Volume of activity required to deliver service priorities, adjusted for case mix (i.e. the mix of types of patients and/or treatment episodes).
- From a plurality of providers.
- On the basis of a standard national price tariff, adjusted for regional variation in wages and other costs of service delivery.

There is a national set of reference costs for each type of service.

The local area commissioning (or planning) body have a responsibility to work closely with LAs to jointly plan (sometimes known as Joint Strategic Needs Assessment) and, in some cases, commission services for shared populations. These plans (sometimes known as local delivery plans) are based on local health, central government priorities, targets (including quality and productivity improvements), and clinical and service standards, e.g. National Service Frameworks (NSFs).

## Contracting for primary care services

A national contracting process underpins the provision of general medical services, local pharmacy, dentistry services, and optician services. In addition, local commissioners can negotiate individual additions with these independent contractors to the NHS (📖 General Practice, p. 13; 📖 Other types of primary care medical services contracts, p. 15; 📖 Other primary health care services, p. 16).

## Further information

NHS in England. Available at: 🔊 www.england.nhs.uk/
NHS Primary Health Care Commissioning. Available at: 🔊 www.england.nhs.uk/resources/resource-primary/
Northern Ireland. Available at: 🔊 www.dhsspsni.gov.uk/index.asp
NHS Scotland. Scottish Health on the Web. Available at: 🔊 www.show.scot.nhs.uk
Health in Wales. Available at: 🔊 www.wales.nhs..lk

# Public health in the NHS

Public health focuses on *health*, as well as *disease*, and *populations* not *individuals* (📖 Key definitions of primary care and public health, p. 4). It seeks to protect health and prevent illness by studying health patterns/trends, and planning to address health needs. Health impact assessment (HIA) is becoming a defining feature of this work. In addition, there are national and local Public Health Department responsibilities for public protection, e.g. investigation and management of communicable disease outbreaks.

## Current public health practice

Uses complementary approaches alongside epidemiology and demography that emphasize:

- *Equity:* fairness and social justice.
- *Cross cutting approaches:* known as partnership or intersectoral work.
- Community participation in the development of services.
- Participation in health service commissioning decisions.

## Health impact assessment

HIA is intended to help make decisions by predicting the health consequences (good and bad) if a proposal is implemented, whether the consequences are the same or different for groups within the population, e.g. socio-economic groups, recommending how to maximize or minimize the consequences. There are different types of policy proposals impact assessments, e.g. equity impact assessments. Public health specialists recommend that health should be considered in all of these.

## Public health strategies and polices

Each of the four countries has separate public health strategies that provide the over-arching targets for health improvement.

## Nurses, midwives, and health visitors

All nurses, midwives, and health visitors (HVs) are expected to contribute to public health. Nurses and HVs on the Nursing and Midwifery Council (NMC) public health register are required to contribute to and influence policies affecting health.

## Further information

Public Health England. Available at: ℘ www.gov.uk/government/organisations/public-health-england
Public Health England. Health Protection Agency. Available at: ℘ www.hpa.org.uk/HPAwebHome/
NHS Scotland. Health Improvement Agency Scotland. Available at: ℘ www.healthscotland.com/index.aspx
Public Health Wales. Available at: ℘ www.publichealthwales.wales.nhs.uk/
Public Health Agency (NI). Available at: ℘ http://www.publichealth.hscni.net/
Public Health England (2013). Network of Public Health Observatories. Available at: ℘ www.apho.org.uk/apho/
Public Health England. (2013). Health Impact Assessment Gateway. Available at: ℘ www.apho.org.uk/default.aspx?QN=P_HIA
NICE. (2013). National Library for Public Health. Available at: ℘ https://www.evidence.nhs.uk/nhs-evidence-content/public-health

# Health needs assessment

Health needs assessment (HNA) processes promote a strategic and evidence-based approach, enabling evaluation of the effectiveness of interventions and promoting equity. HNA is central to public health (📖 Public health in the NHS, p. 10) and to make decisions as to where to apportion resources and funding for health care.

## HNA techniques

HNA techniques range from those that are individual to population focused. Often they combine statistical and participatory methods, e.g. participatory rapid appraisal using lay participation and multidisciplinary teamwork, which takes account of the wider societal determinants of health (📖 UK health profile, p. 2). Public health departments usually undertake population level health needs assessments for strategic planning and commissioning (📖 Commissioning of services, p. 9). HNA is also undertaken at a general practice or local community level. Practitioners should be cognisant of the ethical dimension of HNA and avoid raising expectations if change/services are not going to be available.

### Epidemiological and demographic methods

Statistical data, such as mortality rates, use of services, age of population, incidence, and prevalence of disease/accidents are collated and analysed. Increasingly, these are plotted using geographical health information systems, which can inform needs assessment at a macro-level. Public Health Departments provide local area level information reports, e.g. in Annual Public Health Reports or through Public Health Observatory reports (📖 Public health in the NHS, p. 10).

### Participatory methods

The usefulness of statistical information is enhanced when combined with qualitative data, which explains, e.g.:
- Why people do not attend.
- How services might be developed.
- The impact of services on health.

## References

Health Development Agency (2005). *Health Needs Assessment: A Practical Guide.* Available at: ℘ www.nice.org.uk/aboutnice/whoweare/aboutthehda/hdapublications/health_needs_assessment_a_practical_guide.jsp
Health Development Agency (2002). *Health Needs Assessment: A Workbook.* Available at: ℘ www.nice.org.uk/aboutnice/whoweare/aboutthehda/hdapublications/health_needs_assessment_workbook.jsp

# Overview of services in primary care

There are a wide range of NHS services available to the public, but some local variation. Different types of services have different relationships to the central NHS:
- Some directly managed in NHS structures, e.g. community health services.
- Some are outside NHS management structures, but mainly only provide services under a nationally agreed contract to the NHS, e.g. general practitioners.
- Some are independent of the NHS, but have a nationally agreed contract for NHS payment for particular activities, e.g. community pharmacists.
- Some are locally contracted by the NHS from not-for-profit and for-profit organizations, e.g. some sexual health services.

## Core primary care health service elements

Available to all are:
- 24-hr NHS helplines, e.g. NHS 111, NHS 24.
- General (📖 General practice, p. 13) or personal (📖 Other types of primary care medical services contracts, p. 15) medical services and their out of hours (OOH) services.
- Dentistry, pharmacy, optometry (📖 Other primary health care services, p. 16).
- Community health services based in community clinics, health centres, and GP surgeries. Usually includes:
  - Nursing in the home (📖 District nursing, p. 42).
  - Public health nursing (📖 Health visiting, p. 40, 📖 School nursing, p. 36).
  - Sexual health and contraceptive services (📖 Nurses in primary care, p. 32).
  - Chiropody, dentistry, speech and language therapy, physiotherapy for specific vulnerable groups (📖 Other primary health care services, p. 16).

In addition many primary care organizations (PCOs) have:
- *Walk-in centres:* assessment and treatment of minor injuries and health problems, which are usually staffed by nurses.
- *Multi-disciplinary specialist teams:* e.g. palliative care, rehabilitation, intermediate care, rapid response.
- *Specialist nurses:* e.g. continence, diabetes, TB, special needs (paediatric), child protection.
- *Community hospitals:* admission and clinical management through general practitioners (GPs) and primary care nurses.

## Further information

For each UK country's central government health website, see 📖 The National Health Service (NHS), p. 6.

# General practice

There are 39,920 GPs in the UK in >10,000 practices. About 27% are single-handed GPs. Average practice list size between 5000–6000 patients. The majority of GPs are independent contractors, i.e. not directly employed by the NHS. They work in general practices, which have General Medical Service (GMS) or Personal Medical Service (PMS) contracts with the NHS. GP vocational training includes 1yr as a GP registrar supervised by GP trainer. GPs with special interests (GPwSI) are appointed by their local PCO to provide specialist health care in a generalist setting, e.g. CHD, child protection, ENT.

## The GMS contract

This is a contract between an individual practice and the local NHS organization. All the partners of the practice (one has to be a GP) have to sign the contract. Details and annual changes are on the NHS employers website. It includes:

- Global sum for essential services, some additional services, and adjustments for workload and costs incurred by features of the patient population served.
- Quality and Outcome Framework (□ Quality and outcomes framework, p. 66).
- Direct enhanced services (DESs) are special services that have been negotiated nationally. Practices can choose to provide or not.

In addition PCOs can contract for locally enhanced services (LES) to meet local health care needs, e.g. homeless people.

### Essential services

Must be provided to their registered patients:

- Day-to-day medical care, which includes management of minor and self-limiting illness, referral to 2° services and other services.
- Non-specialist care of people who are terminally ill.
- Chronic disease management.

### Additional services

The practice can opt out of these and receive less payment:

- Cervical screening (□ Cervical cancer screening, p. 337).
- Contraceptive services (□ Contraception: general, p. 359).
- Vaccinations and immunizations, both childhood basic course, those >6yrs, missing the basic course and reinforcing doses (□ Childhood immunization, p. 156).
- Child health surveillance, excluding neonatal check (□ Overview of the healthy child programme, p. 146).
- Maternity services, excluding intrapartum care.
- Minor surgery procedures, e.g. curettage, cautery, cryocautery.

### Directed enhanced services
These are commissioned by the PCO and attract additional payment:
- *Directed enhanced services:* these have national specifications (specific to each country) and have to be provided by the PCO. Examples include:
  - Childhood immunizations for children <2yrs and pre-school boosters <5yrs. 70% coverage to reach lower payment and 90% coverage to reach higher payment (📖 Childhood immunization schedule, p. 158).
  - Influenza immunization for >65yrs and at-risk groups (📖 Targeted immunization in adults, p. 347).
  - More complex minor surgery.
- *National enhanced services:* these have national specifications, but the PCO does not have to provide them in primary care, e.g. anticoagulation monitoring.

### Out of hours
OOH is defined as from 18.30 to 08.00 hours on weekdays, the whole of weekends, Bank holidays, and public holidays. Practices have mostly opted out of this for reduced finance. OOH services are usually provided by GP OOH organization or local PCO.

### Dispensing
Some practices are also dispensing practices, i.e. contracted to provide dispensing of medicines, particularly in rural and remote areas.

### Practice information
Each practice has to produce a practice leaflet detailing services, practice policies, and route for complaints.

### Registration with a practice
People apply to register by handing in their NHS medical card to the reception or completing an application form. The practice informs the PCO and it confirms acceptance with a new medical card to the patient. Temporary registrations can be given if the patients is resident >24hrs and <3m.

### List closures
Practices can only close their lists after negotiation with the PCO. When a list is closed the practice can only accept new patients who are close family relatives of existing patients.

### Removal from practice list
Patients can be removed from practice lists because of violence, or crime and deception to receive treatment, or distance from the surgery.

### Patient's right to change GP
People can choose to change GP without giving an explanation, giving a period of notice, or informing the GP.

## Further information
NHS Employers. Available at: 🔗 http://www.nhsemployers.org/PayAndContracts/GeneralMedical ServicesContract/Pages/Contract.aspx
NHS Primary Care Commissioning. Available at: 🔗 www.england.nhs.uk/resources/resource-primary/
Royal College of General Practitioners Information Sheets. Available at: 🔗 www.rcgp.org.uk/

# Other types of primary care medical services contracts

PMS contract is the local alternative to the GMS contract (🕮 General practice, p. 13). The PMS contract is made with the PCO. >40% of GPs in England have PMS contracts. Some nurses hold PMS contracts with PCOs. It aims to give primary care professionals the freedom to innovate, work more closely as a team to improve services for patients, and address inequalities in health care provision.

## Elements of the PMS contract

Practices are paid to provide a package of services. How it provides those services is up to the practice. Most PMS budgets consist of:
- *Practice costs:* e.g. premises, staffing.
- *Core services:* usually services patients would expect to receive from any GP (equivalent to GMS contract essential services).
- *Additional services:* both those usually expected from a GMS contract (e.g. maternity, minor surgery, contraception), and also can be those usually provided by community services (e.g. community nursing), or 2° care (known as PMS Plus, e.g. endoscopy, ultrasound, etc.)
  - Plus prescribing budget (optional) and QOF (🕮 Quality and outcomes framework, p. 66).

## Specialist PMS contracts

This allows primary care delivery for groups poorly served by other systems by removing the need for patients to be registered for all 'core' primary care services with that practice. Examples include:
- Specific groups, e.g. the homeless, asylum seekers.
- Specific service provision, e.g. services for violent patients, OOH care, teenage contraceptive services, sexual health clinics.

## Alternative provider medical services (APMS)

APMS contracts are used with a wide range of providing organizations to address local population needs and gaps in PMSs, e.g. in areas of under provision, or where it is difficult to recruit or retain GPs. It can be with existing GP practices or groups of practices, private companies, or social enterprises.

## Further information

NHS Employers. Available at: 🖅 www.nhsemployers.org/PayAndContracts/GeneralMedicalServices Contract/Pages/Contract.aspx

# Other primary health care services

A range of services and professionals are available in primary care. This following is a summary (alphabetically) of the most commonly used.

## Chiropodists

Registered chiropodists, also known as podiatrists, are trained in all aspects of care of the feet and lower limbs. Some are also podiatric surgeons undertaking surgery for conditions such as hammer toes. Services are available in consulting rooms, at home, and in care homes, and are paid for privately (Society of Chiropodists and Podiatrists[1]).

*Community chiropody services* NHS-funded services for specified vulnerable groups, e.g. older people, those with diabetes, rheumatoid arthritis, osteoarthritis. Local referral criteria and pathways apply, often requiring GP referral.

## Dentists

Dental practices take private and NHS patients. NHS dentists have agreements to provide NHS dental services. Patients not eligible for free NHS dental treatment (📖 NHS entitlements, p. 8), pay 80% of the cost of treatment, up to a maximum of £384 per course of dental treatment (British Dental Association[2]).

*Community dental service (CDS)* NHS-funded to provide dental treatment to those who have difficulty accessing dental care, e.g. those with learning disabilities, the housebound. Ususally able to provide a domicillary service. Local policies on referral process, e.g. may only be through GP. CDS usually also provides school oral screening for public health.

## Opticians

Provide eye sight tests and examine eyes for abnormalities, e.g. glaucoma. They also fit and supply spectacles to prescription. Dispensing opticians only fit and supply glasses. Free NHS eye tests are available to certain groups (📖 NHS entitlements, p. 8; 📖 Benefits for people with a low income, p. 791). PCO funds screening (mostly by orthoptist) as part of child health promotion programme (📖 Overview of the healthy child programme, p. 146). PCO ensures there is a mechanism for a domicillary service for housebound people (General Optical Council[3]).

## Pharmacists

Community pharmacists, also called chemists, prepare and dispense medicines on prescription to the general public. They may own their business or work for a bigger company. The contract between local pharmacies and PCOs specifies services dispensing medicines, waste disposal of medicinal products, and public health activities, e.g. smoking cessation, emergency contraception, advice about other services, information on self-care. Community pharmacists may also provide other services, e.g. repeat prescribing through electronic transmission of prescriptions, medicine reviews (📖 Principles of medication reviews, p. 135), supplementary prescribing (📖 Medicines management, p. 126), home delivery services, OOH (Royal Pharmaceutical Society[4]).

*Primary care pharmacists and medicines management teams*    Pharmacists employed by the NHS to advise general practice, community health service staff, and local community pharmacists on issues related to supply, storage, legislation concerning medicines, formularies, and prescribing budgets. They are also known as prescribing advisors.

## Physiotherapists

Physiotherapy is concerned with human function and musculoskeletal movement. Physiotherapists deal with a wide range of issues, e.g. sports injuries, incontinence, arthritis, back pain, and work in a range of settings, including private practice (Organization of Chartered Physiotherapists in Private Practice[5]).

*Community physiotherapists*    PCO-funded physiotherapists usually work as part of specialist multi-disciplinary teams (MDTs), e.g. stroke rehabilitation, intermediate care teams, children with special needs, providing clinic-based and domiciliary services. There are local variations in availability and referral pathways.

## Occupational therapists

State registered occupational therapists (OTs) work to enhance a person's ability to participate in everyday activities and reduce avoidable dependency through occupation and environmental changes. Available as a private service from OTs working independently (British Association of Occupational Therapists[6]).

*Community OTs*    Usually employed by LAs to work with specific vulnerable groups, e.g. disabled adults, in community care processes for aids and adaptions (📖 Assistive technology, p. 776). Also in NHS-commissioned services, e.g. community mental health teams, children with special needs teams. Local variation in access and referral routes.

## Speech and language therapists (SLTs)

SLTs work with children and adults with difficulties communicating, or with eating, drinking, and swallowing. Some are in independent practice, paid for privately (Royal College of Speech and Language Therapists[7]).

*Community SLTs*    NHS-employed SLTs may work as part of specialist teams, e.g. children with special needs, or more broadly across a client group, e.g. children or adults. Local variation in access and referral pathways.

## References

[1] Society of Chiropodists and Podiatrists. Available at: 🔊 www.feetforlife.org
[2] British Dental Association. Available at: 🔊 http://www.bda.org/
[3] General Optical Council. Available at: 🔊 www.optical.org
[4] Royal Pharmaceutical Society. Available at: 🔊 www.rpharms.com/home/home.asp
[5] Organization of Chartered Physiotherapists in Private Practice. Available at: 🔊 www.physiofirst. org.uk
[6] British Association of Occupational Therapists. Available at: 🔊 www.cot.co.uk/
[7] Royal College of Speech and Language Therapists. Available at: 🔊 www.rcslt.org

# Services to promote hospital discharge and prevent unplanned admission

A range of time-limited services aiming to achieve one or more of the following:
- Avoid unplanned hospital admissions triggered by a crisis.
- Facilitate discharge from hospital.
- Respite care for parent/carer to help sustain caring relationship.
- Provide rehabilitation and support to enable independent living.
- Intensive care at home otherwise provided by 2° care.

These services are locally determined, and have a range of titles, service providers, and funding. There are overlapping approaches to service provision.

## Intermediate care

The main focus is older people. It is time-limited, normally <6wks, with the explicit goal of maximizing independence, and involves a range of integrated services to promote faster recovery from illness, prevent unnecessary hospital admission or premature admission to long-term residential care, or support timely discharge from hospital. Provided by a MDT on the basis of a comprehensive assessment, a structured care plan often with single professional records and shared protocols, with active therapy and/ or treatment. It can be provided at home (can include being part of a 'virtual ward') or in designated beds in care homes or community hospitals.

## Rapid response teams/hospital at home

This allows people who might otherwise be admitted to hospital or have a prolonged in-patient stay, to be at home, e.g. patients with chest infections, a mild stroke, recovery from elective surgery, or in need of end-of-life care (some areas offer hospice-at-home). Teams may provide IV antibiotics, blood transfusions, nutritional support, and general health and social care till the acute episode of need is over.

## Case managers/community matrons for people at risk

Health or social care professionals who manage a discrete caseload of people who are considered at risk of unplanned hospital admission and/ or are vulnerable. Local organizations have different criteria for admission to this service but often include people with a history of unplanned admissions, falls, or multiple health and social care needs. See also 🕮 Care/case management models, p. 112.

**Partnership initiatives** Locally organized cross-agency projects that aim to reduce demand on 2° care by providing more support for low-level community care, e.g. supporting more people to live at home, e.g. by providing extra care.

**Respite care** See 🕮 Carers assessment and support, p. 412.

## Further information

Intermediate Care (2009). *Intermediate Care – Halfway Home Updated Guidance for the NHS and Local Authorities.* Available at: ℘ http://www.jitscotland.org.uk/publications-1/intermediate-care/
Age UK (2012). *Right Care Right Time* Available at: ℘ www.ageuk.org.uk/Documents/EN-GB/For professionals/Research/ID200060%20Right%20Care%20First%20Time%2028ppA4.pdf?dtrk=true

# Services for children, young people, and families

The UN Convention of the Rights of the Child (1989)[1] is the basis of government policies for children in each country of the UK. These focus on priority outcomes of being healthy, staying safe, enjoying and achieving, making a positive contribution, and achieving economic wellbeing. The policies emphasize multi-agency planning and provision of publicly-funded services for children and families.

In any LA area there is a wide range of state-funded, voluntary organization, and private services for children and families. Sources of information include:
- LA Family Information Services.
- Local public library.

## Early years: social support and play

This provision ranges from groups to one-to-one support. It can be meetings in community centres organized by a paid worker, e.g. parent and toddler groups, 1 o'clock clubs, or purely voluntary meetings in people's homes, e.g. National Childbirth Trust (NCT) groups, Meet a Mum. Organizations such as Family Welfare Association, Home-Start UK, and some Sure Start services offer one-to-one befriending, and practical support schemes for new parents and parents under stress.

## Early years: child care, play, and education

Working parents have a range of options, depending on availability and what they can afford, between one-to-one types of care in the home, e.g. child minders, au pairs, nannies, or group care, e.g. in nurseries. LA Family Information Services provide local information on child care. All child minders and group care for under 8-yr-olds have to be registered and meet national standards. Children in need (📖 A child or young person in need, p. 150) are usually prioritized for state-funded support in day-care facilities. Crêches, pre-schools, and playgroups offer sessions focused on play and encouraging early years development. All 3- and 4-yr-olds are entitled to a free, part-time place in a nursery school.

## Education

Every child has to receive education from 5 to 16yrs, either at a state school, private school, or home. Every LA provides information on its schools and entry procedures. Many schools have breakfast and after-school clubs. Pupil referral units or home tutoring is provided by each LA for children who need alternative provision, e.g. have been excluded from mainstream school or are school phobic. State schools are supported by LA-wide services, such as education welfare officers or social workers, and education psychology services. See also 📖 Children with special educational needs, p. 227.

Education for 16–18-yr-olds is in schools, sixth form colleges, or further education colleges, which also provide vocational and access education to >18yrs.

## Young people's health services

Many areas provide open-access young people's drop-in health clinics, most providing sexual health and contraceptive services. GP services are being encouraged to become more accessible to teenagers.

## Leisure activities and sport

Schools, LA services (e.g. education, youth, and leisure), voluntary organizations (e.g. guides and scouts, Woodcraft Folk, faith organizations,) and the private sector may provide a range of different sports and leisure activities in an area.

## Careers advice

There are LA and national sources of advice for young people on career paths, e.g. Careers Information and Advice for Young People, Careers Scotland.

## Children and young people in need

*Social services* See 📖 Social services, p. 26; also 📖 Looked-after children, p. 235.

*Youth offending team (YOT)* Every LA in England and Wales has a multi-agency YOT to respond to the needs of each young offender and prevent reoffending (℗ https://www.gov.uk/browse/justice/young-people).

## Related topic

📖 Child health promotion, p. 144.

## Reference

[1]UN Convention of the Rights of the Child (1989). Available at: ℗ www.unicef.org/crc/index_30184.html

## Information for professionals and parents

Children in Scotland. Available at: ℗ www.childreninscotland.org.uk
Department of Education (England). Available at: ℗ www.education.gov.uk/childrenandyoungpeople

## Information for children and young people

National Careers Service. Careers information and advice for young people. Available at: ℗ www2.cxdirect.com/home.htm. ☎ Tel: 0800 100 900.
Childline. Available at: ℗ www.childline.org.uk/pages/home.aspx ☎ Tel: 0800 1111.
Careers Scotland. Available at: ℗ http://www.myworldofwork.co.uk/

# Homes and housing

The Office of National Statistics[1] reports:
- 65% UK households are owner occupied (80% of pensioner households).
- 66% lone parents with dependent children households are in rented properties.
- In 2011, 48,510 applicants (households) were accepted as statutory homeless (see 📖 Homeless people, p. 398).
- About 4% of dwellings were classed as unfit for human habitation. Unfit or in serious disrepair dwellings were most likely to be occupied by people on low incomes, those over 75yrs, or young people.

Citizens Advice Bureau (CABs)[1] and Housing Advice Centres are key resources for advice and help on housing issues.

## Help with housing

### Not-for-profit housing
In most areas there is a central waiting list for LA and housing association properties. Each has different systems for accepting applicants and prioritizing people on their waiting lists for housing, usually including factors such as poor health made worse by housing conditions, mobility problems, inadequate number of bedrooms for family size, homelessness, length of time in the area. Medical problems are assessed by an independent advisor.

### Supported housing
This may be available to specific groups of people, e.g. older people or those with physical or mental health problems. This type of housing, e.g. sheltered housing, is often provided by councils, housing associations, or voluntary groups. There may be eligibility criteria and waiting lists. Some supported housing is staffed 24hrs/day, while in others support is only provided intermittantly.

### Rented accommodation
Landlords are responsible for health and safety. LA Environmental Health Services can inspect rented properties and enforce basic living standards. They can assess properties on dampness, disrepair, structural stability, adequate lighting, heating, ventilation, food preparation, and sanitary facilities, and drainage. Houses in multiple occupation are required to have a licence from the LA. Failure to tackle basic problems can result in closure of the premises, legal notices served for improvements to be made, or prosecution of the landlord or agent.

## Help with house maintenance, heating, and security

LAs may provide loans or grants for schemes for people on low incomes for essential repairs, insulation, and adaptations. Specific schemes may be available for older people, e.g. Care and Repair[2] or linked to home accidents and falls prevention schemes, or Keeping Warm in Winter schemes.

*Damp* Dampness, condensation, and mould growth, caused either by water penetration through the fabric of the building or by condensation. Advice for condensation includes increasing insulation, reducing moisture production (do not use paraffin heaters), increasing ventilation to remove moisture. Detailed advice is usually available through LA environmental health office (📖 Environmental health services, p. 23).

*Heating*  There are UK estimates of 30,000 excess winter deaths related to cold. The majority are people over 75yrs. Winter 'Keep Warm' campaigns include information on local sources of heating and insulation grants for low income families, pensioners, and other vulnerable adults.

*Security*  LAs may have schemes for helping low income households, particularly pensioners, and to install or improve home security. Advice on crime prevention, home security and bogus callers is available from local policy forces and their websites.

*Problems with neighbours*  Tackling anti-social behaviour is a crime reduction partnership activity in all LA areas. Most LAs have information and/or staff dealing with this issue. Issues like noise problems are usually dealt with in the first instance by environmental health services (📖 Environmental health services, p. 23).

### Help for homelessness

Each country has a legal definition of homeless, which in England includes:
- No home in the UK or anywhere else in the world.
- Only able to stay in current place on a very temporary basis, or have been locked out of home.
- Can't live at home because of violence or threats of violence.
- Unreasonable to stay in that house, e.g. home in very poor condition.

LAs have a legal duty to provide advice to people who are homeless or threatened with homelessness. They only have a responsibility to help with accommodation if people meet all of the criteria:
- Legally eligible (many groups, e.g. asylum seekers, are excluded).
- Are not intentionally homeless.
- Are in priority need, i.e. is pregnant or has dependent children under 16 or 19yrs if in full-time education, or through an emergency, such as a flood, or aged under 16yrs (not in Northern Ireland). It may also include people vulnerable through illness or disability, at risk of violence, and homeless after leaving prison, hospital, or the armed forces.

The LA may give temporary accommodation while they investigate. The LA has to help those who qualify, but does not have to provide LA properties. Local social services authorities have a duty to provide accommodation for children and young people over 16yrs leaving care, or in need (📖 Children in special circumstances, p. 160) for other reasons.

### References

[1]Citizens Advice Bureau. Available at: 🔊 www.citizensadvice.org.uk
[2]Care and Repair (for older people) England. Available at: 🔊 www.careandrepair-england.org.uk/ Wales www.careandrepair.org.uk/ Scotland. Available at: 🔊 www.care-repair-scot.org.uk/

### Further information

Shelter (Wales). Available at: 🔊 www.shelter.org.uk Wales. Available at: www.sheltercymru.org.uk
Shelter (Scotland). Available at: 🔊 www.shelterscotland.org.uk
UK National Statistics. Publication Hub. Available at: 🔊 www.statistics.gov.uk/hub/people-places/ index.html

# Environmental health services

Practitioners frequently come across environmental health issues that impact on their patients and clients. Each LA has an environmental health department (sometimes called consumer protection department) employing environmental health officers (EHOs). Their role is to prevent, detect, and control environmental hazards that affect human health. The department's core functions are usually:

- Private sector housing.
- Food hygiene and safety.
- Noise and pollution control.
- Pest control.
- Occupational health and safety.
- Notifiable and reportable diseases control (with NHS public health departments).

It may also include other functions e.g. waste disposal and cleansing services, animal wardens for stray dogs. EHOs are also involved in public health and health promotion campaigns.

**Private sector housing** (📖 Homes and housing, p. 21) EHOs can inspect rented properties and enforce basic living standards.

**Food hygiene and safety** Food premises are inspected according to the food safety risk they pose to the public. Premises found to contravene basic food hygiene standards can be closed down and prosecuted.

**Noise and pollution control** EHOs have powers to deal with noise problems from industry, continual neighbourhood noise, e.g. barking dogs, music. They can seize noisy equipment or serve notices to stop. Failure to comply can result in prosecution.

**Pest control** Advice and action to remove ants, bees, mice, rats, wasps, and other pests from homes and business. Fees are usually charged, reduced for those on low income benefits or pension.

**Occupational health and safety** EHOs inspect non-manufacturing premises under the Health and Safety at Work, etc. Act 1974, and can stop work activities immediately, require improvements to be made, and/or prosecute businesses. EHOs also investigate workplace accidents.

### Infectious diseases and food poisoning

LA appoint a 'proper officer' to be notified of legally reportable infectious dissuades. EHOs investigate the causes of notifiable and reportable diseases (📖 Infectious disease notification, p. 103), and food poisoning in conjunction with NHS public health leads for communicable diseases (forming a team for infectious disease outbreak control), as well as other 'reportable diseases'.

### Further information

There is direct access for the public and professionals to these services. Information on the services and how to access them is on every LA website.

# Social support

Social support is the existence or availability of people on whom you can rely, who let you know that you are cared about, valued, and loved. The main source of social support comes from family, friends, and involvement in local organizations, e.g. clubs, schools, trade unions, and faith groups. Even after accounting for various factors that may also affect health, e.g. age, gender, education, and marital status, individuals who say they have family and friends they can count on to help in times of trouble are consistently more satisfied with their personal health. Social support is a concept linked to social capital ( Community approaches to health, p. 302).

### Lack of social support and the experience of loneliness

- Associated with ↑ morbidity and mortality.
- *Socio-economic classification:* those with higher incomes are less likely to report a lack of social support than those with low incomes.
- *Gender:* ♂ more likely to report a lack of social support than ♀.
- *Ethnicity:* contrary to popular stereotypes, people from a range of ethnic backgrounds often report severe lack of social support.
- ~20% of older population is lonely sometimes and another 8–10% is intensely lonely.
- 17% of older people are in contact with family, friends, and neighbours <once a week, and 11% are in contact <once a month.
- 51% of all people aged 75yrs and over live alone.
- Half of all older people (over 5 million) say television is their main company.

Questions to assess levels of social support available to clients and patients include:

- Is someone available to talk with, who will listen?
- Is someone available to help with activities of daily living?
- Is there someone who can provide emotional support?
- What is frequency of contact with those you feel close to and who you trust and confide in?

### Sources of social support

- Local community-based organizations, e.g. faith organizations, political parties, schools, community centres, tenants associations, youth clubs.
- Local support groups for people in same situation, e.g. carers support groups.
- Local branches of national charities and voluntary organizations, e.g. Alzheimer's Society, Gingerbread, Family Welfare Association.
- Local volunteer organizations and good neighbour schemes.
- Online and telephone support, e.g. Childline, Parentline.
- Health and Wellbeing Boards.
- Health, social work, and other public service professionals.
- Campaign to End Loneliness.

Every nurse working in primary care needs to know how to provide clients and patients with information about *local* sources of social support and when appropriate what opportunities there are to become more involved (e.g. volunteering). Good starting points for getting local directories are:
• Local library.
• LA website.
• Local Council for Voluntary Services.

## Related topics
📖 Health needs assessment, p. 11.
📖 Learning to work in primary care, p. 33.

## Further information
Campaign to End Loneliness. Ending loneliness and creating connections in older age. Available at: ℘ www.campaigntoendloneliness.org.uk

Information on volunteering. Volunteer placements, rights and expenses. Available at: ℘ www.direct.gov.uk/en/HomeAndCommunity/Gettinginvolvedinyourcommunity/Volunteering/index.htm

# Social services

Social care departments (England and Wales), social work departments (Scotland), or health and social services board (Northern Ireland) have wide-ranging legal responsibilities to use public funds to provide a range of care, support, and protection services for:
• Children, young people, and their families.
• Vulnerable adults who, by reason of age or disability, need assistance to live an independent life, and their carers.

They are part of the LA (except in Northern Ireland). They work in partnership with health, education, housing, the police, and voluntary sector to meet the needs of vulnerable people. Planned legislation for England aims to focus on increasing people's control over care and integration of services.

## Contacting social services

Social services take direct enquiries from the public, as well as take referrals by professionals. People are assessed by a social worker to determine needs (📖 The assessment of children, young people, and families, p. 148; 📖 Integrated (or single) assessment process, p. 114; 📖 Carers assessment and support, p. 412). Social workers can provide:
• Information about the care and support services that are available.
• An assessment of need.
• Practical help and support for some people according to local eligibility criteria.
• Information about other organizations that may help.

*Note:* most services are charged for, following an individual assessment of ability to pay (varies in each country).

Support for children, young people, and their families includes:
• Protection for children and young people from abuse and neglect.
• Support for vulnerable families to prevent family breakdown.
• Looking after children who cannot live at home.
• Support for families with a child who has a permanent and substantial disability.
• Work to reduce likelihood of young people committing offences.

Services likely to be available include:
• Safeguarding children (📖 Child protection, p. 230).
• Family support.
• Short-term breaks.
• Equipment and adaptations to the home (📖 Assistive technology, p. 776).
• Residential care and support for young people leaving care (📖 Looked-after children, p. 235).
• Youth justice teams.

Support for vulnerable adults include:
- Older people with physical and mental frailty.
- People with physical and/or sensory disabilities or learning disabilities.
- People with mental health needs.
- People with problems of substance misuse (drugs, alcohol, etc.).
- People who have HIV/AIDS.

Services likely to be available include:
- Home care and meals on wheels.
- Day centres and group activities.
- Short-term breaks.
- Equipment and home adaptations (📖 Assistive technology, p. 776).
- Registration for disabled people.

Adult social care services may directly provide services or pay for other providers. Some people may have direct payments to purchase their own care with public funds. If the locally set financial limits for assistance in the community are exceeded, the person is offered residential or nursing home care (📖 Care homes, p. 28).

## Social work teams

Can be organized in different ways:
- Cover a geographical area and work generically.
- Be part of a joint service with health, e.g. community mental health teams.
- Be based in a neighbourhood centre, hospital, or health centre.
- Specialize in:
  - Children and families.
  - Adults services.
  - Specific groups, e.g. people who are blind, deaf, or have dementia.

Most social services have a duty system, whereby designated social workers/teams take new enquiries or referrals.

*Note:* every nurse in primary care needs to identify local referral pro-cesses to adult social care, children's services, and social workers.

## Related topics

📖 Services for children, young people, and families, p. 19.
📖 Homes and housing, p. 21.
📖 Environmental services, p. 23.
📖 Social support, p. 24.

## Further information

Care Quality Commission. Available at: 🔗 www.cqc.org.uk
Scottish Social Care Services Council. Available at: 🔗 www.sssc.uk.com

# Care homes

4% of people >65yrs of age live in care homes and 20% of people >85yrs; ~65% are women[1]. Registered care homes either have on-site nursing care (previously known as nursing homes) or are without on-site nursing care (previously known as residential homes). Care homes are run by not-for-profit voluntary organizations, private companies or, less frequently, LAs and the NHS.

## Registration and inspection

All care homes are inspected to ensure that they comply with national standards, and are registered by the Care Quality Commission (CQC) in England, Care Inspectorate Scotland, and Care and Social Services Inspectorate Wales. Some care homes have specific registration for different groups, e.g. people with learning disability (LD), dementia. Local offices and social service departments provide lists of registered care homes.

## Provision

Care homes can provide:
- Long-term care for adults who, through frailty or disability, need help with personal care and/or have nursing care needs.
- Long-term care for vulnerable groups in need of special/extra care (e.g. children and adults with learning disabilities).
- Respite and intermediate care.
- Continuing NHS care.
- Palliative care.

## Personal care

In care homes, personal care (i.e. not nursing care) is usually defined as:
- Help with washing, bathing, and showering.
- Help with managing continence, including using catheters and stomas.
- Assistance with eating and managing special diets.
- Help to move around indoors.
- Help with simple treatments, e.g. applying creams, lotions, dressings.

## Primary health care

Care home residents are registered with GPs like other citizens (📖 General practice, p. 13) and receive primary care services in the same way. Evidence shows that residents in care homes receive erratic care from NHS services and should have better access to specialist care. District nurses (DNs) provide nursing care for residents in care homes. Some DNs visit care homes with on-site nursing, although local custom and practice may influence the range of services offered. In addition to nursing tasks DNs may have:
- Planned meetings with care home staff to review care, discuss issues of concern.
- Proactive review of residents' health and medication needs.
- Involvement in end-of-life care.
- Education and training of care home staff.

## Public financial assistance for care home fees

The starting point in all countries is the assessment of needs by the LA, usually by a social worker. Social services have a set ceiling for fees and a list of preferred providers. Rules for public financial assistance differ in the four countries and are linked to national eligibility criteria for NHS continuing care, if someone has been assessed as needing fully-funded NHS care (sometimes also called continuing health care), the NHS is responsible for paying all care home fees.

More than half of residents in care homes have fees paid by LAs. Individuals fund their own fees if their financial resources are above the national threshold (e.g. in England residents with over £23,250 of eligible capital will be expected to meet the full cost of their care). *Note:* legislation and guidance is rapidly changing, so check with local adult social care/services and Age UK have regularly updated fact sheets.

## Individual's contribution to care fees

The LA financial assessment includes income, e.g. pension, savings, shares, and property (including the individual's own home) when working out an individual's contributions to fees. The value of a home is excluded:
• For the first 12wks after entry into permanent care.
• If the home is shared by partner, relative >60yrs old, incapacitated relative <60yrs old, carer, or child <16yrs old.
• LA discretion, e.g. someone who was previously a carer.

The LA must leave the individual some money for personal use. If the LA is contributing to care home fees and the person chooses a more expensive care home than the LA ceiling amount, a third party, e.g. a relative, has to contract with the LA and care home to pay the top-up amount.

## NHS contribution to care home fees

A resident in a care home with nursing may have the nursing care element of their fees paid by the NHS. PCOs will have a system for assessing the need for funded nursing care contribution Amounts differ in each country, e.g. in England the NHS contribution for people assessed as requiring the help of a registered nurse is £108.70 per wk at standard rate and 149.60 per wk at the higher band of need for nursing.

## Complaints and concerns

Complaints and concerns not addressed by a care home should be referred to these inspection bodies:
Care Quality Commission (CQC). Available at: ℘ www.cqc.org.uk
Scottish Care Inspectorate. Available at: ℘ www.careinspectorate.com

## Related topics

📖 Social services, p. 26.
📖 People with dementias, p. 438.

## Reference

[1]Office of National Statistics. Available at: ℘ www.statistics.gov.uk

## Further information

Age UK. Available at: ℘ www.ageuk.org.uk (linked sites for all countries)
Counsel and Care. Available at: ℘ http://www.independentage.org/

# Nursing in primary care

# Nurses in primary care

Primary care services are those services that can be accessed directly by the public without referral from another professional (📖 Overview of services in primary care, p. 146). Nurses and HVs work in a variety of primary care settings delivering services that range from public health, preventative, curative, chronic disease management, through to the care of people who are dying. Sometimes the main work roles are categorized as providing first contact services, providing chronic disease management services, and providing public health services. Some groups of nurses focus more on one aspect, e.g. HVs on a public health role while others may combine all three aspects, e.g. practice nurses. The service can be reactive (in response to people seeking them out or referring to them) or proactive (actively seeking out people or particular populations). Nurses in primary care can be generalists, e.g. practice nurses, or specialists (i.e. working with only one type of condition), e.g. people with sickle cell disorders, or only one part of the population, e.g. travellers, or providing only one type of service, e.g. sexual health or contraceptive services.

In the UK over 68,000 (head count) nurses and HVs are employed directly by primary care organizations (PCOs) and other NHS organizations to work in the community and over 26,000 (head count) practice nurses are employed directly by general practices. The numbers are increasing as more health care is delivered in primary health-care settings.

The largest groups of nurses are within:
• District nursing services.
• Practice nursing.
• Health visiting.
• School nursing.

However, there are also significant numbers in specialist services such as family planning, sexual health services, community children's nursing, walk-in centres, OOH centres, and occupational health services. Some specialist nurses also work in primary care as outreach from the hospital consultant led team, e.g. diabetes specialist nurses.

Many services are evolving and changing constantly, sometimes introducing new roles, e.g. community matrons in England. Primary care offers a very dynamic environment for career development. Local as well as national advice should always be sought on educational pathways and competencies required of different roles.

## Further information

NHS Careers Nursing. Available at: ℛ www.nhscareers.nhs.uk
NMC Nursing and Midwifery Council. Available at: ℛ www.nmc-uk.org/Nurses-and-midwives/
See also professional organizations (📖 Useful websites, p. 800)

# Learning to work in primary care

Working in primary care and domiciliary settings (📖 Key definitions of primary care and public health, p. 4) is very different to working in the hospital environment.

❶ Nurses new to primary care, irrespective of prior clinical experience and seniority, become novice practitioners again. This is because:

• The patient/client is in control of all decisions; the nurse/HV is a guest in the home.
• Patients and their carers undertake most of their own care, the overall nursing contribution is small (📖 Key facts on carers and caring, p. 410).
• Many systems and infrastructures support the delivery of health and social care and are locally specific and variable; it takes time to familiarize oneself with the full range of available services (e.g. 📖 Social services, p. 26; 📖 Homes and housing, p. 21).
• Clinical decision-making and care delivery are often done independently and at a physical distance from other colleagues.
• Nurses in primary care work with uncertainty, changing situations, and services; this requires flexibility in approach and assertiveness to work on the patient/client's behalf.

## Orientation to primary care

Nobody knows how long it will take individual nurses to become orientated to working in primary care. Some adapt rapidly, others take much longer. In addition, the different responsibilities of the range of posts mean that nurses need different preparation. Information about professional preparation programmes are given in each of the topics about the different groups of nurses and services. However, all nurses new to working in primary care should ensure that they have:

• An orientation and induction process from their employer (📖 Clinical supervision and appraisal, p. 46).
• A mentor to review and discuss work with (📖 Teaching and mentorship, p. 48).
• Opportunities to work with other nurse role models and to shadow other professionals.
• Access to information (e.g. directories) about the local service environment: the range of local services, referral mechanisms, key contacts, eligibility criteria, and funding mechanisms for different services.
• Knowledge of risk assessment processes for both patient and personal safety (📖 Clinical risk management, p. 72).
• Information on how to get around the area physically.

## Related topic

📖 Useful websites, p. 800, lists all the relevant nursing and professional organizations.

## Reference

Drennan V, Goodman C, Leyshon S. (2005). Supporting nurses new to primary care. Available at: ✏ eprints.kingston.ac.uk

# General practice nursing

The majority of practice nurses are directly employed by general practices ([ General practice, p. 13; [ Other types of primary care medical services contracts, p. 15). They mainly work as self-directing practitioners within the practice organization, often in small nursing teams that may include advanced nurse practitioners and/or health care assistants (HCAs).

## Focus of practice nurses' work

- Provide appropriate care/treatment in conjunction with the GP or independently where care has been transferred to the nurse by the GP.
- Assess nursing needs of patients registered with GP practice.
- Document the process of assessment of need and delivery of care.
- Evaluate the outcome of care, make changes to care plan, and modify practice with patient.
- Liaise with other members of primary health care team (PHCT) to assure appropriate care.
- Provide counselling and health education.
- Contribute to clinical governance, QOF ([ Quality and outcomes framework, p. 66), and risk management of practice.

In addition those working as nurse practitioner (NPs) (also known as Advanced Nurse Practitioner (ANPs)) may:

- Provide telephone triage.
- Receive patients with undifferentiated and undiagnosed problems and makes an assessment of their health-care needs based on advanced level nursing skills and knowledge including physical examination.
- Make differential diagnoses using decision-making and problem-solving skills.
- Provide counselling and health education.
- Work collaboratively with other health-care professionals.
- Provide leadership, management, and consultancy functions as required.

*Note:* the demarcation of roles between NP and practice nurses is fluid.

## Main areas of responsibility and skills

Each practice nurse agrees their responsibilities with their employer. They require a range of clinical skills and knowledge for general patient care developed through experience and training. Depending on their work role, these skills may include:

- Chronic disease management, e.g. diabetes, CHD, hypertension, asthma.
- Cervical cytology ([ Cervical cancer screening, p. 337).
- Travel health ([ Travel health, p. 350).
- Child and adult immunization ([ Childhood immunization, p. 156; [ Targeted immunizations in adults, p. 347).
- Wound care ([ Wound assessment, p. 475).
- Ear care ([ Ear care, p. 544).

- ♀ health, i.e. HRT, contraception (📖 Contraception: general, p. 359), well woman.
- Health education and promotion.
- Triage assessment.
- Audit and record keeping, particularly for QOF indicators.

In addition those working as NPs/ANPs will have additional skills including:
- Physical examination, investigation, initiate treatment, prescribe medications, referral to another health-care professional in either 1° or 2° care.
- Screen patients for disease risk factors and early signs of illness.
- Order necessary investigations; provide treatment and care, individually, as part of a team, and through referral to other agencies.
- Admit and discharge patients from their caseload, and refer to other health-care providers as appropriate.
- Manage the treatment and care of patients with acute and/or chronic illness.

## Education, training, and qualifications

### Practice nurses
- A registered nurse usually with some post-registration experience.
- Will have evidence of ongoing professional and academic education and training.
- Can access degree level education in practice nursing specific degree programmes and modules as well as short courses, e.g. diabetes management, COPD management.

### Advanced nurse practitioners
- Defined by the Royal College of Nursing (RCN) as a registered nurse who has undertaken a specific NP course at 1st degree level (minimum) though currently not regulated or required.
- Debates continue in the UK as to possible future regulation by NMC.

## Further information

NHS Careers Practice Nursing. Available at: ℐ www.nhscareers.nhs.uk
Nurse Practitioner UK. Available at: ℐ www.nursepractitioner.org.uk/
RCGP General Practice Foundation. Available at: ℐ www.rcgp-foundation.org.uk/
RCN Practice Nurse Association. Available at: ℐ www.rcn.org.uk/development/communities/
    rcn_forum_communities/practice_nurses
RCN Advanced Nurse Practitioner Forum. Available at: ℐ www.rcn.org.uk/development/
    communities/rcn_forum_communities/nurse_practitioner

# School nursing

### Focus of work

The main focus of the school nurse (SN) work is enabling children and young people to achieve their potential by staying healthy, staying safe, enjoying and achieving, making a positive contribution, and reaching economic wellbeing. Working towards these priority outcomes is based on joint working with school and other education service staff, professionals from safeguarding children's boards such as social workers, other health professionals, and the voluntary sector. SNs in many areas are known as school health advisers to reflect the change in focus of their work in health promotion and public health.

### Main areas of responsibility

SNs work with school-aged children and young people and their families to:
- Assess health and social care needs, monitor, and refer as necessary.
- Promote healthy lifestyles through health promoting activities (e.g. sex and relationship education (SRE), personal, social, health education (PSHE) and citizenship, healthy schools programmes), either in groups or one to one.
- Identify those in need of protection, monitor, refer, and contribute to safeguarding children in accordance with local/national policies.
- Organize and administer immunization programmes in line with DH guidelines.
- Provide support for those with special/complex needs.
- Provide advice, support and teaching for school staff, parents, carers, children, and young people.

### Team and work organization

School health services are offered mainly in state schools and community settings. It includes school doctors/paediatricians, although other health-care professionals may visit schools as part of their public health work, e.g. community dentists. SNs are organized in a variety of ways according to local needs, e.g.:
- SNs may be named nurses with responsibility for a number of schools (either primary or secondary or both).
- SNs may work in teams with nursery nurses, HCAs, led by a senior SN.
- SNs may work only as part of a school immunization team.

The work of SNs is organized to follow the recommendations from national child health programmes, e.g. the Healthy Child Promotion programme. It may involve specific clinical or health promotion sessions in schools as well as offering open access drop in sessions for school children.

## Education and training for school nursing

SNs are qualified nurses mostly employed by PCOs and Foundation Trusts in the NHS. Independent schools may also employ their own nurses or receive a limited school nursing service from their local health trust. SNs are likely to hold an additional community nursing or public health qualification in the form of:

- Specialist community practitioner public health (school nursing).
- Certificate, diploma in school nursing/public health.
- Other specific training in contraceptive and sexual health, health education, mental health, enuresis, and counselling or others.

## Related topic

📖 Working in schools, p. 38.

## Further information

NHS Careers School Nursing. Available at: ✆ www.nhscareers.nhs.uk

Community Practitioner and Health Visitor Association. Available at: ✆ www.unitetheunion.org/sectors/health_sector/professional_groups__assoc/cphva.aspx

RCN toolkit for School Nurses. Available at: ✆ www.rcn.org.uk/__data/assets/pdf_file/0012/201630/003223.pdf

The Department for Education (Health information on the National Curriculum and the National Healthy Schools Programme). Available at: ✆ www.education.gov.uk

DH (2012). Getting it right for children, young people and family: Maximizing the contribution of the school nursing team (Gateway Ref 17158). Available at: ✆ https://www.gov.uk/government/uploads/system/uploads/attachment_data/file/152212/dh_133352.pdf.pdf

Welsh Assembly (2009). A Framework for School Nursing in Wales. Available at: ✆ http://wales.gov.uk/topics/health/publications/health/reports/nursing/?lang=en

DHSSPSNI (2010). Healthy Futures: The Contribution of Health Visitors and School Nurses. Available at: ✆ http://www.dhsspsni.gov.uk/healthy_futures_2010-2015.pdf

# Working in schools

## Key principles

Health provision for school-aged children is delivered in different ways on a variety of sites in order to meet the needs of young people, their parents, and carers. School nurses work flexible hours, e.g. prior to and after normal school hours. Services are predominantly provided in the school setting, but additionally at other sites, e.g. health centres/clinics, children's centres, youth centres. The SN needs to develop effective communication processes with key school members including:

• The head/deputy head teacher.
• The special educational needs coordinator (SENCO).
• The child protection/safeguarding children coordinator.
• Healthy schools coordinator.
• PSHE and citizenship adviser/coordinator.

A key contact is the school secretary who holds information on both the school organization and details of the children and their families.

SNs identify health needs through school health profiling and plan key health promotion activities with school staff according to local needs and priorities. With policy changes for education and young people, e.g. extended schools, health provision for children may be delivered in different ways in future, e.g. shift working, health assessments on different types of sites, or more work with parents.

The head teacher and school governors are responsible for developing school health-related policies, e.g. ☐ Sex and relationship education, p. 223, health, and safety. School nurses contribute to provide up-to-date evidenced-based information.

### Year and term planning

The academic year dates and most school activities are planned a year in advance. ∴ SNs and other professionals liaise with relevant school staff to contribute towards health promotion and curriculum planning during the summer term for the next school year. Some activities/sessions can be organized on a termly basis, but it would be wise to do this a term in advance. The school terms in most areas are organized as follows:

• *Autumn:* September–December.
• *Spring:* January–April.
• *Summer:* May–July.

### School health records

School health records in some areas are kept in locked filing cabinets on school premises (key access only for SN); in other areas records are kept at the health centre base. Electronic child health records are also used in some areas. Parents and children are encouraged to bring their personal child health record (☐ Client and patient-held records, p. 87) with them to health assessments in school.

### Medicines in schools

There are national and local policies to help education staff and health professionals in meeting the needs of children/young people requiring medicines in schools. Responsibility for giving or supervising medicines is usually undertaken by teachers or classroom helpers who are often trained by school health advisers, children's community nurses, or specialist nurses to carry out that role. The whole process involves careful planning between the MDT, e.g.:

• Training for parents, carers, school staff restorage, administration, and disposal.
• Proper discharge planning from hospital and suitable drug regimens to facilitate smooth administration.
• GP—for review.

## Children with statements of special education needs

Children with special educational needs (SEN) statements have yearly reviews with multi-agency input. Dates for these reviews are planned in advance and a list given to the designated medical officer with responsibility for special needs. It is good practice to try and coordinate health reviews to coincide with the educational reviews. School nurses/doctors attend these reviews and provide medical or nursing reports as necessary.

## Working in special schools

Special schools cater for children and young people with complex needs requiring a multi-disciplinary approach (📖 Children with complex health needs and disabilities, p. 225) involving: allied health professionals—SLTs, OTs, physiotherapists, health professionals, education staff and parents, social services.

Arrangements for nursing cover vary; some areas have nurses on site, while others visit on a regular basis. Nurses will, in most instances, undertake medicine administration, tube feeding, IV, or rectal medicines. Generally, nurses working in special schools will perform a wider range of hands-on nursing care compared to those in mainstream schools. Some members of the school staff may also be trained to undertake some tasks such as feeding, emergency medicines, catheter care, etc.

### Special units

Some children/young people who are excluded from school will attend pupil referral units. Some schools also provide for children with hearing/vision impairment or language difficulties in special units. SNs and the medical team support the families and school in meeting their needs.

## Related topics

📖 Child health promotion, p. 144; 📖 Child protection, p. 230.

## Further information

Department for Education Healthy Schools Programme. Available at: ℘ www.education.gov.uk/schools/pupilsupport/pastoralcare/a0075278/healthy-schools
Department for Education. Managing Medicines in Schools and Early Years Settings (2005 updated September 2011). Available at: ℘ www.education.gov.uk/publications/standard/publicationDetail/Page1/DFES-1448-2005
Medical Conditions at School: A Policy Resource Pack. Available at: ℘ http://medicalconditionsatschool.org.uk/

# Health visiting

## Focus of work

Health visiting is a public health nursing specialism. The focus of the work is the promotion of health and the prevention of ill health. The main principles in health visiting activity are:

- The search for health needs.
- The stimulation of an awareness of health needs.
- The facilitation of health-enhancing activities.
- The influence on policies affecting health.

This public health focus can be with any group in the population and can be with an individual, a family, group, or community. The search for health needs can be through formalized health needs assessment (📖 Health needs assessment, p. 11), of a community, a caseload, or an individual. The locus of the activity may be in the client's home, in health centres, surgeries, in children's centres or community settings. Each country has its own programme and plans for HV services, e.g. DH England has reaffirmed HVs as key professionals in public health delivery and is increasing the numbers trained and employed.

## Main areas of responsibility

The majority of HVs are employed to work with families with young children. Evidence from neuroscience and social sciences shows that the early years are crucial to a child's future development and adult health. HVs lead and deliver on nationally agreed, evidence-based public health programmes for a healthy child starting in pregnancy through early childhood (📖 Child health promotion, p. 11), e.g. the English Health Child Programme (HCP) and four different types of services. These include:

- Health promotion services to improve health and wellbeing, as well as reduce inequalities, may include community development (known as Your Community Services in England).
- Health promotion and support of families with young children, alongside general practice, to access HCP and local services at key points (antenatally (📖 Antenatal education, p. 379)), soon after the birth of the baby (📖 New birth visits, p. 168). This includes:
  - Advice on adult health, including maternal mental wellbeing to enable strong early attachment and infant emotional wellbeing (📖 Emotional development in babies and infants, p. 199).
  - Advice and support on parenting (📖 Support for parents, p. 166) and child development <5yrs to support emotional wellbeing and to develop improved school readiness.
  - Advice and support of nutrition including breastfeeding (📖 Breastfeeding, p. 176), infant nutrition for individual good health and to address rising obesity rates (📖 Food and the under fives, p. 201).
  - Advice and information on child immunization (📖 Childhood immunization, p. 156) for the individual and to achieve population immunity.

- Early identification of health (physical, social, emotional, and mental) needs of babies, children, and adults, and negotiating and agreeing an action plan with clients which may involve more contact with HV team, e.g. for listening visits or referral to other services.
- Expert help from the HV team with more frequent contact in response to an identified need or problem e.g. breastfeeding problems or postnatal depression (known as Universal Plus in England), ongoing support from the HV team and a range of other services to address more complex issues over a period of time. Examples are children with disabilities (📖 Children with complex health needs and disabilities, p. 225), child with child protection needs (📖 Child protection, p. 230).

## Team and work organization

HVs work collegiately with other HVs either from the same base or working with the same GPs. Some share their caseloads (known as 'corporate caseloads') in order to ensure equity in workloads and improve access and services to clients. Caseloads (of clients) are created from either those living in a geographical area or a GP patient population. They proactively make contact, offering services, as well as receiving referrals from other services. They work closely with others, e.g. early years practitioners, midwives, GPs, and social workers, and other agencies both statutory and voluntary. Some HVs have specialist roles to work with specific vulnerable groups (e.g. homeless families, travelers) or specific health promotion programmes, e.g. specialize in community development.

Many HVs lead teams of other staff, e.g. nursery nurses, staff nurses, and health-care assistants to deliver the public health agenda and HCP. HVs may also be part of wider initiatives in multi-agency settings, e.g. public health departments. HVs are active in implementing programmes such as the Family Nurse Partnership and Maternal Early Childhood Sustained Home Visiting (📖 Support for parents, p. 166).

## Education and training for health visiting

All HVs are registered nurses or midwives before commencing specialist practitioner training, a 1yr full-time or 2yr part-time course at degree level or postgraduate level. Usually HV services provide NHS funds for the course and salary through sponsorship. Opportunities for sponsorship are advertised locally and nationally.

Newly qualified HVs are registered on specialist community public health register of the NMC, with an annotation to show they are HVs.

## Further information

NHS Careers Health Visiting. Available at: ℘ www.nhscareers.nhs.uk
Institute of Health Visiting Practice. Available at: ℘ www.ihv.org.uk/
Community Practitioner and Health Visitor Association. Available at: ℘ www.unitetheunion.org/sectors/health_sector/professional_groups__assoc/cphva.aspx
Family Nurse Partnership Programme Scotland. Available at: ℘ www.scotland.gov.uk/Topics/Health/NHS-Scotland/nursing/ModernisingCommunityNursi/MNCBoardMeetings/FNP
DHSSPSNI (2010) Healthy Futures: The Contribution of Health Visitors and School Nurses. Available at: ℘ http://www.dhsspsni.gov.uk/healthy_futures_2010-2015.pdf

# District nursing

### Focus of district nursing work

DN teams will accept direct referrals from, and liaise with, hospitals, health and social care professionals, patients, and carers. They assess, prescribe, monitor, provide, and evaluate nursing care for people in their home, in care homes, and clinics based in primary care settings (e.g. health centres). Increasingly DN services are seen as a key service that can help to reduce numbers of unplanned admissions and readmissions to hospital. The range of the service provided is dependent on local policies and practice and availability of other community specialist services, e.g. IV therapies, specialist palliative care. The majority of provision is to frail older people, adults with long-term conditions, and sometimes children who require nursing care in the home. DN patients are identified either by being registered with a specific GP practice that the DN team works with (GP attachment) or the locality where they live (geographical working). As well as a 'core' daytime service, many DN services provide an 'OOH' service, which includes evening and night nursing care. DN services are free at the point of delivery and can be contacted through the primary care organization and/or GP practices.

### Main areas of responsibility assessment and care for people

- Short-term, self-care education and support, e.g. support and teaching to newly diagnosed diabetic patient.
- Case/care management of people with complex and/or long-term conditions.
- Rehabilitation care and support in recovery.
- Intermediate care and care following discharge from hospital.
- Palliative care.
- Care in collaboration with other clinical nurse specialists (e.g. Macmillan nurses, continence specialists, tissue viability nurses, etc.).
- Carer assessment and support.
- Administration and maintenance of technical therapies in the home, e.g. IV therapy, PEG feeds, continence care, wound care, diabetic care, some injections.
- Assessment and social support: DNs work closely with social care providers and community care agencies.

A DN is a qualified nurse employed by the NHS who is likely to be a nurse prescriber (📖 Medicines management, p. 126) and hold an additional community nursing qualification in district nursing/nursing in the home. Usually works as team leader or member of a skill mixed nursing team (i.e. with community staff nurses and health-care assistants) with responsibility for a specific patient caseload.

## Education and training

- William Rathbone established first training school in Liverpool in 1863.
- DN current training (shortened) degree or postgrad diploma. Entry NMC registered (or expected to be by the beginning of the academic year) with either a diploma or degree as a nurse or midwife. Courses are 1yr full-time or 2yrs part-time, at colleges and universities throughout UK (sponsorship provided through NHS).
- Courses known by a range of titles including Community Health-care Nursing, and Specialist Community Practitioner Award, sometimes referred to as nursing in the home. Comprise 50% theory and 50% practice with practical placements supervised by an experienced DN.
- *Four areas:* clinical nursing practice, care and programme management, clinical practice development, clinical practice leadership.
- Work-based learning courses available for staff nurses entering DN posts/rotation schemes for flexible entry to primary care.
- Short courses and modules for community nurses in specialist topics, e.g. tissue viability, palliative care, case management, chronic disease management.

## Further information

Queens Nursing Institute. Available at: ℘ http://www.qni.org.uk/
NHS Careers. Available at: ℘ www.nhscareers.nhs.uk
Royal College of Nursing. Available at: ℘ www.rcn.org.uk
See also central Departments of Health for current strategies and policies for district nursing.
(☐ Useful websites, p. 800)

# Employment contracts

## The contract

In British law a contract comes into existence on starting to work for an employer, irrespective of whether it is verbal or in writing. The contract is formed where there is:

- An offer of work.
- An acceptance of that offer.
- A promise by the employer to pay the employee in return for the employee's promise to work.

If an offer is withdrawn the employer may be in breach of contract and could be taken to an employment tribunal.

## Statement of terms and conditions

There is a legal entitlement to a statement of the terms and conditions of the post within 2mths of start date provided employment lasts for 1mth or more. Must include by law:

- The names of the employer and the employee.
- The date when the employment began.
- Remuneration and the intervals at which it is to be paid.
- Hours of work.
- The place of work.
- Holiday entitlement.
- Entitlement to sick leave, including any entitlement to sick pay.
- Details of the employer's disciplinary and grievance procedures.
- Pensions and pension schemes.
- The entitlement of employer and employee to notice of termination.
- Any collective agreements affecting employment terms or conditions.
- The date when it is to end if not permanent.

### Fixed-term contracts

Legislation exists to ensure people on fixed-term contracts are not treated unfairly. The non-renewal of a fixed-term contract is a dismissal in law and can be contested as unfair dismissal. There is also an entitlement to redundancy payment. There is a statutory limit of 4yrs on the use of successive fixed-term contracts then the contract is deemed permanent.

## Further information

Gov UK: Employment Contract. Available at: ℘ www.gov.uk/employment-contracts-and-conditions/overview

BusinessLink Employment & Skills. Available at: ℘ http://www.businesslink.gov.uk/bdotg/action/layer?topicId=1073858787

From all professional and trade union organizations 📖 Useful websites, p. 800.

RCN (2005). Nurses Employed by GPs: RCN Guidance on Good Employment Practice. Available at: ℘ www.rcn.org.uk/__data/assets/pdf_file/0006/78621/002435.pdf

# NHS pay and terms

Agenda for Change is the name of the UK NHS pay structure and terms and conditions of service to all staff except doctors. Not all general practice employers or independent employers use this framework (📖 Employment contracts, p. 44) and may have different terms and conditions.

## National job profiles

All nursing, HV, and support posts have national job profiles which have been agreed between NHS employers and Trade Unions[1]. These use the NHS knowledge and skills framework (KSF) and are assigned to an Agenda for Change pay band (1–9). Newly-qualified nurses enter at Band 5 and the first 12mths is referred to as 'preceptorship'. Each post usually has a job description and person specification issued by the employer.

## Terms and conditions

Standard full-time hours of work are 37.5hrs/wk, excluding breaks. Annual leave entitlement and entitlement to sick leave increases with the length of service. All are specified in the NHS Terms and Conditions Handbook found on the NHS employers website.[1]

## Pay

Pay is made up of basic salary then, as applicable, high cost-of-living area supplement, recruitment and retention premiums, enhanced rates for unsocial hours, and on-call payments. Overtime is paid as time and a half (double on public holidays only) or given back as time off in lieu (TOIL).

## NHS occupational pension schemes

The NHS occupational pension scheme is available to all NHS Trusts, GP practices, and other NHS organizations, including some social enterprises providing NHS services.

## Travel costs

All NHS employers reimburse work-related travel expenses on production of receipts and journey logs. Some may have a car lease scheme for staff undertaking domiciliary work.

## Reference

[1] NHS Employers. Agenda for Change Section including KSF, current pay scales, job profiles. Available at: ℘ www.nhsemployers.org/PayAndContracts/AgendaForChange/Pages/Afc-Homepage.aspx

## Further information

NHS Pensions (England and Wales). Available at: ℘ www.nhsbsa.nhs.uk/pensions
Public Pensions (NHS) Scotland. Available at: ℘ www.sppa.gov.uk/
NHS Pensions (N. Ireland). Available at: ℘ www.dhsspsni.gov.uk/index/hsc-pensions.htm

# Clinical supervision and appraisal

## Clinical supervision

Clinical supervision is a practice-focused professional relationship that enables reflection on practice with the support of a skilled supervisor. It is an element of both clinical governance (📖 Quality governance, p. 62), and continuing professional development (📖 Continuing professional development, p. 47). It has some or all of these purposes:

- Normative, i.e. maintaining appropriate standards of practice.
- Educative, i.e. developing competence.
- Supportive, i.e. providing a mechanism for staff to manage the intense pressures of work and to focus on the emotional resources needed to maintain high-quality care.

### Models of clinical supervision

Each work environment and staff group has to develop its own model to fit their needs. Possible models include:

- One-to-one, using line managers of the same discipline as supervisors.
- One-to-one with another, more experienced nurse or other professional, but excluding line managers as supervisors.
- Group supervision, either through peer group or MDT discussions.

### It is important to be explicit about:

- The aims of the supervision.
- The most appropriate model(s) and skilled supervisor.
- Ground rules (including timing, attendance, and confidentiality).
- The mechanism for evaluating the model of supervision.

## Appraisal

Appraisal is a formal opportunity for practitioners to review and develop their performance in the context of their organization's goals, their own job description, and the linked KSF. It is a separate process from clinical supervision. It is a formal system to:

- Review past performance, set new objectives, and identify training and development needs in a personal development plan (PDP).
- Highlight individual potential and discuss short-, medium-, and long-term career development.
- Acknowledge and record employee achievements, as well as performance concerns.

In the independent sector it may link to performance-related pay and bonus systems. In the NHS it links to the Agenda for Change gateways in pay bands (📖 NHS pay and terms, p. 45).

## Further information

Advisory, Conciliation and Arbitration Service (ACAS) Employee appraisal guidance. Available at: 🔗 www.acas.org.uk/media/pdf/o/q/B07_1.pdf

Schon, D. (1983). *The Reflective Practitioner*. London: Temple Smith.

# Continuing professional development

Health care and professional practice are continuously changing. All professionals have to maintain and develop competence through a lifelong learning process known as continuing professional development (CPD). CPD needs should be identified through everyday reflection on practice, clinical supervision (📖 Clinical supervision and appraisal, p. 46), and a personal development plan (PDP) developed during induction and appraisal processes.

## NMC requirements

The CPD element of the NMC Post-Registration Education and Practice Standards (PREP) for 3yrs re-registration, states that each nurse must:

- Undertake at least 35hrs of learning activity relevant to practice during the 3yrs prior to re-registration.
- Maintain a personal professional profile (PPP) of their learning activity.
- Comply with any request from the NMC to audit how they have met these requirements.

Learning may be formal (e.g. through course attendance) or informal (e.g. through reflection on a research paper). The NMC does not accredit courses for PREP and there is no such thing as an 'approved PREP' learning activity. The PPP is used to document the learning activity and how it has influenced practice. A suggested template for the PPP is included in the NMC's PREP handbook[1].

## Sources of support for nurses' CPD

- *National level:* electronic access to NHS Evidence, professional organizations (📖 Useful websites, p. 800), provision of study days and conferences, as well as financial support opportunities.
- *Local level:* may include:
  - Access to health-care libraries in local universities and health promotion/public health departments.
  - Practice PDPs in general practice.
  - PCO-wide general practice and primary care multidisciplinary learning events.
  - In-house PCO and Trust training and development programmes.
  - PCO or Trust learning and development plans that commission places for nurses on formal education courses at universities (*note:* a slightly different mechanism in each country).
  - Employer paying fees and giving time for higher degrees or specialist courses.
  - PCO or Trust sponsorship (i.e. salary plus fees) for specialist community and primary care qualifications.

## Reference

[1]NMC. (2011). *The Prep Handbook.* London: NMC. Available at: ♒ www.nmc-uk.org/Publications/Standards/

# Teaching and mentorship

Primary care nurses provide clinical teaching, mentorship, and preceptorship to a range of nursing and HV students. Some primary care nurses have designated clinical teaching posts for certain types of students, e.g. practice teachers, practice nurse trainers, specialist or community practice teachers for DN, HV, SN. These types of posts may attract additional salary (☐ NHS pay and terms, p. 45) or designated time for teaching. General practices may require payment for practice nurses to act as trainers or provide clinical placements to students. Local Higher Education Institutions (HEIs) provide short courses for clinical teaching roles as well as specific preparation for supporting different types of students.

## Principles of effective teaching and mentorship

*Adult learners*
- Are active in, and respond to, participation in the learning process.
- Have a rich resource of experience to contribute to the process.
- Are aware of their own learning needs linked to work roles and tasks.
- Are competency-based learners wanting to apply or experiment with new knowledge.

*Adult learning*
Best practice in teaching or mentorship suggests:
- Treat students/mentee with respect.
- *Agree:*
  - Clear objectives for the teaching/mentorship, based on what they are trying to learn.
  - Learning/mentoring opportunities based on the objectives.
  - Opportunities for reflection on the learning/mentorship process.
- Facilitate independence and active engagement.
- Provide balanced feedback that highlights areas of good practice as well as aspects for development.
- If applicable, use appropriate, objective, fair, and relevant assessment tasks for competence.
- Learn from students/mentees—evaluate and improve your teaching/mentorship.

## Consent of patients to teaching

The teacher practitioner should gain the full consent of patients/clients before students 'sit in' on consultations or provide clinical/professional services (☐ Consent, p. 77). It is good practice to have public information about the teaching in the practice/service and the right of patients/clients to decline to participate.

## Further information

NMC (2008). *Standards to support learning and assessment in practice.* NMC: London. Available at: ℘ www.nmc-uk.org/Publications/Standards/
RCN (2007). *Guidance for mentors of nursing students and midwives.* RCN: London. Available at: ℘ www.rcn.org.uk/__data/assets/pdf_file/0008/78677/002797.pdf

# Research in primary care

Research is the systematic inquiry to develop or contribute to the development of new knowledge that can be generalizable. It is essential for provision of high quality health care. Methodologies may be quantitative, qualitative, or mixed as appropriate to the question to be answered. Data collection methods range from clinical drug trials through to surveys, questionnaires, ethnographies, and in-depth case studies. All research follows a systematic process (see Fig. 2.1).

All countries' central health departments have research policies, funding for research and research careers, e.g. in England and Wales this is the National Institute for Health Research (NIHR) which can be found on their web pages (📖 Useful websites, p. 800). The UK Clinical Research Network supports the infrastructure for clinical research UK wide.

Many nurses contribute to research in the NHS. Nurses in primary care often undertake some stages of the research process (see Fig. 2.1) as part of educational programmes. Nurses undertaking higher degrees are required to undertake a research study. The number of academic primary care nurses undertaking and leading funded research is a small, but growing group. There have been recent initiatives to support clinical academic career pathways for nurses and AHPs.

## Ethics

Ethical review of research, where research participants are patients (and sometimes staff) of the NHS or users of social care services, is undertaken by one of a network of NHS Research Ethics Committees. UK wide they follow the same procedures and use an electronic application form known as the Integrated Research Application System (IRAS). All details and guidance, e.g. on informed consent on website of the National Research Ethics Service (NRES).[1]

Research outside the remit of these committees and undertaken as a student or in collaboration with an HEI will follow university research ethics procedures.

## Research governance and permissions

This is concerned with setting standards to improve the quality of research and safeguard patients and the public. All research projects have to gain written permission from the organization in which they will take place (usually via a research office). In many NHS organizations the process of approvals uses IRAS. In England there is also a coordinated system for gaining NHS permission NIHR (CSP) in many organizations at the same time.

Turn the issue or idea into a specific question
↓
Search and review the literature to see what is already known
↓
Write a detailed proposal including:

- The research questions
- Rationale (importance of the question and what this study would add)
- Background
- Aim and objectives
- Methods of enquiry
- Ethical and data protection considerations
- Timescale
- Costs and resources required

↓
Obtain funding or resource agreement
↓
Obtain permissions from the health organization
↓
Obtain ethical review
↓
Commence recruitment and data collection
↓
Analyse data
↓
Write report of research and findings
↓
Disseminate findings through publication and presentation

**Fig. 2.1** The research process.

### Reference

[1]National Research Ethics Service (NRES). Available at: ℘ http://www.nres.nhs.uk

### Further information

RCN Research Society. Available at: ℘ www.rcn.org.uk/development/researchanddevelopment
Research and Development Information. Available at: ℘: www.rdinfo.org.uk
NIHR Clinical Academic Careers. Available at: ℘ www.nihrtcc.nhs.uk/cat/
Public involvement in research. Available at: ℘ www.invo.org.uk
Primary Care Research Network. Available at: ℘ http://www.crncc.nihr.ac.uk/about_us/pcrn
International Collaborations in Community Nursing Research (ICCHNR). Available at: ℘ www.icchnr.org/
UKCRN. Available at: ℘ www.crncc.nihr.ac.uk/about_us/uk_wide_working

# Teamwork and innovation

Effective teams in organizational settings are characterized by:

- A defined group of individuals who perceive themselves as members of the team.
- Defined roles within the team respected and understood by all team members.
- Regular interaction and communication between team members.
- Clear, shared team goals.
- Equal participation in decision-making by all team members.

A team approach has been shown to improve patient outcomes in a range of settings.

There are many different types of teams, who may have a leader (📖 Leadership in practice, p. 55) by virtue of a management structure, clinical seniority, or elected by the rest of the team:

- Those that are managed together.
- Those that come together with a shared client/patient group.
- Those that come together to work on individual issues/events/problems.

Primary care nurses may be members of many teams, particularly if they work with a number of general practices or provide specialist input. They need to consider how they become an integrated team member, with at the very least face-to-face communication with other professionals also involved with their patients or clients.

Teambuilding initiatives in health and social care have been shown to have some benefits:

- Developing practitioners' awareness of the benefits of team-working.
- Improving communication.
- Improving shared decision-making.
- Improving problem solving.
- Improving trust and support.

However, innovations resulting from this may be short lived if there is no ongoing support from the wider organization.[1]

## Innovation and introducing change

Any change process has five parts:

- Precipitating factors.
- Team or organization members felt need for change.
- Decisions and plans for instigating change.
- Implementation.
- Outcomes (intended and unintended).

Almost all changes face some resistance, most commonly because of a:

- Desire not to lose something of value.
- Misunderstanding of the proposed change and its implications.
- Belief the change does not make sense.
- Low tolerance for change.

Planning for change has to capitalize on the energy and ideas of those supporting the change as well as reduce the resistance to the change. There are many tools to help plan change, e.g. force field analysis (as described in Iles and Cranfield.[2] Strategies to reduce resistance include:
• Inviting resisters to help plan and implement.
• Widening dissemination of proposals and consultation processes.
• Demonstrate commitment to modify plans taking in resisters' views.
• Develop alternative plans.
• Start small by piloting the change to learn and adapt as necessary.
• Wear down resistance over time.

A number of change models are used in the NHS, e.g. Plan-Do-Study-Act (PDSA) cycles or RAID:
• Review.
• Agree.
• Implement.
• Demonstrate.

Commonest reasons that innovations fail to be implemented and sustained:
• More time was needed than planned for.
• Major problems surfaced that had not been anticipated.
• Coordination of important activities was not effective.
• Competing activities distract the key members.
• Skills and abilities of those involved not sufficient.
• Training and support to lower level and support staff inadequate.
• Powerful external events interfere.

Detailed planning needs to include time, resources, all staff training and involvement, milestones, feedback mechanisms.

### References

[1]NHS Leadership Academy. Available at: ℵ www.leadershipacademy.nhs.uk/
[2]Iles, V, Cranfield, S. (2005). *Developing Change Management Skills. A Resource for Health Care Professionals and Managers.* Available at: ℵ www.netscc.ac.uk/hsdr/files/project/SDO_FR_08-1001-001_V01.pdf

# Principles of successful meetings

Meetings are important as venues for sharing ideas, hearing differing viewpoints and evidence, making decisions, planning, and reviewing actions by a group or team. Meetings are essential to a democratic, efficient organization. Without good planning or forethought they become ineffective both for participants and the organization.

## Terms of reference and ground rules

Groups that are planning to have regular meetings should establish terms of reference to specify:
- The purpose of the meeting.
- The participants required to address the purpose.
- The frequency of meeting to achieve the purpose.
- To name the chair and arrangements for minute taking.
- To state who and where the decisions of the meeting will report to.
- To state a point in time when the terms of reference will be reviewed.

Groups that only meet once or twice may need to establish these points at the first meeting and 'ground rules', e.g. turning off mobiles, confidentiality. This is particularly important if there is a mix of type of participants or the topic matter is likely to be sensitive.

## Meeting prerequisites
- An aim and agenda.
- A Chair, who will lead the meeting.
- A note-taker (secretary), who will take notes.
- All participants should have the agenda and any supporting documents in enough time to read and think about before the meeting.
- An agreed fixed time limit.
- A venue that is accessible for all participants.

## The agenda

Will include most of:
- Welcomes and apologies.
- Minutes of last meeting (and agree at this stage that they are accurate. In a formal situation the Chair should sign them to confirm this).
- Matters arising from the last meeting (that are not on the agenda).
- Items listed for discussion.
- Items to note for information only.
- Any other business (AOB).
- Date and venue of next meeting.

## The notes or 'minutes'
- Should have same headings as the agenda.
- Should note who was present.
- Should note what was decided.
- Should note what actions agreed by who and when.
- Not generally necessary to record all the discussion.

### Role of the Chair

- Ensures group covers agenda in the given time.
- Exercise firm, but sensitive control of the discussion to ensure one conversation happens so that all can participate. *Note:* in formal meetings, people don't speak to each other and all remarks are addressed to the Chairperson.

### After a meeting

- Every member (including those absent) should have a copy of the notes or minutes and know the outcome.
- Every member should know what actions they have to take, and any following meetings.

# Leadership in practice

Acts of leadership can come from anyone. Leadership is a set of skills, qualities, and behaviours, which all nurses and health-care practitioners are expected to demonstrate. Leadership qualities are key to developing services that improve patient experience, health outcomes, and meet population needs. Leadership development should be within continuing professional development (📖 Continuing professional development, p. 47), appraisal processes (📖 Clinical supervision and appraisal, p. 46), and clinical supervision.

## Principles of leadership

The NHS Leadership Qualities Framework (used UK wide) has been developed for specific use with NHS staff. There are five clusters of qualities:

- *Demonstrating personal qualities:* self-awareness, managing yourself, CPD, and acting with integrity.
- *Working with others:* developing networks, building and maintaining relationships, encouraging contribution, working within teams.
- *Managing services:* planning, managing resources, managing people, managing, performance.
- *Improving services:* ensuring patient safety, critically evaluating, encouraging improvement and innovation, facilitating transformation.
- *Setting direction:* identifying contexts for change, applying knowledge and evidence, making decisions, evaluating impact.

## Leadership development

There are many opportunities to develop leadership skills. Primary care nurses can access these opportunities by:

- Identifying development needs in annual appraisal.
- Getting the support of manager/employer for further development and training.
- Looking for courses at university/e-based courses.
- Undertaking a 360° assessment through the NHS Leadership Qualities Framework.[1]
- Attending clinical leadership programmes such as those provided by the RCN or other professional organizations (📖 Useful websites, p. 800).

## Reference

[1] NHS Leadership Academy. Available at: 🌑 www.leadershipacademy.nhs.uk/

# Project planning

Common projects that primary care nurses are involved in include:
- Introducing a new service, e.g. new clinic session, specialist team.
- Introducing or rolling out new clinical activities.
- Reorganizing a team or working practices.
- Introducing new clinical or administrative technologies.

Critical to the success of any new project is the planning phase. This involves:
- Detailed planning done by a small group of key people committed to making it happen.
- Consultation on the overall plan or key elements that involves those interested and those affected by the change (key stakeholders) to gain their ideas, win their approval, reduce their resistance to the plans.

## Project plans

These should include:
- The aim or goal of the project as a broad statement of the problem to be solved or what is to be achieved.
- Objectives derived from the broader aim. They set the realistic targets to achieve during the project. 'SMART' objectives are:
  - *Specific*—clear about what will be achieved.
  - *Measurable*—it's possible to quantify results and measure when they have been achieved.
  - *Achievable*—they can be achieved.
  - *Realistic*—attainable with resources or the resources bid for.
  - *Timed*—attainable within a specified timescale.
- All projects have an element of risk. A risk analysis addresses the following questions:
  - What could possibly go wrong?
  - What is the likelihood of it happening?
  - How will it affect the project?
  - What can be done about it?
- Roles and responsibilities.
- A breakdown of tasks against timescales, deadlines, or milestones.
- Resources required and costs.
- Communication mechanisms.
- Review date after completion with all involved.

### Costing

These should include:
- Staff salary costs for the time involved in the project activity (*Note*: includes employer's contributions to pensions and national insurance).
- Organizational overheads: usually expressed as a percentage of the salary costs and covers central services that keep the organization functioning, e.g. running and maintenance of premises.
- All materials, equipment, non-staff resources to be used.
- Any additional expenses: e.g. hire of rooms, payment for speakers.

*Planning tools*
- Computer software can be bought to aid project planning.
- Tools such as GANTT (named after developer)—charts with detailed steps and time frames in a diagrammatic way (see Fig. 2.2) help identify all tasks, the person responsible for them, and monitor progress.
- Other tools include critical pathway analysis which diagrammatically shows when activities can happen in parallel or are dependent on each other.

| Task | Person Responsible | Week 1 | Week 2 | Week 3 | Week 4 |
|------|-------------------|--------|--------|--------|--------|
| Collect information | Nurse A | × | | | |
| Write draft report | Nurse B | | × | | |
| Revise report | Nurse A and B | | | × | |
| Present report to general practice meeting | Nurse A to speak. Nurse B to answer questions | | | | × |

**Fig. 2.2** A GANTT chart.

## Common problems in project planning
- Focus is too narrowly on the work of one team and fails to consider how it fits into the larger picture.
- Underestimates the time involved for work.
- Failure to warn others external to the project on whom elements depend.
- Failure to identify all the materials, equipment, and staff needed for the project.

The NHS uses a systems approach to planning, scheduling, and controlling high-level, high-risk change involving multiple, large-scale services. IT projects often use the PRINCE2™methodology.

## Further information
NHS Leadership Academy. Available at: ℘ www.leadershipacademy.nhs.uk/

# Using information for practice

A key primary care and community nursing activity is to use data to inform and change their practice and activities. This is often called profiling, although other terms may also be used. Three types of profiling activities are used:

- Community profiling.
- Caseload profiling.
- Workload profiling and resource management.

Nurses working in or closely with general practice may also be using practice patient profiles or QOF (📖 Quality and outcomes framework, p. 66) returns to inform their practice.

## Community profiling

This means using local public health data (📖 Public health in the NHS, p. 10), to understand the health issues of the community/population they work with, combined with LA and community data on resources to help address those needs. Without having to collect additional information, this informs the nurse what the priority issues to be aware of are, and what she should address her practice to. This links to health needs assessment activities (📖 Health needs assessment, p. 11).

## Caseload profiling

Caseload profiling is a technique for understanding the collated health and social care needs of those within the 'caseload' held by the nurse or team of nurses. The purpose is to assist with planning, prioritizing activities, and identifying particular issues/groups/trends that need addressing either by the team or by alerting others to, or making a business case for, more or different resources. Data should only be included on aspects that address issues of importance to planning. It is usually undertaken on an annual basis as a snapshot. Typically caseload profiles collate information on the patients/clients:

- The demographic profile (age, sex, self-assigned ethnicity, first language).
- Presence of morbidity and key health and social issues: e.g.
  - Chronic obstructive pulmonary disease (COPD), CHD, DM, cerebrovascular accident (CVA), cancer.
  - Substance misuse, mental health problems, dementia.
  - Carers, including child carers, lone parents.
  - Violence or neglect to children, older adults, women.
  - Children with special needs.
  - Adults in receipt of services under the Community Care Act.
  - Indicators of socio-economic status, e.g. receipt of state income support.
  - In short-term or temporary accommodation.
  - Asylum seekers and refugees.
- Key public health indicators: e.g. breast-feeding rates, influenza vaccination rates, smoking cessation rates, obesity measures.

- The levels of service offered/received from the nursing service, e.g.:
  - Many DN services have a dependency scale or care objective scale that assigns patients to 1 of 3/4/5 categories that indicates both the objectives of care, but also how much nurse time that involves. *Category examples*—short-term, self-limiting, intermittent support to long-term condition, weekly support to long-term condition, daily (or near) daily support to unstable and fluctuating long-term condition, palliative care at end stage of life.
  - HV services may also assign clients/families to a grouping that indicates that that family receives more support/home visiting than those receiving the locally determined core service (in England Universal Plus services). *Categories*—likely to include families with children who are or have been on the child protection register, families receiving additional supportive/listening visits (e.g. after detection of postnatal depression).
- Any service outcome/performance data in addition to public health indicators, e.g. venous leg ulcer healing rates, outcome measures from coding systems such as the OMAHA system[1], early identification of speech and language problems in children, audit data (📖 Clinical audit, p. 64).
- The total volume of patients/clients that have been admitted to the caseload in a given period, e.g. annual/6mths.
- The total volume of patients/clients that have been discharged/left the caseload through moving or death.

Caseload profile information only becomes meaningful when it is compared to wider information, e.g. local teenage pregnancy rates or compared year on year or against a benchmark. Some areas provide proformas with local public health data inserted for instant comparison. It only becomes useful in terms of workload and resource management with other information added and compared with others or accepted benchmarks.

## Data from clinical/professional records

The increased use of electronic patient/client records and coding systems (📖 IT, electronic records and telehealth, p. 84) allows easier aggregate data analysis for understanding health issues addressed by nurses, their contribution to service delivery and the outcomes of their interventions. American developed coding systems such as the OMAHA[1] provides additional coding for identification of the problems addressed by nurses and outcomes. Many PCOs still use nurse activity only information systems at the nurse (rather than the patient level) to return information to service commissioners and central government statistics. In some areas this is changing so that nurse activity information is derived from computerized patient records held in general practice. In general practice, the implementation of QOF (📖 Quality and outcomes framework, p. 66) has made the level of nurse activity in practice outcomes more visible.

## Workload profiling and resources

There are no national population to number of nursing staff required guidelines because the number of staff required is dependent on the types of nursing work for different populations that is commissioned (📖 Commissioning of services, p. 9). Caseload and workload profiling assist practitioners and managers in determining:

- Equitable distribution of staffing to work.
- Increased or decreased demand on the nursing staff resource.

Beyond the aggregate caseload data, workload includes all the other important activities included in the nursing teams responsibilities, e.g. nurse education responsibilities, attending GP practice/clinical meetings, liaison sessions to other services, travel distances.

All patients/clients/work activities do not have equal demands on nursing time. In order to determine the impact on nursing resource, weighted scoring systems are applied to the caseload and the extra work activities. In district nursing teams, the weighted scoring system is linked to patient dependency on the nursing team (rather than self-care/informal carers or home carers). In health visiting, the score is linked to issues such as child protection although research has shown that receipt of income support can act as a very accurate proxy for high demands on health visiting team time. In school nursing teams, the weighted score is linked to numbers of children in schools with special needs and child protection needs. Weighted scores are also given to issues such as travel distances, number of GP practices or schools linking with the service.

The weighted scoring results are triangulated with the regular monitoring data of nursing activity levels, outcomes, and quality indicators. Experienced staff and managers then also use their expert knowledge in determining manageable workloads and decisions are made including:

- Shifting or changing team staffing or team activity focus (requires change management planning).
- Discussing increased demand on nursing resource with commissioners in contracting rounds.

## Commissioning (contracting) of nursing services

Commissioners are looking to contract, on behalf of the public, nursing services for specified groups of clients, specified activities or specified quality within the NHS reference costs. In the past this has been done by 'block' contracts in most areas, e.g. a district nursing service with a range of new contact visits in a year and this level of clients/contacts throughout the 12mths. Many commissioners are now looking for greater detail.

## Reference

[1]Martin, K. (2005). *The Omaha System. A Key to Practice, Documentation, and Information Management*, 2nd edn. Missouri: Elsevier Saunders.

## Further information

Hurst, K. (2005). *Primary Care Trust Workforce Planning and Development*. London: Whurr Publishers.

# Chapter 3

# Quality and safety

# Quality governance

Quality (or clinical) governance is the term for the quality assurance and continuous quality improvement framework. Country-specific guidance encompassing domains of:

- Clinical effectiveness in patient care.
- Safety in care.
- Positive patient experiences in which they are treated with dignity and respect.

Those responsible for commissioning or planning health services will also use these domains in their specifications ([] Commissioning of services, p. 9). The expectation is that each organization will use nationally available, evidence-based clinical guidelines (e.g. NICE, SIGN), and nationally set quality indicators (e.g. NHS Outcomes Framework) as criteria against which to measure themselves and plan for improvement, through both service change and staff development. In addition, organizations will have named clinicians and managers responsible for quality, safety, and patient experience. There will be an annual plan of activity together with annual reporting to the governing body of the organization and the public (in England called Quality Accounts), which is likely to include:

- Evidence of the patients' experiences, and processes for consulting users.
- The use of information about patient safety and outcomes of patient care.
- Quality improvement activities including:
  - Risk management.
  - Clinical audit programmes.
  - Evidence-based practice and clinical effectiveness.
  - Learning from adverse events/incidents.
  - Learning from complaints.
- The development of a learning organization, e.g. evidence of education and staff development.
- Evidence of leadership and strategic planning in service review and improvement.
- Plans for quality improvements in the coming year.

There are country-specific mechanisms for health organizations to have their patient safety and quality assessed. In England this is the role of the Care Quality Commission in England and Healthcare Improvement Scotland.

## Further information

Care Quality Commission. Available at: ℘ www.cqc.org.uk/public

Department of Health NHS Outcomes Framework 2013 to 2014. Available at: ℘ www.gov.uk/government/publications/nhs-outcomes-framework-2013-to-2014

Department of Health Quality Accounts toolkit 2010/211. Available at: ℘ www.gov.uk/government/publications/quality-accounts-toolkit-2010-11

Healthcare Improvement Scotland. Available at: ℘ www.healthcareimprovementscotland.org/welcome_to_health care_improvem.aspx

Welsh Government. The Quality Delivery Plan for the NHS in Wales. *Achieving excellence - The quality delivery plan for the NHS in Wales 2012–2016.* Available at: ℘ http://wales.gov.uk/topics/health/publications/health/strategies/excellence/?lang=en

# Evidence-based health care

*Evidence-based health care* refers to the use of all valid, relevant information taken into account when making decisions that affect the care of patients, provision of health services, and public health. *Evidence-based clinical practice* is when the professional uses the best evidence available, in consultation with the patient or client, to decide upon the option for action.

*Critical appraisal* is the process of assessing and interpreting evidence by systematically considering its validity, results, and relevance. Evidence is then classified by the source. Results from study type 1 is considered strongest and 4 weakest:

*1:* meta-analyses, systematic reviews of randomized controlled trials (RCTs), or RCTs (including cluster RCTs).

*2:* Systematic reviews of, or individual, non-randomized controlled trials, case-control studies, cohort studies, controlled before-and-after (CBA) studies, interrupted time series (ITS) studies, correlation studies.

*3:* Non-analytical studies (e.g. case reports, case series).

*4:* Expert opinion, formal consensus.

## Guidelines

User-friendly statements to inform decision making, regarding a specific health problem from critically appraised evidence and other information. Increasing numbers are produced to reduce harmful, ineffective and expensive variations in health care. NICE and SIGN are NHS funded bodies producing guidelines.

## Protocols

These usually refer to specific guidelines on evidence-based professional activities and treatments required for particular conditions and situations, and are more directive than guidelines.

## Integrated care pathways

These are statements that amalgamate all the elements of evidence-based care and treatment for a particular patient group, along a patient's journey, that includes 1°, 2°, and social care inputs. The aim is to improve patient-centred health and social care, making explicit what should happen when and how communication should happen between different services.

## Further information

Healthcare Improvement Scotland. Evidence, advice, guidance and standards. Available at: ℬ www. healthcareimprovementscotland.org/evidence.aspx

National Institute for Health and Care Excellence (NICE). Available at: ℬ www.nice.org.uk

NHS Scotland. What are Integrated Care Pathways? Available at: ℬ www.e-p-a.org/index2.html

NICE Evidence Search Health and Social Care. Available at: ℬ www.evidence.nhs.uk

The Cochrane Collaboration. Available at: ℬ www.cochrane.org/cochrane-reviews

# Clinical audit

This is a quality improvement process aimed at improving patient care and outcomes as part of an organization's quality governance programme (🕮 Quality governance, p. 62), which systematically reviews current care (i.e. what is happening?) against explicit criteria (i.e. what should be happening?), identifying deficiencies or problems (i.e. what changes are needed?), implements changes at an individual, team, or service level and monitors to ensure continued improvement in health care delivery. It is often described as the audit cycle or spiral (see Fig. 3.1). Starting points are often significant events, complaints (🕮 Complaints procedures, p. 70), QOF (🕮 Quality and outcomes framework, p. 66) targets, clinical guidelines, or protocols (🕮 Evidence-based health care, p. 63), prescribing data, and an individual's or teams' observations. There are a number of national clinical audits undertaken which are required in England for organizations Quality Accounts (🕮 Quality governance, p. 62).

## Clinical audit in primary care

- Every health care organization has an annual programme of priority areas for audits based on quality standards in service specifications, contracts, QOF, national guidance.
- Most organizations are trying to increase the involvement of service users in the audit process.
- Many larger organizations have audit officers who offer training, advice, and sometimes help undertake audits.
- Many professionals find clinical audit very threatening. The organization or team should ensure that audit is undertaken in a culture of supportive development not punishment.

### Preparing to undertake an audit
Ensure the team and organization support the audit, both in the resources, skills to undertake it, and the commitment to act on findings. Everyone needs to be clear whether audit is conducted at individual practitioner level and how findings will be reported back.

### Choosing a topic for audit
Should be important, manageable, clearly defined, and preferably have data easily available.

### Choosing audit criteria
These should be explicit and evidence-based. Good starting point, are statements in national or local clinical guidance. Statements should be made as to what standard is expected, i.e. whether the criteria should be fulfilled in 100% or a smaller percentage of cases.

### Measuring current performance against the criteria
Methods of gathering data depends on the criteria being measured and available resources. It can include computer and medical records, data collection sheets, and questionnaires. Results should be compared with standards and any other available audit data, e.g. published audits from other practices, teams.

*Planning for improvement*
Identifying changes needed requires a team and organizational approach
(📖 Teamwork and innovation, p. 51) as well as plans for continued
monitoring of change implementation. May also involve addressing issues
in individuals PDPs (📖 Continuing professional development, p. 47).
Following implementation, the cycle leads back into re-auditing.

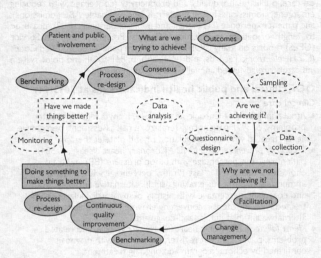

**Fig. 3.1** The clinical audit cycle.

Reproduced with permission of the National Institute for Health and Clinical Excellence (2002)
from *Principles of Best Practice in Clinical Audit*. London: National Institute for Clinical Excellence.

## Further information

NHS England Essence of Care Benchmarks. Available at: 🔗 http://www.tin.nhs.uk/local-networks/
essence-of-care/background/
NICE (2002). *Principles for Best Practice in Clinical Audit*. Available at: 🔗 www.nice.org.uk
Burgess R (2011). *New Principles of Best Practice in Clinical Audit*, 2nd edn. Oxford: Radcliffe Medical
Press.
Health Care Quality Improvement Partnership. National charity promoting quality in health care
and leading national clinical audits. Available at: 🔗 www.hqip.org.uk/
NHS Clinical Governance Support Team (2005). *Practical Handbook to Clinical Audit*. Available
at: 🔗 www.hqip.org.uk/assets/Downloads/Practical-Clinical-Audit-Handbook-CGSupport.pdf

# Quality and outcomes framework

The QOF applies to the GMS and PMS contracts (📖 General practice, p. 13). QOF uses a points system against defined standards, with linked financial incentives (average value per point £156.92 in England 2013/14), to encourage high quality care. QOF indicators fall into four domains: clinical care, public health, quality and productivity (concerned with reducing emergency admissions, hospital referrals, and avoidable A&E admissions), and patient experience (📖 Patient and public experience, p. 69) measured by length of patient consultations. General Practice Extraction Service (GPES) reports on many QOF indicators from patient record Read Codes (📖 IT, electronic records, and telehealth, p. 84). QOF and point system indicators are reviewed annually and results published.

## QOF clinical and public health indicators (as at 2013/14)

*Clinical care*

- *Atrial fibrillation* (📖 Chronic heart failure, tachycardia, and related problems, p. 597): patient register, stroke risk assessment, percentage at risk treated with anti-coagulation or anti-platelet therapy.
- *Secondary prevention of CHD* (📖 Coronary heart disease, p. 584): patient register, percentage with blood pressure (BP) and total cholesterol measured in last 12mths, percentage with influenza immunization, percentage taking aspirin, alternative anti-platelet or anti-coagulant, percentage with history of myocardial infarction (MI) treated with angiotensin-converting enzyme (ACE) inhibitor, aspirin, alternative anti-platelet, or anti-coagulant.
- *Heart failure* (📖 Chronic heart failure, tachycardia, and related problems, p. 597): patient register, percentage with diagnosis confirmed by echocardiogram and ongoing treatment.
- *Hypertension* (📖 Hypertension, p. 589): patient register, record of measurement in previous 9mths and percentage within normal range, assessment of physical activity for those >16yrs and <75yrs, evidence of brief intervention for those scoring less active on the General Practice Physical Activity Questionnaire.
- *Peripheral arterial disease:* patient register, BP and cholesterol measurement in past 12mths, percentage treated with aspirin or an alternative anti-platelet.
- *Stroke* (📖 Principles of rehabilitation following stroke, p. 414) *and transient ischaemic attack (TIA):* patient register, referrals for further investigations, BP, and cholesterol measurement in past 12mths, percentage with non-haemorrhagic stroke or TIA treated with aspirin or an alternative anti-platelet, percentage given influenza immunization.
- *Diabetes mellitus* (📖 Diabetes: overview, p. 611): patient register, percentage with BP, total cholesterol, albumin:creatinine ratio test and IFCC-HbA1c measured in last 12mths, percentage with influenza immunization, retinal screening, foot assessment and dietary review by suitably qualified professional in past 12mths, percentage referred to structured education programme and percentage ♂ asked about erectile dysfunction and record of advice for those with dysfunction.

- *Hypothyroid* (📖 Thryroid, p. 656): patient register and record of thyroid tests.
- *Asthma* (📖 Asthma in adults, p. 566): treated patient register, percentage reviewed including smoking status in past 12mths.
- *Chronic obstructive pulmonary disease* (📖 Chronic obstructive pulmonary disease, p. 574): patient register, percentage diagnosis confirmed with post-bronchodilator spirometry, review, and record of forced expiratory volume (FEV) and Medical Research Council (MRC) dyspnoea grade ≥3 with record of oxygen saturation level.
- *Dementia* (📖 People with dementias, p. 438): patient register, percentage with new diagnosis with record of full blood and organ function screening in past 6mths, percentage with diagnosis record with a face-to-face review in past 12mths.
- *Depression* (📖 People with depression, p. 435): percentage with new diagnosis and assessment of severity using a validated tool.
- *Mental health* (📖 People with schizophrenia, p. 443): patient register of those with schizophrenia, bi-polar affective disorder, psychoses and others on lithium treatment, including practice register and percentage with comprehensive care plan and BP measured, percentage of those >40yrs with measurement of blood glucose, body mass index (BMI), alcohol consumption in previous 12mths, percentage of eligible ♀ had cervical screening (📖 Cervical cancer screening, p. 337).
- *Cancer:* patient register and case review <3mths of diagnosis.
- *Chronic kidney disease* (📖 Renal problems, p. 705): patient register, BP and urine albumin:creatinine ratio in past 12mths, and on treatment
- *Epilepsy* (📖 Seizures and epilepsy, p. 693): patient register, percentage treated and seizure-free in past 12mths and percentage ♀ on anti-epileptic drugs counselled about contraception and pregnancy in past 12mths.
- *Learning disabilities* (📖 People with learning disabilities, p. 408): patient register and percentage patients with Down's syndrome >18yrs with a record of blood thyroid-stimulating hormone (TSH) in past 12mths.
- *Osteoporosis* (📖 Osteoporosis, p. 558): register of patients >18yrs and <75yrs with diagnosis or record of fragility fracture.
- *Rheumatoid arthritis* (📖 Rheumatoid arthritis, p. 555): patient register, percentage with face-to-face annual review, percentage >30yrs and <85yrs with annual cardiovascular disease (CVD) risk assessment, percentage >50yrs and <91yrs with annual fracture risk assessment.
- *Palliative care:* patient register and MDT review at least 3-monthly.

### Public health

- *Cardiovascular disease-primary prevention:* percentage of newly diagnosed with hypertension (>30–<75yrs) treated with statins, given face-to-face CVD risk assessment and percentage with hypertension diagnosis given lifestyle advice in past 12mths.
- *Blood pressure:* percentage >40yrs with record of BP in past 5yrs.
- *Obesity* (📖 Weight management: overweight, obesity, p. 307): patient register >16yrs with BMI ≥30.
- *Smoking:* percentage patients >15yrs with record of smoking status in previous 24mths, percentage patients on a QOF register, e.g. diabetes mellitus (DM) and record in past 12mths of smoking status, percentage offered support or treatment to quit (📖 Smoking cessation, p. 315).

- *Additional services under GMS contract:*
  - *Cervical screening* (☐ Cervical cancer screening, p. 337)—practice protocol (including audit) in line with national guidance, percentage uptake of eligible ♀.
  - *Child health surveillance*—in line with national guidance.
  - *Maternity services*—antenatal care and screening (☐ Antenatal care and screening, p. 380) offered as per national guidelines.
  - *Contraception* (☐ Contraception: general, p. 359)—register of 5 < 54yrs prescribed contraception.

## Further information

NHS Employers. Quality and Outcomes Framework. Available at: ℬ www.nhsemployers.org/PayAndContracts/GeneralMedicalServicesContract/QOF/Pages/QualityOutcomesFramework.aspx

NHS Information Centre. QOF Online GP practice results database. Available at: ℬ www.qof.ic.nhs.uk/

# Patient and public experience

Each country has different mechanisms for ensuring the public voice is heard in decision-making, e.g Health Watch in England (see ⬛ The National Health Service (NHS), p. 6) As part of the policies for continuous service improvement (e.g. Health and Social Care Act 2012), health organizations are required to ensure that the patient and service user experience is a positive one, and find ways of capturing that and learning from negative experiences. This is also a requirement of commissioners and planners of services.

The patient and service user experience has more than one domain including:
- Clinical care and health promoting activities.
- The administrative process supporting those.
- The environment in which these take place in.

Professionals, services, and organizations can capture information about that experience in many different ways and feed it into their quality governance systems (⬛ Quality governance, p. 62). Examples of ways to receive feedback (positive and negative) include:
- Suggestion boxes in reception areas.
- On-line comments and feedback systems both open access and closed, e.g. only to particular service user groups.
- Waiting room kiosks for electronic feedback.
- Patient surveys, including as part of national ones, such as the English GP patient survey, cancer patient experience survey.
- Complaints (⬛ Complaints procedures, p. 70).
- Patient representative groups.
- As part of clinical audit (⬛ Clinical audit, p. 64) and QOF (⬛ Quality and outcomes framework, p. 66) activities.

In addition patient-reported outcome measures (PROMs) are being developed as structured clinical evaluation tools to measure health gain from the patient perspective of clinical care, mainly of 2° care.

## Further information

GP patient experience survey England. Available at: 🖰 www.gp-patient.co.uk/info/

Health and Social Care Information Centre. Patient reported outcome measures. Available at: 🖰 www.hscic.gov.uk/proms

Patients Opinion. A not-for-profit social enterprise. Available at: 🖰 https://www.patientopinion.org.uk/

Public Health England. Cancer Patient Experience England. Available at: 🖰 www.ncin.org.uk/cancer_information_tools/cancer_patient_experience.aspx

# Complaints procedures

Anyone using NHS-provided or -funded services who is unhappy with the treatment or service are entitled to make a complaint, have it considered, and receive a response from the health organization or primary care practitioner concerned. Each country has an agreed complaints procedure that is also written into the GMS contract. Every organization and general practice has to publicize its complaints procedures to the public. Each country has mechanisms for helping the public identify procedure for complaint, e.g. Patient Advice and Liaison Service (PALS) in hospitals and local Health Watch in England (see 🕮 The National Health Service (NHS), p. 6).

People who complain generally want:
• Their complaint to be heard and investigated promptly.
• To be dealt with courteously and sympathetically.
• To receive an apology if mistakes have occurred.
• The problem rectified promptly if possible.
• To be assured that steps will be taken to prevent a recurrence.

## Key principles
• *Timescale:*
  • Complaint can be made by affected individual or someone acting on their behalf with their consent.
  • Complaint should be made within 6mths of event(s) or from time they became aware that they had cause for complaint.
• *Form of complaint:*
  • Can be to any member of staff who may be able to resolve concerns without need for a formal complaint.
  • More formal complaint has to be to local organization concerned in first instance.
  • Can be oral, by email, or in writing.
• *Complaint handling at the local level:*
  • Every organization and practice should have named and publicized manager who receives all complaints, and has to respond in a timely way, also advising of local advice or advocacy service.
  • Complaints manager contacts all involved, investigating facts and actions to be taken.
  • Complaints manager has to respond in writing within locally-specified time period. Can also report progress in investigation if not completed.
  • Complaints manager has to summarize findings, need for apology, actions taken to rectify situation, actions to prevent recurrence. Response to complainant may be by letter or face-to-face meeting. Conciliation should also be offered.
  • All attempts should be made to resolve complaint at local level.
• *Failure to resolve complaint at the local level:*
  • Complainants have right to take their complaint to independent review, e.g. Parliamentary and Health Service Ombudsmen (England).

All organizations use complaints as part of their quality and clinical governance procedures (📖 Quality governance, p. 62) as a way of learning how to improve services. In the same way, they also usually collect positive feedback, such as letters of thanks and appreciation.

## Further information

Citizens Advice Bureau. NHS and local authority social service complaints (all countries). Available at: ✆ www.adviceguide.org.uk/england/health care_e/health care_nhs_health care_e/nhs_and_local_authority_social_services_complaints.htm

NHS Choices. GP complaints. Available at: ✆ www.nhs.uk/choiceintheNHS/Yourchoices/GPchoice/Pages/GPcomplaints.aspx

Patient Advice and Liaison Services (England). Available at: ✆ www.pals.nhs.uk/default.aspx

The Parliamentary and Health Service Ombudsman. Available at: ✆ www.ombudsman.org.uk

# Clinical risk management

It is estimated that 850,000 incidents and errors occur every year in the NHS. All health care and work activities involve risk. Organizations have a duty to manage risks, i.e. identify what harm its activities, environments, and working practices *could* do to patients, staff, and visitors, and assess whether it has taken all possible precautionary measures to reduce the risks to an acceptable level.

Risk management is a key component of quality governance ( Quality governance, p. 62) and there are legal responsibilities for some elements, see  Health and safety at work, p. 88. All health organizations have to have risk registers that document and grade types of risk in the organization, e.g. types of clinical care, hazards to workforce. Clinical risk management aims to:

• Identify what could (and does) go wrong during clinical care.
• Understand factors that contribute to incidents and errors.
• Put systems in place to reduce risks.
• Minimize consequences to patients and staff when errors do occur.
• Learn lessons from any adverse events and implement change.
• Ensure action is taken to prevent recurrence.

There are a variety of tools, such as the Patient Safety Walkrounds, Patient Safety Dashboards, Manchester Patient Safety Frameworks, which can aid patient safety focus (see  Health and safety at work, p. 84).

## Adverse incidents and events

An adverse incident is any event that could have or did lead to unintended or unexpected harm, loss, or damage. It includes accidents and near misses. These may be identified by complaints ( Complaints procedures, p. 70), audits ( Clinical audit, p. 64), or staff reporting of accidents/incidents (see  Health and safety at work, p. 84). All incidents, errors, and adverse events should be accurately documented in patient records ( Record keeping, p. 81).

## Reporting incidents and events

There are three types of reporting.

• All organizations have to have systems for centrally reporting incidents and accidents, and investigating them, so that lessons are learnt. The NHS aims to encourage 'blame-free' culture that acknowledges most adverse events are part of systems failure, rather than individual failure. A blame-free culture does not override the need for disciplinary or criminal processes in the event of negligence or criminal acts.
• Reporting requirements to regulatory bodies for different types of incidents, e.g. Care Quality Commission (England) for serious patient safety incidents, to Medicines and Health Care Products Regulatory Agency (MHRA), Health and Safety Executive, i.e. statutory reporting workplace injuries, diseases, and dangerous occurrences, RIDDOR. In England and Wales there is a National Reporting and Learning System (NRLS) for patient safety problems through the National Patient Safety Agency.[1]

- To local level multi-agency bodies, e.g. notifying the Local Safeguarding Children Boards (England) Child Protection Committee (Scotland) under local agreed procedures when a child dies (or attempts suicide), and where child abuse or neglect was known or suspected. This may trigger a multi-agency case review as specified in child protection legislation of each country (📖 Child protection processes, p. 234).

## Investigating and learning from incidents and events

The NHS makes a distinction between:

- *'Latent conditions'*: inadequate organizational policies or inappropriate decisions that mould environment for active failure to breech safety defences.
- *'Active failures'*: unsafe acts committed by individuals.

Each organization has policies identifying who has responsibility, and the processes, for internal investigations (or may be stipulated in legislation) or review in the case of 'near misses' and for reporting centrally. Specific techniques may be used. such as root cause analysis. The investigation should cover:

- *Immediate events:*
  - *What happened?*—Event and those involved.
  - *Where and when did it happen?*—Location, date, and time.
  - *What action was taken?*—Immediate and longer-term.
- *What impact did the event have?* Harm to patient, others, the organization.
- *Why did it happen?* Sequences of events, work environment, communication processes, levels of supervision, elements of particular task, availability of guidance, factors related to individual patient, family, or household, factors related to individual members of staff.
- *What factors did, or could have, minimized the impact of the event?*

*Note:* multi-agency investigations, e.g. after a child death associated with abuse or neglect, have agreed processes.

## References

[1] National Patient Safety Authority (England). Provides guidance, tools, and reports on patient safety from analysis of incident reporting. Available at: ℘ www.npsa.nhs.uk/
[2] Patient Safety Root Cause Analysis investigation e-Toolkit. Available at: ℘ www.nrls.npsa.nhs.uk/resources/collections/root-cause-analysis/

## Further information

Department of Health, England (2000). *An Organization with a Memory.* London: Stationery Office.
National Patient Safety Authority. Patient Safety practical information and tools. Available at: ℘ www.nrls.npsa.nhs.uk/
Wales 1000 Lives plus: quality and safest health care programme. Available at: ℘ www.1000livesplus.wales.nhs.uk/home

# Professional conduct

Respect for human rights is the basis for all nursing and health care practice. Human rights rest on three key principles:
- Every human has certain rights, which are not conferred on him or her, but which arise in him or her by virtue of their humanity alone.
- A person cannot be deprived of those rights by another or by their own acts.
- Just laws must be applied consistently, independently, impartially (without fear or favour), and with fair procedures.

## The UK Human Rights Act 1998 (HRA)

Incorporates into domestic law certain rights from the European Convention and has three main effects:
- An allegation of a breach of rights can be brought in the UK courts.
- It is unlawful for a public body (including the NHS) to breach rights.
- In situations where courts find that legislation is incompatible with rights set out in the Act, judges can make a 'declaration of incompatibility'. Legislation will be referred back to Parliament for reconsideration.
- Examples of rights set out in the HRA that relate to health care are shown in Box 3.1.

> **Box 3.1  Health care rights in the HRA**
> - *Article 2:* right to life.
> - *Article 3:* prohibition of torture.
> - *Article 8:* right to respect for private and family life.
> - *Article 14:* prohibition of discrimination.
> - *Article 17:* prohibition of abuse of rights.

## NMC code of conduct, performance, and ethics

Beyond practising in ways that respect human rights, the NMC professional code specifies that registered nurses and midwives must:
- 'Make care of people their first concern, treat them as individuals, and respect their dignity.
- Work with others to protect and promote health and wellbeing of those in care, their families and carers, and the wider community.
- Provide a high standard of practice and care at all times.
- Be open and honest, act with integrity, and uphold reputation of the profession (NMC, 2008)'.

A registered nurse, midwife, or HV is personally accountable for their practice, must act lawfully, and be able to justify decisions. Failure to act within the code can bring fitness to practise into question and, with it, registration.

## Further information

Council of Europe Convention for the Protection of Human rights and Fundamental Freedoms (amended 2010). Available at: ℘ http://conventions.coe.int/Treaty/en/Treaties/Html/005.htm

Liberty. Available at: ℘ www.liberty-human-rights.org.uk/index.php

NMC (2008). Code of conduct, performance and ethics for nurses and midwives. Available at: ℘ http://www.nmc-uk.org/Publications/Standards/The-code/Introduction/

Nursing and Midwifery Council. Available at: ℘ www.nmc-uk.org

# Anti-discriminatory health care

The Equality Act 2010, underpinned by HRA, prohibits discrimination, victimization, or harassment of a person on the grounds of age, disability, gender re-assignment, marriage and civil partnership, pregnancy and maternity, race, religion or belief, sex or sexual orientation. This applies to all aspects of professional practice, access to and provision of health services, and employment.

Equality Impact Assessments (EqIA) are required of all organizations to ensure services, policies, and decisions are equitably provided, and do not unlawfully discriminate and advance equality of opportunity.

Detailed guidance for health care professionals and good practice examples to increase equality and decrease sexism, racism, ageism, disability discrimination, and sexuality discrimination are available in each country along with EqIA guidance.

## Further information

England DoH. Available at: ⅌ Equality and diversity: https://www.gov.uk/government/organisations/ department-of-health/about/equality-and-diversity

Equality and Human rights Commission. Available at: ⅌ www.equalityhumanrights.com/

NHS Scotland. Equality and Diversity. Available at: ⅌ http://www.nes.scot.nhs.uk/about-us/ equality-and-diversity.aspx

NHS Wales. Centre for Equality and Human Rights. Available at: ⅌ http://www.search.wales.nhs. uk/search/?q=equality+*+diversity

Northern Ireland HSCNI. Equality and Human Rights Information Bank. Available at: ⅌ www. hscbusiness.hscni.net/services/1798.htm

# Consent

This is voluntary agreement with (or refusal of) an action proposed by another. It is fundamental to human rights and professional practice (📖 Professional conduct, p. 74). It is a continuous process and relates to all aspects of care. Valid consent must have these elements:

- *Voluntary:* i.e. given without undue pressure or coercion.
- *Reasonably informed:* i.e. person must understand:
  - The nature of the act proposed.
  - Its associated benefits and risks.
  - Alternatives (including doing nothing).
  - The associated benefits and risks of the alternatives.
- *Made by a competent person:* i.e. someone who has capacity to understand information and weigh up options to reach a decision. Competency is 'function specific'—someone may have capacity to take some health care decisions, but may lack capacity to decide more complex matters. All adults (≥18yrs old in England and Wales, ≥16yrs old in Scotland) are presumed to be competent, but that presumption can be questioned and refuted.

See also 📖 Contraception: general, p. 359 for information on Fraser Guidelines regarding under 16-yr-olds and consent. See 📖 Mental capacity, p. 424 for information on this issue under the Mental Capacity Act.

## Format of consent

The professional providing the care, treatment, or investigation should seek consent. It can be:

- *Implied consent:* e.g. rolling up sleeve for BP measurement.
- *Express verbal consent:* for minor procedures, such as venipuncture.
- *Express written consent:* for procedures with ↑ risk, e.g. vaccination.

See also 📖 Mental capacity, p. 234, for mentally incapacitated adults.

*Consent forms* act as a record in case of future disputes. Different types should be used if consenting for others.

### Emergencies

Treatment can be provided without consent as long as it is limited to saving life or preventing serious injury, and known not to be contrary to previous wishes of a competent patient.

## Further information

Department of Health (2009). *Reference guide to consent for examination or treatment*, 2nd edn. Available at: ℘ www.gov.uk/government/publications/reference-guide-to-consent-for-examination-or-treatment-second-edition

NHS Choices. Consent to Treatment. Available at: ℘ www.nhs.uk/conditions/Consent-to-treatment/Pages/Introduction.aspx

Office of the Public Guardian. Available at: ℘ www.justice.gov.uk/about/opg

Welsh Assembly Patient Consent. Available at: ℘ http://www.wales.nhs.uk/sites3/page.cfm?orgid=465&pid=11930

# Professional accountability

Accountability means being responsible for someone or something. All nurses are accountable for their professional practice; individually, they are answerable for their actions and omissions. Nurses can be called to account via:

- *Professional regulation:* i.e. the NMC.
- *Criminal law:* e.g. law of assault.
- *Civil law:* e.g. tort of negligence.
- *Employment law:* e.g. through enforcement of contract.

## Duty of care and negligence

Nurses have a legal and professional duty of care for patients and clients. Duty of care means taking reasonable care to avoid acts or omissions that can be reasonably foreseen as likely to be injurious to patients and clients. Patients and clients can make complaints (Ⅲ Complaints procedures, p. 70) to the organization and NMC about negligent care. They can also sue through the civil court. Any court considering a claim of negligence against a nurse would apply the Bolam test, i.e. that the nurse had acted competently as an ordinary nurse in the view of expert opinion. The Bolitho case amended this to state that the expert opinion had to demonstrate a logical basis. Both the employer and the nurse have a responsibility to ensure the nurse is competent.

**Duty of care and new roles** Nurses undertaking roles usually undertaken by other professionally qualified staff would be judged against the ordinary competent other professional performing that role.

## Duty of care and students and junior staff

Students and junior staff actions are also judged against the ordinary competent professional, and not that of a student or junior. Nurses have a duty to ensure that the care that they delegate to juniors or students is carried out at a reasonably competent standard. This means they remain accountable for the delegation of the work and for ensuring that the person who does the work is able to do it.

## Vicarious liability

Employers are vicariously liable for the actions and omissions of their staff, which means that if a patient successfully sues for negligence, the employer will usually pay the compensation, not the nurse. However, this *only* includes those activities within the job description and contract (Ⅲ Employment contracts, p. 44). It does not cover 'Samaritan' acts or acts in roles not specified in the job description. Some employers may seek re-imbursement of compensation paid out from the staff member who committed the negligent act. Most nurses pay for professional indemnity through subscription to a professional or indemnity organization (Ⅲ Useful websites, p. 800).

## Further information

Nursing & Midwifery Council. Available at: ℘ www.nmc-uk.org.uk
NHS Litigation Authority. Available at: ℘ http://www.nhsla.com/Pages/Home.aspx

# Chaperones

All consultations, examinations, and investigations are potentially distressing. Patients can find examinations, investigations, or photography involving the breasts, genitalia, or rectum particularly intrusive (these are referred to as 'intimate examinations'). Also consultations involving dimmed lights, the need for patients to undress, or for intensive periods of being touched may make a patient feel vulnerable.

A chaperone is present as a safeguard for all parties (patient and practitioners) and is a witness to continuing consent (☐ Consent, p. 77) of the procedure. Every health care organization is expected to have a chaperone policy (☐ Quality governance, p. 62).

## Good practice principles

The inquiry into how the NHS handled allegations about the misconduct of Dr Clifford Ayling (Department of Health, 2004) recommended:
- The presence of a chaperone must be patient's decision, but it should routinely be offered by health care professional.
- Trained clinical staff should undertake the chaperone role, rather than unqualified staff (e.g. practice receptionists).
- No family member or friend of a patient should be expected to undertake any formal chaperoning role.

In addition:
- Patients should be made aware of availability of chaperones through notices and practice leaflets.
- If patient does not want a chaperone, it should be recorded that the offer was made and declined.
- If chaperone is present, that should be recorded, including chaperone's identity.
- If, for justifiable practical reasons, a chaperone cannot be offered, this should be explained to patient and, if possible, offer to delay examination to a later date. Discussion and its outcome should be recorded.
- The same principles for offering and use of chaperones should apply in all settings, including home visits and OOH centres.

## Further information

Department of Health (2004). Committee of Inquiry. ndependent Investigation into how the NHS handled allegations about the conduct of Clifford Ayling. Available at: ℘ www.dh.gov.uk

NHS Clinical Governance Support Team (2007) *Guidance on the role and effective use of chaperones in primary and community care settings*. Available at: ℘ www.lmc.org.uk/visageimages/guidance/2007/Chaperone_model%20framework.pdf

# Whistle-blowing

Whistle-blowing is when an employee informs on a fellow employee or their employer, who is either breaking the law or in breach of organizational or professional codes of conduct or policy. It is the exposure of:

• Fraud.
• Negligent actions.
• Abuse by an employee.

It is important for making sure an organization is alert to scandal, danger, malpractice, or corruption and emphasized following the Francis Report.

## Protecting practitioners

Practitioners may be too afraid to report something, because of fear of victimization, being shunned by their peers, or losing their job. The Public Interest Disclosure Act 1998 sets out the mechanisms for promoting whistle-blowing and provides legal protection to people who do this. A qualifying disclosure will be 'protected' if the practitioner:

• Makes the disclosure in good faith.
• Reasonably believes that the information disclosed is true.

## Action to take

If you have a concern, you should:

• *Make an immediate note of your concerns:* e.g. what was said, date, time, and names of people involved.
• *Convey your suspicions to someone with the appropriate authority and experience:* most health organizations have established policies for whistle-blowing.
• *Deal with the matter promptly:* delay may cause your organization or patients to suffer or increase the risk of harm.

If you have a concern, you should *not*:

• Do nothing.
• Forget there may be an innocent or good explanation.
• Be afraid of making your concerns known.
• Approach or accuse any individuals directly.
• Try to investigate the matter yourself.
• Convey your suspicions to anyone other than those with the proper authority.

## Related topic

📖 Clinical supervision and appraisal, p. 46.

## Further information

Public Concern at Work. ☎ 020 7404 6609. Available at: ℅ http://www.pcaw.org.uk/law-and-policy
NHS and Social Care Whistle-blowing Helpline. ☎ 0800 072 4725. Available at: ℅ http://wbhelpline.org.uk/?doing_wp_cron=1372862024.6160550117492675781250
GOV.UK Whistleblowing. Available at: ℅ www.gov.uk/whistleblowing/overview
Health Care Commission. ☎ 0845 601 3012
Francis Report ℅ http://www.midstaffspublicinquiry.com/report

# Record keeping

Good record keeping promotes continuity of care (through accurate communication), acts as a means to demonstrate the quality of care, and provide a resource if nurses are called to account at a later date. (*Note:* it may be more difficult to convince a court it happened if it wasn't recorded.)

**What counts as a record?** Any permanent form of data recorded about a client or patient. This includes both paper and information stored electronically.

## General principles for good record keeping

Records should be:
- Contemporaneous.
- Include date and time information was recorded.
- If paper version, should be legible, using black permanent ink, signed, and name printed.
- Clear, comprehensive, and focused on provision of accurate, objective, factual, and relevant information relating to client's diagnosis/needs and care/treatment.
- Written in collaboration with patients.

Records should not:
- In general, they should not include anything you are not prepared to say or reveal to the client (📖 Access to records, p. 83).
- They should not be altered, except to make corrections to inaccurate information (any alterations should be clearly marked as such and signed/dated).

## Details to include when making entries to patient records

- *Information on which decisions have been based*, i.e. problems/needs presented by the patient/client; relevant information on past history (including health, medication, family, and social history); observations, test results, or examination findings.
- *Impressions of the current situation:* priorities for care/treatment.
- *Action plan:* as negotiated with patient/client (may include referrals made, prescriptions given, tests undertaken).
- *Information shared and advice given:* concerns/worries of patient/client or their family/carers; health advice given to patient; plans for follow-up/next visit.
- *Other essential information:* including details of correspondence with others.

## Storage of records

- When not in use, records should be stored (including laptops and personal digital assistants) under lock and key.
- If records are patient or parent/child held, then reinforce the need to keep information secure.
- *Electronic records:*
  - Do not leave a terminal/laptop unattended and signed-in.
  - Never share passwords.
  - Change passwords regularly.
  - Clear the screen of one patient's information before viewing another patient.
  - Use password-protected screen-savers.
- *Manual records:*
  - Store files closed and in a logical order.
  - Use a tracking system to monitor whereabouts of files.
  - Return files as soon as they are no longer needed.
- *Retention of records:* DH suggests the following as minimum retention periods:
  - *Children and young people*—until their 25th birthday or 26th if young person was 17 at time of conclusion of treatment, or 8yrs after patient's death if death occurred before 18th birthday.
  - *Maternity* (including midwifery and obstetric)—25yrs.
  - *Mentally disordered patients*—20yrs after no further treatment, or 8yrs after patient's death.
  - *Oncology*—8yrs after conclusion of treatment.
  - *General*—8yrs after conclusion of treatment.
  - *GP records*—10yrs after conclusion of treatment.
- Destruction of records should be through secure process organized by the health care organization.

## Further information

Department of Health (2007). NHS Information Governance—Guidance on Legal and Professional Obligations. Available at: ℘ www.connectingforhealth.nhs.uk/systemsandservices/infogov/codes/lglobligat.pdf

# Access to records

It is good practice to write records in collaboration with patients, in order to promote trust and increase communication. Patients and clients have legal rights to privacy in the processing of personal data and rights of access to those data.

## The Data Protection Act 1998 (DPA)

The DPA gives patients/clients (known as 'data subjects') formal rights of access:

- To be informed as to whether personal data are processed.
- To be given a description of data held, purposes for which data are processed, and knowledge of persons to whom details may be disclosed.
- To be given a copy of information constituting data.
- To be given information on sources of data.
- To have errors about them corrected in records.

To gain formal access to records, patients/clients have to write to the organization that holds the records. The responsible manager has 40 days to respond. Access to a record by a data subject is restricted:

- When access would be likely to cause serious harm to physical or mental health of data subject.
- When to give access would reveal identity of a third person (unless consent given to disclosure). Does not apply if third person is a health professional, involved in care of data subject, unless giving access is likely to cause serious harm to that health professional.

## Who can seek access to health records?

- Any competent person (including a competent child/young person) can apply for access to their personal records.
- Person with parental responsibility for a child (<18yrs old in England and Wales, <16yrs old in Scotland). *Note:* a competent child/young person has a right to confidentiality (&#128214; Consent, p. 77).
- Person appointed by a court on behalf of a person who is incapacitated, in order to discharge their duties (&#128214; Consent, p. 77).
- Third party when authorized by data subject. *Note:* family, friends, and carers don't have right of access unless patient consents.
- Executor or administrator of deceased person's estate may apply under Access to Health Records Act 1990.

## The Freedom of Information Act 2000 (FOI)

This gives a general right of access to information recorded by or on behalf of public authorities. The Act requires that all public bodies:

- Publish details of classes of recorded information held routinely.
- Permit individuals access to non-personal records of the organization.

## Further information

Information Commissioners Office. Available at: &#8478; ico.org.uk/

# IT, electronic records, and telehealth

Health care delivery is based on the use and sharing of information. ↑ use of information technology is central to government strategies.

**Resources for professionals** NHSnet is an intranet, giving access to email, electronic choose and book service, electronic transmission of prescriptions amongst other applications, such as mobile worker. All NHS staff should have a work email address and access to the NHSnet.

## NHS electronic patient records

All health organizations are working to have electronic rather than paper, patient records. Each country has different guidance on standards to ensure information is handled legally and securely, e.g. Care Record Guarantee for England. Summary Care Records provide key information on prescriptions and allergies summary care records which can be accessed on by health care staff directly involved or those with Smartcard with a chip and pin code (NHS records). Patients can chose to opt out of this system. By 2015 in England patients will have access to their GP computerized records.

## NHS clinical classification of conditions and activity

A classification (SNOMED CT®) of clinical terms is being introduced across the UK to enable the easy sharing of information and easy production of patient population summary data (e.g. for audit, health needs assessment (HNA)). It is replacing Read Codes™ used in general practice. Codes are given to all types of information—assessment, history (including medical and social), diagnosis, treatment, and professional activities.

## General practice

Most general practices are computerized and many are 'paperless', using electronic patient record systems such as EMIS and TOREX. These allow clinical templates, e.g. diabetes review prompt list, to be developed, which can be opened on-screen during a patient consultation. General practice also uses electronic methods to:

• *Choose and book:* an online method used by GPs and other primary care staff to refer patients and book initial hospital appointments online.
• *Electronic transfer of prescriptions:* an electronic method by which GPs and primary care staff can issue prescriptions and send them to the pharmacist chosen by patient.
• *GPES:* allows GP practices and commissioners to collect QOF information (📖 Quality and outcomes framework, p. 66).

## Community nursing services

Using IT and electronic care records is increasing in community health services, particularly mobile applications (such as digital pens and pads) for use in home visiting. Many GP-attached HVs and DNs record their interactions with patients/clients on the general practice patient electronic record.

## Telehealth and telecare

A wide range of new technology systems are being explored in all countries of the UK, e.g.:

- Assistive technology for supporting people to remain independently in their own homes (📖 Assistive technology, p. 776).
- For home medical monitoring that relays clinical readings through telephone to the health professional.
- For video consulting with other remote health professionals.

## Further information

Health Informatics (2013). Systemised Nomenclature of Medicine. Available at: 🔗 http://healthin-formatics.wikispaces.com/Systemized+Nomenclature+of+Medicine+-+SNOMED+

Kings Fund. Telecare and telehealth. Available at: 🔗 www.kingsfund.org.uk/topics/telecare-and-telehealth

NHS. Summary Care Records. Available at: 🔗www.nhscarerecords.nhs.uk/

RCN. Telehealth and Telecare. Available at: 🔗 www.rcn.org.uk/development/practice/e-health/telehealth_and_telecare

Scottish Centre for Telehealth and telecare. Available at: 🔗 www.sctt.scot.nhs.uk/

3 millionlives. Improving your access to telehealth and telecare. Available at: 🔗 3millionlives.co.uk/

# Confidentiality

Confidentiality is when you ensure that information shared by patients/clients is not disclosed to a third party without permission. Preserving confidentiality is:

- Important for maintaining trust between patient and professional.
- Recognized in statue and UK case law (📖 Access to records, p. 83).
- Stated in the NMC Code of Professional Conduct (📖 Professional conduct, p. 74).
- Stated or implied in your contract of employment.

Although health professionals often routinely share information, this should be with the consent (implied or expressed) of the patient.

### Refusal of consent to share information

The patient/client should be made aware of the implications of this decision. Their choice should be documented and, unless the breach falls into the following categories, respected.

### Circumstances when patient confidentiality can be breached

- When the patient consents (📖 Consent, p. 77).
- *In best interests of the patient:* e.g. in emergency.
- *To protect a child:* Children Act 1989; 📖 Child protection, p. 230.
- Under a court order.
- *Where there are statutory duties to disclose:* e.g. Public Health (Control of Diseases) Act 1984.
- *In the public interest:* however, no definition of 'public interest' has been laid down. Risk should be serious and substantially reduced by disclosure.
- Information disclosed should be limited to that necessary to protect patient/client.

### Caldicott guardians and principles

Caldicott guardians (established under the Data Protection Act 1998) are senior health and social care staff appointed to ensure Caldicott principles of disclosure of patient identifiable information are applied and should:

- Justify the purpose.
- Do not use patient identifiable information unless absolutely necessary.
- Use the minimum necessary patient identifiable information.
- Access to patient identifiable information should be on a strict 'need-to-know' basis.
- Everyone with access to patient identifiable information should be aware of their responsibilities.
- Understand and comply with the law.

### Further information

NHS Scotland Caldicott Guardians. Available at: 🖰 www.knowledge.scot.nhs.uk/caldicottguardians.aspx

# Client and patient-held records

Patients and clients increasingly hold their health and social care records in the UK, although they remain the property of the issuing organization. Employers and health and social care partnerships have local policies as to whether duplicates (e.g. carbon copies) or summaries are held by the organization or if the client/patient-held record is the sole record.

## Benefits
- Facilitates partnership.
- Enables patients/clients ↑ involvement in care.
- Ensures all contact with health and social care providers is recorded in one place.
- Ensures key information is available to the next professional.

Research studies demonstrate that client/patient-held health records do not get lost. In some countries outside UK client/patient-held records are the norm, rather than the exception.

## Types most commonly encountered in primary care
- Personal maternity records or cooperation card.
- DN home records.
- Parent-held child health record.
- School child health record.
- Personal health records of asylum applicants and refugees.
- Local disease-specific patient-held record, e.g. diabetes care.

## Further information
National Personal Child Health Record. Available at ℠ www.rcpch.ac.uk/PCHR

# Health and safety at work

The Health and Safety at Work Act 1974 provides the main legal framework.

## Employers

Employers have a legal duty to ensure staff health, safety, and welfare at work. Employers must consult staff or their safety representatives on matters relating to health and safety at work (often through safety committees, set up to monitor systems). Employers must:

- Assess and address risks to staff health and safety.
- If there are 5 or more staff, record risk assessment and plans, and draw up a health and safety policy available to all.
- Appoint a competent person responsible for health and safety.
- Set up emergency procedures and provide first-aid facilities.
- Ensure workplace satisfies health, safety, and welfare requirements, e.g. temperature, lighting, and sanitary and rest facilities.
- Ensure work equipment is suitable, maintained, and used properly.
- Prevent or control exposure to damaging substances (Control of Substances Hazardous to Health (COSHH) legislation) and protect against danger from flammable, electrical, or explosive hazards, noise, and radiation.
- Ensure no hazardous manual handling operations and reduce likelihood of injury.
- Provide health surveillance as appropriate.
- Provide free personal protective equipment (PPE) (□ Personal protective equipment, p. 98) when risks are not controlled in other ways.
- Ensure there are safety signs.
- Report certain occupational diseases, injuries, and dangerous events to authorities (RIDDOR).

## Employees

Employees also have legal duties:

- Taking reasonable care for their own health and safety and that of others.
- Cooperating with employer on health and safety issues.
- Correctly using work items provided by employers, including PPE, as trained or under guidance.
- Not interfere with or misuse anything provided for health, safety, or welfare.

## Safety representatives

Safety representatives are appointed by trade unions to represent their members on health and safety issues, and may represent entire workforce. They are entitled to paid time off to carry out their role. Unions offers full training and information backup.

## Health, safety, and welfare in the NHS

Key areas of attention in the NHS are reducing accidents and musculoskeletal injuries, reducing stress and violence to staff, providing smoke-free workplaces, tackling bullying and harassment, reducing risk of blood-borne viruses and latex allergies, ensuring occupational health services are offered to all staff, including GPs, ensure sickness absence, and opportunities for rehabilitation and redeployment are managed well.

## Health and safety at work concerns

Concerns should be raised with the employer or manager, or through the safety representative. If they fail to act or respond satisfactorily, the employee or safety representative can contact health and safety inspectors of the enforcing authority. Anyone can get health and safety information confidentially from the Health and Safety Executive's (HSE) Information line

## Further information

Health and Safety Executive. Available at: ℘ www.hse.gov.uk/index.htm

See also Health and Safety at work web pages of main unions and organizations, e.g. RCN, Unison, Unite/CPHVA (🕮 Useful websites, p. 800).

NHS Employers Health & Safety Essential Guide. Available at: ℘ http://www.nhsemployers.org/HealthyWorkplaces/Pages/Home-Healthy.aspx

HSE. RIDDOR - Reporting of Injuries, Diseases and Dangerous Occurrences Regulations 1995. Available at: ℘ www.hse.gov.uk/riddor

# Lone working

Lone working is any situation or location in which someone works without a colleague nearby or when someone is working out of sight or earshot of another colleague. The main factors creating a risk from users/patients to lone workers are impatience, frustration, anxiety, resentment, drink or drugs, and inherent aggression or mental instability. Employers have to assess the risk of violence and put measures in place to avoid or reduce risk to the lowest practicable level (📖 Clinical risk management, p. 72), e.g. ensure seating arrangements in consultation rooms allows staff to reach door without being blocked, appropriate alarm buzzers.

Wherever possible and legally permissible, health and other public sector providers should share information on individuals and addresses known to be a risk.

All services should have a system for keeping staff details required in an emergency, e.g. mobile and home numbers, next of kin, car registration and model, staff photographs.

## Good practice guidance for lone working and home visiting

- *Scheduling appointments and reporting movements:*
  - Ensure colleagues are aware of one another's movements including full addresses, details of home visiting, journey details, telephone numbers, and anticipated arrival and departure times. Some areas use texting to let a colleague know when staff member has safely left after each home visit.
  - All staff need to know procedures if colleagues do not return when expected.
- *If the patient, relative, or carer has a history of violence or the location is considered unsafe:*
  - Do not visit alone.
  - If possible contact should take place at a neutral location or within a secure environment, such as within Violent Patient Scheme in primary care.
- *Key safety equipment to be carried:*
  - ID badge.
  - Mobile phone—keep fully charged and close at hand, emergency contacts on speed dial, check signal before entering lone worker situations, do not use overtly in open spaces.
  - Map of the local area.
  - Personal attack alarm and torch.
  - Emergency telephone numbers.
- *Arriving at and conducting the appointment:*
  - When front door is opened, carry out a 10-s risk assessment.
  - Have an excuse ready should it be deemed necessary not to enter.
  - Request that animals be secured prior to entry.
  - Shut front door and be familiar with door lock.
  - Maintain awareness of entrances and exists.
  - If uncomfortable, do not sit down and do not spread belongings out.
  - If feeling unsafe, make an excuse and leave immediately.

## Good practice principles for travelling

### Lone working and vehicles

- Ensure enough petrol and join a recovery breakdown service.
- Do not leave valuables visible.
- Avoid nurse on call badges, as may this encourage thieves after drugs.
- Hold keys when leaving premises to avoid looking for them outside.
- Lock doors/shut windows at slow speed and at traffic lights.
- Park in well-lit locations, facing the direction you wish to leave.

### Lone working and public transport

- Use a busy stop or station that is well-lit.
- Keep a transport timetable.
- Sit near driver, in an aisle seat and near emergency alarm.
- Avoid upper decks, empty carriages, or carriages occupied by only one other person.

### Lone working and travelling by foot

- Walk briskly and do not stop in unfamiliar areas.
- If carrying equipment, use bags that do not advertise what is carried.
- In event of attempted theft, relinquish property at once without challenge.
- Keep house keys and mobile phone separate from handbag.
- Remain aware of location and surrounding people.
- Avoid waste ground, isolated pathways, and subways.

## Further information

Health and Safety Executive. Lone working. Available at: ℘ www.hse.gov.uk/treework/site-management/lone-working.htm

The Suzie Lamplugh Trust. Information and resources on personal safety. Available at: ℘ www.suzylamplugh.org

NHS Employers. Improving safety for lone workers guides in partnership with the NHS Staff Council for staff and managers. Available at: ℘ http://www.nhsemployers.org/HealthyWorkplaces/Keeping-staff-well/POSHH/Pages/POSHH.aspx

Professional bodies and unions also provide information (see 📖 Useful websites, p. 800)

# Patient moving and handling

Moving patients is a major factor in back injury and musculoskeletal disorders in nursing staff. The manual handling regulations place duties on employers to ensure manual handling is avoided where reasonable and practicable, and if not to carry out an assessment of risk and then minimize risk by implementing measures relating to the working environment such as equipment, uniform, organizational staffing levels, training, written instructions, definition of roles, and communication. Employees have a duty to obey reasonable instructions and cooperate with employers in manual handling procedures. Patient-handling risk assessments and care plans to minimize risk for each type of moving and handling activity should be documented in patient held notes. All staff involved in patient handling should receive training and regular updating, including equipment use.

## Factors that predispose to injury and should be avoided

- Lifting patients.
- Working in an awkward, unstable, or crouched position.
- Undertaking work that requires bending forward, sideways, or twisting.
- Lifting loads at arms length.
- Lifting with a starting or finishing position near the floor.
- Lifting with a starting or finishing position overhead at arms length.
- Lifting an uneven load with the weight mainly on one side.
- Handling an uncooperative or falling patient.

## Issues to consider in the handling risk assessment

- The task: e.g.
  - What task needs to be performed, e.g. move from bed to chair?
  - Where is it to be carried out?
  - Number of people required?
  - Equipment required?
- The patient: e.g.
  - Expectations, wishes, willingness to accept equipment.
  - Potential for rehabilitation to greater independence.
  - Ability to weight bear, history of falls.
  - Pain or arthritis.
  - Level of cooperation.
  - Problems with sight or spatial awareness.
  - Body weight and distribution.
  - Medication that might affect mobility.
- The handler: e.g.
  - Physical capabilities, health, and fitness.
  - Up-to-date in handling training.
  - Suitable clothing and footwear.
  - Heights of people working together.
  - Familiarity with chosen equipment.
- The environment: e.g.
  - Space available.
  - Obstacles that might need to be moved.
  - Type of floor or surface.
  - Gradients or distances involved.

## Handling equipment

Patient handling aids should be used whenever they can reduce the risk of injury. Their selection should be based on individual patient assessment. Physiotherapist's and/or OT's assessment and advice may be required. Special equipment might be needed for bariatric (i.e. clinically obese) patients. Equipment should be regularly maintained and CE marked as per Medical Devices Regulations. Local policies apply to equipment to aid nursing and to aid independent living (🕮 Assistive technology and equipment for home nursing, p. 778). Equipment to consider includes:

- *Aids for greater patient independent movement:*
  - Dutch lifting poles or rope ladders in bed.
  - Patient hand blocks.
  - Transfer boards.
  - Bath boards and rails.
  - Raised toilet seats and rails.
  - Swivel seats.
  - Leg lifters.
  - Variable height beds.
  - Stair lifts.
- *Aids for movement assisted by others:*
  - Handling belts, and slings.
  - Standing turntables.
  - Variable height beds.
  - Hoists (mobile, freestanding, and ceiling mounted) and slings.
  - Sliding aids.

If the patient refuses equipment, negotiation skills become important. Staff need to report refusal to line manager as the risk of injury to staff has to weighed up against the risk to the patient if a particular procedure is not carried out.

## Essential reading

Smith, J. (ed.) (2011). *The Guide to the Handling of People—a systems approach* (6th edn). Teddington: Backcare. Available at: 🔊 www.backcaretrading.org.uk/

## Further information

HSE Manual Handling. Available at: 🔊 www.hse.gov.uk/msd/manualhandling.htm
National Back Exchange. Available at: 🔊 www.nationalbackexchange.org/
Professional organizations and unions also provide information (see 🕮 Useful websites, p. 800)

# Hand hygiene

Hand washing is the single, most important practice to prevent health care-associated infection. All health organizations will have policies on hand hygiene for staff to follow.

## Risk assessment

To help decisions about when to wash your hands and what to use before patient contact. Assess:

• Risk of infection to the patient.
• The susceptibility of the site to infection.
• The nature of the activity.

After patient contact, assess:

• The risk of infection to self and others, e.g. family members.
• The extent and type of contamination resulting from the activity.

## Types of hand washing

### Soap and water and hand sanitizers (alcohol hand gels)

Use to remove transient micro-organisms, dirt, and organic matter.

Wash palm to palm, then:

• Right palm over left dorsum and left palm over right dorsum.
• Palm to palm, fingers interlaced.
• Backs of fingers to opposing palms with fingers interlocked.
• Rotational rubbing of right thumb clasped in left palm and vice versa.
• Rotational rubbing, backwards and forwards with clasped fingers of right hand in left palm and vice versa.
• Wet hands transfer micro-organisms more effectively than dry ones.
• Disposable paper towels should be used.

*Alcohol hand rub* use to disinfect *clean hands*. Rub hands together vigorously, covering all surfaces, until all the alcohol has evaporated. Useful in the patient's home where hand-washing facilities are limited.

### Additional factors to reduce cross-infection

• *Finger nails:* keep short; do not wear false nails.
• *Rings:* staff who wear rings have higher numbers of organisms on their hands than those who do not. Ensure wash under ring as often heavily colonized with Gram-negative organisms.
• *Cuts and abrasions:* cover with waterproof dressings.
• *Staff with skin infections:* e.g. boils and exfoliative skin conditions (e.g. psoriasis, eczema)—seek advice from occupational health (OH).
• *Hair:* wear so it does not need readjustment ∴ avoiding contaminating hands.
• *Carers/relatives:* remind them to wash their hands on completion of care and after contact with a patient with an infection.

## Further information

Royal College of Nursing (2012). Essential practice for infection prevention and control. Guidance for nursing staff. Available at: ℘ www.rcn.org.uk/__data/assets/pdf_file/0008/427832/004166.pdf
WHO. Five moments for hand hygiene. Available at: ℘ www.who.int/gpsc/tools/Five_moments/en/

# Cleaning, disinfection, and sterilization of equipment

GPs and other community employers are responsible for assessing risks to health in the workplace and implementing effective but safe decontamination practices. Consult with local health organization policy and procedures.

## Cleaning

The physical removal of dirt and organic matter (e.g. blood). Single-use cloths with neutral detergent in water is recommended, but a detergent wipe may also be used. Cleaning essential before disinfection or sterilization is carried out. Dry all cleaned equipment thoroughly before storage.

- *Manual cleaning:* wear gloves, plastic apron, and face and eye protection if splashing a possibility. Use detergent and hot water in a deep, dedicated sink (not hand basin). Dry thoroughly (air or paper towels).
- *Automated cleaning:* an ultrasonic cleaner is preferred. Change cleaning solution after each sessional use.

## Disinfection

↓ the numbers of micro-organisms. Most disinfectants are effective against a limited range of micro-organisms. Spores are not usually destroyed. Little advantage in the routine use of chemical disinfectants as micro-organisms can be removed through cleaning with a detergent solution. For disinfectants to be effective must use at the right concentration, and store in appropriate conditions and used safely. *Note:* increasing use of disinfectant wipes to decontaminate low-risk equipment is not supported by the available evidence. Dirt removal should be seen as the main purpose of a wipe.

Heat disinfection is preferred to chemical disinfection, which is unreliable. Disinfectants should be used for disinfecting heat-sensitive items.

## Sterilization

↓ numbers of micro-organisms, including spores. Use autoclaves if possible/practical or single-use disposable instruments. The choice of method depends on conditions and the sterility assurance level required (Table 3.1). If practicable and cost-effective, obtain sterile items from a Central Sterile Services Department (CSSD).

## Bench top autoclaves (sterilizers)

Appropriate for use in clinics and GP practices. Must comply with Safety and Medical Device Regulations of the Medicines and Health care products Regulatory Agency (MHRA). They must be validated before use by a 'test person', have their performance monitored on a daily, weekly, quarterly, and annual basis by the owner, and be regularly maintained in accordance with the manufacturer's programme. All results must be documented in a log book, available for periodic inspection. There are two types:

- *Bench top steam sterilizers:* use for sterilization of unwrapped, solid instruments for immediate use.
- *Bench top vacuum steam sterilizers (preferred type):* use for sterilizing bagged instruments (for future use), and items with narrow lumens and cavities.

### General principles
- Clean instruments (as in 'Cleaning') first.
- Ensure there is sufficient water (distilled or water for irrigation) in the sterilizer chamber.
- Open hinged/ratchet instruments to allow steam penetration. Place items in bag with handle nearest the closure.
- Label bag with contents, date, and sterilizer.
- Arrange items on tray/in basket to allow steam to circulate freely. Invert bowls and gallipots.
- Use an appropriate process indicator.
- Close door, select, and start cycle. Enter date, time, cycle details, etc., in the log book.
- Examine cycle printout to ensure satisfactory cycle and keep record.
- *Unpackaged items:* use immediately or keep clean and dry and covered with a sterile field until needed.
- *Packaged items:* check integrity of packaging; store clean and dry.
- Ensure stock rotation.

## Decontamination prior to inspection, service, and repair
All medical equipment must be decontaminated before being sent for inspection, service, or repair. A certificate must be completed detailing the method of decontamination prior to work being carried out.

*Single-use items* must not be re-processed unless the reprocessor can ensure the integrity and safety of the item.

**Table 3.1** Risk categories of decontamination

| Risk category | Indication | Examples | Decontami-nation level | Method |
|---|---|---|---|---|
| Minimal | Not in close contact with the patient or their immediate surroundings | Consultation room | Clean | Manual or automated cleaning<br><br>Damp dusting<br><br>Wet mopping<br><br>Vacuum cleaners |
| Low | Items used on intact skin | Wash bowls, commodes | Clean | Manual cleaning using detergent and water and dry<br><br>Automated cleaning/disinfection<br><br>Disinfectants |
| Medium | Items that have contact with mucous membranes or are contaminated with micro-organisms that are easily transmitted or items to be used on highly susceptible patients or sites | Vaginal specula | Cleaning and disinfection and/or sterilization | Autoclave or single-use<br><br>Low temperature steam washer/disinfectors |
| High | Items that penetrate skin or mucous membranes or that enter sterile sites | Surgical instruments, needles, syringes | Sterile | Hospital CSSD; bench top autoclave and use sterile; purchase of single-use disposables |

## Further information

Control of Substances Harmful to Health. Available at: &#8471; www.hse.gov.uk/coshh/.
Medicines and Health care Products Regulatory Authority. Available at: &#8471; www.mhra.gov.uk/
MHRA (2010). Sterilization, disinfection and cleaning of medical equipment: guidance on decontamination from the Microbiology Advisory Committee (3rd edn). *The Mac Manual.*
National Patient Safety Agency (NPSA) (now part of NHS Health England. Available at: &#8471; www.england.nhs.uk/ourwork/patientsafety)/

# Personal protective equipment

Personal protective equipment (PPE) is worn to protect nurses' clothing, skin, and mucous membranes from contamination with the patient's blood, body fluids, secretions, or excretions, and to reduce the transmission of micro-organisms between patients and staff. The Control of Substances Hazardous to Health Regulations (2002) require employers to

- assess any substances hazardous to health, including biohazards within blood and body fluids (such as blood-borne viruses) and reduce the risk of exposure. Where exposure cannot be avoided, PPE, including gloves should be used. All must be provided by the employer, including aprons, gloves, masks, eye visors/goggles. *Use:* based on an assessment of the risk of contamination.

## Plastic aprons

Plastic aprons must be worn when assisting patients with toileting, bathing, when a patient has a known or suspected infection, or any activity that could disperse pathogens and/or procedures, which cause splashing of blood or body fluids. The apron should be changed as soon as soon as the individual task is completed. Dispose of as per local waste policies.

## Gloves

*Never a substitute for appropriate hand washing.* Use only when required. Inappropriate use can lead to:

- Weakened hand hygiene initiatives.
- Development of skin problems: e.g. contact dermatitis or exacerbation of existing skin problems.

The purpose is to protect the skin against hazardous substances, e.g. chemicals. Gloves must be worn for invasive procedures, contact with sterile sites, and non-intact skin or mucous membranes, and all activities that have been assessed as carrying a risk of exposure to blood, body fluids, secretions, or excretions, or to sharp or contaminated instruments. Used correctly, they can:

- Prevent gross contamination of nurses' hands.
- Reduce transmission of micro-organisms to patients during invasive or other patient care (e.g. wound care).
- Protect the skin against hazardous substances, e.g. chemicals.

### Types of gloves

Rubber, latex, nitrile neoprene, vinyl, sterile, and unsterile. Powdered gloves and polythene gloves should **not** be used for health care activities. Double-gloving is recommended for procedures associated with a high risk of glove tear or percutaneous injury.

- *Latex:* some resistance to puncture and resealing properties, more appropriate for procedures involving the handling of sharp instruments.
- *Vinyl gloves:* can be used to perform tasks, but may not be appropriate with handling blood/body fluids, high risk substances. Check local policy.

*After gloves removed*
Hands must be washed because:
- They do not eliminate hand contamination completely.
- They may be punctured.
- Hands are easily contaminated as gloves are taken off.

Natural rubber latex (NRL) proteins in latex gloves can cause severe reactions in staff and patients with existing allergies. In sensitized individuals it can lead to contact dermatitis and occupational asthma. Under the Reporting of Injuries, Diseases and Dangerous Occurrence Regulations (RIDDOR) it is a legal requirement to report occupational asthma or dermatitis related to NRL to the HSE. If latex gloves are selected must be low protein and single use (HSE 2011).

Alternatives = neoprene and nitrile.

## Disposal of aprons and gloves
- Aprons and gloves are single-use items that must be disposed of at end of individual patient care.
- Depending on procedures being performed, may need to be changed in between care activities on same patient.
- Gloves and aprons must be discarded as clinical waste.
- Gloves must never be washed or disinfected and reused as soap solution can cause glove damage.

## Tabards
They are not water repellent and, when wet, micro-organisms pass through them easily. If worn, they must be laundered to prevent cross-infection.

*Fluid-repellent gowns* Full-length, fluid-repellent gowns must be worn where there is a risk of extensive splashing of blood, body fluids, secretions or excretions onto the skin.

## Face masks and eye visors/goggles
Should be worn when there is a risk of blood, body fluids, secretions or excretions splashing into the face and eyes, e.g. respiratory suction. Eyewear should be fitted correctly.

## Respiratory protective equipment
A particulate filter mask must be used when clinically indicated, e.g. caring for a patient with highly infectious respiratory disease. Staff should be trained in their use

High-efficiency respirator masks are occasionally needed when caring for patients with infections transmitted by droplet nuclei in the air, e.g. multi-drug resistant tuberculosis (MDRTB).

## Work clothes/uniforms

• Contamination occurs from nurses' uniforms, but estimated one-third of organisms present originated from wearer due to normal bacterial skin flora being in contact with uniform.

• During patient procedures clothes/uniforms can become contaminated by organisms such as methicillin-resistant *Staphylococcus aureus* (MRSA), *Clostridium difficile*, and glycopeptide-resistant enterococci (GRE). Even if not visibly soiled, contact transfer of bacteria from clothes/uniforms to patients is possible.

• To minimize risks of cross-infection, uniforms and own clothes should be washed at temperatures to achieve thermal disinfection in the laundering process, i.e. 65°C for first part of wash cycle. Lycra or polyester fabrics may not withstand such temperatures. Dry quickly and iron. *Note:* if employer does not provide a free laundry service for uniforms, nurse can claim tax relief for cleaning costs.

• Shoes should envelop the feet, be non-slip, and provide support. Sandals and clogs may be inadequate protection against sharp objects.

## Related topic

📖 Methicillin resistant *Staphylococcus aureus*, p. 674.

## Further information

Health Safety Executive (HSE) (2011). Selecting latex gloves. Available at: ℘ http://www.hse.gov.uk/skin/employ/latex-gloves.htm

Royal College of Nursing (2012). Essential practice for infection prevention and control. Guidance for nursing staff. Available at: ℘ www.rcn.org.uk/__data/assets/pdf_file/0008/427832/004166.pdf

# Occupational exposure to blood-borne viruses

Occupational exposure to blood-borne viruses is unnecessarily common and most frequently associated with hepatitis B, hepatitis C, and human immunodeficiency virus (HIV). Many exposures result from a failure to follow recommended procedures, including safe handling and disposal of needles and syringes, or wearing personal protective eyewear where indicated (📖 Personal protective equipment, p. 98). All nurses and health care assistants should be vaccinated against hepatitis B (📖 Viral hepatitis, p. 676).

Accidental exposure to blood and body fluids can occur through:

- *Percutaneous injury:* e.g. used needles (📖 Sharps injuries, p. 107), bone fragments, significant bites that break the skin.
- *Exposure of broken skin:* e.g. abrasions, cuts, eczema.
- *Exposure of mucous membranes:* including the eyes and mouth.

Increased risk of exposure associated with:

- Deep injury.
- Visible blood on the device which caused the injury.
- Injury with a needle, which had been placed in the source patient's artery or vein.
- Terminal HIV-related illness in the source patient (📖 HIV, p. 686)

Not associated with saliva, urine, vomit, or faeces *unless* blood is present. There is no risk of HIV transmission where intact skin is exposed to HIV-infected blood. Every employer should have a policy on the management of occupational exposures to blood-borne viruses. All nurses must have immediate, 24-hr access to advice through either:

- An occupational health service.
- OOH cover provided by accident and emergency departments.

## Post-exposure prophylaxis (PEP)

Following accidental exposure to blood and body fluids, regardless of whether the source is known to pose an infection risk, you should:

- Immediately stop what you are doing and attend the injury.
- Encourage bleeding of the wound by applying gentle pressure. Do not suck.
- Wash well under running water.
- Dry and apply a waterproof dressing as necessary.
- If blood and body fluids splash into eyes, irrigate with cold water.
- If blood and body fluids splash into your mouth, do not swallow, rinse out several times with cold water.

Report the incident in line with local policy and complete an accident/incident form. If the injury is from a used needle or instrument, risk assessment should be carried out by an OH adviser, virologist, or other suitable professional. Consent is required if blood needs to be taken.

Nurses who have acquired HIV infection because of exposure to HIV-infected material in the workplace may be able to claim Industrial Injuries Disablement Benefit (📖 Benefits and support, p. 789).

PEP following exposure to HIV consists of a combination of antiretroviral drugs that, ideally, should be started within the hour. PEP may still be considered up to 2wks have elapsed since the exposure. Exposed nurses should be encouraged to:

• Provide a baseline blood sample for storage up to 2yrs and a follow-up sample for testing.
• Seek psychological support.
• Report any sickness absence associated with adverse effects of PEP drugs following an occupational exposure does not contribute to an individual's sickness absence record.

## Further information

Royal College of Nursing (2012). Essential practice for infection prevention and control. Guidance for nursing staff. Available at: ℘ www.rcn.org.uk/__data/assets/pdf_file/0008/427832/004166.pdf

# Infectious disease notifications

Since the beginning of the 19th century certain infectious diseases have been notifiable (see Box 3.2). The statutory process aims to ensure:
• Speed in identifying possible outbreaks and epidemics.
• Prevention of spread of infectious disease.

The specific diseases are selected for notification because they are:
• Potentially life-threatening.
• Spread rapidly.
• Cannot be easily treated.

Occasionally, notification is used to monitor success of immunization programmes and the development of localized outbreaks.

If a GP becomes aware/suspects that a patient has a notifiable disease or is suffering from food poisoning there is a statutory duty in England and Wales to notify the 'Proper Officer' (usually the Medical Consultant for environmental health or Consultant in communicable disease control): for local contact details (Health Protection Agency (HPA)).

The information must include (form available from LA, PCO, if urgent action required information should be phoned/faxed):
• Name, age and sex of patient.
• Address where patient is.
• Details of disease or poisoning, and date of onset.
• Other relevant information (e.g. if individual has been abroad).

---

### Box 3.2  Notifiable diseases

• Acute encephalitis
• Acute poliomyelitis
• Anthrax
• Cholera
• Diphtheria
• Dysentery
• Food poisoning
• Leptospirosis
• Malaria
• Measles
• Meningitis
  • Meningococcal
  • Pneumococcal
  • *Haemophilus influenzae*
  • Viral
  • Other specified
  • Unspecified
• Meningococcal septicaemia (without meningitis)
• Mumps
• Ophthalmia neonatorum
• Paratyphoid fever
• Plague
• Rabies
• Relapsing fever
• Rubella
• Scarlet fever
• Smallpox
• Tetanus
• Tuberculosis
• Typhoid fever
• Viral haemorrhagic fever
• Viral hepatitis:
  • Hepatitis A
  • Hepatitis B
  • Hepatitis C
• Whooping cough
• Yellow fever.

NB Leprosy is also notifiable, but directly to the Health Protection Agency.

In Scotland, health care providers and other agencies should report to NHS organizations who are required to notify the Common Services Agency who inform Health Protection Scotland.

## Schools

OFSTED the inspectorate for children and learners in England, should be notified of:

- Any food poisoning affecting two or more children.
- Any child having meningitis or the outbreak on the premises of any notifiable disease identified as such in the Public Health (Control of Disease) Act 1984 or because the notification requirement has been applied to them by regulations (the relevant regulations are the Public Health (Infectious Diseases) Regulations 1988).

(See also 🕮 Table 7.2, p. 286 Infectious diseases exclusion times).

## Further information

Health Protection Agency. Available at: ℘ www.hpa.org.uk
Health Protection Scotland. Available at: ℘ www.hps.scot.nhs.uk

# Managing health care waste

## Disposal of clinical waste

Part of an employer's overall health and safety management system. Staff training is essential. The organization should have access to a dedicated qualified waste manager. Hypodermic needles and other hazardous health care wastes should never be disposed of in the domestic waste stream. Nurses have a responsibility to protect the health of their patients *and* the natural environment (see Table 3.2 for categories of waste).

Local policies and guidance should be followed:
• Clinical waste is classified as 'hazardous waste' and should be transported as an infectious substance.
• An 'offensive' waste stream describes non-infectious wastes.

## Identification of infectious waste

Only waste generated from health care practice undertaken by a suitably qualified health professional will be considered infectious waste. Soiled waste, e.g. sanitary products, plasters are not considered to be infectious.
• *Bodily fluids that may be infectious:* blood, semen, vaginal secretions.
• *Non-infectious bodily fluids:* faeces, nasal secretions, sputum, tears, urine, vomit. *Note:* these may be considered infectious if they contain visible blood or the source patient has been assessed as having an infection that might be transmitted via the waste, i.e. an infection pathway exists, e.g. faeces known/suspected of contamination with enteric pathogens such as *Salmonella* spp., or *Shigella* spp., or vomit from patient with acute vomiting virus.

## Collection of waste

• *Frequency of collection:*
  • *Infectious waste*—weekly.
  • *Sharps bins*—no less than 3mths.
• *Waste transfer note:* required to keep track of the waste.
• *Producer notification:* all sites producing hazardous waste including health care centres and GP practices, are required to notify the Environment Agency. Can be done through the PCO.
• *Registered waste carriers:* community nurses and those working in home health care; health care providers' vehicles carrying waste generated by them are exempt from registration procedures.
• If patients are treated in their home by a community nurse or a member of the NHS profession, any waste produced as a result is considered to be the health care professional's waste.

**Table 3.2** Categories of waste and receptacles

| Waste category | Receptacle/colour coding | Examples of contents |
|---|---|---|
| Domestic waste | Bag Black | General refuse incl. newspapers, flowers, etc. |
| Infectious waste | Bag Orange | Infectious and potentially infectious waste, e.g. soiled dressings. Autoclaved laboratory waste |
| Offensive waste | Bag Yellow with black stripes | Incontinence pads, nappy bins, sanitary wastes etc. from human hygiene; animal faeces; non-infectious disposable equipment, bedding, gowns, plaster casts |
| Sharps | Yellow bin | Not contaminated with cytotoxic products. Sharps from phlebotomy |
| Sharps | Yellow bin with blue top bin | Contaminated with cytotoxic and/or cytostatic medicinal products |

Should aim to promote the following:
• Waste reduction and prevention.
• Reusable/recyclable products.
• Reduction of disposal of waste to landfills.
• The use of cleaner technologies.
• Energy recovery.
• An integrated network of waste management facilities.

*Think Green. What can you do to minimize waste?*

## Further information

Royal College of Nursing (2012). Essential practice for infection prevention and control. Guidance for nursing staff. Available at: ℗ www.rcn.org.uk/__data/assets/pdf_file/0008/427832/004166.pdf

Health & Safety Executive (HSE). Available at: ℗ www.hse.gov.uk

Department for Environment Food and Rural Affairs Health care waste. Guidance on the correct disposal of potentially hazardous clinical waste. Available at: ℗ www.gov.uk/health care-waste

# Sharps injuries

Employers are required to assess the risk of sharps injuries and, where possible, eliminate the use of sharps. Sharps include needles, blades, suture cutters, broken glass. Sharps injuries are a major cause of transmission of blood-borne viruses and should be treated as a serious event; however, many go unreported.

❶ All staff at risk of sharps injuries should have up-to-date hepatitis B vaccination.

## Prevention of sharps injuries
- Ensure workforce has received training and focus on systemic factors. rather than individual mistakes.
- Never assume there is no risk following a sharps injury.
- Keep sharps handling to a minimum.
- Needle safety devices (devices built into the needle manufacture to reduce risk of needlestick injuries, e.g. by creating a barrier between needle and user's hand) provide safer systems of working for nurses.
- Sharps containers are close as possible to the point of use.
- Sharps must not be passed directly from hand to hand. Handling should be kept to a minimum.
- Needles must not be recapped, bent or broken, or disassembled after use or disposal.
- Containers in public areas must be located in a safe position, and must not be placed on the floor.
- Used sharps must be disposed of into a sharps container at the point of use by the user.
- Containers must not be filled above the mark that indicates that they are full.
- Where a patient uses sharps as part of their self-treatment they are responsible for safe disposal. They can arrange for LA to collect sharps bins for disposal.

## Carriage of sharps containers in cars by community staff
No specific guidance available but the employer should agree practice with the infection control committee. The car should be securely locked when unoccupied and the sharps container kept out of site.

*Disposal* Containers must be disposed of by the licensed route in accordance with local policy.

## Sharps injuries
Immediately following *any* exposure, whether or not the source is known to pose a risk of infection:
- The site of exposure, e.g. wound or non-intact skin, should be washed liberally with soap and water, but without scrubbing.
- Free bleeding of puncture wounds should be gently encouraged, but wounds should not be sucked.

- If there has been a splash into mucous membranes, including conjunctivae, these should be irrigated copiously with water, before and after removing contact lenses.

The nurse must know how to access urgent advice about occupational exposure and PEP for HIV (see 🕮 Occupational exposure to blood-borne viruses, p. 101).

- Accidental exposure to blood or body fluids must be reported through the employers incident/accident reporting system (🕮 Health and safety at work, p. 88).

### Related topics

🕮 Occupational exposure to blood-borne viruses, p. 101; 🕮 HIV, p. 686; 🕮 Viral hepatitis, p. 680.

### Further information

Royal College of Nursing (2012). Essential practice for infection prevention and control. Guidance for nursing staff. Available at: ℘ www.rcn.org.uk/__data/assets/pdf_file/0008/427832/004166.pdf

# Approaches to individual health needs assessment

See also 📖 The assessment of children, young people, and
   families, p. 148

# Individual health needs assessment

The purpose of assessment at an individual level is to establish a baseline of the health and wellbeing of the person and create an agreed care/action plan. In addition, aggregated data informs population health needs (📖 Health needs assessment, p. 11) and service commissioning (📖 Commissioning of services, p. 9). High quality comprehensive assessment is the means by which individuals' access care and services are tailored to their needs. Assessment strategies are influenced by:

- Problem-solving framework of the nursing process (i.e. assessment, planning, implementation, evaluation).
- Nursing models, theories, and values (e.g. focus on activities of daily living (ADLs), self-care, health promotion).
- Specialism (e.g. HV, DN, general practice nurse (GPN), SN) and client group (older people, adult, children).
- National and local policy, e.g. single assessment process for assessing older people, common assessment frameworks for assessing a child and family in need, the Carers Act.
- Electronic patient/client records and databases often dictate how assessment data is collected, recorded, and shared.

## Principles

- Assessment is one part of case/care management (📖 Care/case management models, p. 112).
- Assessment should incorporate a sense of a person's own rating of health status and focus on the needs of the individual and their carers. What is available from the service should *not* limit assessment.
- Objective, quantifiable plus subjective, client-focused data are important for a rounded assessment.
- Assessment includes extent and ways identified needs/problems are already addressed, plus factors that ameliorate or reduce impact of problems/needs. It is important that assessment does not solely focus on what the individual *cannot* do.
- It should lead to identification of agreed needs/problems for which an action/care plan is agreed with patient/client.
- Assessment and needs/problems identification provides basis for selection of nursing interventions and referrals to other professionals or organizations.
- The ability to take a nursing health history depends on level of training, clinical experience and highly developed communication and interpersonal skills (📖 Principles of good communication, p. 117).
- After implementation of care/action plan, further assessment serves to evaluate outcome and effect, as well as identify new problems/needs.

Most individual health needs assessment will include biographical profile, physiological, psychological, sociocultural, developmental, and spiritual domains.

## Values models and in assessment

At an individual level, theories of need have largely provided the basis for primary care nurses to understand how patients respond. These include:

- Maslow's hierarchy of needs[1] suggest lower level needs must be met before higher. Physiological → safety → belonging → esteem → self-actualization.
- Bradshaw's[1] typology of the perceptions of need. Identified as:
  - Normative (that accepted as the 'norm' in society) needs.
  - Felt (as stated by the individual) needs.
  - Expressed (felt and acted upon in some way be the individual) needs.
  - Comparative (compared with others) needs.

Models for directing assessments by nurses in primary care include:

- Activities of Daily Living (ADL) Model[2] uses the 12 activities of living as units of assessment to encourages a focus on health, rather than ill health.
- Self-care model[2] widely used in areas of disease prevention and health promotion. Assessment based on self-care requisites and self-care deficits.
- Biomedical or diagnostic[2] model comprises history taking, physical examination and requesting clinical investigations to arrive at a clinical judgement about disease/illness and an individual's response to that. More commonly used in advanced and first-contact roles.
- 📖 Models and approaches to health promotion, p. 298.
- Child and family assessment frameworks (📖 The assessment of children, young people, and families, p. 148).

## Standardized assessment tools

Standardized assessment tools for adults (📖 Standardized assessment tools for adults, p. 116) are often used for identification of specific problems e.g. mini-mental state examination[3] for dementia.

## References

[1]Harris A. (ed.) (1997). *Needs to know: Guide to Needs Assessment in Primary Care*. London: Churchill Livingstone.
[2]Pearson A, Vaughan B, FitzGerald M. (2005). *Nursing Models for Practice*, 3rd edn. Edinburgh: Butterworth Heinemann.
[3]Folstein MF, Folstein SE, McHugh PR. (1975). 'Mini-mental state'. A practical method for grading the cognitive state of patients for the clinician. *J Psychiat Res* **12**(3): 189–98.

# Care/case management models

A systematic, proactive, and cyclical care approach to caring for people who have highly complex care needs (📖 Generic long-term conditions model, p. 5).

Approach characterized by one person (e.g. nurse, social worker, key worker) having the designated responsibility to coordinate and oversee care to ensure care is actively managed and 'joined up'.

The concept originated in USA and developed in UK in the contexts of:

- *Community care:* under the NHS & Community Care Act 1990 case managers (later referred to as care managers by DH) coordinated the care of individuals with complex, multi agency needs.
- *Care programme approach and the Mental Health Act 1983:* where mental health worker (mental health nurse or social worker) acted as case manager or key worker for patients leaving in-patient care, and needing monitoring and support.
- *Management of long-term conditions:* government's framework includes appointment of case managers/community matrons to case manage those with the most complex needs. People identified as likely to benefit include:
  - Those suffering with chronic disease and/or long-term conditions.
  - People with learning disabilities or enduring mental illness.
  - Older people with high health service use, and/or co-morbidity and polypharmacy.
  - Older people at risk of hospitalization.

A case/care management approach involves:

- *Targeting/case finding:* based on proactive outreach and set referral criteria. Identifies individuals likely to benefit from case management.
- *Assessment of individual's problems and need for services:* using information from patient, carers, and other services involved in care. May include physical assessment and diagnosis.
- *Care planning and securing care:* to address agreed needs and formation of action plan involves coordinating interventions, making referrals; may have a clinical input.
- *Implementation of plan:* either by direct or coordinating care.
- *Monitoring and review of plan:* regular review, monitoring, and consequent adaptation of care plan leading to either discharge from care or continuing care.

## Models of case management

- *Brokerage model:* where case manager is an independent client advocate, purchasing or commissioning services to needs.
- *Cultural tradition, and focus of a discipline and/or clinical specialty:* e.g. district nursing, rehabilitation.
- *Social entrepreneurship model:* where case manager is agency based and holds a budget for purchasing tailored packages of care for clients. Emerged as a social care model.
- *Clinical and/or care coordination model:* where case manager is a member (or members) of an existing MDT, and assumes responsibility for arranging and monitoring care for specific clients. Often preferred health model.
- *In legislatively agreed systems:* led by social services/social work.
- *As specialist posts:* for the case management of people with multiple conditions, e.g. community matrons.
- *As clinical specialists:* with dedicated caseloads that support people with particular diseases and/or conditions e.g. diabetes, multiple sclerosis (MS).

### Nurses assuming a case management/community matron role
Additional preparation and mentoring may be needed in:
- Advanced clinical and diagnostic skills.
- Independent/supplementary prescribing and medicines management.
- Management of exacerbations of illness.
- Information management.
- Coordination across 1° and 2° care.
- Management of cognitive impairment.
- Management of care at end of life.
- Health promotion and patient empowerment.

DH/Skills for Health have produced competency statements for case managers and community matrons available on the DH (England) website in the long-term conditions section (📖 Useful websites, p. 800).

### Related topic
📖 Integrated (or single) assessment processes, p. 114.

### Further information
Case management competences framework for the care of people with long term conditions. Available at: 🔗 www.dh.gov.uk/en/Publicationsandstatistics/Publications/PublicationsPolicyAndGuidance/DH_4118101

Department of Health (2010). Improving care for people with long term conditions: 'at a glance' information sheets for health care professionals. Available at: 🔗 www.dh.gov.uk/en/Publicationsandstatistics/Publications/PublicationsPolicyAndGuidance/DH_121603

# Integrated or single assessment processes

For child and family assessment, see 📖 The assessment of children, young people, and families, p. 148.

## Assessment of need for social care

Under the provision of the NHS and Community Care Act 1990, assessment of need for community care is the duty of local authorities and specifically social services (📖 Social services, p. 26). Note: there is not an equivalent duty to provide services. Locally-determined finite resources determine availability of public funding for services. The purpose of the assessment is to establish needs for the provision of means-tested services according to eligibility criteria, which may be provided by a range of LA, voluntary and/or private providers. Provision of services may include:

- Support to people in their home: by providing domiciliary care (e.g. social home carers), day care (e.g. day centres), and respite care.
- Services for carers (📖 Carers assessment and support, p. 412).
- Provide adaptations to housing (📖 Homes and housing, p. 21).
- Assessment for long-term care and related funding (📖 Care homes, p. 28).

## Integrated health and social care assessment processes

Integrated health and social care assessment processes for adults in need are being promoted by all UK countries, i.e. integrated between disciplines, agencies, and organizations. The procedures are similar to England where it is called the single assessment process (SAP). The purpose is:

- To ensure that older people receive appropriate, effective, and timely responses to health and social needs.
- The scale and depth of the assessment is kept in proportion to older people's needs.
- To ensure that agencies do not duplicate each other's assessments.
- Ensure professionals contribute to the assessment in the most effective way.

Many areas are developing shared electronic records to aid the assessment between health services and social services.

## Four types of assessment

- *Contact:* where significant needs are first identified or suspected, a simple/or single need is addressed.
- *Overview:* if a more rounded assessment is required.
- *In-depth or specialist:* specific problems explored in detail.
- *Comprehensive:* exploration of most or all domains (📖 Individual health needs assessment, p. 110) and level of support required will be intensive or complex.

*Nurse's role*
May contribute to all four types of assessment, and may have an important role in coordinating assessment and care planning, where a number of agencies are involved. Nurses may also be a named case/care manager (see ⬚ Care/case management models. p. 112).

*Assessment tools and accreditation*
Organizations are free to develop their own shared assessment tools. The domains will include the user perspective, clinical background, disease prevention, activities of daily living, relationships, housing and environment, physical wellbeing and senses, mental health, safety, and current resources. There are six accredited tools that can be used for assessment, in NHS and Social Care in England:

- *CAT:* Cambridgeshire Assessment Tool.
- *EASY Care:* University of Sheffield.
- *FACE:* Functional Assessment of the Care Environment of Older People.
- *MDS:* Minimum Data Set for Home Care.
- *NOAT:* Northamptonshire Overview Assessment Tool.
- *STEP:* Standardized Assessment of Elderly in Primary Care.

These assessment tools may incorporate or add on specialized assessment tools. All assessment processes lead to a statement of agreed needs/problems and statements about the agreed care plan/action plan, with review dates (see ⬚ Care/case management models, p. 112).

Each LA (and PCO) publishes information about services and eligibility for services. Since 2009 DH has been moving towards a common assessment framework, adopting the SAP model for all patient groups.

## Related topics
⬚ Generic long-term conditions model, p. 5; ⬚ IT, electronic records and telehealth, p. 84; ⬚ Standardized assessment tools for adults, p. 116.

## Further information
Centre for Policy on Ageing Professional Development and Learning Materials for SAP. Available at: ℘ http://www.cpa.org.uk/sap/sap_about.htmlSingle Assessment Process website includes links to accredited tools and examples of best practice. Available at: ℘ www.dh.gov.uk/en/Publicationsandstatistics/Publications/PublicationsPolicyAndGuidance/DH_4008389
NHS Networks Common Assessment Framework Network. Available at: ℘ www.networks.nhs.uk/nhs-networks/common-assessment-framework-for-adults-learning

# Standardized assessment tools for adults

A range of tools, scales, and interview schedules can inform clinical practice. Standardized assessment tools for specific problems can:

- Help identify their severity, associated risk, and need for health and social care services, aiding equitable allocation of resources.
- More accurately inform the commissioning of services.
- Ensure problems and conditions cannot be missed, e.g. depression and early onset of dementia, diabetes, hypertension, carer stress, etc.

Tools should be:

- Valid, reliable, and culturally sensitive. Shorter versions preferable where available.
- In the public domain (or available via licence holder).
- Designed for use in clinical practice (*Note:* some scales developed for research do not perform well in practice).

These tools can be used as part of an integrated (or single) assessment process, in nursing assessments (see 📖 Individual health assessment, p. 111) and health promotion consultations (📖 Healthy ageing, p. 325). *Note:* specific assessment tools are also referenced in relevant topics.

## Other useful standardized adult assessment tools

### Mental health assessment

- *Depression* (📖 People with depression, p. 435): 15-item geriatric depression scale (GDS). Geriatric Depression Scale is available at: 🖰 http://www.stanford.edu/~yesavage/GDS.english.short.html. Easy to administer, well validated in home and clinical environments, and for evaluating the clinical severity of depression, and ∴ for monitoring treatment.
- *Dementia* (📖 People with dementias, p. 438). Mini-mental State Examination (MMSE) available at: 🖰 http://www.oocities.org/travelnair/mini-mentalStateExamination.pdf:
  - Screening test for cognitive impairment that estimates severity of cognitive impairment at a given point.
  - Useful in following course of cognitive changes in individual over time.
  - Documents an individual's response to treatment.

### Assessment of ADLs and physical dependency

Barthel Index is a measure of physical ability developed in hospital, but widely used to assess ability to perform ADL (*Note:* underestimates impact of cognitive impairment). Scored out of 20 where 14 indicate some disability. See example of use at: 🖰 www.strokecenter.org/trials/scales/barthel.pdf.

## Further information

Social Care Institute for Excellence has information on relevant mental health standardized tools for older people. Available at: 🖰 http://www.scie.org.uk/publications/guides/guide03/process/sap.asp

# Principles of good communication

Communicating is a fundamental social need, important in developing and maintaining client and patient trust, and confidence. Patient-centred care and shared decision-making are key NHS objectives and the following principles help achieve them:
- Know the subject.
- Know the audience.
- Get the message across effectively.
- Look for and act on responses.

The following are important:
- The way in which you greet patient and introduce yourself sets level at which your relationship will continue.
- Maintain reasonable eye contact and sit comfortably towards your patient.
- People differ in ways that they communicate. Some may need more time from you than others.
- Read and acknowledge both verbal and non-verbal cues patient sends.
- People sometimes find it hard to face facts or to hear clearly what you are saying. It may be necessary to say clearly what the situation is and what needs to be done.
- People remember most accurately the first thing that you say, and 20% of what they hear overall. If you have something particularly important to say, this may need to be highlighted or repeated.
- Illustrations or diagrams may help improve understanding.
- Sharing your thoughts with patient is one of the skills that can be helpful in a shared decision-making process.
- Consider lighting and if people can see your mouth easily, people with hearing loss often lip read to interpret what they are hearing
- People with cognitive impairment may find simple statements easier to follow. Avoid multiple questions and ask questions that require a 'yes' or 'no' response if that aids conversation and understanding

## With children
- Adjust how you communicate to take account of child's age, ability, and maturity.
- Open-ended communication works best with the young—more information is elicited by asking 'tell me about…', rather than asking direct questions like 'what did you…?'.
- Prompt, nod, smile, and encourage as necessary.

## Written information for service users

Written information for service users, patients and carers falls into three broad categories:
- Information about services provided and how to access them.
- Health promotion and information about conditions, illnesses, and treatment.
- Copies of letters, assessments, and reports written about them by NHS staff.

It may be produced in print versions, electronic, web-based information, or apps for mobile technology. PCOs and Trust communication units may have standards to which information should comply and may have an accessible information policy.

Written information can:
• Reinforce information given in consultations and help people remember it.
• Give more details than can be given verbally.
• Be kept for future reference.
• Be shown to others, helping patients to share the information.

For service, health promotion, and condition-specific information consider:
• Target audience (age, sex, disability, ethnic and cultural background).
• How it fits in with other information being provided.
• Formats in which it should be offered, e.g. apps for mobile technologies, texts, audio for those visually impaired, web based, large print, translated.
• How information will be distributed.
• Make sure that factual content is accurate, up-to-date, and unambiguous.
• *Prioritize information:* include essentials, but not unnecessary or confusing details.
• Involve service users and patients in developing information, e.g. some organizations have 'Patient Reading Groups' who will consider the suitability of information produced for public use.

**Further information**

NHS Choices language hub provides health information other languages, e.g. Punjabi, Urdu, Bengali, Chinese, French, Gujariti, Somali, Arabic, Turkish, Spanish, Portuguese, and Polish. Available at: ℜ www.nhs.uk/aboutNHSChoices/aboutnhschoices/Aboutus/Pages/languageshub.aspx

NHS Evidence Information for the Public is available on every public health and clinical topic. Available at: ℜ www.evidence.nhs.uk/

Royal National Institute for the Blind. Accessible information. Available at: ℜ www.rnib.org.uk/professionals/Pages/professionals.aspx

The Plain English Campaign produces guides and resources to help make communications with the public crystal clear. Available at: ℜ www.plainenglish.co.uk/

# Adults and children with additional communication needs

Information is a crucial part of any patient journey and central to their experience of care. The form and medium can vary with service user, or patient's needs and preferences—verbal written, signed, Braille, audio, pictorial, drama, translated, etc. It is good practice to reinforce verbal communication with another method, e.g. a leaflet.

## Communicating with adults and children with additional communication needs

Identify with the individual what, if any, ccmmunication support is needed and organize, e.g. induction loops, palantypists (speech-to-text reporting for hearing impaired readers), Makaton (using gestures/signs with language), signers (for hearing impaired) touch signers (deaf blind patients), lip speakers (deaf person who lip reads), Braille (read by touch), interpreters. See also 🕮 People with learning disabilities, p. 408.

*Good practice points*
- Find a suitable place to talk, with good lighting and away from noise and distractions.
- Speak at a moderate pace, directly to patient, even when using communication support. Don't shout.
- Use natural facial expressions and gestures.
- Use clear, simple language, avoiding jargon, ambiguity, and medical terminology.
- Check throughout that you are being understood.
- Use illustrations/pictures where suitable. A useful resource is available at: ℘ www.photosymbols.com.
- If the patient needs to do something, make this obvious.
- Ask whether they want to be copied in to reports and letters about them and in what format.

*Children*
In addition to that listed for adults:
- Address them as individuals.
- Use plenty of illustrations.
- Try to adjust your language to their age.
- Do not talk down to them.

## English as a second language

Many of those with English as a second language (ESL) are fluent. However, there will also be clients and patients:
- Without any knowledge of English.
- Who speak it well, but may understand comparatively little.
- Who understand a great deal, but may be unable to speak much English.

*Good practice points*
- *Health service environments:* well-designed, legible signage systems can benefit everyone.
- *Additional considerations in verbal communication:*
  - Try to ascertain how much English the patient actually understands. Consider using an interpreter or an advocate.
  - Address patient directly.
  - Check whether concepts and terminology, if used, can be directly translated into another language.

*Interpreters and advocates*
- *Official interpreters for the NHS* translate without adding, changing, or omitting anything, and:
  - Will ask for clarification when needed.
  - Will not enter into discussion, give advice, or express opinions.
  - Will not take on additional work on behalf of staff/patients.
  - Are bound by rules of confidentiality.
- *Advocates* provide advice and support, and:
  - Facilitate linguistic and cultural communication.
  - Voice patients' concerns and expectations.
  - Advise how to access health care.
  - Help patients to become informed and make choices.
  - May be provided by the NHS for some groups or community organizations.
- Telephone interpreting may be available, e.g. Language Line available at: ℜ www.languageline.co.uk/. This provides a confidential telephone interpretation service available in over 150 languages, 24hrs/day, every day.
- Best practice suggests that 'official' interpreters are most appropriate.
- Check whether a gender-specific interpreter is required.
- Some patients, e.g. political refugees, may not trust or want 'official' interpreters, preferring initially to use informal interpreters.
- Some parents may prefer to use their children as interpreters, desiring family privacy. In general, this should be discouraged because burden of responsibility may be too great for children.

## Further sources of information

The Royal National Institute of Blind People. Available at: ℜ www.rnib.org.uk/ ☎ Helpline 0303 123 999

The Royal Association for Deaf People. Available at: ℜ www.royaldeaf.org.uk/

The Royal National Institute for the Deaf. Available at: ℜ www.actiononhearingloss.org.uk/ Local interpreting/advocacy services.

The Patient Information Bank in NHS net available to NHS staff only contains over 100 patient information leaflets and factsheets. Covers common health conditions and available in 12 other languages: Punjabi, Urdu, Bengali, French, Gujariti, Somali, Arabic, Turkish, Spanish, Portuguese, Korean, and Polish. Available at: ℜ www.nhs.uk/aboutNHSChoices/aboutnhschoices/Aboutus/Pages/languageshub.aspx

# Telephone consultations and triage

Many nurses are involved in telephone calls with clients or patients, this may be for a full consultation, follow up on a consultation, results giving, advice giving, or for triage. As there are no visual clues about body language or physical problems, e.g. rashes, particular care must be taken in communication and recognizing your own telephone style.

## Good practice points

*Phase 1: the introductions*

- For incoming calls answer promptly or have a system that lets caller know what is happening or where they are in a queue or leave a message.
- Introduce or answer with your full name, title, and service, practice, or clinic.
- Check, obtain, and use caller's or person's name you've called. Check whether it is the patient/client or someone calling on their behalf. *Note:* issues of confidentiality (📖 Confidentiality, p. 86).
- Sound friendly, interested, and empathetic.

*Phase 2: getting and giving information*

- Listen carefully and sympathetically.
- Use good questioning techniques.
- Open questions help the person give more information.
- Avoid using two questions in same sentence.
- Speak clearly, distinctly, and vary voice timbre.
- Avoid jargon and emotive words.

*Phase 3: next steps and goodbye*

- Summarize call.
- Negotiate and agree actions.
- State what you are going to next.
- Check the client or patient has understood, agreed, and given consent if necessary (see 📖 Consent, p. 77).
- Always give client or patient permission to call back or other safety net, giving types of reasons, e.g. if advice doesn't work.

*Phase 4: writing up*

Make a record just as in a face-to-face consultation (📖 Record keeping, p. 81).

## Telephone triage

Triage is a type of consultation increasingly used in OOH and general practice to address patient problems with the appropriate priority. The telephone call may result in either self-management with advice, face-to-face consultation (might mean a home visit or same day appointment) with the nurse, GP, OOH, other health professional, e.g. optometrist, or, more urgently, at A&E. Many nurses will be working to agreed protocols and decision algorithms (computerized or paper).

*Good practice points*
As previously listed plus the following.

*Phase 1*
- Always try and speak directly to patient as first-hand information will be more accurate.
- Anxiety may make caller's tone sound more prickly/aggressive than intended.
- A second call about the same problem within a short period may be best dealt with face-to-face either because problem is escalating or there are communications difficulties for whatever reason.

*Phase 2*
- Give the person enough time to explain in their own words without interruption.
- Question to establish what the problem is, where it occurs, when does it happen, what makes it worse or better, when did it first happen.
- Ask questions to establish if problem has occurred before and whether person is currently receiving treatment for it.
- Acknowledging emotion can help diffuse anger and hostility, e.g. 'I can hear that you are angry' or 'I am sorry that you feel…'.

## Further information

Males T. (2007). *Telephone Consultations in Primary Care: A Practical Guide*. London: RCGP.

# Counselling skills

Counselling provides an opportunity to talk about any matter, which may cause concern. The aim of the process is to help an individual understand their situation to the point where they can see for themselves the most appropriate course of action.

Many nurses and HVs in primary care use the skills of counselling in their consultations. Some (usually with additional training/support) actively use brief counselling interventions over a number of contacts, e.g. 'listening visits' with women identified with postnatal depression, solution-focused brief interventions with couples with relationship problems, bereavement visits (see also ☐ Talking therapies, p. 429).

## Model of counselling

Two main models are used by nurses and HVs:
- Client-centred or non-directive counselling, associated with the writings of Carl Rogers[1]. See also ☐ Motivational interviewing, p. 124. Emphasis on:
  - Unconditionally acceptance of the person.
  - Being a genuine person in the relationship.
  - Having empathic understanding of the person.
  - Being able to communicate acceptance, genuineness, and empathy in such a way that the other person can receive them.
- Problem management models associated with writings of Gerard Egan[2]. Emphasis on helping person answer three main questions:
  - What is going on? (What's the story? Where are the blind spots?)
  - What do I want instead? (Preferred scenario? Realistic goals?)
  - How might I get to what I want? (What will work for you and how to get there?)

## Skills in counselling

These include:
- Respect and acceptance of individuals in a non-judgemental manner.
- Active listening (includes positive non-verbal body language, checking for understanding).
- Paraphrasing and summarizing.
- Reflecting and ensuring concreteness.
- Able to allow silence.
- Able to deal with the others distress.
- Able to help individual plan actions.
- Awareness of own abilities and limitations, when to refer on to others.
- Strategies for dealing with own stress.

## References

[1]Rogers C. (2003). *Person Centred Therapy*. London: Constable and Robinson.
[2]Egan G. (2010). *The Skilled Helper—a problem management and opportunity development approach to helping*, 9th edn. Wadworth: Cengage Learning Belmont.

## Further information

British Association of Counselling and Psychotherapy. Available at: ℘ www.bacp.co.uk/

# Motivational interviewing

Motivational interviewing is a person-centred counselling method. It both explores and resolves ambivalence to change and also amplifies motivational processes within a person to change their behaviour. It is based on three elements:

- *Collaboration (not confrontation):* between professional and client/patient.
- *Evocation:* drawing out of the individuals ideas rather than imposing ideas about change, motivation, and commitment.
- *Autonomy of the individual:* as power to change rests with them not others.

## The principles of motivational interviewing

- *Express empathy:* i.e. client/patient experiences the counsellor as seeing the issues from their perspective.
- *Support self-efficacy:* by highlighting previous successes, skills, and strengths the person already has.
- *Roll with resistance:* counsellor avoids engaging with resistance to change statements, respecting autonomy of the individual.
- *Develop discrepancy:* helping the client/patient become aware of how current behaviours lead them away, rather than take them from values and goals important to them.

OARS[1] is the mnemonic used to remember the counselling techniques used (📖 Counselling skills, p. 123) used:

- **O**pen-ended questions.
- **A**ffirmations.
- **R**eflections.
- **S**ummaries.

## Talk of change

The more someone talks of change the more they are likely to change. The counsellor seeks to guide client/patient to expressions of change as a pathway to behaviour change. Techniques include asking evocative questions, which require answers likely to be about change, exploring values and goals, and exploring the future.

## Reference

[1]Miller WR, Rollnick S. (2002). *Motivational Interviewing: Preparing People for Change,* 2nd edn. New York: Guilford Press.

## Further information

Motivational Interviewing. Available at: ℘ www.motivationalinterview.org/index.html

# Medicines management and nurse prescribing

# Medicines management

The legislation for the prescription, dispensing, safe custody, and administration of medicines applies across the UK, but each country's department of health determines some aspects, e.g. non-medical prescribing.

## Nurse prescribing

A non-medical prescriber is a health care professional other than a doctor, with a registered first level qualification and a recordable prescribing qualification with their regulatory body. Three types available for nurses:

- *Nurse independent prescribers:* can prescribe any licensed drug which lies within their field of competency from anywhere in the BNF including some controlled drugs (CDs). Can also prescribe unlicensed drugs if they are competent, have considered the risks and benefits, have the support of their employing organization, and can justify their actions in the light of the patient's best interests (NMC 2009). Extended formulary nurse prescribers are now known as nurse independent prescribers.
- *Community practitioner nurse prescribers:* nurses, with or without a community specialist practice qualification (CSPQ), with a NMC recorded prescribing qualification, can prescribe from a limited formulary (see 📖 British National Formulary (BNF), p. 800).
- *Supplementary prescribers:* nurses, pharmacists, and designated allied health professionals with recordable qualification can prescribe with a doctor or dentist (as independent prescriber) to a patient specific clinical management plan (CMP). This includes CDs and unlicensed medicines where the doctor agrees within a patient's CMP. CMP template at DH non-medical prescribing programme (2006).

All NHS employers have to keep a list of specimen signatures of their non-medical prescribers. Good practice for private sector employers to do the same. Those not employed by a general practice are issued prescription pads by their employers.

## Prescriptions

NHS prescriptions are made on FP10 (GP10 in Scotland) forms or computer generated, FP10(C). Nurses have to add their NMC number and, if not GP employed, the patient's general practice code. NHS Business Services Authority (NHSBSA) records the costs from each prescription by practice and prescriber. It provides reports for monitoring and auditing prescribing. See 📖 Prescribing, p. 130.

## Dispensing medication

Medicines are usually dispensed (supplied as a response to a prescription by local pharmacists (or a dispensing GP) and are the property of the patient. Nurses working in specialist services may also supply medicines provided by the organization, e.g. family planning clinics, sexually transmitted infection (STI) clinics. All dispensed or supplied medicines must be labelled with patient's name and accompanied by patient information leaflet. Local policies apply.

## Administration of medicines

- In primary care most people administer their own medicines.
- Vulnerable and frail adults at home may be assisted in taking medicines by both nursing and home care services. Local guidance applies on division of responsibilities, accountabilities, and mechanisms for shared record keeping.
- See 📖 School nursing, p. 26, for administration of medicine in schools.
- Directions for administration by nursing staff are given in 1 of 2 ways:
  - A written patient-specific direction (PSD) for a named patient. Either as directed on the patient's pharmacy supplied medicine label or through a written direction by an independent prescriber, e.g. GP request. See 📖 Controlled drugs, p. 137.
  - Patient group directions (PGD) provide a legal mechanism for medicines to be supplied and/or administered by named registered health professionals to groups of patients without prescriptions having to be written. There is specific guidance on the authorization process by a senior doctor and pharmacist. Common examples in primary care are for immunizations, travel vaccines, contraceptives. PGDs: ℘ www.nelm.nhs.uk/en/Communities/NeLM/PGDs/

Prescribed, supplied/administered medicines and appliances should be recorded in clinical and any personally held records.

## Errors in medication dispensing or administration

- Report to the prescriber and consult doctor with responsibility for clinical care, e.g. GP.
- Take an appropriate action advised with regard to the patient.
- Report incident to line manager, complete incident and accident form in line with local policies (see 📖 Clinical risk management, p. 72).

## The monitoring of adverse drug reactions

Any prescribers or patients can report suspected adverse drug reaction (ADRs) to any drug, including those self-medicated by the patient, reactions to blood products, vaccines, radiographic contrast media, and herbal products to the Medicines and Health Care products Regulatory Agency online ℘ www.mhra.gov.uk (details for NI, Scotland, and Wales also given there) or yellow card in BNF.

## Further information

Beckwith S, Franklin P. (2011). *The Oxford Handbook of Prescribing for Nurses and Allied Health Professionals*, 2nd edn. Oxford: Oxford University Press.

BNF Nurses Prescribing Formulary in Appendices. Available at: ℘ www.bnf.org/bnf/bnf/current/

Department of Health (2006). *Medicines Matters: a guide to mechanisms for the prescribing, supply, and administration of medicines*. London: Stationery Office.

Medicines and prescribing support from NICE. Available at: ℘ www.nice.org.uk/mpc/index.jsp

NICE Medicines Information Resources. Available at: ℘ www.evidence.nhs.uk/nhs-evidence-content/medicines-information

NHSBSA. Available at: ℘ www.nhsbsa.nhs.uk/PrescriptionServices.aspx

NMC (2009). Nurse and midwife independent prescribing of unlicensed medicines. Available at: ℘ www.nmc-uk.org/Documents/Circulars/2010circulars/NMCcircular04_2010.pdf

# Medicine concordance and costs

NHS prescriptions cost >£6 billion/yr. Estimated that people take medicines as directed to reach therapeutic effect less than half the time. Reasons include:

- Lack of information about their condition and the importance of treatment.
- Beliefs about medicines, e.g. unnatural or should be able to manage without.
- Unwilling to tolerate side effects.
- Practical difficulties, such as getting the prescription filled, remembering to take medicines, opening containers.
- Costs of filling prescriptions.

## Concordance

Concordance is defined as a partnership process between professional and patient that addresses the beliefs, experiences, and wishes of the patient as well as other factors that contribute to successful prescribing and medicine taking. Patients are more likely to take medicines as prescribed when they:

- Have had their condition explained so they understand and accept it, and recognize consequences of not treating it.
- Agree with course of action and the proposed treatment.
- Have had any concerns or questions about the medicines answered.
- Have the simplest regimen, e.g. od or bd that can fit with their routine.
- Have clear verbal instructions, reinforced with written instructions they can read (e.g. appropriate font size and language).
- Have an opportunity for a follow-up discussion with a professional in 2–3wks if a long-term regimen or difficult technique, e.g. inhalers.
- Have an opportunity for medication review if long-term use.

See 📖 Principles of medication reviews, p. 135; 📖 Principles of good communication, p. 117.

## Help with costs of medicines

NHS prescriptions are free in Scotland, Wales, and NI but not England. Some medicines are cheaper bought over-the-counter (OTC) than with the NHS prescription charge. There is also help with the cost of prescription items for people on low incomes, particular conditions, and multiple medication costs.

### Free prescription entitlement

Information on NHS leaflet HC11 (England) see 📖 Benefits and support, p. 789.

Box ticked on reverse of prescription for:

- Contraception.
- >60yrs, <16yrs, or 16–18yrs if in full-time education.
- Patient or family receiving income support or income-based job seeker allowance.

## Payment exemption certificates

- Maternity Exemption certificate (MatEx) for pregnant women, for 12mths after the EDD or women who gave birth <12mths ago.
- Medical Exemption Certificates (Medex) certificate for certain conditions, using form FP92A signed by doctor (or authorized member of practice staff). The conditions are:
  - Diabetes insipidus or other forms of hypopituitarism.
  - Forms of hypoadrenalism (e.g. Addison's disease) for which specific substitution therapy is essential.
  - A permanent fistula (e.g. caecostomy, colostomy, laryngostomy, or ileostomy) requiring continuous surgical dressing or requiring an appliance.
  - Diabetes mellitus except where treatment is by diet alone.
  - Hypoparathyroidism.
  - Myasthenia gravis.
  - Myxoedema.
  - Epilepsy requiring continuous anticonvulsants.
  - A continuing physical disability so person cannot go out without the help of another person. Temporary disabilities do not count even if they last for several months.
  - Treatment for cancer or the effects of treatment for cancer.

## Pre-payment certificate

May be cheaper for patients who have to pay for >3 prescription items in 3mths or 14 items in 12mths to buy pre-payment certificate (PPC).
- Can only be used by applicant for own prescriptions.
- Cost of PPC (2012) £29.10 for 3mths, £104 for 12mths.
- Apply to NHSBSA online or by phone 0845 850 0030 or form FP95 available in surgeries and pharmacies. Apply for refunds to issuer.

Claiming for payments made while awaiting certificates can be made with for FP57 with official receipts from pharmacist to NHSBSA.

## Further information

Beckwith S, Franklin P. (2011). *The Oxford Handbook of Prescribing for Nurses and Allied Health Professionals*, 2nd edn. Oxford: Oxford University Press.

NHS Choices. Help with Health Costs. Available at: ℘ http://www.nhs.uk/nhsengland/Healthcosts/pages/Prescriptioncosts.aspx

NHSBSA. Help with health costs including prescriptions. Available at: ℘ http://www.nhsbsa.nhs.uk/HelpWithHealthCosts.aspx

# Prescribing

Prescribing a product or medicine is a complex process. The NHS National Prescribing Centre (NPC) has a 7-step model for prescribing considerations:

*Step 1 Examine the holistic needs of the patient.*
- A thorough assessment may show that a non-drug therapy is indicated.
- A full medical, including allergies, social history, and drug history including prescribed items, OTC items, homely remedies, homeopathic and herbal remedies, and any ADRs.

*Step 2 Consider the appropriate strategy.*
- Is the diagnosis established or a GP referral indicated?
- Is a prescription needed at all (e.g. guidance on antimicrobial resistance) or is patient expectation a factor?

*Step 3 Consider the choice of product.*
- Critically appraise evidence to assess a product's effectiveness.
- Consider appropriateness. Check BNF for ADRs, contraindications, special precautions, or drug interactions.
- Consider dose, formulation, and the duration of treatment.
- Does the patient require specialist consideration?
- Is there a non-proprietary (generic) named suitable product?

*Step 4 Negotiating a contract and concordance.*
- Shared decision-making between the patient and health care professional is known as concordance.
- The patient needs to understand: what the prescription is for, how to take it, at what dose and for how long, how long it will take to work, and any side effects.
- How and who to contact if they have any concerns.

*Step 5 Reviewing the patient—consider:*
- Is treatment still needed, working, and still the best choice?
- Is any adjustment in the treatment needed?
- Have there been any adverse effects?
- Is the patient taking any treatment you were unaware of?
- Does the patient understand their treatment, are they taking it correctly and is the next review planned?
- To avoid ADRs, the NPC recommend you:
  - Use as drugs concurrently as possible and lowest effective dose.
  - Check if patient is breastfeeding or of either extreme of age.
  - Know all medication being used by patient including OTCs and family remedies.
  - Check for contraindications such as renal or hepatic impairment.
  - Check if the patient has experienced a previous ADR.

*Step 6 Accurate, up-to-date records.*

*Step 7 Reflecting on your prescribing.* Reviewing and reflecting on prescribing decisions and prescribing analysis and cost (ePACT) data and Scottish Prescribing Analysis (SPA; available through PCOs and practices) will help prescribing practice and knowledge base.

## Prescription writing

Prescriptions should be completed as per specimen given on the 📖 inside cover of this book ensuring either the words 'no more items on this prescription' are written immediately after last item or unused space is deleted with Z. Each prescription requires nurses NMC PIN number and patient's GP code (for costing to NHS prescribing budget). An example of how to complete a prescription is given in the inside cover of this book.

### Handwritten prescriptions

• Write legibly, sign in ink.
• State patient's full name, address, preferably include their age and date of birth (DOB; legal requirement for a child <12yrs) and date.
• The BNF recommends:
  • Avoidance of unnecessary decimal point, e.g. 3mg not 3.0mg, put zero in front of unavoidable decimal point, e.g. 0.5mL. Use units that give whole numbers where possible, e.g. paracetamol 500mg rather than paracetamol 0.5g.
  • Units, micrograms, and nanograms should not be abbreviated.
  • Use the term millilitre (mL) not cubic centimeter, cc, or $cm^3$.

### Computer-generated prescriptions

• Must print the date of issue, the patient's surname, one forename, any other fore names as initials, address, age of those <12yrs or >60yrs.
• The prescriber's name, surgery address, telephone contact number, and reference number should be printed.
• Must be signed in ink.

See specific advice on prescriptions for CDs (📖 Controlled drugs, p. 137).

## Security of NHS prescriptions

• Must be kept in locked drawer, not left in cars or unattended.
• Record serial numbers of prescriptions held so that these can be circulated if a pad is stolen
• Blank prescriptions should not be signed in advance.
• Any loss or suspected theft must be reported immediately to line manager and police.

## Further information

Health Protection Agency. Antimicrobial Resistance: Guidelines for primary care. Available at: ℅ www.hpa.org.uk/Topics/InfectiousDiseases/InfectionsAZ/AntimicrobialResistance/Guidelines/
Medicines and prescribing support from NICE. Available at: ℅ www.nice.org.uk/mpc/index.jsp
NICE Medicines Information Resources. Available at: ℅ www.evidence.nhs.uk/nhs-evidencecontent/medicines-information

# Prescribing for special groups

Particular consideration needs to be given to the altered pharmacokinetics and pharmacodynamics of the old, very young, pregnant and breastfeeding ♀, people with reduced renal function, and people with liver disease. BNF gives prescribing guidance for all groups.

## Older people

- Important to recognize the diversity and individuality of older people.
- Important to assess not only the presenting problem, but also:
  - Altered pharmacodynamics and kinetics (natural ageing process)
  - Any underlying pathologies and/or polypharmacy (4 or more medicines) ↑ the risk of drug interaction and ADRs, implicated in 5–17% of hospital admissions of people >65yrs.
  - The use of alternative therapies, herbal remedies, 'homely remedies', and OTC.
  - Check for possible drug interactions and food–drug interactions.
- Common to initially prescribe at the lower end of a range of adult doses.
- Consider mental capacity, physical dexterity required to undo medication containers, the need for large print labels on containers, ability to swallow solid dosage forms, etc.

### Altered pharmacokinetics

That is, altered ways the body processes the drug.

- *Altered elimination:*
  - It is recommended to assume at least mild renal impairment when prescribing for older people. ↓ renal clearance results in slower drugs excretion and ↑ susceptibility to nephrotoxic preparations.
  - ↓ in renal clearance exacerbated by routine illnesses, such as UTI. Results in adverse effects or overdose in a patient previously stabilized on a drug with a narrow therapeutic margin (e.g. digoxin).
- *Altered absorption:*
  - Total body water ↓ = ↑ plasma levels of water soluble drugs.
  - ↓ body mass, ↓ saliva production, atrophy of intestinal epithelium, slower gastric emptying.
- *Altered distribution:*
  - ↓ cardiac output, ↓ renal mass, ↓ renal blood flow.
  - ↓ plasma proteins = ↑ in 'active' free protein binding drugs.
- *Altered metabolism:*
  - ↓ hepatic blood flow, first pass metabolism ↓.
  - Liver size ↓, blood flow ↓, enzyme production ↓, ↑ likelihood of toxicity with repeated doses.

*Altered pharmacodynamics*

That is, altered number, specificity, and responsiveness of receptors to the drug.

- ↑ sensitivity to drugs due to changes in the responsiveness of target organs, commonly ↑ sensitivity to: opioid analgesics, benzodiazepines, antipsychotics, anti-hypotensives, and non-steroidal anti-inflammatory drugs (NSAIDs).
- Common adverse reactions affecting older people are GI and haematological in nature.

## Infants and children

Pharmacokinetics and pharmacodynamics are often different for children.

*Key points*

- Always refer to the latest edition of the *BNF for Children*. Consult with senior clinician or specialist if in doubt.
- Many drugs are not licensed for children so independent prescribers must be working within scope of practice, have an evidence-based rationale, and support of employer (⊞ Medicine Management, p. 126).
- Doses are generally calculated using child's body weight in kilograms.
- Prescribe sugar-free solutions.
- Legal requirement to write the child's age if <12yrs.
- Advise parents not to add the drug to the child's feed (there may be an interaction or the child may not complete their feed).

## Pregnant women

*Key points*

- Only prescribe for pregnant women when it is essential.
- Where possible, avoid prescribing for pregnant women during the first trimester.
- Prescribe drugs that have been tried and tested as safe in pregnancy.
- BNF (current edition) identifies drugs known to be harmful and not harmful in pregnancy.

## Breastfeeding women

*Key points*

- Only absolutely necessary drugs should be taken when breastfeeding as may harm infant or inhibit sucking reflex or suppress lactation.
- BNF (current edition) identifies drugs that should be used with caution or are contraindicated in breastfeeding; and drugs present in milk but not known to be harmful.

## People with renal disease

Reduced renal function effects ability to excrete drugs, increase sensitivity reduce effectiveness of drug.

*Key points*

- Problems can be avoided by reducing dose or using different drugs.
- Dose adjustment depends on grade of renal failure (mild, moderate, severe) measured by creatinine clearance.
- BNF (current edition) provides prescribing guidance on drugs to be avoided or used with caution/dose reduction.

## People with liver disease

Liver disease may impair drug metabolism, and alter the body's response to drugs, e.g. increase toxicity, and increase sensitivity. Drug prescribing kept to a minimum in severe liver disease. See current BNF[1,2].

**Related topic** 🔲 Prescribing, p. 130.

## References

[1]BNF. Available at: ℛ www.bnf.org
[2]BNF for Children. Available at: ℛ www.bnfc.org

# Principles of medication reviews

Prescribing medication is the most common medical intervention in the UK and 80% of drugs prescribed are repeat prescriptions. QOF medicines management section includes recorded medicines reviews within last 25mths for all on repeat prescriptions and on >4 medicines (📖 Quality of framework, p. 66). NSF for older people recommends those aged >75yrs medicines should be reviewed annually and 6-monthly if >4yrs.

A medication review is: 'a structured, critical examination of patient's medicines with the objective of optimizing the impact of therapy, minimizing the number of medication related problems and reducing waste' (National Medicines Management Collaboration).

There are 4 levels of medicine review
- *Level 0: an* ad hoc *opportunist review.* Done by anyone without access to patient's notes and without the patient. Perhaps to verify name or dose of medication or as a triage to indicate patients requiring prioritization for higher level review.
- *Level 1: prescription review.* This can be either a *prescription intervention,* where patient not present and no access to their notes, or *medicines use review* with patient present, but with no access to their notes. These are undertaken by a community pharmacist, practice technician, or practice nurse.
- *Level 2: full medication review.* Full access to the notes, but the patient is not present. Undertaken by a doctor, pharmacist in specific practice schemes, nurse prescriber, or specialist nurse.
- *Level 3: clinical medication review.* Full access to patient's notes, patient present and consulted, all medications and all conditions reviewed. Undertaken by a doctor, nurse prescriber, or specialist nurse.

Only levels 2 and 3 count in QOF for reviews of repeat medication.

## Principles of medication review
- Seeks to optimize the treatment for an individual patient.
- Is undertaken in a systematic way, by a competent person.
- Any changes resulting from the review are agreed with the patient.
- The clinical medication review gives patients an opportunity to ask questions and highlight problems regarding their medicines.
- Review is documented in the patient's notes (READ codes Medication Review–8B3S or Medication review done–8B3V).
- Impact of any change is reviewed.

## NO TEARS tool[1]

The first principle is *Do no harm!*

N—Need and indication of the medicine. (Why prescribed? Are they still needed?)

O—Open questions (gain patients' views on how medicines used, side effects, and intended effects).

T—Testing and monitoring. (Are doses at the appropriate level?)

E—Evidence and guidelines. (Any changes in evidence base since prescription started?)

A—Adverse events (check for interactions, duplications, or contraindications).

R—Risk reduction and prevention (update opportunistic screening, e.g. risk of falls, blood pressure).

S—Simplification and switches. (Can bd or tds be replaced with od?)

## Setting up a medication review system

- Often local guidance available from pharmacist advisors and medicine management teams for the conduct of medication reviews.
- NICE medicines information site.
- Documentation important for auditing for:
  - Clinical outcomes.
  - Patient views.
  - Cost effectiveness indicators.
  - Quantitative data, e.g. number reviewed.
  - QOF (📖 Quality and outcomes framework, p. 66).

## Reference

[1]Lewis T. (2004). No Tears Tool Student. *Br Med J* **12**: 349–92.

## Further information

Beckwith S, Franklin P. (2011). *The Oxford Handbook of Prescribing for Nurses and Allied Health Professionals*, 2nd edn. Oxford: Oxford University Press.

DoH (2001). *Medicines for Older People: Implementing medicines-related aspects of the NSF for older people*. London: DoH.

# Controlled drugs

Under the Misuse of Drugs Regulations (2001) and subsequent amend-ments CDs are divided into five categories or schedules depending upon their potential use and misuse:

- *Schedule 1:* have no medicinal use and ∴ cannot be possessed or prescribed, e.g. coca leaf, mescaline.
- *Schedule 2:* includes major stimulants, opiates, e.g. secobarbital and amphetamine (additions to schedule 2—amineptine and tapentadol).
- *Schedule 3:* minor stimulants and drugs less likely to be misused than those in schedule 2 (some can be stored on open dispensary shelves).
- *Schedule 4:* split into 2 parts by the 2001 legislation:
  - *Part 1*—benzodiazepines plus eight other substances.
  - *Part 2*—anabolic steroids.
- *Schedule 5:* preparation of CDs, such as morphine and codeine at lower strengths.

All aspects of the management of CDs are underpinned by the Health Act 2006 and CDS (Supervision of Management and Use) Regulations 2006. Every health care organization or designated body has to appoint an accountable officer (AO) responsible for the safe management, supply, disposal, and administration of CDs, plus right of entry and inspection of CD records. All organizations have to have standard operating procedures (SOPs) for responsibilities and procedures for total management of CDs. Local procedures apply for reporting to AO any concerns regarding a health care professional and their use of CDs.

## CD registers

- All GP practices and primary care premises where CDs are stocked for dispensing or used in 'Doctor's Bag' are required to have CD Registers (CDRs).
- It is recommended that care homes have a CD register and obligatory for care homes providing nursing services to have a CD register if nurse in charge of the home requisitions CD stock.
- Original paper or electronic CDRs must be preserved for 2yrs.
- Community nursing services do not hold CDs registers.

## Prescribing controlled drugs

Only nurse independent prescribers can prescribe from limited list of CDs for specific indications (see Table 5.1), identified in Part XVIIB (ii) NHS Drug Tariff (England and Wales) and in Scottish non-medical prescribing policy.

Prescriptions must be written legibly, indelibly, and include:
- Name, address, and age or date of birth if under 12yrs of age); if patient is homeless, 'no fixed abode' is an acceptable address.
- NHS number or Community Health Index number (Scotland).
- Name and form drug, even if only one form exists.
- The strength, dose interval, and the dose to be taken.
- The total quantity of the preparation ≤30 days, or the number of dose units, to be supplied in both words and figures.
- The NMC PIN and UK address of the prescriber, plus date.

❶ Nurse prescribers cannot prescribe CD and another drug for mixing in syringe driver. 📖 Syringe drivers, p. 521.

**Table 5.1** Nurse Independent Prescribers CD list only for indicated medical condition (England & Wales)(see NHS Drug Tariff)

| Drug | Route | Indication |
|------|-------|------------|
| Buprenorphine | Transdermal | Palliative care |
| Chlordiazepoxide hydrochloride | Oral | Treatment of initial or acute withdrawal symptoms of alcohol in one habituated |
| Codeine phosphate | Oral | n/a |
| Co-phenotrope oral | Oral | n/a |
| Diamorphine hydrochloride | Oral or parenteral | Palliative care, pain relief in suspected MI, acute/severe pain post trauma or surgery |
| Diazepam | Oral, parenteral, rectal | Palliative care, initial or acute withdrawal symptoms of alcohol in one habituated, tonic-clonic seizures |
| Dihydrocodeine tartrate | Oral | n/a |
| Fentanyl | Transdermal | Palliative care |
| Lorazepam | Oral or parenteral | Palliative care, tonic-clonic seizures |
| Midazolam | Parenteral or buccal | Palliative care, tonic-clonic seizures |
| Morphine hydrochloride | Rectal | Palliative care, pain relief in suspected MI, acute/severe pain post trauma or surgery |
| Morphine sulphate | Oral, parenteral, rectal | Palliative care, pain relief in suspected MI, acute/severe pain post trauma or surgery |
| Oxycodone hydrochloride | Parenteral | Palliative care |

## Administration of controlled drugs

CDs are only administered under specific written, not verbal directions, of an independent prescriber. Details of prescription must always be record in patients' records. There is no legal requirement for administration to be witnessed by a second person. See ▣ Syringe drivers, p. 521; ▣ Storage, Transportation and Disposal of Medicines, p. 140.

## Further information

DH (2013). Controlled Drugs (Supervision of management and use) Regulations 2013. Available at: ℘ www.gov.uk/government/uploads/system/uploads/attachment_data/file/141407/15-02-2013-controlled-drugs-regulation-information.pdf.pdf

Medicines and prescribing support from NICE. Available at: ℘ www.nice.org.uk/mpc/index.jsp

NICE Medicines Information Resources. Available at: ℘ www.evidence.nhs.uk/nhs-evidencecontent/medicines-information

National Prescribing Centre (2009). *A Guide to Good Practice in the Management of Controlled Drugs in Primary Care in England*, 3rd edn. Liverpool: NPC.

NHS Drug Tariff (England & Wales). Available at: ℘ http://www.ppa.org.uk/ppa/edt_intro.htm

Scottish Government Nurse Prescribing Policy. Available at: ℘ www.scotland.gov.uk/Topics/Health/NHS-Scotland/non-medicalprescribing/nurseprescribing/policy

# Storage, transportation, and disposal of medicines

In the course of using medicines for therapeutic benefit it is important to comply with current legislation, follow guidance issued by the Health Departments and other Government Departments, e.g. Home Office, and manage the risks to patients and staff arising from the use of medicines. PCO pharmacist advisors or medication management teams provide up-to-date local guidance.

## Storage on community sites and general practice
*Key principles*
- Each service should have SOPs (including designated responsible person) for the safety and security of medicines used in it.
- Medicines that are not required for the treatment of anaphylaxis or resuscitation should always be kept locked in a cupboard or refrigerator (designated for the storage of medicines) as applicable.
- The cupboard or refrigerator must conform to British Standards (BS) 2881 (1989) NHS Estates and Building note No. 29.
- Maximum/minimum thermometers should be used to monitor the temperature of the refrigerator (usually 2–8°C). These temperatures should be recorded each working day and records kept for 6mths.
- Medicines held for clinical emergencies should be in packs labelled as such and available in those clinical sessions, otherwise securely stored.
- CDs held as stock, e.g. GP practice, legally require CD register, and to be held in fixed, locked cupboard sited away from the public. The key should be secured, and never left in the cupboard door.

## Storage in the patient's home
Patients' medicines are their property. Key messages to promote to patients and carers are that they should:
- Keep medicines in cool, dark place away from light, heat (including steam), or as directed on instructions, e.g. fridge.
- Always read medicine information leaflets for storage instructions.
- Keep in original container as it has instructions, expiry date, etc. If choose to use compliance devices they should label contents. Some drugs are unsuitable for compliance devices if they are affected by light, moisture, or temperature.
- Keep out of reach and sight of children.
- They should return all unused drugs, including CDs, to pharmacy for destruction, rather than domestic disposal as may harm environment.

*Administering home stored medicines*

- Nursing staff should be aware of individual medicine storage requirements. If drug potency is compromised by poor storage, new supplies need to be obtained for administration or prompting.
- Local guidelines apply to involvement of nursing staff in filling and prompting from medicine reminder devices. Many types available, but widespread safety concerns re: labelling, opportunities for mix-ups particularly if person has cognitive impairment or there are multiple carers helping with medication. Many areas now have schemes for pharmacist to dispense into sealed monitored dosage systems, e.g. blister packs.

## Transportation

*Key principles for professionals*

- Wherever possible patient, their carer or agent should collect any prescribed items from pharmacy. Some pharmacists have local delivery systems.
- If nursing staff are transporting medicines or vaccines, key points are:
  - Do not leave medicines in the car overnight or for long periods.
  - Consider safety issues.
  - Ensure temperature sensitive preparations are transported in conditions to maintain the appropriate temperature range (i.e. preserve the cold chain).
  - Cool boxes and bags should be monitored and maintained at the correct temperature, e.g. for vaccines between 2–8°C.
- Legally, nurses can transport prescribed CDs from pharmacy (requires ID and signature) to a named patient f unable to collect or return unwanted prescribed medicines. Only done if there is no alternative. If necessary to transport CDs, these should be in locked bag/box and kept out of sight.

## Disposal

Disposal into the sewerage system is an environmental hazard.

*Key principles*

- Patients/carers/agents should be encouraged to return unwanted and out-of-date medicines to supplying pharmacy for safe disposal.
- Patients/carers can return unused CDs to any pharmacy. A nurse can do this if no alternative.
- Local guidelines should be followed on the disposal of out-of-date or unwanted medicines or medicinal products for clinic/surgery held stocks. This includes records of disposal.

See 📖 Managing health care waste, p. 105.

## Further information

NHS Choices. All About Your Medicines. Availab.e at: 🖱 www.nhs.uk/medicine-guides/pages/default.aspx

Patient Information Leaflets for every medicine licensed in the UK at the electronic Medicines Compendium (eMC). Available at: 🖱 www.medicines.org.uk

Royal Pharmaceutical Society (RPS) (2005). *The safe and secure handling of medicines: a team approach.* (revision of 1988 Duthie Report). Available at: 🖱 www.rpharms.com/support-pdfs/safsechandmeds.pdf

# Child health promotion

# Child health promotion

The UK ratified the UN Convention on the Rights of the Child in 1989. The Children Act 2004 created children's commissioners to promote the views and rights of children. The Act also places a responsibility on practitioners to work together to help a child:
• Be healthy.
• Stay safe.
• Enjoy and achieve.
• Make a positive contribution.
• Achieve economic wellbeing.

## Children in the UK

There are 11.6 million children <16yrs in UK. Some key statistics from the Office of National Statistics[1] and *Health for All Children*[2]:
• 3.5 million live in households with income poverty.
• Infant mortality rate 70% higher in social class 5 than social class 1 in 1993–5.
• Approximately 400 babies die each year in the UK from sudden unexpected death of an infant (SUDI).
• International comparisons show the UK has some of the highest rates of children 2–15yrs diagnosed with asthma (21%), eczema (24%), hay fever (9%).
• Approximately 36,000 children are on child protection registers.
• 11% boys/young men and 5% girls/young women <20yrs have a severe disability. Disabilities are more frequent in children from families with lower incomes.
• Boys and young men age 11–20yrs are the group at highest risk of committing suicide.

## National child health promotion programmes

These emphasize preventive health care and promotion of good health for children and young people in the context of their families and communities. In each UK country, the programme is based on the evidence in *Health for All Children 4* (HFA4)[2] and country-specific policies, e.g. Healthy Child Programme England[3]. The programme:
• Acknowledges the social, as well as biological determinants of health.
• Emphasizes importance of community-based services for families, such as Sure Start (📖 Community approaches to health, p. 302; 📖 Public health in the NHS, p. 10), approaches to improving child health.
• Is delivered in partnership with parents to help them make healthy choices for their children and families.
• Is an additional service under the GMS contract (📖 General practice, p. 13).
• HVs, public health nurses, and SNs are key health service providers.

The main elements of the programmes are:
- Every child and parent should have access to a universal or core programme of preventative pre-school care (📖 Overview of the healthy child programme, p. 146) based on:
  - Delivery of agreed screening procedures.
  - Delivery of health promotion and support for parenting programmes.
  - Need to establish which families have more complex needs and respond appropriately to those following full assessment.
- Formal screening is confined to those activities agreed by the National Screening Committee (📖 UK screening programmes, p. 321).
- Professionals elicit and respond to all parental concerns with appropriate assessment and action.
- Health promotion (📖 Models and approaches to health promotion, p. 298) activities should include:
  - Supporting breastfeeding (📖 Breastfeeding, p. 176).
  - Prevention of infectious diseases (📖 Childhood immunization, p. 156).
  - Encouraging good nutrition and prevention of obesity (📖 Nutrition and healthy eating, p. 304).
  - Encouraging dental care and caries prevention (📖 Development and care of teeth, p. 185).
  - Reducing the risk of sudden infant death (📖 Sudden infant death syndrome, p. 295).
- The personal child health record should be used (📖 Client- and patient-held records, p. 87).
- There are clear care pathways for children with health or development problems.
- Statutory responsibilities are fulfilled in respect of child protection (📖 Child protection, p. 230), looked-after children, adoption procedures (📖 Looked-after children, p. 235), and children with special educational needs (SEN, 📖 Children with special educational needs, p. 227).
- Health professionals working with adult patients should recognize the impact of adult problems on children (📖 Children in special circumstances, p. 160) and also enquire about them.
- Health care for children and young people in school should include:
  - Support of children with problems and special needs.
  - Participation in public health programmes, e.g. Healthy Schools.
  - Provision of agreed screening and immunization programmes.
  - Promotion of personal, social, and sexual health including emotional literacy (📖 Sex and relationship education, p. 223)

## References

[1]Office of National Statistics. Available at: ℘ www.ons.gov.uk/ons/index.html

[2]Hall DMB, Elliman D (eds) (2009). *Health For All Children*, 4th edn. Oxford: Oxford University Press.

[3]Healthy Child Programme England. Healthy Child Programme: Pregnancy and the First 5 Years of Life. Available at: ℘ www.gov.uk/government/publications/healthy-child-programme-pregnancy-and-the-first-5-years-of-life

## Further information

Commissioner for Children and Young People: England. Available at: ℘ www.childrenscommissioner.gov.uk/; NI. Available at: ℘ http://www.niccy.org/; Scotland. Available at: ℘ www.sccyp.org.uk/; Wales. Available at: ℘ www.childcom.org.uk/

# Overview of the healthy child programme

Each UK country has produced its own version of a healthy child programme and should be checked for updates[1,2,3,4]. Table 6.1 provides an overview of the currently recommended programme.

**Table 6.1** Overview of the currently recommended healthy child programme

| Age | Intervention |
|---|---|
| Soon after birth <72hrs | General physical examination including inspection of eyes and red reflex, Ortolani and Barlow tests for developmental dysplasia of hips (DDH), examination of the heart, and testes |
| 5–8 days (ideally 5 days) | Newborn bloodspot screening |
| By 14 days | New baby review to assess child and family needs. Information/support to parents on key health issues |
| Within 4–5wks of birth | Semi-automated hearing screening |
| 6–8wks | General physical examination including inspection of the eyes and red reflex, Ortolani and Barlow tests for DDH, examination of the heart and testes |
| | Review of general progress and delivery of key health promotion messages. Usually at the same time as the first set of immunizations |
| 2mths (8wks) | 1st set of immunizations |
| 3mths (12wks) | 2nd set of immunizations |
| 4mths (16wks) | 3rd set of immunizations |
| By the 1st birthday | Overall review of the child and family |
| 12–13mths | First measles, mumps, and rubella vaccine (MMR) vaccine and boosters of Hib, Men C, and PCV vaccines |
| 2–3yrs | Review of child and family (not necessarily a face-to-face contact) |
| 3–4yrs | Pre-school booster and second MMR vaccine. Review of child's progress and delivery of key health promotion messages |
| 4–5yrs | Assessment of visual acuity |
| School entry | General review |
| | Hearing screening |
| | Height and weight measurement |

(Continued)

**Table 6.1** (Continued)

| Age | Intervention |
|---|---|
| Throughout school years | Ongoing support by the school health service—no further routine screening procedures recommended. Where there are vision screening programmes in place, in the absence of good evidence, those apart from vision screening at 7yrs old may continue as long as they are properly evaluated |
| Girls 12–13yrs | Human papillomavirus (HPV) vaccine |
| 13–14yrs | Teenage booster and Men C vaccines |

## References

[1]Healthy Child Programme England. Healthy Child Programme: Pregnancy and the First Five Years of Life. Available at: ℛ www.gov.uk/government/publications/healthy-child-programme-pregnancy-and-the-first-5-years-of-life

[2]Scotland Child Health Programme. Available at: ℛ http://www.isdscotland.org/Health-Topics/Child-Health/Child-Health-Programme/Child-Health-Systems-Programme-Pre-School.asp

[3]National Service Framework for Children, Young People & Maternity Services in Wales. Available at: ℛ http://www.wales.nhs.uk/sites3/home.cfm?OrgID=441

[4]Healthy Child, Healthy Future: A Framework for the Universal Child Health Promotion Programme in Northern Ireland. Available at: ℛ http://www.dhsspsni.gov.uk/healthychildhealthyfuture.pdf

# The assessment of children, young people, and families

The promotion of children's and young people's health involves consideration of:

- Their developmental needs.
- The quality of parental care.
- The circumstances and environment in which they grow up in.

Each of these three dimensions has a number of elements as shown in Fig 6.1.

These dimensions form the basis for structuring and recording in parent-held child health record (PHCHR), assessments of children in routine practice as part of the Healthy Child Programme[1,2]. The dimensions are also essential in determining whether a child or young person is 'in need or suffering significant harm' ( A child or young person in need, p. 150).

All assessments should be carried out in partnership with parents and young people to identify strengths, problems, and opportunities for health promotion. HFAC4 emphasizes that child health promotion has to assess and address the needs of the parents, as well as the children. Having jointly agreed problems and areas for health promotion, the next step is to provide as necessary, information, advice, supporting resources, practical help and referral to other services as appropriate. Like all individual health needs assessments ( Individual health needs assessments, p. 110), the plan, and its outcome should be jointly reviewed and amended as the child develops.

In England, the Common Assessment Framework (CAF) is the term used more formally for procedures and forms used across all services for children who may be vulnerable or at risk in some way ( A child or young person in need, p. 150). The CAF provides for identifying a child's or young person's needs, early, assessment, decision-making, coordinated service delivery in response and review.

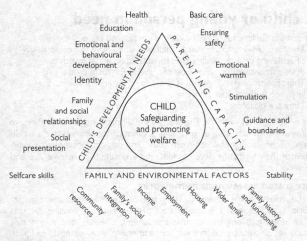

**Fig. 6.1** The assessment framework.

Reproduced under the Open Government Licence for public sector information from the *Framework for the assessment of children in need and their families*. Department of Health, Department of Education and Employment, Home Office (2000). London: Stationery Office.

## References

[1] Healthy Child Programme England. Healthy Child Programme: pregnancy and the first five years of life. Available at: www.gov.uk/government/publications/healthy-child-programme-pregnancy-and-the-first-5-years-of-life

[2] Scotland Child Health Programme. Available at: http://www.isdscotland.org/Health-Topics/Child-Health/Child-Health-Programme/Child-Health-Systems-Programme-Pre-School.asp

## Further information

England Common Assessment Framework. Available at: http://www.education.gov.uk/childrenandyoungpeople/strategy/integratedworking/caf

Scotland. Available at: www.childreninscotland.org.uk

# A child or young person in need

Under the Children Act 1989 a child is considered in need if:
• They are unlikely to achieve or maintain, or to have the opportunity of achieving or maintaining, a reasonable standard of health or development without provision of services for them by the LA.
• Their health or development is likely to be significantly or further impaired without such provision.
• They are disabled.

This Act together with the Children Act 2004 provides a comprehensive framework for the safeguarding and promotion of the welfare of children, i.e. protecting children from abuse and neglect, preventing impairment of their health or development, and ensuring they receive safe and effective care.

## Integrated assessment frameworks

All UK countries are developing integrated or common assessment frameworks (and records) for use by staff of all agencies providing services to children. It is emphasized that assessment, planning, and monitoring processes should be undertaken in partnership with parents, children, and young people. England has developed a pre-assessment checklist (pre-CAF) to help professionals determine vulnerable children requiring full assessment. It asks whether the child or young person appears:
• Healthy?
• Safe from harm?
• Learning and developing?
• To have a positive impact on others?
• Free from the negative impact of poverty?

Children identified as vulnerable and in need are referred to specialist and targeted services (📖 Social services, p. 26; 📖 Children with special educational needs, p. 227). Local child protection procedures are followed if there is risk of harm (📖 Child protection, p. 230).

Full common assessment frameworks cover:
• General health.
• Physical development.
• Speech, language, and communications development.
• Emotional and social development.
• Behavioural development.
• Self-esteem, self-image, and identity.
• Family and social relationships.
• Self-care skills and independence.
• Understanding, reasoning, and problem-solving.
• Participation in learning, education, and employment.
• Progress and achievement in learning.
• Aspirations.
• Basic care, ensuring safety, and protection.
• Emotional warmth and stability.
• Guidance, boundaries, and stimulation.

- Family history, functioning, and wellbeing.
- Parents' health, ill health, or disability, and impact on child.
- Wider family.
- Housing, employment, and financial considerations.
- Social and community elements and resources, including education.

## Impact of adult health problems on children

HFAC4 emphasizes that professionals should assess the impact and needs of children and young people when working with adults with health problems particularly if they are:

- Parents with mental health problems.
- Parents with long-term conditions and disabilities.
- Parents with addictions.

## Care planning, management, monitoring, and evaluation

Assessment should be part of a care management process with an identified lead professional, key worker, or care manager who will work closely with the family to help coordinate:

- A plan to address the identified and agreed needs.
- The delivery of services and support (☐ Services for children, young people, and families, p. 19).
- The monitoring and review of the plan.

## Further information

Children in Scotland. Available at: ℘ www.childreninscotland.org.uk

England Common Assessment Framework. Available at: ℘ http://www.education.gov.uk/childrenandyoungpeople/strategy/integratedworking/caf

Healthy Child Programme England. Healthy Child Programme: Pregnancy and the First Five Years of Life. Available at: ℘ www.gov.uk/government/publications/healthy-child-programme-pregnancy-and-the-first-5-years-of-life

Scotland Child Health Programme. Available at: ℘ http://www.isdscotland.org/Health-Topics/Child-Health/Child-Health-Programme/Child-Health-Systems-Programme-Pre-School.asp

# Child screening tests

Nationally agreed child screening tests are carried out on the whole population (□ UK screening programmes, p. 321). Where there is professional or parental concern additional interventions may be appropriate. Children who are at high risk of a condition may need extra investigations despite a normal screening test. Other topics have been considered at one time or another for inclusion in screening programmes, but have not satisfied the criteria. These include screening tests for developmental and behavioural problems.

Throughout the four countries of the UK, there are different policies on screening for dental disease. Screening is no longer recommended. Surveillance takes place to assess the level of dental disease.

Fully informed consent (□ Consent, p. 77) should be sought from a person with parental responsibility before any screening test or immunization is undertaken.

## Physical examination

### What

- *Eyes:* 20–30 per 100,000 babies have eye problems requiring treatment (□ Eyes and vision screening, p. 154).
- *Hearts:* 500 per 100,000 have CHD needing treatment (□ Congenital heart defects, p. 256).
- *Hips:* DDH—dislocated/dislocatable (120 per 100,000).
- *Testes:* undescended (6000 per 100,000).
- Growth.

### Why

Early treatment can reduce disability:

- Early surgery for cataracts improves visual outcome.
- Surgery for CHD before symptoms develop is beneficial in more severe forms.
- Early treatment (splinting) of DDH reduces need for surgical intervention.
- Early surgery (referral by 1yr of age) for undescended testes may improve fertility and facilitate early diagnosis of malignancy.
- Birth weight and head circumference at birth act as a baseline for future measurements.
- At 6–8wks weight can provide reassurance that a baby is growing appropriately during a period of rapid growth.

### How and by whom

All form part of routine physical examination carried out by a competent practitioner, this might be a nurse or a doctor. Weight should be measured using appropriately calibrated scales, head circumference using a tape measure around the occipitofrontal circumference.

### When

By 72hrs old and again between 6–8wks old.

## Neonatal blood spot screening

*What*
- *Phenylketonuria:* 1 in 10,000 births.
- *Congenital hypothyroidism:* 1 in 4000 births.
- *Cystic fibrosis:* 1 in 2500 births.
- *Sickle cell disease:* depending on ethnicity: overall 1 in 1900,
  West African 1 in 80 live births, West Indian 1 in 200 live births.
- *Medium-chain acyl-CoA dehydrogenase deficiency (MCADD):* 1 in 10,000
  live births.

*Why*
Preventive treatment reduces the risk of disability.

*How and by whom*
Heel prick blood sample usually by midwife.

*When*
At 5–8 days (ideally 5 days). Standards for performance have been agreed nationally and are available on the website. All results from laboratories are sent to child health record departments who are responsible for monitoring coverage and informing HV/GP. HVs are responsible for informing parents of negative results and recording them in PHCHR. Positive results are reported to hospital paediatrician and GP by the laboratory for follow-up and copied to Child Health Records Department.

### Further information
Public Health England. Newborn and Infant Physical Examination. Available at: ℜ http://newborn-physical.screening.nhs.uk/

Public Health England. NHS Sickle Cell and Thalassaemia Screening Programme. Available at: ℜ http://sct.screening.nhs.uk/

Public Health England. The UK Newborn Blood Spot Screening Programme. Available at: ℜ http://newbornbloodspot.screening.nhs.uk/

Public Health England. UK National Screening Committee. Available at: ℜ www.screening.nhs.uk

Northern Ireland. Available at: ℜ www.dhsspsni.gov.uk/index/phealth/php/screening.htm

Scotland National Screening Programmes. Available at: ℜ www.nsd.scot.nhs.uk/services/screening/

# Eyes and vision screening (children)

This is the currently agreed UK screening programme. See 📖 Child screening tests, p. 152 for background information on UK screening test policies for children.

## Congenital ocular opacities

*What and why*

Looking for cataracts (incidence 30 per 100,000 live births), retinoblastoma (40–50 cases in UK per year) and congenital glaucoma (1 in 10,000 births per year). Early treatment leads to improved prognosis.

*How and by whom*

Inspection, including red reflex, as part of the neonatal and 6–8wks physical examinations. Carried out by a health care professional trained to do this.

*When* Within 72hrs of birth and again at 6–8wks.

## Impaired visual acuity

*What and why*

Amblyopia—suppression of vision in a healthy eye due to different images falling on the two retinae—and other causes of impaired visual acuity. Early intervention with glasses and/or patching may lead to improved visual function.

*How and by whom*

• Visual acuity of both eyes assessed separately using standard charts in an appropriately lit environment.
• Carried out by trained personnel, ideally an orthoptist or as part of an orthoptic-led service.

*When* At 4–5yrs or on school entry.

## Related topic

📖 Overview of the healthy child programme, p. 146.

## Further information

UK National Screening Committee. Available at: ℛ www.screening.nhs.uk

# Hearing screening

This is the currently agreed UK screening programme. See 📖 Child screening tests, p. 152 for background information on UK screening test policies for children.

## Neonatal

*What and why* Congenital sensorineural hearing impairment (100–200 per 100,000). Early detection allows implementation of optimal management (hearing aids and parental interaction) with improvement of language development.

*How and by whom* Semi-automated techniques. Oto-acoustic emissions (OAE) and auditory brain responses (AABR), by specially trained personnel.

*When* Either in first days in hospital or by a trained person in the community in the first 5wks of life.

*Targeted ongoing surveillance*
Irrespective of newborn screen outcome if:
• Parental or professional concern.
• Meningitis, chronic middle ear effusion. and craniofacial
  abnormalities (CFA).
• High levels of ototoxic drugs.
• Other risk factors for late-onset, progressive, or acquired deafness.

## School entry

*What and why* Acquired hearing impairment and some cases of congenital sensorineural hearing loss not already identified. A further 50–90 per 100,000 cases of sensorineural deafness will be identified and many more cases of conductive loss. Most commonly acquired conductive loss due to secretory otitis media (glue ear). Hearing loss may contribute to problems with learning, appropriate management can minimize this.

*How and by whom* Pure tone audiometry by trained personal, usually audiometricians or SNs. Involves using a regularly tested and calibrated audiometer in a quietened room and presenting tones (usually at each octave between 125 and 8kHz) through headphones at amplitudes related to expected thresholds for a normal hearing person. The child indicates when they can hear the tones and this is charted. Local protocols specify referral pathways for identified hearing loss. British Society of Audiology[1] produces recommended procedures (in procedures section).

*When* Primary school entry.

## Reference
[1]British Society of Audiology. Available at: ℘ www.thebsa.org.uk/

## Further information
National Services Division, Scotland. Available at: ℘ www.nsd.scot.nhs.uk/services/screening/unhearingscreening/index.html
Newborn Hearing Screening Wales. Available at: ℘ www.newbornhearingscreening.wales.nhs.uk
Northern Ireland. Available at: ℘ www.dhsspsni.gov.uk/screening
Public Health England. NHS Newborn Hearing Screening Programme: England. Available at: ℘ http://hearing.screening.nhs.uk

# Childhood immunization

Childhood immunization is important for both the individual and public health[1]. It is an essential part of the healthy child programme (📖 Overview of the healthy child programme, p. 146).

Information (including leaflets) about immunization programmes is usually given to parents at new baby review and opportunities offered for parents to discuss any issues or concerns.

Fully informed (i.e. including process, benefits and risks) consent (📖 Consent, p. 77) should be sought from a person with parental responsibility before immunization is undertaken.

Each PCO should have a named person who has oversight of the programme. This person should act as a source of expert advice and, if they cannot answer clinical queries, be able to call on a local clinician.

There are national targets for immunization uptake.

PCO child health record departments act as a repository for immunization data, recording consent or refusal to be considered for a course, and administration of immunizations. In some areas they also provide parent and professional reminder systems, although this is done independently by many GP practices. The 1° course of immunization is part of the GMS contract global sum (📖 General practice, p. 13), but may also form enhanced services or PMS contracts for areas or populations with particular challenges in reaching coverage targets.

Immunization should be offered as in the UK immunization schedule (📖 Childhood immunization schedule (UK), p. 158).

## Vaccines

- The routine childhood vaccines are purchased nationally and are available free. Information on suppliers of vaccines is also available on the 'Green Book' website[2].
- Vaccines must be stored at 2–8°C and must not be frozen. The cold chain must be preserved if transported to other sites or on domiciliary visits (📖 Immunization administration, p. 345).

## Addressing parents' concerns

- *Safety and side effects:*
  - All vaccines are carefully tested, both for their efficacy and safety, before being introduced.
  - Each batch of vaccine is tested and close post-marketing surveillance is initiated. Part of this is the 'Yellow Card' system[3].
- *MMR:* much research has been conducted on the vaccine and it has been shown to have a good safety profile with evidence of no link with autism or chronic bowel disease.
- *Thiomersal:* some vaccines used to contain thiomersal, a mercury-containing preservative. No research has shown it to be toxic in doses contained in vaccines but, based on 'precautionary principle', it is being phased out and none of the routine childhood vaccines contain any.

## Homeopathy

Increasing numbers of people are turning to alternative forms of health care. There is no evidence that any of these are effective in preventing the diseases against which vaccines are used.

## References

[1] Health Protection Agency (HPA). Protecting the health of the Nation's children: the benefit of vaccines. Available at: www.hpa.org.uk/Topics/InfectiousDiseases/InfectionsAZ/VaccinationImmunization

[2] Public Health England. Immunization against infectious diseases (The Green Book). Available at: www.gov.uk/government/organisations/public-health-england/series/immunisation-against-infectious-disease-the-green-book

[3] MRHA. Yellow Card Scheme Medicines and Health care Products Regulatory Agency. Available at: www.mhra.gov.uk/Safetyinformation/Howwemonitorthesafetyofproducts/Medicines/TheYellowCardScheme/

## Further information

Great Ormond Street Hospital/Institute of Child Health Immunization. Available at: www.gosh.nhs.uk/parents-and-visitors/general-health-advice/immunisation/

Health Protection Scotland. Immunization and vaccine preventable diseases. Available at: www.hps.scot.nhs.uk/immvax/index.aspx

HPA Publications on Training. Available at: www.hpa.org.uk/webw/HPAweb&Page&HPAwebAutoListName/Page/1204012992964

NHS Choices. The NHS vaccination schedule. Available at: http://www.nhs.uk/Conditions/vaccinations/Pages/vaccination-schedule-age-checklist.aspx

Public Health. Immunisation and vaccines. Available at: www.wales.nhs.uk/sitesplus/888/page/43510

Royal College of Paediatrics and Child Health. *Immunization of the Immunocompromised Child.* Available at: www.rcpch.ac.uk/sites/default/files/asset_library/Publications/I/Immunocomp.pdf

# Childhood immunization schedule (UK)

The immunization schedule, as at 2013, is given in Table 6.2. Other vaccines or extra doses may be indicated for high-risk individuals. These include: pneumococcal polysaccharide vaccine, influenza vaccine, hepatitis B vaccine, and Bacille Calmette–Guérin vaccine (BCG; 📖 Tuberculosis, p. 680).

BCG is only offered to high-risk groups:
- Infants in areas where tuberculosis (TB) ≥ 40/100,000.
- Infants and children <16yrs old, whose parents or grandparents were born in a country with a TB incidence ≥ 40/100,000.
- Previously unvaccinated new immigrants <16yrs old from high TB prevalence countries.
- Children and young people who are going to stay or have stayed in close contact with the indigenous population in high TB prevalence countries for at least a month.

Note: infants, i.e. those under 12mths old do not need Mantoux test prior to BCG. For older groups, consult the 'Green Book'.[1]

## Where and by whom

Routine vaccines for young children are usually given in primary care and for older children by the school health service (see Table 6.2 for UK schedule). Given by someone trained in the administration of vaccines and a high level of knowledge about vaccines and immunization. Nurses and HVs often administer vaccines under PGDs (📖 Prescribing, p. 130). Anyone administering vaccines should be competent in cardiopulmonary resuscitation (CPR) and dealing with anaphylaxis according to local policies.

## Contraindications

- Anaphylaxis to a previous dose of vaccine or a component of vaccine.
- In children who are moderately or severely systemically unwell with a fever, vaccination should be delayed.
- In addition, live vaccines such as MMR may be contraindicated in some immunosuppressed individuals. Before withholding a vaccine from such patients, consult patient's specialist.

**Travel vaccines**  (See 📖 Travel vaccinations, p. 356.)

**Table 6.2** The UK childhood immunization schedule—2013

| Age | Vaccine | Mode of delivery | Site |
|-----|---------|------------------|------|
| 8wks | Diphtheria, tetanus, acellular pertussis, inactivated polio vaccine, *Haemophilus influenzae* type b (DTaP/IPV/Hib) | One injection | IM thigh<br>Same time, different limb or different site (2.5cm apart) |
| | Pneumococcal conjugate vaccine (PCV) | One injection | |
| | Rotavirus vaccine (rota) | Oral | |
| 12wks | DTaP/Hib/IPV | One injection | IM thigh |
| | Meningococcal group C (MenC) | One injection | Injections guidance as 8wks |
| | Rota | Oral | |
| 16wks | DTaP/Hib/IPV | One injection | IM thigh |
| | PCV | One injection | Injections guidance as 8wks |
| 12–13mths | Hib/menC | One injection | IM upper arm or thigh |
| | MMR | One injection | |
| | PCV | One injection | Injections guidance as 8wks |
| 2yrs (just before the 'flu season) | Influenza | Nasal spray | Intranasal in each nostril |
| Pre-school 3yrs 4mths | DTaP/IPV or dTaP/IPV (Pre-school booster) | One injection | IM upper arm Injections guidance as 8wks |
| | MMR (second dose) | One injection | |
| 12–13yrs girls only | HPV | Three injections over 6mths | IM upper arm |
| 13–14yrs | Tetanus, low dose diphtheria, IPV (Td/IPV; teenage booster) and MenC | One injection | IM upper arm Injections guidance as 8wks |

## Essential reference

[1]Public Health England. Immunization against infectious diseases (The Green Book). Available at: ᐟ᠍ https://www.gov.uk/government/organizations/public-health-england/series/immunization-against-infectious-disease-the-green-book

## Further information

NHS Choices. The NHS vaccination schedule. Available at: ᐟ᠍ http://www.nhs.uk/Conditions/vaccinations/Pages/vaccination-schedule-age-checklist.aspx
Health Protection Agency (HPA). Vaccination Immunisation. Available at: ᐟ᠍ www.hpa.org.uk/Topics/InfectiousDiseases/InfectionsAZ/VaccinationImmunisation/

# Children in special circumstances

Children who live in special circumstances may need particular attention to ensure they receive the full child health promotion programme and any particular and exceptional needs are addressed.

## Children as young carers

See also 🕮 Carers assessment and support, p. 412. 6% of children in need are registered because of parental illness or disability. Young carers often miss time from school, have little time for peers and friendship, and may experience stigma by association, e.g. parent has mental health problems. Young carers have the right to a full assessment of their needs and support in their caring role (🕮 The assessment of children, young people, and families, p. 148). Some areas have specialist projects and groups to support young carers.

## Unaccompanied asylum seekers and refugees

See also 🕮 Asylum seekers and refugees, p. 396. Unaccompanied children <18yrs have the right to be 'looked after' (🕮 Looked-after children, p. 235), to have somewhere to live, and to education and health care. They are identified as children in need (🕮 A child or young person in need, p. 150) and should have a full integrated assessment to develop a specialized care plan that includes emotional needs. Their health problems will reflect those of the region they come from, e.g. malaria is endemic in parts of Africa. In addition, they may come from an area with no child surveillance programme and have missed immunizations (🕮 Childhood immunization schedule (UK), p. 158). Psychological distress may be related to separation from family but also from experiences, e.g. war and some may need referral to 🕮 Child and adolescent mental health services, p. 229.

## Homelessness

See also 🕮 Homeless people, p. 398. Children and young people may be part of a family that is homeless or may be homeless as a single person. They are often placed in temporary accommodation, such as hostels, and bed and breakfast accommodation. This is often unsuitable with limited opportunities for play, shared and cramped space for cooking and food storage, and shared toilet and bathroom facilities. Accidents, behaviour problems, and minor infections are common. In some areas, close liaison with housing departments, designated HVs, and primary care teams ensure that families and young people are identified soon after moving in. Priorities are to ensure:

• They have information as to registering with a GP.
• They have information about local health, early years, education, social, and community support services.
• The child promotion programme is up-to-date and a plan to address any problems is made.
• Immunization is up-to-date.
• The PHCHR is used for all contacts or the young person is given a record of all contact and referrals.

## Children, young people, and prison

All children and young people whose lives are touched by prison have special needs. The circumstances may be:

- *Baby born in prison may stay with mother:* however, there are few mother and baby units (only four in England and Wales). Babies can stay until 9 or 18mths depending on unit. Local HVs provide child health promotion programme to these units. When mothers and babies cannot stay together, early opportunities for bonding and psychological attachment are lost (💭 Emotional development in babies and children, p. 199).
- *A parent may be imprisoned:* the children are separated and experience significant loss. Particularly painful if mother is imprisoned, as not only is there separation, but many children have to live with relatives or be looked after by LAs. Visiting may be difficult as there are few women's prisons so can be at great distance. Emotional and psychological consequences for children and young people of all ages.
- *Young people detained in their own right:* vulnerable young people. The prison health service is currently transferring to local primary care organizations and identifies health needs at an entry assessment.

### Further information

Action for Prisoners Families. Available at: 🖱 http://www.prisonersfamilies.org.uk/
CarersTrust Young Carers – for professionals. Availab e at: 🖱 http://www.youngcarers.net/
Prison Reform Trust. Available at: 🖱 http://www.prisonreformtrust.org.uk/ProjectsResearch/Childrenandyoungpeople
Safe Network. Support for unaccompanied asylum-seeking children and young people. Available at: 🖱 http://www.safenetwork.org.uk/help_and_advice/best_safeguarding_practice/Pages/unaccompanied-asylum-seeking-children.aspx

# Child injury prevention

Accidental injury to children is a major public health and inequalities issue. Accidental injury is one of the biggest killers of children, second only to cancer. The patterns and types of injury are closely linked with child development stages and steep socio-economic gradients persist:

- Over 2.3 million under 10-yr-olds attended emergency departments (EDs) in England between 2010 and 2011.
- 105,000 children and young people under 18 were admitted to hospital as a result of unintentional injuries in 2007–2008.
- In 2010, 172 children and young people under 15yrs died in accidents in England and Wales, and an additional 302 in the 15–19-yr-old group.
- Death rate from accidents for children of parents classified as never having worked or long-term unemployed is 13 times that for children in higher managerial/professional occupations.

## Types of accidents

- Road traffic accidents (RTAs) are the most common cause of accidental death (single biggest cause of accidental death in children aged 12–16yrs) including:
  - *Child pedestrian*—most common in boys aged 5–9yrs.
  - *Child passengers in vehicles*—particularly if unrestrained.
  - *Bicycle accidents*—1 in 80 boys have a chance of admission to hospital through a cycling accident.
- *Falls and head injuries:* minor head injuries common with little long-term effect, but 1 in 800 of these develop serious problems.
- *Burns and scalds:* 2nd most common cause of death from accidents (includes from house fires).
- *Drowning:* 3rd most common cause of accidental death. Most victims are young children, 3 times more common in boys than girls.
- *Choking, suffocation, strangulation:*
  - Babies and small children choke on small toys, food, or vomit.
  - Accidental strangulation on curtain cords, bedding, and necklaces.
- *Dog bites:* 1 in 100 children present in ED with dog bites.
- *Accidental poisoning:* peak age 30mths, ingesting medicines, household cleaning products, eating plants.

## Emotional, family, and relationships consequences

These can be far reaching, leading to parents/carers experiencing acute stress disorder or significant traumatic stress symptoms for 6mths or more after the initial injury. Caring for a child who has been seriously injured can stop a parent from returning to education or work, or plunge an already disadvantaged family further into poverty.

## Action for prevention

- Accident prevention is most successful at a public health (📖 Public health in the NHS, p. 10) and legislative level, e.g. traffic calming measures, child-resistant medication containers, compulsory use of seat belts in all parts of car.
- Individual parents also need to be aware of:
  - Risks at different child developmental stages and preventative action.
  - Use of home safety equipment and schemes that loan equipment e.g. stairs gates, or provide for free, e.g. smoke detectors (particularly for low income families). Often run by LA, Sure Start, or in case of smoke detectors, local fire brigade.
  - Risks associated with different leisure and sport activities and preventative action, e.g. cycling and the use of helmets.
  - Use of in car safety equipment correctly for the age group.
- There are also opportunities for education for children and young people on safety, e.g. crossing road, learning to swim from an early age, cycling proficiency courses. These types of learning opportunities may be provided by parents, local leisure organizations, early years education, PSHE in schools.

## Related topic

📖 Child health promotion, p. 144.

## Futher information

Child Accident Prevention Trust. Available at: ℘ www.capt.org.uk/
Royal Society for the Prevention of Accidents. Available at: ℘ www.rospa.org.uk
ROSPA website on child car sea safety. Available at: ℘ www.childcarseats.org.uk/
Making the Link. Available at: ℘ www.makingthelink.net/ supports senior practitioners and policymakers working to prevent unintentional injury to children and young people in England
Think Road Safety. Available at: ℘ think.direct.gov.u</index.html includes resources for teaching children, cycle safely etc

# Working with parents

This might involve parents expecting a first child or those living with adolescents. Work might be preventative ( Support for parenting, p. 166) or in response to significant problems defined by the parents, school, or the wider society, and all points between, such as sleep problems, aggression towards other children, and theft.

## Overall aim

The aim is to work with parents to achieve 'good enough parenting', protecting the child, and promoting physical, intellectual, emotional, and social development. Different approaches exist, which may have various theoretical underpinnings:

- *Behavioural modification:* concentrates on the behaviour to be changed, e.g. attention seeking or bed wetting, by rewarding acceptable behaviour.
- *Parent advisory models:* seek to understand individual context in which child and parent live. Helper–parent relationship is seen as central, with helper an active listener, followed by negotiated plan to meet individual family's needs.
- *Brief interventions:* short-term interaction focused on a particular issue.
- *Child development programme:* sees developmental achievements of child as central. Considering what child can do, the parents develop ideas for care and stimulation, including health factors such as diet.

Many draw from different perspectives, humanistic, counselling, social learning, and active listening. Integrating these views can lead to an approach specific for the family. Widely used models include the Solihull Approach[1], Mellow Parenting[2], Triple—P.[3]

## Current and most effective approaches

### Relationship building

Central to this is the spirit of partnership based on informal interactions, respect, mutual esteem, and recognition. Health workers need to demonstrate genuineness, humility, empathy, qualified enthusiasm, and confidence building as they seek to empower the parent. Shared records are likely to be part of this. Parents and professionals need to make clear what they can contribute to the relationship, frequency, and duration of the interaction, if the focus is to be the individual, group, or community, and if meetings will take place in the home or a health centre.

### Two-way sharing of knowledge experience and responsibility

The health worker draws on their expertise in child development, health promotion, or adolescent health. The parents know the child, family circumstances, and the sociocultural context in which the family lives. Both contributions are valued as neither can 'solve' the problem alone. Interactions will lead to the development of skills of both parent and professional. Reflection on the situation clarifies the issues and establishes the priorities for action.

### Getting parent (and child or young person) to set own goals and together working out a strategy

The family need to 'own' the issue, define what they want to achieve and what is manageable. This may be different from the professional or parents' views. Professionals will advocate for the parents, often lobby with them, and help them provide the best opportunities for their children.

### Recognizing and celebrating success

Small positive developments need to be noted and celebrated, this builds up the confidence of all involved, develops self-esteem, and increases expectations of success.

### Accessing other parenting support if necessary

This may include early years provision, regular attendance at school, after school facilities, and activities in the community or extended school.

## Impact of other issues

Parents may have problems or issues that impact on parenting. Interventions in terms of domestic violence (📖 Domestic violence, p. 402), family breakdown, mental illness (see 📖 People with depression, p. 435; 📖 People with schizophrenia, p. 443), and overuse of alcohol (📖 Alcohol, p. 319), substance misuse (📖 Substance misuse, p. 433) health issues, housing (📖 Homes and housing, p. 21), and income support (📖 Benefits and support p. 789) may be appropriate.

## Parenting and child mental health

Parenting may be linked with child mental health work. SNs, HVs, GPs, nursery nurses, teachers, and youth workers should be involved at the first level, promoting sound parenting and child mental health. Entrenched difficulties may need the involvement of mental health teams and specialist multidisciplinary teams. Building good parenting skills needs to begin early in life, and so can feature in personal social and health education, and citizenship in schools, together with youth organizations, pre-conceptual care and early antenatal interventions (📖 Health promotion in schools, p. 217).

## References

[1] Solihull Approach. Available at: 🖱 http://www.solihullapproachparenting.com/
[2] Mellow Parenting. Available at: 🖱 http://www.mellowparenting.org/
[3] The Triple P – Positive Parenting Program. Available at: 🖱 http://www.triplep.net/glo-en/home

## Further information

Care for the Family aims to promote strong family life and to help those who face family difficulties. Available at: 🖱 http://www.careforthefamily.org.uk/
Institute of Health Visiting Practice. Available at: 🖱 www.ihv.org.uk/
Mumsnet is an on line community and social network. Available at: 🖱 http://www.mumsnet.com/
Netmums is an online parenting organization with local networks. Available at: 🖱 http://www.netmums.com/home/about-us.

# Support for parenting

All national polices on children have support for parenting as a key standard. 'Good enough parenting' providing love, care, and commitment, can act as a buffer against adversity, e.g. poverty. It contributes to emotional wellbeing reducing the need for later reactive intervention. Good parenting will include:

- Provision of resources to facilitate growth and development.
- Meeting child's needs for love and security.
- Realistic expectations of child linked to their development and maturity.
- Provision of appropriate stimulation and opportunities for social development.

A quality environment, providing appropriate accommodation and nutrition, good nursery provision, play spaces, maternity/paternity leave, family friendly working patterns, and financial support; also supports parenting.

## Support for parenting

### Family and networks

Traditionally extended families provided practical and emotional encouragement. This still exists with some groups, but when families are spread throughout the country/world, support may come from community links and faith/cultural groups. Those without support may not be obvious and may include lone parents, father or mother, and those whose previous focus was on career development.

### Home visits

Visits by health workers or volunteers are effective in developing parenting skills, promoting the child's development, improving breastfeeding rates, and reducing unintentional injury. Health care organizations promote the use of specific techniques and programmes such as Brazleton approach[1], the Solihull Approach[2], Mellow Parenting[3], Triple—P.[4]

### Peer support

Support is available in groups facilitated by HVs and SNs, such as postnatal support groups, parent drop-ins, and parenting groups. These seek to build parental confidence and local networks. Mother and Toddler groups and local branches of organizations, such as the National Childbirth Trust and Meet a Mum may have similar aims.

### Programmes and centres

A variety of programmes to groups and communities seek to support parenting, some are local, some nationally based. They include:

- *First parenting programmes:* for new mothers and fathers as they make transition to parenthood.
- *Home-Start:* voluntary organization providing informal support for families with young children in their own home. Friendship and practical support is given with reassurance that their childcare problems are not unusual or unique. Encouragement is given as parents try to get the fun back into family life. Support is free, confidential, and non-judgemental. Almost 25% of families refer themselves to Home-Start.

- *Children's Centres:* e.g. Sure Start, government-funded services for pre-school children and their families. These bring together early education, childcare, health, and family support. Services provided include advice on health care and child development, play schemes, parenting classes, family outreach support, and adult education and advice.

These and other groups may include play and space for children, peer support for parents, talking and listening, valuing of parents, help with setting boundaries and whatever parents find useful.

Teenage parents may draw on any of the above support listed, but may need further support to continue or re-enter education or employment. Specialist programmes and extra childcare may all facilitate this.

The programmes listed here, as well as others will generally aim to:
- Take a partnership approach.
- Raise parents' self-esteem.
- Build up parent support networks.
- Take a positive approach to discipline, setting clear boundaries.
- Understand how families see issues.
- Recognize there are different parenting styles.

Setting up such programmes should involve partnership with parents in the planning, development, and monitoring of services. They might be involved in the writing of the mission statement, recruitment and appraisal of staff, design and evaluation of the service, contributing to new ways of working for both staff and users.

## References

[1] Brazelton Approach: promoting an understanding of infant behaviour. Available at: http://www.brazelton.co.uk/

[2] Solihull Approach. Available at: http://www.solihullapproachparenting.com/

[3] Mellow Parenting. Available at: http://www.mellowparenting.org/

[4] Triple P – Positive Parenting Program. Available at: http://www.triplep.net/glo-en/home

## Further information

Find a Sure Start Children's Centre. Available at: https://www.gov.uk/find-sure-start-childrens-centre

Home Start is an organization that supports families in local communities across the UK. Available at: www.home-start.org.uk

Institute of Health Visiting Practice. Available at: www.ihv.org.uk/

National Childbirth Trust local Branches. Available at: http://www.nct.org.uk/branches

Netmums is an online parenting organization with local networks. Available at: http://www.netmums.com/home/about-us.

Parenting UK is membership body for parenting support and education. Available at: http://www.parentinguk.org/

Positive Parenting: focuses on being parent to parent support rather than expert to parent. Available at: www.parenting.org.uk/

TOPSE A tool to measure parenting self-efficacy University of Hertfordshire. Available at: www.topse.org.uk/

Wales Flying Start Programme. Available at: http://wales.gov.uk/topics/childrenyoungpeople/parenting/help/flyingstart/?lang=en

# New birth visits

A new birth visit is the first contact (usually at home) with a family with a new baby made by the health visiting service 10–14 days after birth. Ideally by the HV rather than other members of team. It is part of the child health promotion programme (📖 Child health promotion programme, p. 144). The HV may already know the mother from antenatal contacts, classes, or from contacts with previous children.

## Information about a new birth

Every maternity unit provides the details of all births to the child health department in the PCO where the mother resides. The child health department informs the health visiting service, which covers that mother's home address or the GP that the mother is registered with. Any change of address is logged in the child health system and, on moving out of the area, the child's records are forwarded to the next child health department and/ or appropriate HV or SN. The community midwife will usually contact the HV and pass on a summary of the delivery and midwifery care, highlighting any particular problems and maternal or baby needs.

## Key principles of the new birth visit

- To introduce themselves, HV and child health promotion programme (📖 Child health promotion programme, p. 144) to family, particularly mother.
- To begin to establish relationship of trust with mother and family so client feels safe to raise issues or problems they are experiencing, and be prepared to receive information and support in dealing with them.
- To encourage and support all aspects of learning to nurture baby, and being a parent, often through using techniques such as Brazleton approach[1] to sensitizing parents to newborn abilities.
- To encourage and support all aspects of ensuring good physical and emotional health in mother (see also 📖 Postnatal depression, p. 393).
- To encourage and support all aspects of ensuring good physical and emotional health in baby.
- To assess and identify any maternal, baby, or family health (physical, mental, and emotional) or social problems, and offer advice and agree steps to addressing the problems, such as onward referral to another service.
- To identify children in need (📖 A child or young person in need, p. 150) and plan appropriate action with parent.
- To provide information on the child health promotion programme (📖 Child health promotion programme, p. 144), particularly child immunization (📖 Childhood immunization schedule (UK), p. 158) and seek written consent to the inclusion of the child in the computerized call and recall system for immunization and child health screening by the child health department.

- To provide information about local services, e.g. local parent and child networks, including children's centres, general medical services, birth registration, child benefit, state support for families and children, as required.
- To agree a pattern of future contact and provide information about how to contact the health visiting service.

## Key topics

Local health care organizations have guidelines and standards on this important contact which is informed by NICE guidance and the agreed child health promotion programme[2]. These will include: establishing infant feeding, especially (📖 Breastfeeding, p. 176, promoting sensitive parenting and parent–baby relationship (📖 Working with parents, p. 164), prevention of SIDS (📖 Babies and sleeping, p. 189), maternal mental health (📖 Postnatal depression, p. 393), parents relationships, sex and contraception (📖 Contraception general, p. 359), and keeping the baby safe (📖 Child injury prevention, p. 162, including passive smoking (📖 Smoking cessation, p. 315).

## Style of contact

HVs usually conduct the visit conversationally, with open-ended questions, using PHCHR and inviting the parents to raise issues that concern them. HVs often start by asking what the birth was like as a way into understanding the experience so far (see NICE guidance[3]). Many PCOs or PHCHRs provide specific checklists for assessing the baby and the family setting, but most HVs use these as an *aide memoire* in their conversations, rather than as a yes/no checklist.

## Records

All health care organizations have record keeping (📖 Client and patient held records, p. 87) guidance. PHCHR may be given out by HV or midwife according to local guidance. All contacts are recorded in PHCHR and noted in the health care organizations records, which are usually held electronically and sometimes also in the patient records held in general practice. Integrated child health e-records and systems are being developed.

## References

[1]Brazleton Approach: promoting an understanding of infant behaviour. Available at: ℘ www.brazelton.co.uk/
[2]Health Child Programme. (2009). Healthy Child Programme: Pregnancy and the First 5 Years of Life. Available at: ℘ www.gov.uk/government/publications/healthy-child-programme-pregnancy-and-the-first-5-years-of-life
[3]NICE (2006). *Postnatal Care: routine postnatal care of women and their babies*. Public version. Available at: ℘ www.nice.org.uk

## Further information

Directory of Community Health Services (Pavilion Publications) is published annually providing full contact details of all child health departments and health visiting services in the UK. Available at: ℘ www.pavpub.com/c-19-directories.aspx
Institute of Health Visiting Practice. Available at: ℘ www.ihv.org.uk/
NHS Choices. Pregnancy and Baby Guide. Available at: ℘ www.nhs.uk/Conditions/pregnancy-and-baby/pages/pregnancy-and-baby-care.aspx
NHS Information Service for Parents. Available at: ℘ www.nhs.uk/InformationServiceForParents/pages/home.aspx

# Child development 0–1 years

Child development is the interaction between heredity and the environment (📖 Overview of the healthy child programme, p. 146). In assessing development as part of the assessment of children, young people, and families (📖 Assessment of children, young people, and families, p. 148) it is often subdivided into four areas:

- Gross motor.
- Fine motor and vision.
- Speech, language, and hearing.
- Social, emotional, and behaviour.

## Developmental progress

Is about the sequential acquisition of skills. It is important to remember:

- There is a wide timescale within normal range, e.g. children walking unaided 25% by 11mths, 90% by 15mths, 97.5% by 18mths.
- Median ages indicate when half a standard population should have acquired the skill (see Table 6.3 for children 0–1yrs).
- Pre-term babies are assessed from expected date of delivery (EDD) up until 2yrs of age.

Refer for more in-depth assessment if:

- Failure to meet acquisition by upper limits of age need more detailed assessment, and investigation often through referral to community or hospital paediatrician, e.g.:
  - No responsive smile by 8wks.
  - Not achieved good eye contact by 3mths.
  - Not sitting unsupported by 9mths.
- Also refer if:
  - Parents concerned.
  - Discordant levels of development between areas.
  - Regression of previously acquired skills.
  - Development plateaus.

Development can be delayed or sub-optimal:

- Indirectly from adverse environmental factors or ill-health.
- Directly from neurological or neurodevelopmental problems.

## Further information

Sheridan M. *From Birth to Five Years: children's developmental progress*, 3rd edn. Revised and updated by Sharma A, Cockerell H. (2008). London: Routledge.

Hall D, Williams J, Elliman D. (2009). *The Child Surveillance Handbook*, 3rd edn. Abingdon: Radcliffe Publishing.

**Table 6.3** Overview of median age of development in children 0–1 years

| | Newborn | 6–8wks | 3–4mths | 6–7mths | 8–10mths | 11–12mths |
|---|---|---|---|---|---|---|
| Gross motor | Limbs flexed, symmetrical postures; marked head lag on pulling up; primitive reflex Moro and stepping | Raises head to 45° | 3mths: holds head up while lying prone | Sits without support 6mths, with rounded back; 8mths straight back | 8mths crawling, 10mths furniture walking | Walking unsteadily, broad gait, hands apart |
| Fine motor and vision | Reflex grasp; follows face in midline | 6wks: follows moving object by turning head | 4mths: reaches out for objects | 6mths: palmar grasp; transfers objects from one hand to other | Pincer grip | At least one word with meaning and understands some words |
| Language, speech, and hearing | Startles and blinks to loud noises | 4–6wks gurgles in response; notices sudden sounds and pauses to listen | Vocalizes alone, or when spoken to; laughs, squeals, blows between lips; quietens or smiles to voice of parent | Coos and babbles uses syllables—da, ba, ka; 7mths: turns immediately to parent's voice; turns to soft sounds out of sight if not preoccupied | Two-syllable babble; sounds used discriminately, e.g. dada, mama | |
| Social, emotional, and behaviour | Soon after birth flickers eyes when spoken to; after 2wks recognizes parent | Smiles responsively, responds to conversation through movements | Responds in conversations with smiles, gurgles, movements; finger feeds from 6mths | Curious about all sights, sounds, people; 6mths: puts arms out to be picked up: may be shy of strangers; 7mths: looks for dropped items | 8mths: separation anxiety; familiar with routines; 10mths waves bye-bye, plays peek-a-boo; looks for hidden items | Drinks from cup; gives kisses |

# Pre-term infants

Pre-term describes infants born <37wks. Estimated that 42,500 pre-term babies are born annually in UK. Infants born at 23–26wks gestation have 17–50% chance of survival. They have many problems (e.g. respiratory distress, hypotension, metabolic problems), require many weeks in intensive and special care, and have high levels of mortality. Very low birth weight (<1500g) babies ↑ risk of neurodevelopmental problems (5–10% have severe problems), including visual impairment, hearing loss, cerebral palsy, and learning difficulties. Those born after 32wks have good prognosis with few problems.

## On returning home from hospital

- Parents may need extra reassurance and support.
- Very premature and low birth weight babies ↑ risk of hospital readmission in first year.

Key areas of support and advice from primary care professionals may be:

*Bonding* May have been difficult while in hospital and added to by fear of baby dying (📖 Child development 0–1yrs, p. 170).

*Feeding* Pre-term babies are 'suck and swallow' poor so need frequent feeding (📖 Breastfeeding, p. 176). Breast milk (sometimes with calorie supplements) or special low birth weight formula is used. Vitamin and iron supplements are routine. Weaning advice for each baby will be different so parents should ask for advice from paediatric team.

*Clothes that fit very small babies* Advice from BLISS[1] (charity).

*Temperature control* May be poor at first. Needs controlled temperature (~18°C/65°F) and adequate insulation with clothes and blanket.

*Respiratory problems* Sometimes sent home on oxygen via nasal cannulae (📖 Oxygen therapy in the community, p. 581). ↑ Risk from respiratory infections. Possibly advise use of apnoea monitor at home.

*Vision problems* As a result of ↑ partial pressures of oxygen in special care. May need follow-up in primary care.

*Hearing* ↑ Risk of hearing problems. Should have neonatal screening and follow-up.

*Sudden infant death* Pre-term babies have ↑ risk. Foundation for Sudden Infant Death Syndrome (FSIDS)[2] have produced a leaflet for parents. See also 📖 Babies and sleeping, p. 189, for prevention advice.

## References

[1]BLISS : for babies born too soon, too small and too sick. Available at: ℘ www.bliss.org.uk
[2]FSID (the cot death charity) Baby Zone How to keep your baby safe and healthy ℘ http://fsid.
org.uk/page.aspx?pid=419

## Further information

BLISS Parent support helpline ☎ 0500 618140 (Monday to Friday 09.00–21.00 hours).
Lullaby Trust. Safer Sleep for Babies Available at: ℘ www.lullabytrust.org.uk/new-design/
safer-sleep/safer-sleep

# New babies

Many parents, particularly first-time ones, need reassurance, and advice about the changes and minor problems that arise in their new baby.

## Head

May appear elongated or misshapen as a result of the bones moving during the birth process. Resolves spontaneously during the first weeks.

## The umbilicus

After birth, the umbilicus dries, becomes black, and separates at about 1wk of age. Problems:

* *Stump can become infected:* offensive odour, pus, malaise; refer to GP for antibiotics.
* *Sometimes a granuloma forms:* refer to GP for silver nitrate cautery.
* *Hernia:* weak abdominal wall allows intestines to bulge out. This is common and usually resolves by 1yr.

## Skin

The vernix protects against minor skin problems, such as peeling and flaking. Peeling (common in those born after due date) is best dealt with by a non-irritant moisturizer, e.g. olive or baby oil, aqueous cream (📖 Baby hygiene and skin care, p. 183). Skin may be blotchy as blood vessels are unstable. Babies of black parents are often light skinned at birth, then produce melanin and reach permanent skin colour by 6mths.

### Birth marks

* *Strawberry (stork) marks:* pink areas, may grow, but fade. Sometimes raised bumps that shrivel and go by 2nd year.
* *Spider naevi:* network of dilated vessels, usually go by 2nd year.
* *Port wine stains:* found anywhere; can be treated with lasers or camouflaged.
* *Mongolian blue spots:* dark-skinned children often have harmless bluish black areas on back or base of spine; fade by 2yrs.

### Common skin problems

* *Milia:* tiny pearly white papules on the nose and face, blocked sebaceous ducts. Disappear spontaneously.
* *Neonatal urticaria:* red blotches with a central, white vesicle. Common in first week. Disappear spontaneously.
* *Heat rash:* small, red spots on face. Encourage not to overwrap or overheat rooms.
* *Harlequin colour change:* one side of body flushes red, while the other stays pale; harmless vasomotor effect.

## Hair

The baby may be bald or have full head of hair. Hair colour may change. Lanugo (downy hair on body) will fall off soon after birth.

### Eyes

- May have broken blood vessels following birth; this is harmless and resolves within a couple of weeks.
- *Sticky eyes:* common, usually due to blocked tear duct. Treated by swabbing with boiled water at each nappy change. Purulent discharge requires referral to GP and swabs for microscopy, culture and sensitivity (MC&S; <21 days to exclude ophthalmic neonatorum caused by *N. gonorrhoeae*).

### Nose

Sneezing and snuffling are very common to clear amniotic fluid. Reassure parents.

### Genitals

Many babies, male and female, may appear to have enlarged genitals and swollen 'breasts' shortly after birth, due to maternal hormones in their bloodstream. Advise to leave alone as this will subside spontaneously.

### First nappies

- *Bowel movements:* meconium (blackish-green) is the first bowel movement passed within 24h. Stools then change to greenish-brown then yellow semi-solid. Stools of bottle-fed babies often resemble scrambled eggs. Most babies have bowel movements soon after feeding (&#x1F4D6; Baby hygiene and skin care, p. 183).
- *Red-stained nappy:* common usually due to urinary urates, but may be due to blood from vagina through oestrogen withdrawal. Reassure parents.

**Feeding** See &#x1F4D6; Breastfeeding, p. 176; &#x1F4D6; Bottle feeding and weaning, p. 178.

**Weight gain** See &#x1F4D6; Growth 0–2yrs, p. 181.

### Related topics

&#x1F4D6; Overview of the Healthy child programme, p.146; &#x1F4D6; New birth visit, p. 168.

### Further information

NHS Choices Pregnancy and Baby Guide. Available at: &#x1F6F8; www.nhs.uk/Conditions/pregnancy-and-baby/pages/pregnancy-and-baby-care.aspx

NHS Information Service for Parents. Available at: &#x1F6F8; www.nhs.uk/InformationServiceForParents/pages/home.aspx

NICE (July 2006). Postnatal Care: routine postnatal care of women and their babies. Professional version. Available at: &#x1F6F8; www.nice.org.uk

# Twins and multiple births

Twins occur in 1:80 pregnancies, triplets 1:8000, quadruplets in 1:73,000. Multiple pregnancies more common in ♀ treated for problems with fertility (📖 Problems with fertility, p. 735).

## Special considerations
- Pregnancy can be more tiring, anaemia and fluid retention more common, and may need extra prenatal care and monitoring.
- Babies are often born earlier or smaller (📖 Pre-term infants, p. 172). May result in death of one or more babies (📖 Bereavement, p. 528).
- Coping with two or more newborn babies can seem an overwhelming task and financially problematic.
- Multiples may experience language delay, behavioural disorders, excessive rivalry, or dependency.

*Extra help*
Extra help is usually needed at first not just to cope with physical demands but also to give time to each baby and to the parents' own needs. HVs are able to provide local information on child care support (📖 Services for children, young people, and families, p. 19). Sometimes local nursery nurse courses are looking for placements for students, but these can only help with child care under direct supervision.

*Feeding*
Breastfeeding (📖 Breastfeeding, p. 176) should be encouraged, particularly in premature babies and because two babies can be fed and held close at once. Bottle feeding allows others to help. Guidance from Multiple Birth Foundation.[1]

*Sleeping* Twins, particularly premature twins, placed in the same cot are often more contented then when alone. Usual advice is given on sleeping (📖 Babies and sleeping, p. 189).

*Equipment* TAMBA provides advice on equipment such as buggies and sources of secondhand equipment.[2,3]

*Development and treating each baby and child as an individual*
Parents should be encouraged to remember that each baby has their own needs and they need to create time to spend with each. Identical twins need to be treated as individuals, rather than merged and will have different developmental progress (📖 Child development 0–1yrs, p. 170). Elements to help treating them as individuals are different clothes, feeding equipment, bed clothes, etc.

## References
[1] Multiple Births Foundation (MBF) Information for both professionals and parents. Available at: 🌐 www.multiplebirths.org.uk
[2] Twins and Multiple Birth Association (TAMBA). Available at: 🌐 www.tamba.org.uk
[3] TAMBA parent helpline: ☎ 0800 138 0509 (7 days a week).

# Breastfeeding

Breastfeeding is the optimum method for at least the first 6mths of life. Levels of acceptability differ between social classes and cultures in the UK. While two-thirds of mothers initiate breastfeeding, this rapidly drops off. Nearly 90% of mothers in social class I start breastfeeding compared with <50% from social class V. Many health organizations have breastfeeding support and peer support co-coordinators. UNICEF Baby Friendly UK initiatives promote environments and the training of professionals to support breastfeeding. Public health guidance promotes peer to peer support (NICE 2008[1]).

## Benefits

- Provides the right nutrients for a growing baby (baby >6mths advise to give vitamin drops).
- Convenient, at the right temperature, needs no preparation, and cheap.
- Helps develop intimate, loving relationship between mother and baby.
- ↓ gastrointestinal (GI) problems, chest and ear infections in babies, and ↓ inflammatory bowel disease (IBD), DM in later life.
- Breastfeeding promotes mother's uterus and pelvis to return to pre-pregnant state.
- Some protective effect against breast and ovarian cancer in mother.

## Issues to be aware of

- Certain diseases can be transferred in breast milk, e.g. hepatitis B, HIV. *Note:* HIV+ mothers should not breast feed as it is a route of viral transfer. See ▦ HIV, p. 686 for more information on preventing mother-to-child transfer.
- Some drugs/medicines can pass from mother through breast milk to baby or inhibit sucking reflex. Full list in BNF Appendix 5. COC contraindicated in breastfeeding mothers (▦ Contraception: missed rules COC, p. 364).

## Establishing breastfeeding

Every woman and baby needs to learn how to breastfeed together:
- *First 72h breasts produce colostrum:* ↑ protein and immunoglobulin. ↓ in volume, but no supplement formula feeds or water required. Supplements interfere with milk let-down reflex. Milk comes in 3rd or 4th day.
- *Let-down reflex:* sucking action on breast stimulates pituitary gland to release prolactin, for milk manufacture, and oxytocin lets down milk from glands to reservoirs behind the areola.
- *Latching-on:* use rooting reflex to ensure baby opens mouth wide enough to take large part of areola, as well as nipple in mouth (see Positions for breastfeeding ▦ p. 177).
- Baby needs frequent small feeds to start with, usually about every 2hrs including night; as weight increases spacing widens. Let-down reflex means that breasts produce milk on demand for breastfeeding. By about 6wks night feeds are reduced.

- Breastfeeding mothers are advised to have a good diet and take vitamin D (10 micrograms/day; Scientific Advisory Committee on Nutrition (2007).[2]

## Positions for breastfeeding

- Mother should be comfortably seated or lying down.
- NCT saying 'tummy to mummy—chest to chest—nose to nipple—chin to breast' to remind women of right position for baby to latch-on well.
- *Three positions:*
  - *Sitting up, cradling baby in front*—support baby on pillows so high enough to face breast.
  - *Underarm*—baby on pillow at side with legs pointing behind mother. Right hand cradles head while at right breast. Often a good position for women starting to breast feed for first time, for feeding twins, and those who have had Caesarians.
  - *Lying down*—on side facing baby. May need pillow behind to prevent backache and towel under rib to support breast.

## Common problems

- *Sore/cracked/bleeding nipples:* caused by poor positioning. Check baby latching-on correctly, check position, try different one. Feed from least sore side first.
- *Full, hard, lumpy breasts:* engorgement when milk first comes in or when baby drops a feed later on. Use warm flannels, shower, or bath before feeding to help milk flow. Express by hand first so baby can latch-on.
- *Small tender lump in breast:* blocked duct may be because bra is too tight or having slept awkwardly. Hand massage and warm flannels, etc. as above to help milk flow.
- *Red, inflamed areas on breast and flu-like symptoms:* mastitis, needs rest, pain killers, fluids, warm massage as above, continue breastfeeding, offer sore side first, and advise to see GP if continues, as may need antibiotics.

## Expressing milk

Expressing milk allows someone else to feed breast milk by bottle. Can be expressed by hand, hand pumps, or electronic pumps (e.g. mums with babies in special care units). Milk can be frozen (using special bags) and defrosted as required. Bottles and milk should be treated as for bottle feeding (🕮 Bottle feeding and weaning, p. 178).

## References

[1]NICE maternal and child nutrition (PH11) 2008. Available at: 🕭 http://www.nice.org.uk/PH11
[2]Scientific Advisory Committee on Nutrition (2007). Update on Vitamin D. London: Stationery Office.

## Further information

The Breastfeeding Network and helpline. Available at: 🕭 http://www.nationalbreastfeedinghelpline.org.uk

Breastfeeding Helpline Line. ☎ 0300 100 0212

National Childbirth Trust. Available at: 🕭 www.nct.org.uk

NCT breastfeeding line. ☎ 0300 330 0771

UK UNICEF Baby Friendly Initiative (information, training, accreditation). Available at: 🕭 www.unicef.org.uk/BabyFriendly/

# Bottle feeding

## Bottle feeding

Feeding a baby with a bottle is an opportunity for close, intimate relationships to develop. The parent should be in a comfortable position with the baby well supported in his or her arms.

If not breastfed, infants require formula milk modified to ~ the composition of human milk, with added iron and vitamins. A formula based on cows' milk that has the casein to non-casein ration modified by addition of demineralized whey, provides an amino acid profile more like breast milk. There is no evidence that any one brand is superior to another. Families on low incomes may be entitled to free formula milk for their babies (📖 Benefits for mothers and those with responsibility for children, p. 793). Formula-fed babies do not need additional vitamins.

### Preparing bottles

- Advise parents to make up formula exactly to the manufacturer's instructions and not to add extra powder. Formula milk is available ready-made in cartons (↑ expensive) and in powder form.
- Feeding bottles and teats should be well washed, correctly sterilized until >6mths of age (sterilizing tablets or steam units), to prevent sickness and diarrhoea.
- Good hygiene is important when making up feeds.
- Feeds should be made up, one at a time, as the baby needs them (to reduce risk of infection).
- Boiled water, at a temperature of 70°C, should be used (will kill any harmful bacteria). Feed then be allowed to cool before given to baby.
- Any infant formula left in bottle after a feed should be thrown away, also unused feed that has been kept at room temperature for >2hrs.

### Soya-based and other types of formula milk

- Other artificial formulas are available for babies intolerant of cows' milk. Such babies are usually under the care of a paediatric consultant and formula milk is prescribed as advised.
- There are concerns that if babies drinking soya-based formula they may absorb high levels of phyto-oestrogens (shown to affect rats' reproductive systems).
- Modified goats' milk is not approved for use in Europe.

### Introduction of whole, pasteurized cows' milk

Not recommended until the baby is >1yr old as this is less digestible and deficient in vitamins A, C, D, and iron. Breast or first formula milk should be used until 1yr, then switched to whole cows' milk. A 'follow-on' formula is not necessary.

## Further information

NHS Choices. Available at: 🔊 http://www.nhs.uk/Conditions/pregnancy-and-baby/Pages/bottle-feeding-advice.aspx
NICE maternal and child nutrition (PH11) (2008). Available at: 🔊 http://www.nice.org.uk/PH11

# Weaning

Weaning is the gradual shift from a milk-based diet to family food. WHO[1] recommend that milk only is sufficient until 6mths. The child is likely to be ready for mixed feeding when s/he can sit up, wants to chew (putting objects in mouth, rather than pushing out), reaches and grabs accurately. Weaning prior to 6mths should be discouraged and if started early advise sterilizing bowls and spoons, and avoid foods likely to cause allergies—wheat-based foods and others containing gluten, eggs, fish, shellfish, nuts, seeds, and soft and unpasteurized cheeses.

## How to start weaning

- Offer just a few teaspoons of food, once a day,
- Use a little of usual milk to mix food to desired consistency.
- Give baby a range of foods and textures to taste, trying new foods one at a time, allow them to touch food in the bowl or spoon.
- Encourage the baby to feed themselves using their fingers as soon as they show an interest. Use bibs and covers to catch the mess.
- If baby doesn't want solids then wait and try again later.
- Do not add any foods (including rusks, cereal or sugar ) to infant formula feeds.
- Suitable weaning foods can be:
  - *Soft, cooked and mashed*—e.g. baby rice mixed with baby's usual milk, mashed soft fruits, e.g. banana, cooked and mashed, peeled vegetables, e.g. potato, carrot, and peeled hard fruit, e.g. apple, pear.
  - *Finger foods*—e.g. carrot sticks, cooked and cooled green beans, cubes of cheeses, peeled fruit (chop small ones, e.g. grapes to avoid choking), all types of breads (see baby-led weaning[2]).
- Foods to avoid:
  - Salt should not be added to any food.
  - Do not add sugar to foods; try naturally sweet foods, e.g. bananas.
  - Avoid honey until >1yr, as some contains bacteria that causes infant botulism and contributes to dental caries.
  - Avoid raw eggs and cook eggs well.
  - Avoid whole nuts until >5yrs in case of choking.
  - Low fat foods are not suitable for <2yrs as fat needed for calories and vitamins.
- Where there is a family history of allergies may make a baby more prone to allergies. Advise to:
  - Breastfeed to 6mths.
  - *Introduce foods that commonly cause allergies one at a time*—eggs, milk, wheat, nuts (not whole until >5yrs), seeds, fish, and shellfish).
  - *Peanuts*—advice has been changed in recent times[3]. Only if child has a diagnosed food allergy, eczema, or immediate family have diagnosed allergy then child may have a higher risk of peanut allergy. Parents are advised to discuss with GP or medical allergy specialist before trying peanut foods for the first time.

### Established meals

- Eating family foods together at meal times promotes good eating habits, offers opportunities for interaction, seems to develop less 'fussy' eaters. Keeping meal times free of arguments about eating contributes to this. Commercially produced foods in jars and packets should not replace family food altogether (📖 Food and the under-fives, p. 201).
- By 9mths the baby should be eating three meals a day, which include protein, carbohydrates, and fruit and vegetables (vitamin C is important for absorption of iron).
- Intake of milk is reduced as solid food increases, but child still needs at least 600mL/day of milk (*note:* cows' milk not suitable until 1 yr).

### Vitamin supplements

- All children should take vitamin drops with vitamins A, C, and D from the age of 1 to 5yrs old (📖 Food and the under-fives, p. 201).
- Breastfed babies, and those drinking less than 500mL of infant formula milk per day, should begin vitamin drops at 6mths (📖 Breastfeeding, p. 176).
- Vitamins (and vouchers for infant formula) may be available via schemes such as Healthy Start[4] for low income families (📖 Benefits for mothers and those responsible for children, p. 793).

### References

[1]WHO (2002). *Infant and young child nutrition.* Geneva 2002: WHO. Available at: ℘ http://apps.who.int/gb/archive/pdf_files/WHA55/ea5515.pdf

[2]Baby led weaning. Available at: ℘ www.babyledweaning.com/

[3]Food Standard Agency. Available at: ℘ www.food.gov.uk/multimedia/pdfs/acm762a.pdf

[4]Healthy Start. Available at: ℘ www.healthystart.nhs.uk

### Further information

NHS Scotland Ready Steady Baby –Weaning your baby. Available at: ℘ www.readysteadybaby.org.uk/growing-together/looking-after-your-growing-baby/weaning-your-baby/index.aspx

NHS Choices. Available at: ℘ http://www.nhs.uk/Conditions/pregnancy-and-baby/Pages/bottle-feeding-advice.aspx

NICE maternal and child nutrition (PH11) (2008). Maternal and child nutrition. Available at: ℘ http://www.nice.org.uk/PH11

NHS Information Service for Parents. Available at: ℘ www.nhs.uk/InformationServiceForParents/pages/home.aspx

# Growth 0–2 years

Growth starts *in utero* and ends after puberty.

## Infant growth

- Dependent on nutrition, good health, happiness, pituitary growth hormone, thyroid hormone, and vitamin D.
- *Definitions:*
  - *Low birth weight*—<2.5kg.
  - *Very low birth weight*—<1.5kg.
  - *Small for gestational age*—length or weight at birth <2nd centile.
  - *Large for gestational age*—birth weight >90th centile.
- All babies lose weight in first week of life and 80% reach birth weight by 2wks.
- Growth measurement should only be undertaken by those trained to do so or others supervised by them.

## When to weigh and measure

- Babies are weighed in first week to help assess feeding and thereafter as needed.
- If parents wish, or there is professional concern, babies can be weighed at 6–8, 12, and 16wks, 12–13mths at time of routine immunizations.
- If there is concern, weigh more often but no more frequently than:
  - Once a month from 2wks to 6mths.
  - Once every 2mths from 6 to 12mths.
  - Once every 3mths from >1yr.
- Length is measured if there are any worries about a child's weight gain, growth, or general health.
- Head circumference is measured at birth, at 6–8-wk check, and any time after, if concerns about child's head growth or development.

## How to measure

- *Weight:* remove baby's clothes and nappy, weigh only on a Class III clinical electronic scales.
- *Length (until 2yrs):* supine, without clothes, nappy or shoes, using approved measuring board or mat and two people measuring.
- *Head circumference:* remove all headwear, use thin plastic or paper tape measure where head circumference is greatest.

## Recording

Plotted as single dot in pencil on UK WHO 0–4 boy or girl growth charts[1] (see Fig. 6.2) and PHCHR:

- *Full-term infants:* birth weight (and, if measured, length and head circumference) plotted at age 0 on the 0–1 year chart.
- *Healthy infants born after 32wks and before 37wks:* all measurements plotted in pre-term section until 42wks then on the 0–1-yr chart using gestational correction (plot at actual age with arrow back to weeks since birth).
- Pre-term born before 32wks or hospitalized neonate: a separate low birth weight chart is used.

*Interpretation*
- The charts show the growth range of children in the UK. The centile indicates the expected number of children below, e.g. 50% below the 50th.
- Plotting a weight or length within a quarter of the space above or below a centile is described as 'on the centile', otherwise it described as between two centiles, e.g. 50th–75th. Weight usually tracks within one centile.
- The term 'faltering weight gain' refers to slow weight gain and may indicate a feeding problem (📖 Breastfeeding, p. 176; 📖 Bottle feeding, p. 178).
- Rates of growth vary but review by GP or child health doctor if:
  - Birth weight not regained by 2wks (possible illness).
  - Weight graph sustained downwards or crossing down 2 centile lines.
  - <0.4th centile or >99.6th centile.
- <5% faltering weight due to organic causes. Non-organic failure to thrive (NOFTT) refers to poor growth from psychosocial factors. A full assessment and care plan will address more than just improved nutrition (📖 The assessment of children, young people and families, p. 148).

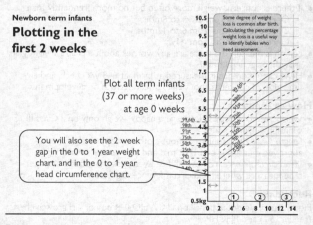

**Fig. 6.2** Plotting in the first 2wks.
Reproduced with permission from the Royal College of Paediatrics and Child Health.

## Key reading and resources

[1]UK-WHO 0–4 years growth chart resources: charts, training materials, fact sheets. Available at: ℅ www.rcpch.ac.uk/child-health/research-projects/uk-who-growth-charts-early-years/uk-who-0-4-years-growth-charts-initi

# Baby hygiene and skin care

Many new parents need reassurance and advice about hygiene and skin care. Parents can be reminded that these activities create good opportunities for talking and playing with the baby and creating a good attachment.

## Key principles

*Skin cleaning*

- A daily bath is not essential, although with an older baby it is helpful as part of an evening routine.
- Face, hands, and neck creases need washing as necessary, but at least once a day.
- Eyes should be washed in the newborn with wet cotton wool balls, avoid poking around in ears and nostrils.
- Skin in nappy area needs protecting at every nappy change by:
  - Washing (can be with a wipe).
  - A barrier cream applied to protect against nappy rash if required.
- Nappy changing should happen at least after every feed and more frequently as necessary.
- In girls, nappy area cleaning should be from front to back, i.e. towards the anus, without opening vulva. In boys, it is not necessary to pull back foreskin.
- Skin care products should be non-perfumed to avoid irritation and dryness.

*Bathing babies*

Key principles involve concern for safety (📖 Child injury prevention, p. 162), maintaining body temperature, and having a pleasurably interactive time together.

- Bath in warm room with no draughts.
- Make sure all equipment is to hand before starting.
- Cold then hot water to shallow depth (5–8cm for new baby), temperature should always be checked with elbow, inner wrist, or bath thermometer. A non-perfumed bath lotion can be used.
- Talk, smile, and reassure baby through whole process. Introduce water toys as child gets older.
- Wrap baby in towel, wash and dry face before placing in bath. In young babies also wash and dry hair/top of head before lowering baby in.
- Always support a young baby in water, with adult's arm under its back grasping furthest away baby's arm. Bath seats are available for older babies but babies should never be left alone in them.
- On lifting out, immediately wrap in towel and dry to maintain body heat.

*Hair care*
- Hair washing is easiest as part of bath routine using bath lotion water.
- After about 3–4mths, hair is thicker and a small amount of baby shampoo (i.e. non-stinging if gets in eyes) is better at cleaning.
- Soft baby hair brushes are available.
- Cradle cap (a form of seborrhoeic dermatitis) common in young babies with thick, yellow scales over scalp. Daily gentle shampooing may help. Also rubbing olive oil into scalp, leave overnight to soften scales, then shampooing out and rubbing scales off with fingers. If becomes inflamed may need antibiotic or steroid treatment.

*Nail care*
- Best trimmed after a bath when soft.
- Blunt-ended baby scissors are available.
- Some parents find it so unnerving to use scissors on a small baby, they prefer to bite off nails.

*Nappies*
- Parents choose disposable (biodegradable ones available) or cloth nappies according to their circumstances, finances, and available information.
- LAs and Real Nappy Campaign (see Women's Environmental Network (WEN)[1] provide detailed comparative information on types of nappies. New types of cloth nappies are both cheaper and more environmentally friendly than disposables. Some LAs provide trial packs.
- Cloth nappies now come in much easier designs, e.g. using Velcro™ that use disposable or washable liners. They do not need soaking if washed in machines at 60°C. Some areas have nappy laundering services.
- *Preventing nappy rash:*
  - Good skin care, regular and prompt changing of nappies.
  - Correct washing of nappies in non-irritant powder if washables.
- *Managing nappy rash:*
  - More frequent changing and cleaning.
  - Exposure to air.
  - Different barrier cream (see BNF 13.2.2).
  - If associated with fungal infection e.g. *Candida albicans*, an antifungal should be prescribed (see BNF 13.10.2).

**Reference**
[1] Women's Environmental Network (WEN). Available at: ℘ www.wen.org.uk/

**Further information**
NHS Information Service for Parents. Available at: ℘ www.nhs.uk/InformationServiceForParents/pages/home.aspx
NHS Choices Nappy Hygiene. Available at: ℘ www.nhs.uk/conditions/pregnancy-and-baby/pages/nappies.aspx
UK Nappy Helpline details of local cloth nappy contacts: ☏ 0845 850 0606
The Real Nappy Information Service. Available at: ℘ www.goreal.org.uk/

# Development and care of teeth

The age at which teeth cut through the gum and appear varies enormously. Most start around 6mths, but very occasionally babies are born with a tooth (sometimes removed if loose or badly positioned) and some don't cut teeth until after 12mths. Primary teeth are important as they guide adult teeth into the correct position. Erosion and loss of primary teeth affect placement of adult teeth.

Twenty primary teeth cut through gum in the same order:
- The lower then upper 2 incisors (6–12mths).
- The lower then upper canines (6–18mths).
- The 1st molars (12–20mths).
- The 2nd molars (18–24mths).

## Teething

Signs of teething are:
- Dribbling.
- Wanting to chew or gnaw.
- Often irritable, grizzly, and/or fretful.
- Red cheeks.

Discomfort may be relieved by:
- Giving something hard to gnaw on, e.g. carrot, teething ring.
- Use of OTC teething gels (see BNF 12.3.1).

## Teeth care: prevention of caries and misalignment

- Teeth need to be cleaned twice a day as soon as they appear with a smear of fluoride baby toothpaste on a soft brush.
- For <2yrs, British Dental Association recommends toothpaste with least 1000ppm (parts per million) fluoride and >3yrs a pea-size blob of toothpaste with 1350–1500ppm, and for >7yrs 1350ppm fluoride toothpaste or above.[1]
- Encourage tooth brushing as a game or copycat activity.
- Children need help and supervision in teeth cleaning until about 7yrs:
  - Clean babies teeth with them sat on lap or in chair and head slightly tilted for a good view inside mouth.
  - Adults need to stand behind older children to clean teeth.
  - Spit not rinse. Children should spit out water after teeth cleaning with fluoride toothpaste. Advise *not* to rinse so the fluoride remains around teeth.
- *Encourage:*
  - Water and milk-only drinks.
  - Savory and calcium-rich diet.
  - Use of cup, rather than bottle when weaning to promote good alignment of teeth.
  - Sugar-free medications.
- *Discourage:*
  - Sweetened drinks.
  - Dummies and sucking on thumb to avoid misalignment of teeth.
  - Use of bottle for drinks other than water and milk to avoid sugary liquid held in mouth.

- Babies should be registered with a dentist from birth if possible. First appointment with a dentist should be when first teeth break thorough.
- Country-specific advice on frequency of check-ups varies. Usually 6-monthly in <18yrs, but may be more or less frequently according to individual assessment. <18yrs exempt from payment for NHS dental check-ups and treatment.
- Dentists may advise pit and fissure sealants (plastic coating) for adult molars and pre-molars to prevent caries (see British Dental Health Foundation[2]).

## Use of fluoride supplements

- Each PCO area will have a policy on the need for fluoride supplements in view of levels of fluoride in drinking water.
- PCO community dental service provides advice.
- Use of fluoride supplements should only be on the advice of a dentist and at recommended dosage (see BNF 9.5.3).
- Dental fluorosis can occur when too much fluoride is taken, e.g. when water supply is already fluoridated and supplements are taken, or when children 'eat' toothpaste. Fluorosis can lead to pitting or flecking of tooth enamel.

## Fluoride varnish

- Fluoride varnishes are effective in preventing caries.[3]
- Prescribed by dentists and applied by dental staff 2–4 times a year to children aged 2yrs and over.
- May be part of NHS dental public health programme.
- *Post-application advice:* not to eat or drink for 30min, soft food for rest of day, don't brush teeth that day, may temporarily discolour teeth.

## Dental health promotion programmes

Some PCOs and countries have targeted dental health programmes, which may include distribution of toothbrushes, fluoride toothpaste, and leaflet at fixed times for under 5's plus supervised tooth brushing in nurseries (see, e.g. Childsmile[4]).

## Related topic

📖 Dental health in older children, p. 214.

## References

[1]British Dental Association. BDAsmile available at: ✆ www.bdasmile.org/index.cfm
[2]British Dental Health Foundation. Available at: ✆ www.dentalhealth.org.uk/
[3]Marinho VCC, Higgins JPT, Logan S, Sheiham A. (2008). Fluoride varnishes for preventing dental caries in children and adolescents. *Cochrane Rev.* Available at: ✆ http://summaries.cochrane.org/CD002279/fluoride-varnishes-for-preventing-dental-caries-in-children-and-adolescents
[4]Childsmile (Dental health promotion programme for children in Scotland). Available at: ✆ www.child-smile.org.uk/index.aspx

# Crying babies

All babies cry and some babies cry a great deal. Some parents need support to recognize that this is the baby's way of alerting adults of a need for attention, comfort, or care. A crying baby can be exhausting and stressful. Early evening is the most common time for this to happen. When they cry during the night it can be particularly stressful. Parents, particularly first time, may need help recognizing the causes and developing strategies that work for them and the baby. Dealing with babies that cry a lot can be very frustrating and parents and carers need to be aware that shaking a baby is particularly dangerous. While crying is normal there is usually a reason for excessive crying.

## Soothing babies

As a general rule, most babies are soothed by movement, contact, and sound, e.g. rocking, mobile over cot, cuddling and walking, holding them at the same time as talking or crooning. Having babies in baby slings or closely wrapped on the parent's back creates contact and movement. Some babies are more 'sucky' than others and might calm with a feed, or thumb in mouth or dummy.

Parents learn to recognize signs in their own babies of the causes and address them:

- *Hunger or thirst:* offer a feed or boiled water, check for problems with feeding (🕮 Breastfeeding, p. 176).
- *Tired, but fighting sleep:* lay them down either in quiet darkened place or in buggy to go out for a walk.
- *Discomfort with wet or dirty nappy:* change it (🕮 Baby hygiene and skin care, p. 183).
- *Discomfort as too hot or cold:* remove or add clothes or covering.
- *Lack of contact:* lift and cuddle, stroke, talk to.
- *Pain:* through a physical cause, e.g. wind after feeding, colic, or teething (🕮 Development and care of teeth, p. 185).

Parents need to be alert that the crying and associated behaviour may be unusual for their baby, and it is a sign of illness or infection that requires medical attention.

### Colic

Colic affects about 1 in 4 babies in first 3–4mths. Inconsolable crying, drawing up of knees can last for hours and occurs mostly in the evenings. Cause is unknown, it is benign, but distressing for parents. No evidence that gripe water, herbal remedies, or changing mother's diet are of benefit. Reassure parents, work through possible list of causes, and suggest soothing strategies.

*Older babies*
As babies get older, the causes change, can include:
- *Boredom:* needs company and distractions, such as rattles, toys, talking to, playing with.
- *Frustration:* as they start to crawl and cruise, items have to be put out of the way (☐ Child injury prevention, p. 162) leading to great frustration, distraction tactics become important.
- *Fear of separation and strangers:* usually between 6 and 8mths. Give lots of reassurance, cuddling, comfort, gradual periods of separation, gradual familiarity with new surroundings help.

## When the crying becomes too much
Sometimes, parents feel overwhelmed and frustrated by a baby who will not stop crying. Any health professional working with parents, who say that their babies cry a lot, should help them work through coping strategies to ensure they don't over-react, lose their tempers, or become rough with the baby. These include:
- Getting help from other adults.
- Having someone else look after the baby for an hour or so.
- Creating time to think through other causes and strategies to stop baby crying by putting baby down safely and leaving room.
- Putting baby down safely and leaving room if they feel it is all too much, and getting another adult or using a helpline.
- Talking to someone about how you feel, such as the HV or Cry-sis helpline.
- Remember, this difficult time won't last forever, it is only for a short time.

## Further information
Cry-sis for support to families with excessively crying, sleepless, and demanding babies. Available at: ℘ www.cry-sis.org.uk. ☎ 08451 228 669.
NCT Coping with colic. Available at: ℘ www.nct.org.uk/parenting/coping-colic
Institute of Health Visiting Practice. Available at: ℘ www.ihv.org.uk/
NHS Choices. Colic. Available at: ℘ http://www.nhs.uk/conditions/Colic/Pages/Introduction.aspx

# Babies and sleeping

A newborn baby's sleep pattern is determined by their weight and feeding requirements. When they are not feeding, most babies are asleep, although some are active and alert for long periods. As a rough guide:
- 2kg baby awake for 7–8 feeds.
- 3kg baby awake for 5–6 feeds.
- 4.5kg baby awake for 4–5 feeds.

However, every baby is individual and patterns will vary. Some sleep for long periods, some in short snatches. Most babies are able to sleep for longer periods through the night without feeds by 6wks. The periods of wakefulness during the day extend as they get older. Older babies need morning and afternoon naps during the first year.

## Safe sleeping

The safest place for a baby to sleep is in a cot beside the parents' bed for the first 6mths. To reduce the incidence of SIDs (📖 Sudden infant death syndrome, p. 295) the baby put down to sleep should:
- Be on their back.
- Have their head uncovered.
- Feet to foot of the cot.
- Not get too hot or too cold. Advice includes:
  - Cotton sheets and blankets not duvets, baby nests, or sheepskins.
  - No pillows, wedges, or cot bumpers.
  - Never placed with hot water bottles, electric blankets, or next to radiators, fires, or in direct sunshine.
  - Ideal room temperature is about 18°C (65°F).
  - Only need to wear nappy, vest, and sleep suit.

Other advice to prevent SID includes parents to stop smoking and no smoking in same room as baby.

### Co-sleeping

While there are many advocates of sharing there are real risks to the baby (📖 Child injury prevention, p. 162; 📖 Sudden infant death syndrome, p. 295) and potential for disrupted sleep patterns for both parents.

Parents should never share a bed or bring the baby into the bed if:
- Either parent smokes (risk of SUDI 📖 Sudden infant death syndrome, p. 295).
- They have been drinking or taking illegal drugs or medication that increases drowsiness.
- They are unwell or extra tired so it might affect their ability to arouse or respond to the baby.
- If the baby was premature (born before 37wks) or was of low birth weight (less than 2.5kg).

❶ Parents or carers should never fall asleep with a baby on an armchair or sofa as there are real dangers of the person shifting and suffocating the baby.

## Sleeping and settling routines

Bed time sleep routines help babies and parents establish good patterns of separating to sleep. Around 6wks is a good time to start and they are usually established by 3–6mths. Most routines tend to include some or most of the following:

- A bath.
- A feed.
- A quiet time.
- Placing in bed, lullaby, later story.
- Cuddle and kiss goodnight.
- Leaving them in a darkened room, with a night light, baby listener switched on, and gentle music, e.g. part of a mobile.

### Night waking babies 0–6mths

- Any night feeds still required should be very low key, with little eye contact or words; all signals that this is not the time to be awake.
- Check for all causes of crying (📖 Crying babies, p. 187) and settle.

### Night waking babies 6–12mths

Babies who wake at night or only go back to sleep with lots of parent attention/feeds can usually be persuaded to change their behaviour by the checking routine (also used for older children). Over a 2-wk period when the baby wakes:

- Leave to cry for 5min.
- Parent goes in checks him, tucks in, and leaves.
- Parent does not cuddle, give drink, or 'reward' in any way.
- This process is repeated often with increasing intervals until baby recognizes night time waking produces no results and stays or quickly returns to sleep.

Parents need to be convinced of the value of this process and not undermine their own efforts by re-starting to 'reward' night waking.

### Further information

Cry-sis for support to families with excessively crying, sleepless, and demanding babies. Available at: 🕸 www.cry-sis.org.uk ☎ 08451 228 669

Department of Health/FSID (2009). 4 Reducing the risk of cot death: an easy guide. Available at: 🕸 www.Dh.gov.uk

Lullaby Trust. Safer Sleep for Babies Available at: 🕸 www.lullabytrust.org.uk/new-design/safer-sleep/safer-sleep

# Promoting baby development safely 0–1 years

Health professionals, particularly HV teams, are in a good position to advise parents on how to help their babies develop (📖 Child development 0–1yrs, p. 170), at the same time providing health promotion advice on injury prevention (📖 Child injury prevention, p. 162) particularly as they become mobile.

## Key principles to promote with parents and carers

- Babies are learning from the first day and their abilities quickly develop.
- New parents often need to learn to play and talk to their babies.
- Interacting with the baby in every activity promotes attachment or bonding, learning, and speech development:
  - Talking to them with eye-to-eye contact, with face up close when newborn, and responding to their noises at every opportunity.
  - Holding them to feed, holding on lap, carrying, cuddling, singing nursery rhymes, games like peek-a-boo.
- Help babies find out about the world around them, e.g.:
  - From 6wks babies can be propped up against pillows or in bouncing chairs (always on floor not tables).
  - Out and about to parks, friends' houses, shops in buggies.
- To have realistic expectations of the developmental stage, e.g. babies explore through their mouths so don't try to stop them, just make sure the things they take to their mouths are clean, safe, and can't be swallowed or are small enough to cause a blockage.
- Simple toys are the best—people are better than toys early on.
- *Encouraging movement safely:*
  - *Learning to crawl*—needs opportunities on tummy on the floor, once able to roll never leave alone except on floor in clear space without objects that could hurt or be swallowed.
  - *Once independently moving by rolling, crawling, furniture cruising*—remove poisonous substances from reach level, fit safety gates, remove glass topped items, protect sharp-edged furniture (📖 Child injury prevention, p. 162).
  - *Discourage parents from using baby walkers*—they cause more accidents than any other baby equipment.

## Resources to support development

- Many HV and children's centre teams have produced resource packs or have drop-in sessions to support parents in helping the development of their babies.
- HV teams in many areas (England, Wales and NI) distribute book packs from the Bookstart.[1]
- Toy libraries often provide packs and ideas for 0–1yrs (📖 Services for children, young people, and families, p. 19).

*Promoting accident prevention*

All baby equipment should be to British Standard or European Standards.

**!** *Baby car seats* New babies should be in rear facing car seats and never placed in the front seat if the car has air bags.

Accident prevention for babies includes:

- *Falls:* e.g. rolling off changing mats, etc. Promote strapping in buggies, placing on floors, and safe places.
- *Burns and scalds:* e.g. too hot bath water, spilt hot drinks. Promote cold water then hot in bath, testing bath water, not having hot drinks near baby.
- *Fires in the home:* e.g. distracted parent leaves chip pan over heat. Promote smoke alarms.
- *Drowning:* e.g. in bath. Highlight danger in leaving baby alone in, or near, water.
- *Choking:* highlight danger of prop feeding and small items sticking in trachea.

Many HV teams and children's centres provide first aid classes for parents.

## Reference

[1]Bookstart. Available at: ✍ www.bookstart.org.uk

## Further information

British Association for Early Childhood Education. Available at: ✍ www.early-education.org.uk
National Literacy Trust. Talk to Your Baby. Available at: ✍ http://www.literacytrust.org.uk/talk_to_your_baby
British Literacy website for parents. Available at: ✍ www.wordsforlife.org.uk/
Sure Start Children's Centers finder. Available at: ✍ childrenscentresfinder.direct.gov.uk

*Prevention of injury*

Child Accident Prevention Trust. Available at: ✍ www.capt.org.uk
Royal Society for the Prevention of Accidents and Department of Transport dedicated site on child car seats. Available at: ✍ www.childcarseats.org.uk/

# Child development 1–5 years

Child development is the interaction between heredity and the environment (📖 Child health promotion, p. 144). Development is assessed as part of the healthy child programme (📖 Overview of the healthy child programme, p. 146).

## Developmental progress

This is about the sequential acquisition of skills. It is important to remember that:

- There is a wide time scale within the normal range, e.g. children walking unaided: 25% by 11mths, 90% by 15mths, 97.5% by 18mths.
- Median ages indicate when half a standard population should have acquired the skill (see Table 6.4 for children aged 1–5yrs).
- Pre-term babies are assessed from EDD up until 2yrs of age only.

### Referral for more in-depth assessment

Failure to meet acquisition by upper limits of age need more detailed assessment and investigation, often through referral to community or hospital paediatricians, e.g.:

- Not walking unaided by 18mths.
- No pincer grip by 18mths.
- Not saying single words with meaning by 18mths.
- No 2- or 3-word sentences by 30mths.

More detailed and in-depth assessment is also required if:

- Parents concerned about an aspect of development.
- Discordant levels of development between areas.
- Regression of previously acquired skills.
- Development plateaus.

### Development can be delayed or suboptimal

- Indirectly from adverse environmental factors or ill-health.
- Directly from neurological or neurodevelopmental problems.

## Further information

Sheridan M. *From birth to five years: children's developmental progress*, 3rd edn. Revised and updated by Sharma A, Cockerell H. (2008). London: Routledge.

Hall D, Williams J, Elliman D. (2009). *The Child Surveillance Handbook*, 3rd edn. Abingdon: Radcliffe Publishing.

Cowie H. (2012). *From birth to sixteen: children's health, social, emotional and linguistic development*. London: Routledge.

**Table 6.4** Overview of median age of development in children 1–5 years

|  | 15mths | 18mths | 2yrs | 3yrs | 4–5yrs |
|---|---|---|---|---|---|
| Gross motor | Walks alone steadily | Bends to pick up without toppling | Kicks a ball without toppling; runs; 2½: jumps with both feet off the ground | Up and down stairs without holding on; pedals trikes | Hops, skips, catches ball |
| Fine motor and vision | Scribbles with pencil | Turns pages in books; feeds himself with spoon; able to put on some clothes; builds tower of 3 bricks | Builds tower of 6 bricks; able to take off most clothes and put some on | Builds bridge with 3 bricks; draws O (copies 6mths earlier); does up buttons | Builds copy of 6 bricks in steps; draws x at 4; at 4½yrs, △; at 5yrs uses scissors |
| Language, speech, and hearing | Shows 2 parts of body; follows simple instructions, single words | 10–20 words, usually nouns, hums | Uses 2 or more phrases to make simple sentences; 2½: talks constantly in 3–4-word phrases | Vocab 200–300 words; starts asking 'why?' frequently; begins to grasp concept of numbers; knows age and a few colours | Talks a great deal, boasts, tells stories |
| Social, emotional, and behaviour | Imagination appears in doll play | Symbolic play; imitates adults; plays alongside (parallel) others | Learning to play with others but often rivalries; dry by day and bowel control, later, night; starts saying 'no' often | Interactive play with other children; takes turns; dry by night, later | Expanding sense of self, growing confidence, wants to be grown up |

# Growth 2–4 years

Growth starts *in utero* and ends after puberty. It is good practice to record height and weight in any child about whom there is concern, who has chronic ill-health, or requires prolonged follow-up for any reason.

## Growth

- Dependent on nutrition (📖 Food and the under-fives, p. 201), good health, happiness, pituitary growth hormone, thyroid hormone, and vitamin D.
- Growth measurement should only be undertaken by those trained to do so or others supervised by them.

## When to weigh and measure

- *Weight:*
  - At routine visit for review or immunization (i.e. 24mths, between 3 and 4yrs (📖 Overview of the healthy child programme, p. 146).
  - If requested by a parent or if a professional is concerned, but no more frequently than 3-monthly as can be misleading.
- *Height:*
  - If requested by parent, charts have adult height prediction section.
  - Whenever concerns about weight gain, growth, or general health.
  - If weight <0.4th centile or >99.6th centile.
  - If there is rapid weight gain.
- *Head circumference:* if concerns about growth or development.

## How to measure

- *Weight:* toddlers in vest and pants, older children in light clothing on a on a Class III clinical electronic scales.
- *Height:*
  - Without footwear using a rigid rule with T piece or stadiometer, bottom, back, and heels touching apparatus, and ears and eyes at 90° to the apparatus.
  - Measure on expiration.
- *Head circumference:* use thin plastic or paper tape measure where head circumference is greatest.

## Recording

- Plotted as a small dot on UK WHO boy or girl growth charts (see Key reading and resources[1]) and PHCHR.
- Also plotted on BMI conversion section of chart if concern about growth (see Fig. 6.3).

### Interpretation
- A child whose weight is average for their height will have a BMI between the 25th and 75th centiles, whatever their height centile.
- Review by GP or child health doctor if:
  - BMI >91st centile suggests overweight and > 98th centile is clinically obese.
  - BMI < 2nd centile may reflect under-nutrition.
- Acute illness may cause weight loss, but usually re-gained within 2–3wks. Prolonged failure to gain weight or continuing weight loss may indicate other illness or NOFTT. See 📖 The assessment of children, young people and families, p. 148.

Infants and toddlers
## Body Mass Index (BMI) lookup

- Read off the weight and height centiles from the growth chart.
- Plot the weight centile (left axis) against the height centile (bottom axis)
- Read off the corresponding BMI centile from the slanting lines.
- Record centile with date in the data box
- Accurate to ¼ centile space

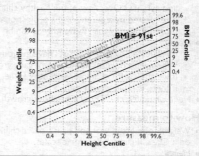

**Fig. 6.3** BMI conversion chart.
Reproduced with kind permission of the Royal College of Paediatrics and Child Health.

### Key reading and resources
[1]UK-WHO 0–4 years growth chart resources: charts, training materials, fact sheets. Available at: ℛ http://www.rcpch.ac.uk/child-health/research-projects/uk-who-growth-charts-early-years/uk-who-0-4-years-growth-charts-initi

# Promoting development in the under-fives

Health professionals, particularly HV teams are in a good position to advise parents on how to help their young children develop (🕮 Child development 1–5yrs, p. 193), at the same time providing health promotion advice (🕮 Models and approaches to health promotion, p. 298) on child injury prevention (🕮 Child injury prevention, p. 162). They are encouraged to work in partnership with parents, and with early years providers of child care and education. All UK countries have policies emphasizing support for early years and child development in the under-fives in readiness for primary school. This includes frameworks for activities and curriculum in pre-school child care and education providers, part-time places at nursery schools for 3- and 4-yr-olds, and early years providers' statements of individual child development at 2yrs given to parents.

## Key principles to promote with parents and carers

- Young children are curious and learning about life, their family, and their home all the time.
- They learn by being part of everyday life in their family life, playing, and asking questions.
- Parents, family, and carers help children develop by:
  - Encouraging and rewarding all efforts, attempts, new achievements, and good behaviour with touching, smiling, words of praise, listening, cuddles.
  - Including them in daily activities, e.g. shopping and family events.
  - Talking to them, singing with them, reading together.
  - Playing games and providing opportunities for different types of games, e.g. outdoor running games, wet play in the bath, imaginative play with dressing up clothes, manipulation games with puzzles.
- Social skills are developed through opportunities to meet other children and adults, e.g. drop-ins, play groups (🕮 Services for children, young people, and families, p. 19).
- Children need the opportunity to be outside, to run about, let off steam and get fresh air every day.
- Most of all relax and enjoy children—they won't be this age long.

## Resources to support development

- Many HV and Children's Centre teams have produced resource packs or have drop-in sessions to support parents.
- Libraries and toy libraries often provide packs and ideas for under-5s.

Local children's or early years services may provide a range of resources about play groups, drop-ins etc. 🕮 Services for children, young people and families, p. 19.

*Promoting injury prevention 1–5yrs*
- Many Sure Start, HV teams, or local children's services provide first aid classes for parents.
- Young children need constant supervision as very curious.
- ↑ mobility ↑ risk of:
  - *Falls*—think about window safety catches, safety gates.
  - *Burns and scalds*—keep hot drinks and saucepans out of reach.
  - *Drowning*—never leave <4yrs in bath alone, fill in or fence off ponds, empty paddling pools.
  - *Poisoning*—keep household cleaners, medicines in locked cabinets out of reach.
  - *Cuts and bruises*—protect sharp edges in home, fit safety glass, use door guards to prevent trapped fingers.
  - *Out and about*—teach road safety to children (see Child Accident Prevention Trust[1]), use age appropriate car seats (see ROSPA[2]), think sun safety (🕮 Skin cancer prevention, p. 331).

## Related topics

🕮 Working with parents, p. 164; 🕮 Support for parenting, p. 166; 🕮 Services for children, young people and families, p. 19.

## References

[1]Child Accident Prevention Trust. Available at: ℘ www.capt.org.uk
[2]Royal Society for the Prevention of Accidents dedicated site on child car seats. Available at: ℘ www.childcarseats.org.uk/

## Further information

British Association for Early Childhood Education. Available at: ℘ www.early-education.org.uk
British Literacy Association. Talk to Your Baby. Available at: ℘ www.literacy-trust.org.uk/talktoyourbaby
Department of Education Early Years Foundation Stage (EYFS). Available at: ℘ www.education.gov.uk/schools/teachingandlearning/curriculum/a0068102/early-years-foundation-stage-eyfs
Scottish Government Early Years Framework. Available at: ℘ www.scotland.gov.uk/Topics/People/Young-People/Early-Years-and-Family/Early-Years-Framework
Sure Start Children's Centers finder. Available at: ℘ http://childrenscentresfinder.direct.gov.uk/
The Foundation Years From Pregnancy to 5. Information and resources for parents and early years and health practitioners. Available at: ℘ www.foundationyears.org.uk
Department of Transport. Road safety resources for teachers, pupils and parents. Available at: ℘ think.direct.gov.uk/education/early-years-and-primary/parents/3-to-5s/

# Emotional development in babies and children

## General

Significant and critical brain and intelligence development occurs during the first 3yrs of life. It is influenced by nutritional and health status, also by interactions developed with people and objects. Key points:

- Highly dependent upon adequate nutrition, stimulation, and optimal care.
- During first years, key brain pathways for lifelong capabilities are established. Once developed, the brain is much harder to modify.
- Adequate attention to the first months and years (including pre-natally) of a child's life are crucial in determining lifelong outcome.
- Duet relationship created by caregiver, and baby builds and strengthens brain architecture and creates relationship in which a baby's experiences are affirmed and new abilities nurtured.
- By school age, a lot of key language abilities, physical capabilities, and cognitive foundations have been set in place.
- While a focus on primary education is important, 5yrs is too late to start paying attention to children's emotional development needs.
- Sensitive and responsive parent–child relationships is also associated with stronger cognitive skills in young children and enhanced social competence and work skills later in school.

## Developmental guideline

Think in terms of stages not ages. The following ages are *guidelines only*.

- *1mth:* voice recognition, express interest—attend to pictures, visual focus.
- *6mths:* senses pleasure: smiling, mouthing objects important, different communication methods—pointing, vocalizing, crying; also words and pictures.
- *9mths:* facial expressions reflecting emotions, e.g. fear, comfort objects.
- *<2yrs:* attachment vital, self-centred, gaining personal identity, change resistant.
- *3yrs:* conforms, more secure, adventuresome, enjoys music, imaginative play, regulation of emotion and self-distraction beginning.
- *4yrs:* sure of self, tests self, often negative, needs controlled freedom.
- *5yrs:* self-assured, stable, self-adjusted, enjoys responsibilities, capable of self-criticism, likes to follow rules.
- *By 6yrs:* learnt which emotions are socially (un)acceptable.
- *Middle childhood:* aware actions lead to (dis)approval, internalize standards of conduct.

## Basics for positive emotional health

- *Unconditional love from family*: praise, firm, but realistic goals, honesty, encouragement.
- Safe and secure surroundings.
- Supportive caregivers, encouraging teachers.
- Self-confidence and self-esteem.
- Appropriate discipline.
- Make time for play.
- Set good example/role model.
- Opportunity to play with other children.

## Key principles for parents

- Think of stages not ages, social and emotional milestones harder to pinpoint than signs of physical development.
- Early support and intervention may prevent damaging patterns being established within families.
- Significant events in adult carer and family life impact on children too, e.g. deaths of grandparents, birth/illness of siblings, family break-up.

## Related topics

📖 Emotional problems in children, p. 268; 📖 Behavioural disorders in children, p. 246.

## Further information

Association of Infant Mental Health. Available at: 🖰 www.aimh.org.uk
Child Psychotherapy Trust. Available at: 🖰 www.childpsychotherapytrust.org.uk
Young Minds. Available at: 🖰 www.youngminds.org.uk
Zero to Three. Available at: 🖰 www.zerotothree.org

# Food and the under-fives

Good nutrition in pre-school children is important because it:
• Ensures optimum growth and functional development.
• Impacts on health in the present and in adulthood.
• Encourages a taste for healthy foods in preference to fatty, salty, and sugary foods.

Under- and over-nourishment are public health issues, influenced by factors such as poverty and inappropriate feeding practices. By 5yrs children should be eating family food that is a balanced healthy diet (☐ Nutrition and healthy eating, p. 304).

## Nutritional requirements

1–5-yr-olds have high energy and nutrient requirements relative to their size and need nutritious snacks between meals as part of a fixed routine (not constant snacking). Estimated average requirements (EAR) for energy:
• *Boys 1–3yrs:* 1230 kcal/day, 4–6yrs 1715 kcal/day.
• *Girls 1–3yrs:* 1165 kcal/day, 4–6yrs 1545 kcal/day.

The developing body, in particular bones and teeth, need a good supply of protein, calcium, iron, and vitamins A and D.

## Diets of pre-school children

Parents should be encouraged to offer children the family meals which follow these guidelines:
• Variety in foods each day from four food groups:
  • Cereals
  • Fruit and vegetable.
  • Meat, egg, pulses
  • Milk and milk products.
• Contain full fat cows' milk until 2yrs when semi-skimmed can be substituted provided the diet is otherwise nutritionally adequate. Skimmed milk not suitable <5yrs.
• Plenty of fluids, preferably plain tap water, to prevent constipation.
• Contain no more than 10% of dietary energy in sugars.
• Are low in salt, avoid salty foods and the addition of salt at table.
• Avoid excessive fibre intake—compromises energy and mineral intake.
• Avoid tea and coffee to ensure mineral (especially iron) bioavailability.
• Promote dental health by keeping sugary foods and drinks to meal times only.
• Supplement with vitamins A, C, and D, from 6mths, unless adequate vitamins through diverse diet and moderate exposure to sunlight.

## Vegetarians and vegans

Children need to be offered a mixture of plant proteins (e.g. cereals, pulses, seeds, ground-up nuts) to ensure the combinations complement each other in forming high quality protein ≥ animal protein. Iron from plant sources is better absorbed with vitamin C, e.g. fruit juice. Children on vegan diets may need supplements of fortified foods to achieve enough calcium, vitamins D and B12, and riboflavin.

## State provided nutrition support for children

- Healthy start schemes for families on low incomes provide vouchers for milk, fruit, and vegetables as well as vitamin drops (📖 Benefits for mothers and those responsible for children, p. 793).
- Day care providers can claim for ⅓ pt for each child attending >2h each day they attend through the Nursery Milk Scheme.
- School fruit and vegetable scheme gives all children aged 4–6yrs in LA maintained schools a free piece of fruit or vegetable each school day.

## Eating: a social skill

Food and eating offers opportunities for learning and interaction with adults, such as helping to shop, cooking, laying the table, washing up. Specific skills include:
- How to feed themselves more skillfully in accordance with family practices, including using utensils.
- How to participate in a social occasion that requires certain ways of behaving.

Children have to be given opportunities to feed themselves, to sit at a table to eat with others and to enjoy mealtimes. Parents need to be:
- Prepared for messy mealtimes with toddlers.
- Consistent about the expected behaviour at the meal table and realistic in what is manageable for the child's age,

## Food problems

Food preferences and refusal are common <5yrs. They are part of growing up and asserting independence, but are also often a source of great tension at meal times. Parents may need advice on positive behaviour management. Key advice for parents:
- Children will not harm themselves if they do not eat for a short while.
- No one food is essential, but don't allow child to stop eating an entire food group, e.g. fruit and vegetables.
- If a food is rejected try:
  - Another in the same food group.
  - Presenting it cooked in a different way.
  - Presenting it in a more fun way.
- If child refuses to eat, don't insist, and don't substitute with snacking.

*Food allergies* See 📖 Allergies, p. 647.

### Foods for children to avoid

- Whole nuts in case of choking.
- Shark, swordfish, and marlin because levels of mercury may affect development of nervous system.
- Raw shellfish to avoid risk of food poisoning.
- *Infants and toddlers:* raw or runny eggs to avoid risk of food poisoning.

## Further information

NHS Choices. Food and Diet pages. Available at: ℘ http://www.nhs.uk/LiveWell/Goodfood/Pages/Goodfoodhome.aspx

Vegetarian Society. Information leaflets on food and children. Available at: ℘ https://www.vegsoc.org/infobooklets#.UeUUU43qnTo

# Toilet training

Most children can do without nappies by day from 2–3yrs and by night from 2–5yrs. How to approach toilet training will vary from child to child.

## General principles

- *Wait until the child is ready:* usually means that child can indicate to parent that they are going to the toilet and has shown an interest in using potty or toilet. It is helpful to have a potty or child's toilet seat to put on normal toilet for child to become familiar with before starting toilet training.
- *Pick a good time*: when child can have a few days at home without nappies in an environment where accidents don't matter. Make sure child has plenty of spare clothes available.
- *Keep the potty handy or stay within easy reach of the toilet:* when child says they wish to go, sit them immediately on toilet. Reward any result with praise. Don't punish child for any accidents—advise parent to ask child to help clear up any mess and reinforce that it would be better to use potty/toilet next time.
- *Until the child (and parent) are confident in the child's ability to use the toilet continue using nappies when out and at night:* take child to toilet at night before bed time. When dry nappies are consistently noted in the mornings, try child without nappies at night—a plastic sheet on the mattress is a good idea. Even when a child has been dry day and night for some time, accidents are common if child is tired, unwell, or unsettled—whether excited or unhappy.

**❶** If the child does not succeed within a few days then either try training pants or revert to nappies and try again at a later date.

## Toilet training for children with developmental delay

The same basic principles apply only at a later chronological age. Parents usually advised to watch for signs of child becoming aware of need to go to toilet, e.g. fidgeting, and for signs of physical readiness, e.g. dry for an hour or two and during naps. Parents may be advised to institute a toileting programme, i.e. a structured daily programme around that child's toileting habits, supported by visual signs to indicate each activity, e.g. take down pants, flush toilet, and reinforced with rewards.

## Related topics

📖 Constipation and encopresis, p. 260; 📖 Nocturnal enuresis, p. 290.

## Further information

Education and Resources for Improving Childhood Continence (ERIC) Potty Training Pages. Available at: ℘ www.eric.org.uk/PottyTraining/potty_training

National Autistic Society web pages on toileting training. Available at: ℘ www.nas.org.uk

National Child Birth Trust Advice on Potty Training. Available at: ℘ www.nct.org.uk/parenting/potty-training

# Understanding behaviour 1–5 years

Developing from a helpless baby to a relatively independent 4-yr-old is a time of great learning and emotion that can often feel very difficult for parents and carers. Toddlers and children are at an egocentric stage in their development, seeing themselves at the centre of the world, ready to be involved in everything, but often overwhelmed with feelings that they can't manage yet. Children react individually and very differently to the triumphs and set backs of each day, needing different types of support and understanding from parents and carers.

Children may become:
- *Bossy:* it's one way of covering up that they are still small and there are things they can't do. Often irritating to other children and adults, but they still need love and support.
- *Fussy:* e.g. fads and rituals. It's one way of asserting independence against adults. Adults need to demonstrate how to give in gracefully over things that are less important, e.g. wearing odd clothes. Sometimes, child is anxious or worried, but unable to talk about it so it's easier to control what goes on the plate than control the anxious feeling. These feelings come and go, but if behaviour becomes particularly difficult consider if there is a particular stress and address that.
- *Clingy and fearful:* it's one way of saying they still feel small, but can be trying to parents and carers. Like all children they need support, love, encouragement, but also more time to take those steps to independence. Important to take new things slowly, e.g. settling into play group, meeting new people.

## Key principles for parents
- Give positive attention (e.g. active listening, smiling, talking to, hugging) to the child in daily activities so they feel encouraged, supported, loved (📖 Promoting development in the under-fives, p. 197).
- Reward efforts, attempts, and good behaviour with smiles, words of praise, cuddles, etc.
- Help build self-esteem by letting children have a go at things.
- Relax and enjoy your children, do fun activities together.
- Reduce your own stress, e.g. create time away.
- When things get tense over behaviour:
  - Don't reward misbehaviour and encourage its continuation with lots of attention.
  - Make sure you stay in control of your own behaviour, leave the room if you are not.

See also 📖 Working with parents, p. 164 and 📖 Support for parenting programmes, p. 166.

## Temper tantrums

Children are coping with strong feelings all day. A temper tantrum is a display of how it feels on the inside at a point when they can no longer cope, are feeling exhausted, and haven't got the words to describe or deal with the feelings. In dealing with a tantrum parents should be advised to:

- Count to 10 before doing anything, unless child is putting themselves in danger.
- Stay calm, acknowledge child's feelings.
- Recognize child is beyond reasoning and do not get into an argument.
- Don't ask more of them than they can manage.
- Try to avoid saying hurtful things that you don't mean.
- Trying to hold or hug the child may make it worse. After it subsides cuddling may help reassure, while explaining it was not acceptable behaviour.

## New siblings

More than one child brings additional complexities to family life. A new baby is the choice of the parents not the siblings. Key principles of advice for parents:

- Prepare other child(ren) during the pregnancy.
- Recognize that the older child may feel sad, angry, or upset as they are no longer the centre of attention.
- The older child needs attention, reassurance, expressions of love, and time alone with parents.
- Find small, manageable ways for the older child to help with the new baby.

## Further information

Child Psychotherapy Trust Information Series of Leaflets on understanding childhood. Available at: ℘ www.understandingchildhood.net/

Familylives a national charity providing support and advice on all aspects of family life. Available at: ℘ http://familylives.org.uk/ Helpline: ☏ 0808 800 2222 24-h, 7 days/wk.

National Family and Parents Institute Family Information Publications. Available at: ℘ http://www.familyandparenting.org/All-Our-Publications/For-Families

# Speech and language acquisition

Children follow a systematic path to the effective use of language and communication skills (see 📖 Child development: 0–1 years, p. 170; and 📖 Child development: 1–5yrs, p. 193). Speech and language development is multidimensional, including speech, vocabulary, syntax, expression, and verbal comprehension. Speech, language, and communication difficulties can affect future learning and achievement, literacy, behaviour and social emotional functioning, confidence, and independence.

Speech and language is developed through parents and carers talking and listening to babies and young children. Primary care nurses and HV teams promote good interactive practice by advising parents to:
• Talk to the child when playing or doing things together.
• Have fun with nursery rhymes and songs, especially those with actions.
• Encourage the child to listen to different sounds, such as birds, animals.
• Gain child's attention when you want to talk together.
• Encourage child to communicate in any way, not just through words.
• Increase vocabulary by giving choices, e.g. 'Do you want an apple or banana?'.
• Talk about things as they happen, e.g. when bathing, shopping.
• Listen carefully and give child time to finish talking. Take turns to speak.
• Always respond in some way when the child says something.
• Help child to use more words by adding to what is said, e.g. if they said 'car' adult responds 'Yes, it's a red car driving down the road'.
• If child says something incorrectly, repeat it correctly, e.g. 'Goggy bited it'. 'Yes, the dog bit it, didn't he?'
• Try and have a special time with the child each day to play with toys and look at picture books together.

(Adapted from Royal College of Speech and Language Therapists, 2002[1]).

HV teams in most parts of UK are also involved in distributing free Bookstart packs of books to babies with guidance materials for parents and carers:

Interactive practice skills are also promoted in parenting skills programmes (📖 Support for parenting, p. 166), as well as in other types of group settings for parents and babies, e.g. mother and baby groups, postnatal groups, infant massage groups.

Babies and young children in bilingual families should be encouraged to speak both family languages and English. Bilingualism does not delay speech and language acquisition.

## Speech and language delay

Primary speech and language delays are those not attributed to other conditions such as hearing loss (📖 Hearing screening, p. 155) or other more general developmental disabilities. Difficulties may arise with receptive language, expressive language, social communication, speech, fluency, or voice. Estimated at 6%, but higher in some areas. Such delays are important as:

- Cause concern to parents.
- Often associated with behavioural and other difficulties in pre-school period.
- Constitute a risk factor for subsequent poor school performance, and for a wide range of personal and social difficulties.
- More common in ♂ than ♀.

Up to 60% of speech and language delays may resolve without treatment between the ages of 2 and 3yrs. However, we are unable to predict which children will spontaneously resolve at time of identification.

### Identification and action

- No universal screening test (📖 Child screening tests, p. 152), but nurses and HV teams should be alert to parental concerns and observe children's communication behaviours for evidence of delay (see also 📖 Overview of the healthy child programme, p. 146).
- On identification of speech or language delay nurses and HVs:
  - Check no other related problem, e.g. hearing.
  - Refer to speech and language therapy services according to local policy.
  - Offer advice on improving interactive communication. In some areas, nursery nurses in HV teams run learning to play sessions for parents and children.
  - Suggest or introduce parent/carer and child to socializing and play opportunities, e.g. one o'clock club, playgroup, mother and children group, childminder group (📖 Services for children, young people and families, p. 19).

## Reference

[1]Royal College of Speech and Language Therapists (2002). *Help Your Child To Talk*. Available at: 🌐 http://www.literacytrust.org.uk/assets/0000/1596/Helpyourchildtotalk.pdf

## Further information

Talking Point (Information and resources on children's communication for parents and professionals). Available at: 🌐 www.talkingpoint.org.uk/Parent.aspx

Talk to Your Baby Campaign with resources. Available at: 🌐 www.literacytrust.org.uk/talktoyourbaby/

Bookstart. Available at: 🌐 www.bookstart.org.uk

# Child development 5–11 years

Child development is the interaction between heredity and the environment (📖 Child health promotion, p. 144). Development is assessed as part of the child assessment framework (📖 The assessment of children, young people, and families, p. 148). Developmental progress is about the sequential acquisition of skills, and there is a range of time within which children acquire the skills indicated in Table 6.5.

Children are expected to achieve nationally defined skills and knowledge in a range of subjects specified in the national curriculums for state schools. In England and Wales: Key Stage 1 by age 7 and Key Stage 2 by age 11. Standard Assessment Tests (SATs) are taken in reading, writing, and mathematics in school year 2 (age 6–7yrs) and school year 6 (age 10–11yrs). In Scotland, each subject is described at 6 levels, starting at Level A. The majority of children are expected to reach Level B by the end of primary year 4.

Puberty follows a well-defined set of stages starting between 8.5 and 12.5yrs in girls and between 10 and 14yrs in boys. The first stage is breast development in girls and testicular development in boys (see 📖 Puberty and adolescence, p. 215). Girls with early onset of puberty while in primary school may need particular support in dealing with their difference from their peers. (See Table 6.5 for median age of development.)

## Further information

Cowie H. (2012). *From Birth to Sixteen: children's health, social, emotional and linguistic development.* London: Routledge.

Department for Education England. Available at: ℜ www.education.gov.uk

Education Scotland. Available at: ℜ www.educationscotland.gov.uk

Learning Wales. Available at: ℜ www.learning.wales.gov.uk.

**Table 6.5** Overview of median age of development in children 5–11yrs

|  | 5–7yrs | 7–11yrs |
|---|---|---|
| Gross motor | Increasing strength, e.g. running faster, jumping higher.<br>Increasing agility, e.g. stand on one leg longer, walk a narrow beam.<br>Increasing coordination, e.g. learns to ride a 2-wheel bike, learns to swim. | Strength, agility, stamina, and coordination continue to develop. Increasingly able to play in team sports. |
| Fine motor and vision | Fine motor skills further developed in manipulating smaller objects with more precision. Able to dress and undress. | Fine motor skills increasingly developed. Dressing, undressing and self-care skills much more developed. |
| Cognitive development | Increased linguistic skills. Conversations more complicated. Learning to read, write, and problem-solve.<br>Dominant mode of thought is tied to immediate circumstances and specific experiences. Beginning to grasp more abstract ideas, like numbers, time, and distance. | Abilities described in 5–7yrs continue to develop. Egocentrism reduces—greater ability with language leads to greater socialization.<br>More objective view of world and causes of physical events and their relationships. |
| Social, emotional, and behavioural | Increasing independence from adults and personal confidence.<br>Able to wash and bath with less supervision. Still needs help in brushing teeth properly.<br>Plays games with simple rules and many fantasy games.<br>Identifies with same-sex friends.<br>Peer acceptance and approval begins to become important. | Increased desire for independence at the same time as a continued need for parental support.<br>Friends still primarily of the same gender, but interest in opposite gender beginning.<br>Increasing joining into groups and sometimes cliques. Exclusion can feel devastating.<br>Increasingly competitive and self-conscious. Peer approval and acceptance continues to grow in importance. |

# Growth and nutrition 5–11 years

Growth is dependent on nutrition, good health, happiness, pituitary growth hormone, thyroid hormone, and vitamin D. 2–12yrs contributes about 40% of adult height, often in rapid growth spurts during puberty (📖 Puberty and adolescence, p. 215). Obesity is a major public health issue with a fifth of children in England aged 4–5yrs overweight or obese, rising to 1 in 3 by 10–11yrs.[1]

All those involved in measuring children should receive training, and understand local policies and guidance.

## Reasons for measuring school aged children?
- Indicator of health.
- Identify disorders in growth.
- Identify individual overweight and obesity.
- Monitor population levels of obesity in children as part of public health programmes, e.g. national child measurement programme.[2]

## When to weigh and measure
- *Height and weight:*
  - At school entry age 4–5yrs as part of child health promotion programme (📖 Overview of healthy child programme, p. 146).
  - National policies then apply, e.g. England as part of national child measurement programme in reception year (4–5yrs) and year 6 (10–11yrs).
  - Good practice as part of reviews of children with chronic illness, concerns about growth, or with special educational needs.

## How to measure
- *Weight:* remove heavy clothing and shoes on Class III clinical electronic scales.
- *Height:*
  - Without footwear using a rigid rule with T piece or stadiometer.
  - Bottom, back, and heels touching apparatus, ears and eyes at 90° to apparatus.
  - Measure on expiration.

## Recording
- Plotted as a small dot on UK WHO 2–18yrs boy or girl growth charts[3] and PHCHR.
- Also plotted on BMI conversion and on parental height comparator sections of chart if concern about growth.
- Adult height predictor can be plotted if child or parent wishes.

## Interpretation
- A child whose weight is average for their height will have a BMI between the 25th and 75th centiles, whatever their height centile.
- Most children are within 2 centile spaces of the mid-parental height centile.

- BMI >91st centile suggests overweight.
- Review by GP or community paediatrician if:
  - BMI > 98th centile (clinically obese).
  - BMI < 2nd centile may reflect under-nutrition, but may simply reflect a small frame or low muscle mass.
  - Child height centile more than 3 centile spaces below mid-parental centile.

## Nutrition

Estimated average requirements for energy: boys 7–10yrs 1970kcal/day, girls 7–10yrs 1740kcal/day. All children should be eating family food in a balanced healthy diet, i.e. 47–50% carbohydrates (preferably complex), 15% protein, 5+ portions of fruit and vegetables a day, some fats, and low in salty and sugary foods. Vegetarian diets need to ensure adequate protein, iron, and selenium, as well as adequate B12 for vegans. See also 📖 Nutrition and healthy eating, p. 304.

### Overweight

Overweight children should be encouraged to remain at a constant or slow increase, while their height increases through healthy eating and increased exercise. 📖 Overweight children and adolescents, p. 291.

### Food in schools

Parents can buy reduced cost milk daily for children in primary schools via the EU school milk subsidy scheme. Children whose parents receive low income benefits (📖 Benefits for mothers and those responsible for children, p. 793) are eligible for free school meals and sometimes free milk. Government set standards for nutrition in school provided meals. Many schools now have whole school food policies, incorporating a range of activities throughout the curriculum and school day.

### Food allergies   See 📖 Allergies, p. 647.

### Foods for children to avoid

- Shark, swordfish, and marlin because levels of mercury may affect development of nervous system.
- Girls should limit the portions (portion = 140g) of oily fish to 2 a week because of potential build-up of dioxins and polychlorinated biphenyls (PCBs) that may affect the development of any fetus in later life.

## Reference

[1]Health and Social Care Information Centre (2012). *Lifestyles Statistics National Child Measurement Programme: England, 2011/12 school year*. Available at: 🔎 www.hscic.gov.uk/home

## Key resources

[2]UK-WHO 2–18 years growth chart resources: charts, training materials, fact sheets. Available at: 🔎 www.rcpch.ac.uk

## Further information

British Nutrition Foundation. Available at: 🔎 www.nutrition.org.uk
Childrens Food Trust. Available at: 🔎 www.childrensfoodtrust.org.uk/
Food Standards Agency. Available at: 🔎 http://www.food.gov.uk/multimedia/pdfs/publication/eat-well0708.pdf

# Communication and learning problems

Around a fifth of school children require extra help at some point in their schooling, ♂ > ♀. Poor progress at school can be caused by a range of physical, social, and emotional problems, as well as problems in school or home environment. Children may also have specific communication and learning problems that require individual assessment, and support, that may include special education needs statements (📖 Children with special educational needs, p. 227).

## Dyslexia

Dyslexia is a combination of abilities and difficulties that affect the learning process in one or more of reading, spelling, and writing. Term often used interchangeably with 'specific learning difficulties' (SpLDs). It affects 3–5% of population, ♂ > ♀. It is a persistent condition, affecting children across the ability range. Accompanying difficulties often in areas of:

- Spoken language and motor skills.
- Speed of processing information and short-term memory.
- Organization and sequencing items.

If suspected, teachers consider specific educational support and involve SENCO. May requires assessment and recommendations for educational support by educational or chartered educational psychologist.

## Dyscalculia

Dyscalculia is the mathematical equivalent of dyslexia, i.e. difficulty in conceptualizing numbers, number relationships, outcomes of numerical operations, and estimation. If suspected, teachers consider specific educational support and involve SENCO. The child may require assessment and recommendations for educational support by educational or chartered educational psychologist. S/he may require speech and language therapy.

## Dyspraxia

Dyspraxia is the impairment of the organization of movement, may be associated with other problems of language, perception, and thought. It used to be known as clumsy child syndrome, developmental coordination disorder, or motor learning difficulties. It affects <2%, ♂ > ♀. Common features include:

- *Pre-school was late in reaching milestones:* e.g. rolling over, sitting, standing, walking, and speaking.
- Clumsiness, poor body awareness, poor posture, awkward gait.
- Difficulty hopping, skipping, riding bike, catching things.
- Reading and writing difficulties.
- Unable to remember or follow instructions, poorly organized.
- Better in one-to-one than group teaching situation.
- Speech production difficulties (developmental verbal dyspraxia).

If suspected, teachers consider specific educational support and involve SENCO. The child may require assessment and recommendations for educational support by educational or chartered educational psychologist. Also s/he may require speech and language therapy, physiotherapy, occupational therapy support.

## Dysfluency (stammering)

About 5% of all children will have some difficulty with their fluency during the development of their speech. About 80% of these will achieve normal fluency. Causes are multi-factorial. The problem can fluctuate from mild to severe depending on the situation, the time of day, or for some other unidentifiable reason. Often embarrassing or distressing to speaker so child will often adopt strategies to minimize or hide problems, e.g. not speaking in class or avoiding words that they stammer on. General advice for adults:

• Don't say the word or finish the sentence for the child.
• Be patient, don't ask multiple questions, give time for child to talk.
• Don't tell child to slow down or take a deep breath (becomes part of struggle to speak).
• Praise child for things that they are doing well.

General advice for child/young person:
• Take time, rather than rushing, speak a bit more slowly.
• Pause for a moment before starting to speak.
• Remember to think well done for having a go.

If parent and child agree there is a cause for concern then refer to speech and language therapist according to local policy.

## Further information

Afasic Information and resources for unlocking speech and language in each UK country. Available at: ℘ www.afasicengland.org.uk/
British Dyslexia Association. Available at: ℘ www.bdadyslexia.org.uk
Dyspraxia Foundation. Available at: ℘ www.dyspraxiafoundation.org.uk/
Action for Stammering Children. Available at: ℘ www.stammeringcentre.org

# Dental health in older children

Most children start to lose their primary teeth and gain their adult teeth at about 6yrs. By 12yrs most children will have 28 adult teeth. The four molars or wisdom teeth usually appear at 16–22yrs.

Surveys show that caries levels in 5-yr-old children show a marked geographic gradient with caries prevalence lowest in England, rising in Wales then Scotland, and highest in Northern Ireland. In each country, children from disadvantaged groups have the poorest dental health, and are more likely to have dental caries. There are country-specific dental public health programmes (see e.g. Child smile[1]).

Caries prevention: see 📖 Development and care of teeth, p. 185.

## Sports injuries and accidents

- Dentists can make mouthguards to protect teeth during contact sports, e.g. rugby.
- *Knocked out teeth:* advise to hold by tooth not root, if dirty rinse in milk or water, push gently back into socket or keep moist (in milk, water, or inside of mouth) until they can get to a dentist (NHS helplines can help with finding dentists OOH).

## Orthodontic treatment

Common dental problems include protruding upper front teeth, crowding, asymmetrical alignment, bite problems, impacted teeth. Children are referred by their dentist to a specialist for orthodontic treatment. NHS-funded if the need for treatment is sufficient. This may start in primary school years, but more commonly in teenagers.

### Treatment

- May include removable, fixed, and functional braces, removal of teeth, use of orthodontic headgear, retainers (for ensuring teeth remain in place after treatment).
- Takes between 18 and 24mths with appointments every 4–6wks.

### Day-to-day management

- Orthodontists give advice on managing discomfort when appliances altered (painkillers and soft diet for a day or two) and on dental hygiene (special toothbrushes and mouthwash).
- It is recommended that removable appliances are removed for contact sports, and that mouthguards should be worn over fixed appliances.
- Teenagers often feel very self-conscious about having to wear appliance. Adults need to be very supportive and encouraging not to become shy or withdrawn. Be alert to signs of teasing or bullying.

## Reference

[1]Childsmile (Dental health promotion programme for children in Scotland). Available at: 🔗 www.child-smile.org.uk/index.aspx

## Further information

British Dental Association. Available at: 🔗 www.bdasmile.org/index.cfm
British Dental Health Foundation. Available at: 🔗 www.dentalhealth.org.uk/
British Orthodontic Society. Available at: 🔗 British Orthodontic Society. Information for teenagers. Available at: 🔗 http://www.bos.org.uk/orthodonticsandyou/orthodonticsforteenagers

# Puberty and adolescence

## Adolescence

The period between childhood and adulthood broadly corresponds with the teenage years, a time of rapid physical development and deep emotional changes. These are exciting times, but also can be confusing and uncomfortable for child and parents. Young people:

- Become more independent, learn how to get on with other people, and gain a sense of identity that is distinct from that of the family.
- Make close relationships outside family, with friends of their own age. Friends and peer group identity very important to most.
- Parents become less important in their children's eyes as their life outside the family develops. They develop views of their own that are often not shared by their parents.

**Puberty** The period when 2° sexual characteristics develop and sexual organs mature. In healthy children starts 9–14yrs in ♂; 8–13 yrs in ♀.

### Girls

Oestrogens stimulate growth and development of reproductive organs, deposition of fat (to produce narrow shoulders, broad hips, breasts, external genitalia), body hair, softer texture skin. Sequence of changes:

- *Breast development:* is the first sign. Breast buds are the initial phase followed by breast growth with smooth contoured areola, then areola projects above the breast and breast tissue grows to adult shape.
- *Pubic hair growth and rapid height spurt:* (☐ Growth and nutrition 12–18yrs, p. 221) occur almost immediately after breast buds appear. Then axillary hair.
- *Menarche (first menstruation):* occurs between 9 and 16yrs, on average 2.5yrs after start of puberty, and signals end of growing (on average another 5cm height remain).

### Boys

Androgens, primarily testosterone, stimulate growth and development of the reproductive organs, body hair pattern, enlargement of the larynx, and muscles. Boys will begin to experience erections as soon as they start to mature sexually, often unconsciously. Sequence of changes:

- Testicular enlargement: the first sign.
- *Pubic hair growth:* follows testicular growth.
- *Testicular enlargement:* accompanied by growth in length then circumference of penis, darkening of scrotal skin.
- *Husky voice:* often first indicator of larynx enlargement that lowers pitch of voice by an octave.
- *Sequence of hair growth:* pubic, axillary, facial, thoracic, scapular, pinnal, nasal.
- *Height spurt:* occurs later and of greater magnitude than in girls (☐ Growth and nutrition 12–18yrs, p. 221).

Up to a ⅓ of boys around 12–14yrs will start to develop breasts that disappear later on. This is caused by lag in production of testosterone allowing female hormones to act, and can be a great worry and embarrassment. As soon as testosterone increases, the breast growth goes.

Most experience unconscious erections and ejaculation during their sleep ('wet dreams'). For the first time, sexual feelings become strong urges, which require conscious control.

**Both sexes** The development of body odour, acne, and mood changes.

*Body odour*
Two types of sweat glands:
• Eccrine glands produce sweat used to control body temperature.
• Apocrine glands only start working at puberty. Secrete a different type of odourless sweat in response to stress, excitement, and sexual excitement. When bacteria start decomposing it, a strong distinct smell is released, thus causing body odour.

*Sleep*
• Sleep patterns changed by both behaviour and hormonal changes.
• Enough sleep essential because hormone to stimulate growth spurt is released during sleep.
• Lack of sleep contributes to moodiness, impulsiveness, and depression.

*Spots*
• 80% of teens suffer to some degree. Boys more than girls because testosterone increases spots, whereas oestrogen prevents them.
• The face most common area, but can appear on the neck, upper back, shoulders, and chest.
• The cause is overactive sebaceous glands (🕮 Acne vulgaris, p. 240).

*Mood changes*
Teenagers experience mood swings. This could be the effect of raging hormones (particularly for girls in premenstrual hormone fluctuations), but also response to physical and emotional changes that leave them feeling uncertain and self-conscious. Moodiness changes as teenagers become more confident.

*Early or delayed puberty* See 🕮 Growth disorders, p. 280.

## Further information

BBC Science and Nature, Body and Mind Information on Puberty. Available at: ℘ www.bbc.co.uk/science/humanbody/body/interactives/lifecycle/teenagers/
Connexions provides careers advice and other information. Available at: ℘ www.connexions-direct.com
Directgov's section for teenagers. Available at: ℘ www.direct.gov.uk/en/YoungPeople/index.htm
Royal College of Psychiatrists Leaflet Surviving Adolescence—a toolkit for parents. Available at: ℘ www.rcpsych.ac.uk/expertadvice/youthinfo/parentscarers/growingup/adolescence.aspx
Teenage Health Freak. A site aimed at teenagers but relevant for health and youth workers. Available at: ℘ www.teenagehealthfreak.org
Youth Health Talk. Young people's real life experiences of health and lifestyle. Available at: ℘ www.youthhealthtalk.org/

# Health promotion in schools

Promoting health is part of the school curriculum in each country of the UK, although the emphasis varies in local areas. The science curriculum, which is a statutory requirement, includes a range of topics such as sexual health and substance abuse. Substance abuse includes the abuse of alcohol, tobacco, cannabis and other drugs, and solvent and volatile substance abuse. Sexual health includes issues related to contraception, pregnancy and sexually transmitted infections. School health services may contribute to this and Healthy Schools Programmes[1], as requested by the school (ￂ Working in schools, p. 38). In England and Wales, Sex and Relationship Education are statutory, but not in Scotland (ￂ Sex and relationship education, p. 223).

PSHE in England brings together personal, social, health education, work-related learning, careers, enterprise, and financial capability. There are two non-statutory programmes of study at Key Stages 3 and 4: personal wellbeing, and economic wellbeing and financial capability based on policy aims specified in the Childrens Act 2004 (ￂ Child health promotion, p. 144). In Wales and Scotland, themes are similar, but there are differences to the Personal Social Education programmes.

The PSHE health objectives for children 5–7yrs include:
- How to make simple choices that improve their health and wellbeing.
- To maintain personal hygiene.
- About process of growing from young to old and how people's needs change.
- The names of the main parts of the body.
- That all household products, including medicines, can be harmful.
- Rules for and ways of keeping safe, including basic road safety, and about people who can help them to stay safe.

The PSHE health objectives for children 7–11yrs include:
- The components of a healthy lifestyle, including the benefits of exercise and healthy eating.
- The importance of hygiene in stopping the spread of diseases.
- How the body changes approaching puberty.
- Substances and drugs that are legal and illegal, their effects and risks.
- To recognize the different risks in different situations and then decide how to behave responsibly, including sensible road use.
- How to recognize and resist pressures to behave in an unacceptable or risky way and how to ask for help.
- Basic emergency aid procedures.

The PSHE health objectives for children 11–14yrs include:
- To recognize and manage the physical and emotional changes that take place at puberty.
- How to keep healthy and what influences health, including the media.
- That good relationships, and a balance between work, leisure, and exercise can promote physical and mental health.

- Basic facts and laws about alcohol, tobacco (by 15yrs, 24% are regular smokers), illegal substances (experimentation starts around 13–14yrs), and the risks of misusing prescribed drugs.
- SRE (see ⬛ Sex and relationship education, p. 223) links with strategies to reduce teenage conceptions.
- To recognize and manage risk, and make safer choices about healthy lifestyles, different environments, and travel.
- How to recognize and resist pressures to behave in an unacceptable or risky way, and how to ask for help.
- Basic emergency aid procedures.

The PSHE health objectives for children 14–16yrs include:

- To think about the alternatives, long- and short-term consequences when making decisions about personal health.
- The causes, symptoms, and treatments for stress and depression, and to identify strategies for prevention and management.
- About the link between eating patterns and self-image, including eating disorders.
- About the health risks of alcohol and other substances.
- Making safer choices/understanding risk taking behaviours.
- SRE links with strategies to reduce teenage conceptions and STIs.
- To seek professional advice confidently and find information about health.
- Develop the skills to cope with emergency situations that require basic aid procedures, including resuscitation techniques.

## Reference

[1]National Healthy School Programme (England): Healthy Schools. Available at: ℘ www.education. gov.uk/schools/pupilsupport/pastoralcare/a0075278/healthy-schools

## Further information

PSHE Association. Available at: ℘ www.pshe-association.org.uk

England PSHE resources. Available at: ℘ www.education.gov.uk/schools/teachingandlearning/ curriculum/secondary/b00198880/pshee

Wales PSE. Available at: ℘ www.wales.gov.uk/psesub/home/resources/documents/ pseframework/?lang=en

Scotland PSE. Available at: ℘ www.scotland.gov.uk/Topics/Education/Life-Long-Learning/cld

Scotland Health promoting schools. Available at: ℘ www.healthpromotingschools.co.uk/

Welsh Network of Healthy School Schemes (WNHSS). Available at: ℘ www.cmo.wales.gov.uk/ content/work/schools/wnhss-e.htm

Drug Education Forum. Available at: ℘ www.drugeducationforum.com/

Family Planning Association factsheet on SRE. Available at: ℘ http://www.fpa.org.uk/professionals/ factsheets/sre

# Working with teenagers

Teenagers are coping with the ambiguity of not being a child or an adult. Professionals need to assess their biological, psychological, and social development so they interact relevantly and give appropriate responsibility without unacceptable risk. This is reflected in what they can do at particular ages:
- *Be held criminally responsible:* age 10yrs.
- *Buy cigarettes:* age 16yrs.
- *Drive a moped:* age 16yrs.
- *Join the armed forces:* age 16yrs.
- *Drive a light motorcycle or car:* age 17yrs.
- *Vote in an election:* age 18yrs.
- *Order alcohol in a public house:* age 18yrs.

## Teenage health care
Significant because:
- Health indicators for age group have improved very little in past 20yrs.
- Patterns of behaviour and use of services acquired at this point carry on into adult life.
- Teenagers are represented in key target areas of sexually-transmitted disease and teenage pregnancy.
- Adolescents assess risk differently from health professionals; peer pressure is more significant than long-term consequences.

## Services
Services should be age appropriate, responsive to their needs. Teenagers use general services in hospitals, surgeries, and health centres, and those designed specifically for them, SN drop-ins, child and adolescent mental health services, and young people's sexual health clinics. Encouraging teenagers to take responsibility for their own health, professionals face the challenge of encouraging teenagers to use mainstream services—peer educators, teenagers who work along side those of a similar age and background may facilitate this. Ideally, they appreciate different health services in one relaxed setting without appointment systems.

### Any contact needs to
- Foster a spirit of partnership identifying needs of the young person (e.g. stress, body piercing and menstruation), as well other high profile issues (nutrition, sexual health, mental health, and substance misuse).
- Have confidentiality explained and guaranteed except in case of child protection issues, when it might be broken.
- Let the young person increasingly take decisions appropriate to his/her age and development. Consenting to health interventions (Fraser competencies) is dependent on age and understanding of the issues. See also ⃞ Consent, p. 77; also in ⃞ Contraception: general, p. 359.
- Focus on communication, establishing rapport and an honest open relationship by listening, questioning, understanding, responding, explaining, and summarizing. Teenagers value staff being approachable and positive in attitude.
- Empower young people to set and achieve their own goals.

Individual contact with teenagers needs to go alongside national and community approaches. This might include banning of smoking in public places, the wider availability of contraception, and whole school approaches impacting on nutrition in the school canteen.

## Further information

Teenage Health Freak. A site aimed at teenagers but relevant for health and youth workers. Available at: ℰ www.teenagehealthfreak.org

The Connexions site that gives information and advice to help young people make decisions and choices. Available at: ℰ www.connexions-direct.com/

Viner R. (2002). *ABC of Adolescence*. London: BMJ Books.

UK's free, confidential helpline service for young people under 25 who need help, but don't know where to turn. Available at: ℰ www.getconnected.org.uk/

# Growth and nutrition 12–18 years

The pubertal growth spurt is the 4th phase of human growth. Sex hormones cause the back to lengthen, adding 15% to final height, and fuse the epiphyseal growth plates. If puberty is early (not uncommon in girls) the final height is reduced because of early fusion of epiphyses.

## Nutrition

All young people should eat a balanced healthy diet. Short-term this helps appearance (shiny hair, healthy skin) and in the long-term protects against cardiovascular disease and osteoporosis. Energy requirements ↑:

- Boys: 11–14yrs 2220kcal/day; 15–18yrs 2755kcal/day.
- Girls: 11–14yrs 1845kcal/day; 15–18yrs 2110kcal/day.

Protein requirements ↑ by approximately 50%. Calcium requirements higher than adults: ♂ 1000mg; ♀ 800mg a day as skeletal development is rapid. Once menstruation starts girls need 14.8mg of iron a day compared to 8.7mg for boys.

### Key issues in teenagers

- About 60% regularly skip breakfast (breakfast cereals and breads are fortified with vitamins and minerals).
- Inadequate nutrients (particularly vitamins and minerals) in diet, and fats feature highly for energy sources. About 50% ♀ 15–18yr do not have adequate nutrients (especially iron and calcium) in diet.
- 46% ♂ and 69% ♀ 15–18yrs spending less than recommended 1hr/day in activities of moderate intensity.
- Increasing use of unsuitable methods control weight, e.g. skipping meals, very low energy dieting, and smoking.
- Vegetarianism more common among teenagers (more ♀), but with a poor understanding of how to achieve a balanced diet with adequate protein, iron, selenium.

### Monitoring

Routine monitoring of weight and height beyond reception class entry (4–5yrs) and year 6 (England only) is not recommended. Good practice to record height and weight in any young person over whom there is a concern, or has chronic ill health. Use UK-WHO 2–18yrs growth charts to assess growth and any problem.[1]

## Key nutrition and obesity prevention messages

Best delivered through media that reach young people, in peer settings, through PSHE curriculum and healthy schools initiatives. Includes:

- Base your meals on starchy foods.
- Eat lots of fruit and vegetables (at least 5 portions a day).
- Eat moderate amounts of protein, iron-rich foods, low-fat diary produce, more fish.
- Don't skip breakfast.
- Get active and minimize sitting activities.
- Cut down on saturated fat and sugar.
- Try to eat less salt: no more than 6g/day.
- Drink plenty of water.

*Foods for young people to avoid*
- Shark, swordfish, and marlin because levels of mercury may affect development of nervous system,
- Girls should limit portions of oily fish to 2/wk because of the potential build-up of dioxins and PCBs that may affect the development of any fetus in later life.[2]

## Other nutrition issues

*Food in schools*
- <16yrs whose parents receive state benefits for low income are eligible for free school meals (📖 Benefits for mothers and those responsible for children, p. 793).
- Many schools now have whole school food policies, incorporating a range of activities throughout the curriculum and school day.

*Food allergies* See 📖 Allergies, p. 647.

*Weight management* See 📖 Overweight children and adolescents, p. 291.

*Eating disorders:* See 📖 People with eating disorders, p. 431.

## Further information

British Nutrition Foundation. Available at: ℘ www.nutrition.org.uk
Vegetarian Society Young Veggie. Available at: ℘ www.youngveggie.org
NHS Choices. When your child is overweight. Available at: ℘ www.nhs.uk/Livewell/loseweight/Pages/child-overweight.aspx
NICE guideline 43. Obesity: the prevention, identification and management of overweight and obesity in adults in children guidance. Available at: ℘ www.nice.org.uk/CG43

## Key resources on growth measurement in young people

[1]UK-WHO 2–18 years growth chart resources: charts, training materials, fact sheets. Available at: ℘ www.rcpch.ac.uk
[2]Food Standards Agency. Available at: ℘ www.food.gov.uk

# Sex and relationship education

SRE takes place in schools and may involve health professionals, particularly SNs and sexual health outreach nurses. Given that some children are not in school because of exclusion or truancy, or are withdrawn by parents from this potentially sensitive subject, educational input in other settings (e.g. home, youth group, or a community group) is to be encouraged. Government guidance states SRE should be part of PSHE and citizenship. All schools (primary and secondary) must have a written policy on sex education developed with parents and agreed by the school governors. Opinions are often strongly held as to how SRE should be taught or if it should be taught at all. Any SRE has to be as stated within the school policy. Most agree that SRE should begin before children reach puberty. Discussion of relationships in its widest sense is appropriate from school entry and before.

SRE seeks to help and support young people through their physical, emotional, and moral development. SRE is about the importance of stable and loving relationships, respect, love, and care, as well as teaching about sex, sexuality, and sexual health. SRE is seen as important in contributing to a reduction in the number of teenage conceptions.

## Elements of SRE
- *Attitudes and values including:*
  - Issues of individual conscience.
  - Value of family life.
  - Nurturing of children.
- *Personal and social skills including:*
  - How to manage emotion.
  - Developing respect for self and others.
  - Realizing the consequences of own choices.
  - Recognizing and avoiding exploitation and abuse.
- *Knowledge and understanding including:*
  - Physical development at particular stages.
  - Understanding human sexuality, reproduction, sexual health, emotion, and relationships.
  - Contraception, avoidance of pregnancy, and protection from sexually transmitted diseases.
  - Reasons for choosing to delay or commence a sexual relationship.

## Delivery of SRE
Whoever is involved in providing SRE, the following contribute to positive evaluations:
- Established skills in facilitating groups.
- Relevant and up-to-date knowledge in relation to sexual health and supporting resources.
- Motivation to lead the session.
- Positive attitudes and values in relation to sexual behaviour.
- The use of discussion as a teaching strategy. Young people do not like the emphasis on physical aspects of reproduction, preferring the opportunity to discuss feelings, relationships, and values.
- A safe environment facilitated by agreed ground rules and depersonalization of the issues.

## Issues to consider

- *Single sex groups:* single sex groups more appropriate for some issues at some points.
- *Confidentiality* (📖 Confidentiality, p. 86): a statement of confidentiality needs to be discussed with whole class, exhibited and adhered to by all involved.
- *Age of consent:* sexual activity with <16yrs is illegal yet the average age of onset of sexual activity is now about 17yrs with 20% commencing before 16yrs. Concerns will be raised by sexual activity involving a young person <13yrs or a significantly older partner.
- *Sexual orientation:* some teaching staff have been concerned they will be accused of promoting homosexuality. Good practice requires that questions are dealt with honestly and sensitively, but there should not be direct promotion of any sexual orientation.

## CPD

SN and HV education programmes will have prepared staff to work with groups of young people. CPD programmes in PHSE are available to nurses.[1]

## Reference

[1]National PSHE CPD Programme. Available at: ℘ www.babcock-education.co.uk/4S/PSHE-CPD

## Further information

Sex Education Forum at the National Children's Bureau, is the national authority on sex and relationship education. Available at: ℘ www.sexeducationforum.org.uk

Personal Social Health & Economic Education Association. Available at: ℘ www.pshe-association.org.uk/

NHS Choices Sex and Young People. Available at: ℘ www.nhs.uk/Livewell/Sexandyoungpeople/Pages/Sex-and-young-people-hub.aspx

# Children with complex health needs and disabilities

About 6% of UK children are disabled and the prevalence of severe disability is increasing[1]. Up to 6000 children living at home are dependent on assistive technology. A number of issues have still to be addressed to ensure these young people reach their full potential, e.g. 29% of disabled children live in poverty, educational achievements are lower than their peers, only 4% of disabled children are supported by social services. The term disabled children is used here to include children and young people with learning disabilities, autistic spectrum disorders, sensory impairments, physical impairments, and emotional/behavioural disorders. The aim as specified in country policies (see 🕮 Child health promotion, p. 144) is to ensure children with disabilities and complex health needs and their families:

- Are supported to participate fully in family and community life.
- Receive integrated multi-agency assessments, leading to timely, responsive care plans and interventions that support the child to reach their full potential.
- Children, young people, and their families are actively involved in those decisions.

## Integrated assessment and care planning

Increasingly local areas have integrated health, education, and social care services, e.g. specialist children services (community based involving a variety of LA and health teams), child development centres (multi-disciplinary assessment and treatment centres often in hospital premises), and child development teams (community-based MDTs). The rationale is to provide a coordinated assessment and care plan. Child development teams commonly include:

- Community paediatricians specializing in child development.
- Specialist HVs.
- SLTs, OTs, and physiotherapists.
- Home-based learning support teachers and nursery nurses, e.g. Portage.
- Orthoptist.
- Educational psychologist.
- Social worker.

## Key principles for working with children and families

- Early identification through antenatal screening (🕮 Antenatal care and screening, p. 380), child health promotion programme (🕮 Overview of healthy child programme, p. 146), response to parental concern, follow-up of high-risk newborn babies.
- Integrated diagnosis and assessment processes.
- Early interventions through home-based learning services, e.g. Portage, as well as interventions to support optimal physical and cognitive development, while promoting child and family's inclusion in community.

- Coordination between primary, secondary, and tertiary health care.
- Provision of a key worker/care manager recognized by others in multi-disciplinary service environment to ensure delivery of services is coordinated, family has access to all services, and becomes first point of contact if problems arise.
- Supporting parents and families as carers (☐ Carers assessment and support, p. 412).
- *Promote social inclusion by:*
  - Ensuring family have knowledge about all benefits (☐ Benefits and support, p. 789), and charities that can help, e.g. the Family Fund.
  - Access to mainstream public services and children services including social services, therapy services, and Child and Adolescent Mental Health Services (CAMHS) as these children are more vulnerable to mental health problems than others.
  - Reduce impact of multiple health care appointments on school and family life.
  - Access to suitable housing, equipment, and assistive technology.
  - Access to play, sport, leisure, and holiday facilities.
- Access to appropriate educational opportunities.

In addition:
- All professionals need to be aware that these children are at greater risk of abuse than other children, particularly if they live away from home (☐ Child protection, p. 230).
- Transition from child to adult services needs particular care in planning as, in many cases, it is poorly coordinated resulting in a decline in support and deterioration in health and social inclusion.

For some children their condition may require adequate consideration of palliative care needs (☐ Palliative care in the home, p. 509) and additional support to family and carers through this period and on a child's death (☐ Bereavement, grief, and coping with loss, p. 528).

## Planning for children and families
Under the Children Act 1989, the LA must keep a register of all children with disabilities in that area. However, it is a voluntary decision whether the child or young persons details are added.

## Reference
[1] Office for Disability Issues, Disability prevalence fact sheet. 2012. ℳ http://odi.dwp.gov.uk/disability-statistics-and-research/disability-facts-and-figures.php

## Further information
Contact a Family UK for families with disabled children. Available at: ℳ www.cafamily.org.uk/
Disabled Living Foundation advice on daily living equipment for children. Available at: ℳ www.livingmadeeasy.org.uk/children/
Family Fund Charity for disabled children and their families. Available at: ℳ www.familyfund.org.uk/
Office for Disability Issues. *Disability prevalence fact sheet 2012.* Available at: ℳ http://odi.dwp.gov.uk/disability-statistics-and-research/disability-facts-and-figures.php

# Children with special educational needs

Children with SEN are defined as having considerably greater difficulty in learning than others of the same age, as well as children who cannot use the educational facilities their peer group use because of their disability. Children under school age who fall into either category without extra help are also included.

## Codes of practice (UK)

Each country sets out the key principles for identifying, assessing, and reviewing children with SEN and the role of different agencies. Codes of practice are slightly different in each country and are under review, but all follow similar principles:

- All emphasize working in partnership with parents and child/pupil involvement.
- Emphasis on early identification (but full assessments <2yrs rare).
- Places emphasis on inclusion of children with SEN in mainstream schools.

## Involvement of health services

- *In early years:* the child health services must alert the parents and the local education authority (LEA) to the child's potential difficulties. A child development centre or team may provide a multi-professional view at an early stage.
- All education settings need to know how, with parental consent, to obtain information and advice on health-related matters, using school health service, GP, or a relevant member of child development centre or team.
- Each health area has to designate a medical officer (usually a community paediatrician) to work with LEA on behalf of children with SEN and to lead the health services contribution to the statutory assessment process.

## Graduated educational assessments for children >2yrs

*3 levels*

- *Early years and school action:* early years staff or teachers identify child who needs extra support. Parents and SENCO consulted, agree a plan for extra support. Written in individual education plan (IEP), reviewed twice a year with parents.
- *Early years and school action plus:* this level involves outside support services or more specialist advice being sought to help a child's development or additional needs. Requested after meeting with parents.
- *Requests for a statutory assessment:* if levels above not adequate to additional needs. The education provider, with the parents and anyone else involved with the child, should consider a request to the LEA for a statement. Request can be made by a parent. LEA may consider request and decide not to proceed. Parents have right of appeal.

## Statutory assessment

A detailed multi-professional examination includes educational, medical and psychological advice, and advice from social services and from other agencies. Parents are also asked to give a report and given a named LEA officer to help record their views and information. An assessment also includes, where possible, the views of the child.

## Statement of SEN and provision

If a child needs extra provision to meet his/her SEN, a proposed statement is made and sent to parents. Statement includes: proposed educational provision (e.g. extra help, school placement, extra equipment) and non-educational provision (e.g. SLT and social services). Parents have the right to negotiate, put their views forward, and appeal if they disagree. Once proposed statement is agreed, LEA issues a final statement, which the LEAs must provide from the date of statement. The Special Educational Needs and Disability Tribunal (SENDIST) is an independent tribunal, which hears parents' appeals against LEA decisions affecting children with SEN and disabilities.

## Annual review

All statements must be reviewed at least annually (>5yrs every 6mths), involving parents, and the child or young person. The LEA requests the review, usually coordinated by SENCO. A medical advice form has to be completed by designated medical officer, specialist doctors, CAMHS if involved. Two reviews are of particular note:

- Year 6 timed so parents know by February which secondary school their child will attend.
- Year 9 annual review is used to develop transition plan for moving into further education, training or employment. It is multi-agency, including services, such as Connexions Service and other agencies with a major role in the young person's post-school life, such as health and social services.

## Further information

Department of Education Northern Ireland Special Educational Needs. Available at: ℘ www.deni. gov.uk/index/support-and-development-2/special_educational_needs_pg.

DfE England Special Educational Needs and Disability. Available at: ℘ http://www.education.gov. uk/childrenandyoungpeople/

Scottish Government Manual of Good Practice in meeting Special Educational Needs. Available at: ℘ www.scotland.gov.uk/Publications/2004/02/19009/33932

UK government overview of children with special educational needs. Available at: ℘ www.gov.uk/ children-with-special-educational-needs/

# Child and adolescent mental health

Psychological wellbeing in children and young people is well recognized as essential for health, development, and resilience. Mental health problems can be observed in difficulties in capacity for play and learning, personal relationships, psychological development, and in distress and maladaptive behaviour. Mental health problems affect about one in 10 children and young people. When they persist, are severe, and affect functioning they are defined as mental health disorders. Approximately 10–15% of 15-yr-olds have a diagnosable mental health disorder, e.g. depression, psychosis. Similar numbers are thought to have less serious mental health problems. It is important to be especially aware of these problems in three groups:

- Looked-after children are 5x more likely to have mental health disorder than peers (💭 Looked-after children, p. 235).
- Children and young people with learning disabilities (💭 Learning disabilities, p. 144).
- About 40% of young offenders found to have a diagnosable mental health disorder.

It is recognized that everyone has a role in ensuring the environment in which children grow up in promotes their mental health. Policies encourage health, education, and public services to:

- Tackle bullying and racism.
- Increase awareness of mental health issues.
- Improve the recognition of children's emerging needs.
- Provide support for those children with particular needs.

Child health promotion (💭 Child health promotion, p. 144) policies make it explicit how HV, SN, and primary care services should promote child mental health and link to specialist services:

- *Primary level of care (tier 1):* includes all services contributing to mental health care of children and young people, e.g. GPs, HVs, SNs, social workers, teachers, juvenile justice workers, voluntary agencies. Focus on the initial assessment and identification of difficulties, may include advice or the provision of therapeutic help not requiring specialist training.
- *Specialist individuals, teams and in-patient services (tiers 2–4):* likely to include child and adolescent psychiatrists, clinical psychologists, nurses, psychotherapists, OTs, SLTs, art, music, and drama therapists, family therapists.

All policies emphasize the need for clear, coordinated care pathways for referrals as well as training and support to primary care professionals.

## Further information

Anti-bullying alliance resources and links for public and professionals across UK. Available at: 🖰 www.anti-bullyingalliance.org.uk

Child and Adolescent Mental Health for professionals, young people and parents. Available at: 🖰 www.camh.org.uk/

Young Minds charity provides information for public and professionals on mental health and mental problems of children and young people. Available at: 🖰 www.youngminds.org.uk/

# Child protection

Protecting (or safeguarding) children is a duty of care for all organizations who are required to have criminal records checks through the Disclosure and Barring Service (DBS) on all volunteers and employees coming into contact with children.

In the UK, inquiries into child deaths from abuse and neglect show that:
- Most occur in what is perceived to be a context of low-level need (📖 The assessment of children, young people, and families, p. 148).
- The agency most likely to be involved is the health service.
- Common professional failings include:
  - Inadequate sharing of information.
  - Poor assessment processes.
  - Lack of clarity about roles and responsibilities.
  - Poor recording of information.
  - Failure to keep the child in focus.

## National frameworks

*Working Together to Safeguard Children—England*, sets out the parameters of good practice:
- Be alert to indicators of abuse or neglect (📖 Identifying the child in need of protection, p. 232).
- Be alert to the risks that individuals may pose to children.
- Share information that relates to concerns about child safety and welfare (📖 Confidentiality, p. 86).

❶ Familiarize yourself with:
- The government guidance.[1]
- The local child protection procedures agreed through the local Safeguarding Children Board (England) or Area Child Protection Committee.

These detail exactly what individuals and agencies must do when abuse is suspected.

### Sources of advice and support

Every health provider has to have a safeguarding team, named doctor and nurse, to offer advice and support to employees with regard to children about whom they have concerns.

Every Local Safeguarding Children Board (LSCB)/ LA area has a designated doctor and nurse to offer advice and support regarding children at risk of harm, and to support commissioning services.

❶ Find out the names of the specialist nurse and designated doctor for child protection and how to contact them.

## What nurses should do in cases where abuse is suspected

- *Discuss* with senior colleagues as appropriate.
- *Decide* whether the child needs:
  - Immediate protection; and/or
  - Urgent medical attention.

*If the answer to either is yes*
- Contact social services or the police, and relevant medical service.
- Discuss concern with parent/carer and child, unless it is unsafe to do so. In some cases it could ↑ risk to child.
- Record all relevant information and action taken.

*If the answer is no*
- Discuss concern with parent/carer.
- Listen carefully to the child.
- Consult colleagues who know the child/family, such as social worker, GP, HV, or teacher. There may be earlier or ongoing concerns.
- Record suspicions and evidence that supports them.
- Decide whether to refer to social services.
- Seek advice if necessary from one of the named or designated child protection nurses or doctors or other experienced colleague.

## Referral to social services

Social services have the statutory responsibility for making enquiries into child protection referrals and coordinating the inter-agency response (📖 Child protection processes, p. 234).

*When making a referral to social services*
- Discuss concerns with social worker and confirm referral in writing within 48h.
- Record whether parent has been informed and, if not, why.
- Follow-up outcome to referral to establish that it has been understood and responded to appropriately.

## Reference

[1]HM Government (2013). *Working Together to Safeguard Children*. Available at: ℘ www.education. gov.uk/publications/standard/publicationDetail/Page1/DFE-00030-2013

## Further information

Barker J, Hodes D. (2004). *A Child in Mind, A Child Protection Handbook*. London: Routledge.
DFE England. Working together to safeguard children. Available at: ℘ www.education.gov.uk/ aboutdfe/statutory/g00213160/working-together-to-safeguard-children
NI DHSSPS Child Protection. Available at: ℘ www.dhsspsni.gov.uk/index/hss/child_care/child_ protection.htm
NSPCC online child protection resource. Available at: ℘ www.nspcc.org.uk/inform/
Powell C. (2011). *Safeguarding and Child Protection for Nurses, Midwives and Health Visitors: A Practical Guide*. Maidenhead: Open University Press.
Scottish Government Child Protection. Available at: ℘ www.scotland.gov.uk/Topics/People/ Young-People/protecting/child-protection
Welsh Government Child Protection. Available at: ℘ http://wales.gov.uk/topics/childrenyoun gpeople/health/protection/?lang=en

# Identifying the child in need of protection

Sustained abuse or neglect can have a major impact on all aspects of a child's health, wellbeing, and development. Assessment should be made within the child assessment framework (📖 A child or young person in need, p. 150).

## Factors that ↑ risk of abuse or neglect

- If parent/carer has a history of any of the following:
  - Drug and/or alcohol misuse.
  - Domestic violence.
  - Mental health problems.
  - Learning difficulties.
  - Abuse in their own childhood.
- The risk is further ↑ if:
  - Poor attachment to child, e.g. intolerant and/or indifferent.
  - Non-compliance, e.g. parent denies there is a problem and/or refuses to engage with professional network.
- If child is:
  - A premature or low birth weight infant.
  - A multiple birth (e.g. twins) or <18mths between siblings.
  - A child with a disability.
  - Born unwanted and/or unplanned.
  - A child not attending school.
  - A looked-after child.

## Evidence of harm

Harm means ill-treatment or the impairment of health or development. Ill-treatment is classified under four categories of abuse and neglect.

Evidence that a child is being harmed is obtained by:
- *Observation of signs in child*, e.g.
  - Unexplained bruising or bruising in unusual places.
  - Injuries with inconsistent explanations or inappropriate to developmental age.
  - Appears afraid, quiet, withdrawn.
  - Appears constantly tired, hungry, or dirty.
- *Observation of perpetrator* acting aggressively, violently, or in a sexual manner to child or young person.
- *Allegation* from a child or another person.
- *Disclosure* from a child or someone who says they are harming a child.

## Ill-treatment

### Physical abuse

Physical abuse is violence directed towards children, including hitting, shaking, suffocating, burning, poisoning. *Points to remember:*
- The younger the child the ↑ risk from physical abuse.
- Sometimes minor injuries signal something more serious.
- Domestic violence (📖 Domestic violence, p. 402) and child abuse coexist in most cases and can begin in pregnancy.

### Child sexual abuse

Child sexual abuse is sexual molestation of children by adults or older children. It involves forcing or enticing a child or young person to take part in activities that lead to the sexual arousal of the perpetrator. *Points to remember:*

- It is an abuse of power that often relates to age difference.
- Perpetrator is usually known to child, probably a family member.
- Most perpetrators deny abuse and refuse treatment programmes.

### Emotional abuse

Emotional abuse is a relationship between a child and parent that is characterized by harmful interactions that convey to the child that they are worthless or unloved. Integral to all forms of abuse and neglect, but also occurs alone. *Points to remember:*

- Under-reported, despite easily identifiable negative parent/child interactions.
- Sustained abuse has impact on long-term mental health, self-esteem, and behaviour.

### Neglect

Neglect is the persistent failure to meet a child's basic physical and emotional needs (🕮 Child health promotion, p. 144), and the failure to provide or respond to the changing needs of a growing child. *Points to remember:*

- Neglect is the most prevalent form of child maltreatment.
- Neglect is usually chronic and rarely a single incident.
- Mental health problems, learning difficulties, and substance misuse are common in the histories of the parents (🕮 Children in special circumstances, p. 160).

## Further information

NSPCC online child protection resource. Available at: 🖱 www.nspcc.org.uk/inform

Powell C. (2011). *Safeguarding and Child Protection for Nurses, Midwives and Health Visitors: A Practical Guide.* Maidenhead: Open University Press.

### Information and advice for children

ChildLine: ☏ 0800 1111.

### Information and advice for adults

Familylives: ☏ 0808 8025544.
NSPCC helpline: ☏ 0808 800 5000. Available at: 🖱 www.nspcc.org.uk

# Child protection processes

All countries have legislation and agreed frameworks for these processes. Following a referral reporting a concern about a child, social services will:
• Carry out an initial enquiry and assessment.
• Decide whether to hold a child protection conference.

## The child protection conference

Convened by social services, it is a confidential meeting of parents, social workers, health and other professionals involved with the family, and the police. Its purpose is:
• To share information and assess risk to the child.
• To decide whether to place child's name on the child protection register. If the decision is 'yes', then a review conference has to be held within 6mths.
• To draw up a protection plan to safeguard the child, including:
  • Support and services to be provided to child and family.
  • Changes required to ↓ risk.
  • How social services will monitor the child's welfare.

## Information sharing and confidentiality

Sharing confidential information is essential (📖 Confidentiality, p. 86). In many cases, it is only when information is shared that it becomes clear that a child is at risk.

*Points to remember*
• Disclose information relevant to safeguarding the child. This will be about:
  • Health and development of a child and her/his exposure to harm.
  • A parent/carer who is unable to care adequately for a child.
  • Other individuals who may present a risk to the child.
• Share information on a 'need-to-know' basis.
• If in doubt, consult one of the named or designated nurses or other experienced colleague.

## Further information

Powell C. (2011). *Safeguarding and Child Protection for Nurses, Midwives and Health Visitors: A Practical Guide*. Maidenhead: Open University Press.

NSPCC online child protection resource. Available at: ℘ www.nspcc.org.uk/inform/

DFE England. Working together to safeguard children. Available at: ℘ www.education.gov.uk/aboutdfe/statutory/g00213160/working-together-to-safeguard-children

The Scottish Government Child Protection. Available at: ℘ www.scotland.gov.uk/Topics/People/Young-People/protecting/child-protection

The Welsh Government Child Protection. Available at: ℘ http://wales.gov.uk/topics/childrenyoungpeople/health/protection/?lang=en

NI DHSSPS Child Protection. Available at: ℘ www.dhsspsni.gov.uk/index/hss/child_care/child_protection.htm

*Advice and information for parents and children*
ChildLine: ☎ 0800 1111.
NSPCC helpline: ☎ 0808 800 5000. Available at: ℘ www.nspcc.org.uk

# Looked-after children

Children in the care of LAs are described as 'looked-after children'. They live in a variety of settings, including foster care, residential care homes, kinship care, residential school, or young offender units. Children who are looked after generally have greater health needs than their peers. Many of them (62%) will have become looked after as a result of abuse or neglect, and a further 20% are looked after because of family dysfunction or distress. They are among the most vulnerable children in the UK:

- High percentage have mental health problems 4× higher than for all children.[1]
- High percentage parents by the age of 20yrs.
- High percentage of young women become mothers before the age of 18yrs.

The aim is to support children back into care of families where that is possible. About 40% return home within 6mths, but 60% are looked after for longer.

Recent substantial criticism that public authorities are failing these children. Current policy aims to:

- Improve the stability of placements and continuity of at least one carer.
- Increase adoption orders and special guardianship orders.
- Improve educational attainments of those looked after longer >6mths.
- Improve health and access to health care, particularly CAMHS.

## Health needs

Many of these children have increased health needs in comparison to those with their families from comparable socio-economic backgrounds. These may arise from:

- Living in families affected by alcohol, domestic violence, or drugs.
- A disability or special needs.
- Having a highly mobile family.
- Poorer access to universal services, such as dental services, immunizations, routine child health surveillance, and health promotion.
- Grief and loss through experience of leaving family and being placed in care.

## Improving health care

The LA should notify the relevant health organization of each child moving in or leaving area. Each area has a designated community paediatrician(s) and designated nurse(s) for looked-after children. They are responsible for ensuring:

- A holistic health assessment (including health promotion) by a doctor as soon as practicable after a child starts to be looked after.
- The health assessment is recorded, a health plan is included in care plan for the child; child and/or carer holds a personal health record.
- Subsequent health reviews undertaken by nurse, 2–5yrs at least every 6mths, >5yrs at least annually.

- Children/carers are able to access universal health (e.g. GP) and health promotion services and records are 'fast tracked' if moving placement.
- All young people leaving care should have access to a leaving care health service, which includes access to a GP and dental services.
- Issues of particular risk in this group, i.e. unsafe sex, self-harming, substance and alcohol misuse, are addressed for each young person.

Each health professional who comes into contact with children or young people in this situation is expected to consider the widest range of health and health promotion needs of the young person.

## Adoption

Up to 5000 children are waiting for permanent new families at anytime. Fostering is a temporary arrangement, although sometimes it may be the plan until the child grows up. An Adoption Order severs all legal ties with the birth family and confers parental rights and responsibilities onto the new adoptive family (can be married, single, unmarried couple of any sexuality). Adoption is through an adoption agency, usually social services, but also voluntary agencies, e.g. Barnardos.

### Applicants
- Screened for suitability (including requesting information from GP).
- Matched to children (via the Adoption Register in England and Wales).

### Proposed matches
- Presented to an adoption panel, who decides whether to proceed with placement.
- Child moves to live with new parent/s after planned period of introductions, with support of social worker.
- Court cannot make an adoption order until child has lived with adopters for at least 13wks (19wks if newborn).
- A number of organizations provide support for new adoptive parents and children e.g. British Association of Fostering and Adoption.

All adopted children receive the usual child health promotion programme (📖 Overview of health child programme, p. 146) and any additional services in response to particular needs.

Note: international adoption has different regulations.[2]

## References
[1]NICE. Looked after children and young people (PH28). Available at: 🔗 http://guidance.nice.org.uk/PH28
[2]Intercountry Adoption Centre. Available at: 🔗 www.icacentre.org.uk/

## Further information
British Association of Fostering and Adoption. Available at: 🔗 www.baaf.org.uk/
DfE Children in Care Guidance. Available at: 🔗 www.education.gov.uk/childrenandyoungpeople/families/childrenincare/regs
NSPCC online looked after children resource. Available at: 🔗 www.nspcc.org.uk/inform/
Scottish Government. Looked after Children. Available at: 🔗 www.scotland.gov.uk/Topics/People/Young-People/protecting/lac

# Child and adolescent common health problems

# The sick baby and child

Minor illnesses, e.g. viral URTI, are commonplace. Most <5yrs have at least five viral URTI a year. Parents need to be reassured, as well as informed on how to manage minor illness and recognize signs for seeking medical attention. Ill babies and children become pale, listless, and do not want to eat.

## Advice for parents on managing minor illness

- Ensure plenty of fluids, wake babies to offer feeds if sleeping a lot.
- Ensure does not overheat, particularly babies, remove clothing and tepid sponge if necessary.
- Use paediatric liquid paracetamol (BNF 4.7.1) to address discomfort and keep temperature down.
- Use a digital thermometer in the armpit to monitor temperature (37°C normal).
- Keep monitoring how they look, their breathing, how much they are drinking, and how much fluid they lose, e.g. how often they vomit, or have wet nappies.

Ill babies <6mths may deteriorate rapidly. Parents should be encouraged to seek medical advice promptly.

## Advice for parents on when to seek medical attention promptly for a baby

- High pitched or weak cry.
- Much less active or more floppy than usual.
- Looks very pale all over.
- Grunts with each breath or has dips in upper abdomen or between ribs when breathes.
- Has not taken fluids in 8hrs.
- Has less wet nappies than usual, i.e. urine output ↓.
- Repeated vomiting or vomits bile (green fluid).
- Passes blood in stool.
- High fever or sweating a lot.
- Temperature >38°C for a baby <3mths or >39°C for a baby >3–6mths.
- Fontanelles bulging or sunken.
- Neck stiffness.
- A spotty, purple-red rash anywhere on the body (may be meningitis).

Any practitioner consulted about a sick baby or child should refer for medical opinion if significant signs as listed.

## Advice for parents on when to seek *urgent* medical attention, i.e. ring 999 for an ambulance

- Stops breathing or goes blue.
- Is unresponsive.
- Has glazed eyes and does not focus on anything.
- Cannot be woken.
- Has a fit, even if recovers without medical attention (📖 Febrile convulsions and epilepsy, p. 272).

Any practitioner consulted or first on scene when a baby or child has these symptoms should request an ambulance is called, if in surgery or clinic call for medical help, and then assess and commence CPR if required (📖 Child BLS, p. 748).

### Further information

NHS Choices. Spotting signs of serious illness in babies. Available at: ℅ www.nhs.uk/Conditions/pregnancy-and-baby/pages/spotting-signs-serious-illness.aspx

NHS Direct (England). A digital health and advice service, available at: ℅ www.nhsdirect.nhs.uk

NHS111 (England). 24-h helpline when medical help is needed fast but it's not a 999 emergency.

NHS Direct (Wales). 24-h helpline ☎ 0845 46 47. Available at: ℅ www.nhsdirect.wales.nhs.uk/

NHS 24 (Scotland). 24-h helpline ☎ 08454 242424. Available at: ℅ www.nhs24.com/

# Acne vulgaris

A disease of the pilo-sebaceous units that can occur on the face, chest, or back. Most commonly occurs between 13 and 20yrs. Everyone gets some acne. May continue into the 20s or 30s and occasionally into later life. Often has an emotional impact on confidence and self-esteem.

## Causes
- Genetic factors are important in the severity, duration, and clinical pattern.
- Rarer causes include endocrine problems, chemicals, steroids.

## Factors
There are four 1° pathogenic factors in the development of acne:
- Increased sebum production.
- The presence of proprionibacterium acnes bacteria.
- Abnormal keratinization.
- Inflammation.

Stress, heavy sweating, and premenstrual hormonal changes may have an impact. Some beauty products, e.g. pomades, de-frizzing agents, sun-tan oils may also impact. Misconceptions that diet or poor hygiene have impact on the development or severity of acne.

## Clinical features
- *Comedones (or blackheads):* plug of keration and sebum extrudes from pilo-sebaceous orifice.
- Whiteheads, papules, pustules, nodules, cysts, and scars may also be present.

## General advice on management
- *Skin care:* wash bd with soap and water and apply moisturizer.
- *Squeezing:* don't squeeze red or yellow pustules.
- *OTC preparations* (BNF for children 13.6.1): use lowest concentrations and consult health professional if no improvement within 2mths.
- *Make-up:* avoid using thick, oil-based types.

## Treatment (BNF for children 13.6)
Treatment is commenced early to prevent scarring.
- *Comedonal acne:* azelaic acid or benzoyl peroxide (OTC).
- *Mild inflammatory acne:* topical retinoid and topical antibiotic or benzoyl peroxide plus topical antibiotic.
- *Moderate inflammatory acne:* long-term tetracycline plus topical retinoid or other antibiotic (doxycycline, erythromycin, lymecycline, minocycline). For females oral anti-androgen plus topical retinoid.
- *Severe inflammatory acne:* referred to dermatology specialist. Treated with oral isotretinoin or high-dose oral antibiotic plus topical retinoid.

*Refer to dermatology specialist* if severe, any scarring or associated with fever, arthritis or no improvements to treatments.

## Related topics

📖 Growth and nutrition 12–18yrs, p. 221: 📖 Bacterial skin infections, p. 632.

## Further information

Teenage Health Freak. Spots. Available at: ℘ www.teenagehealthfreak.org/spots
NHS Choices. Acne. Available at: ℘ www.nhs.uk/Conditions/Acne/Pages/Introduction.aspx
NICE. Clinical Knowledge Summaries guidance on acne vulgaris (includes patient information sheets). Available at: ℘ http://cks.nice.org.uk/acne-vulgaris#azTab

# Asthma in children

Asthma is a lung disease, with intermittent narrowing of the bronchi, causing shortness of breath, wheezing, cough, and tightness in the chest. During an asthma attack the muscles in the bronchi contract and the lining swells, becomes inflamed, and produces excess mucus.

Affects about 5% of children. Ratio $2\sigma$:1$\female$ in childhood, but equal numbers in adolescence. Breastfeeding ( Breastfeeding, p. 176) has preventative effect for wheezing. The majority of children who present with asthma aged <2yrs are free of symptoms by age 6–11yrs. Asthma accounts for 10–20% of acute hospital admissions. Although detection and treatment is improved, it is still a major cause of school absenteeism, major anxiety in children and families, and over 20 children die from asthma in the UK each year.

## Predisposing factors
Both genetic predisposition and environmental:
- Family history of atopy (i.e. allergies, eczema, rhinitis, hay fever).
- Co-existence of atopic disease.
- Bronchiolitis in infancy.
- Parental smoking.
- Prematurity.

## Common precipitating factors
- Infection, exercise, emotion.
- Household allergens including house mites, fur, and feathered pets.
- Weather (fog, cold air, thunderstorms), air pollutants (smoke and dust).

## Symptoms
- Recurrent wheeze.
- Noisy breathing.
- Dry cough particularly at night.
- Breathlessness.

## Diagnosis
Diagnosis made on history and clinical examination. In children >5yrs: bronchodilator responsiveness, peak flow variability and spirometry are used to confirm diagnosis as for adults ( Measuring lung function, p. 562). Height of children is the only determinant of PEFR (see predicted PEFR table  Normal spirometry and peak flow values, p. 564). Often referred to specialists for diagnosis and establishment of treatment. Often referred for skin allergy testing also.

## Management and treatment
*Aims*
- To allow child to lead as normal life as possible.
- To minimize need for relieving medication.
- To prevent severe attacks or exacerbations.

Treatment is by stepwise approach (BNF for children 3.1,  Asthma in adults, p. 566) that includes short-acting inhaled bronchodilator therapy (relievers), e.g. salbutamol or tetrabutaline, and prophylactic therapy (preventers), e.g. regular inhaled steroids. As the severity and frequency of symptoms increase so do the addition of therapies until good control reached then treatment is stepped down. Advice on other measures is also given, e.g. parental smoking cessation, restricting access to fur or feathered animals, reducing house mites.

## Types of chronic asthma and management

- *Infrequent episodic:* i.e. <4 episodes/yr (75% of asthmatic children), need no regular treatment only inhaled bronchodilators as required.
- *Frequent episodic:* i.e. symptoms every 2–4wks (20%), need regular inhaled prophylactic therapy, initially with low-dose steroid, plus an inhaled bronchodilator as required.
- *Persistent asthma:* <5% need prophylaxis with inhaled steroids, also may need long-acting bronchodilator and oral steroids. Usually treated and monitored in specialists clinics.
- *Exercise-induced asthma:* mild symptoms controlled by bronchodilator before exercise. Warm up exercises important.

## Structured proactive review and monitoring

Regular, structured patient review of symptoms, level of symptom control, and use of medications should be organized and delivered by nurse or doctor in primary care with asthma management training. Review should include asthma education, parent/child self-management, and action plans as well as use of symptom diaries. Adolescents in particular are high users of emergency departments with acute asthma. Encourage parents and young people to seek review if:

- Needing more and more reliever treatment.
- Waking at night coughing, wheezing, shortness of breath (SOB).
- Non-attendance at day care, nursery/school because of asthma.
- Unable to do usual physical activities, sports.

## Inhalers

Inadequate technique may be mistaken for drug failure. Children <15yrs should have a pressurized metered-dose inhaler and spacer device. <5yrs with face mask if necessary, if not effective nebulized therapy is considered. Advice on inhalers and spacers includes:

- Shake inhaler well before fitting to spacer, press inhaler once and without delay allow child to take 5 slow breaths in and out of the spacer (tidal breathing).
- Remove inhaler, shake well, and repeat as prescribed.
- Spacers should be cleaned monthly in mild detergent as per manufacturer's instructions, replaced every 6–12mths (BNF for children 3.1.5).

See also ☐ Asthma attacks, p. 572.

## Further information

Asthma UK. ☎ Advice line 0800 121 62 44. Available at: ⌕ www.asthma.org.uk
SIGN Booklet. Managing Asthma in Children for parents and carers. British Thoracic Society British guideline on the management of asthma (revised 2012). Available at: ⌕ www.brit-thoracic.org.uk/guidelines/asthma-guidelines.aspx

## Essential reference

British Thoracic Society/SIGN British guideline on the management of asthma (revised 2012). Available at: ⌕ www.brit-thoracic.org.uk/guidelines/asthma-guidelines.aspx

# Autistic spectrum disorder

Autistic spectrum disorder is a developmental disorder with no known cause or underlying condition. It is rare: 3/10,000 children, commoner in boys than girls. It presents in early childhood, usually <3yrs, but is a lifelong condition. Only about 15% live independently in adulthood.

Children with developmental difficulties associated with autistic spectrum disorders are identified during the child health promotion programme (📖 Overview of the healthy child programme, p. 146). Key areas are failure of social interaction skills, e.g. no gestures like waving 'bye' by 12mths, and lack of speech skills, e.g. no babbling by 12mths. Some professionals use the Checklist for Autism in Toddlers (CHAT from the National Autistic Society[1]) to assess gaze monitoring, pretend play, and proto-declarative pointing. The absence of these is strongly associated with an autistic disorder.

Autistic children have a triad of difficulties:
- *Social interaction:* a profound difficulty in relating to other people, e.g. extreme indifference to others and failure to meet gaze.
- *Communication:* a severe language disorder—about half never speak at all.
- *Imagination:* marked routines and rituals associated with minimal imagination, e.g. insistence on the same foods, sameness of environment. Imposing change often precipitates violent temper tantrums.

In addition, odd physical patterns such as flapping hands and walking on tiptoe are common. Some children have hypersensitivity, e.g. to noise or light. About ⅔ have a general learning disability. About ¼ have epilepsy (📖 Febrile convulsions and epilepsy, p. 282). Many children with autism have very challenging behaviour.

## Management

No specific treatment available. Referred to specialist services and will need assessment for special educational needs (📖 Children with special educational needs, p. 227). Parents need a great deal of support as with all families with children with disabilities (📖 Children with complex health needs and disabilities, p. 225). Behaviour modification techniques are often used to teach social skills and reduce difficult behaviour. Education usually within special school environments. Those with moderate symptoms usually grow up to live independent lives. These with severe symptoms usually need to be supported in adulthood.

### Key advice for parents on communication with child with autism
- Have child's full attention when speaking to them, reduce background noise.
- Keep language simple, direct, specific, and literal (e.g. no 'frog in the throat' type phrases).
- Use pictures to reinforce words if possible.
- Provide thinking time to process words.
- Use positive, rather than negative language, e.g. what to do rather than what not to do.

*Key advice for parents on behaviour management*
- Be consistent and keep your word.
- Try to develop routines through the day and help your child understand what will happen next, e.g. through pictures.
- Try to recognize patterns or events that are upsetting for child and trigger tantrums and move in early to distract from or remove these.
- Encourage child to go somewhere safe when they become upset or angry.
- Find ways of positive encouragement for good behaviour.

The National Autistic Society[1] provide a range of information leaflets to help parents with particular issues, e.g. toilet training.

## Asperger syndrome

Asperger syndrome is a mild form of the social impairments of autism in the presence of near-normal speech development. Difficulties in social encounters, stilted language, narrow interests often not shared with others.

## Related topic

📖 People with learning disabilities, p. 408.

## Reference

[1]National Autistic Society. Helpline: ☎ 0808 800 4104(Mon–Fri, 10am–4pm). Available at: ℘ www. autism.org.uk

# Behavioural disorders in children

Behavioural disorders are also known as 'externalizing' disorders. Includes oppositional defiant disorder (ODD), attention-deficit hyperactivity disorder (ADHD), and conduct disorder (CDD). Behaviours are usually noticeable by others: aggression, hyperactivity, distractibility, and defiant behaviours.

## Attention-deficit hyperactivity disorder

*Prevalence suggested by Royal College of Psychiatrists[1]*
- Affects 3–5% school-age children.
- Ratio of boys to girls 4:9 ♂:1♀.

*Presentation*
All children can be overactive and behave impulsively, find it hard to concentrate sometimes. With ADHD, this behaviour is persistent, occurs wherever the child is, not just in one place, e.g. school or at home. Varying degrees of severity, sometimes found together with other conditions, e.g. dyslexia. ADHD is a distinct condition that includes:
- Associated with impairment in social and/or academic functioning compared to individuals at a comparative level of development.
- Developmentally inappropriate degrees of inattention.
- Impulsivity.
- Hyperactivity.
- Present before 7yrs.
- Present in 2 or more settings.
- Not better accounted for by another disorder.

Need to ensure behaviours not due to other problems, e.g. hearing loss, epilepsy, Tourette syndrome, etc.

*Aetiology*
- Strong evidence of genetic contribution.
- High maternal consumption of alcohol during pregnancy.

*Treatment/management*
- Early identification important.
- Identify and address any other medical or social problems.
- Important that all involved with child work together to assess and agree on ways of managing.
- Referral to specialists or CAMHS for:
  - Parental education.
  - Behavioural management.
  - Parenting skills work.
  - CBT for school age or psychological therapies for teenagers.
  - Medication for severe ADHD if >5yrs, e.g. methylphenidate (Ritalin®).

*Outcome*
- Family disturbance contributes to continuity of childhood ADHD into adolescence, 50–80% cases.
- ⅓ hyperactivity decreases after adolescence; ⅓ mildly impaired as adults; ⅓ persist into adult ADHD with worsening of functions.

*Associated problems*
Difficult interaction with peers; delayed social and educational development; more psychological problems, low self-esteem; evokes cycle of 'negative parenting'.

## Conduct disorders

Conduct disorders are characterized by excessive levels of fighting, bullying, cruelty, destructiveness, stealing, lying, truancy, temper tantrums, disobedience. They are severe and persistent (>6mths). Delinquency is antisocial law-breaking behaviour.

*Prevalence* About 5% with an excess of boys.

*Aetiology*
- Adverse psychosocial environments.
- Child's temperament.
- Poor physical health.

*Treatment/management*
Referral to specialists or CAMHS for:
- Problem-solving skills training.
- *Family therapy:* parent management training.

*Outcome if not 'treated'*
- Delinquency, offending, and criminality.
- Emotional disorders.
- Substance misuse.
- Teenage pregnancy.
- Early violent deaths.

*Note:* most antisocial disorders do not progress to adulthood, but many aggressive antisocial adults had the pattern of behaviour in childhood.

## Related topics

📖 Understanding behaviour 1–5yrs, p. 204; 📖 Working with teenagers, p. 219.

## Reference

[1]Royal College of Psychiatrists. Available at: ℅ www.rcpsych.ac.uk/expertadvice/youthinfo.aspx

## Further information

National Attention Deficit Disorder Information and Support Service. Available at: ℅ www.addiss. co.uk/
Young Minds. Available at: ℅ www.youngminds.org.uk
NICE (2008). Attention deficit hyperactivity disorder (ADHD) Guideline 72. Available at: ℅ guidance.nice.org.uk/CG72

# Birth injuries

Babies may be injured at birth if they are too large for the pelvic outlet or malpositioned. Rarer are injuries from assisted vaginal deliveries, e.g. using forceps.

## Soft tissue injuries

- Bruising and swelling to face, after face delivery, or to buttocks after breech delivery. Resolves in a few days.
- *Caput succedaneum:* bruising and oedema of the presenting part of the body. Resolves in a few days.
- *Cephalhaematoma:* rare. Haemorrhage beneath the periosteum. Resolves over a few weeks.

Parents need reassurance as child can look very alarming.

## Nerve injuries

Nerve injuries can occur during breech deliveries or with shoulder dystocia (shoulder trapped behind pelvic bone) during birth. Damage is to cervical nerve roots in brachial plexus. Palsy (loss of control of muscles) according to which cervical nerve damaged. Most common types:

- *Erb's palsy:* upper nerve root injury. One arm abducted, rotated in and fingers flexed.
- *Klumpke's palsy:* lower nerve root injury causing hand weakness and fingers don't move.
- *Complete brachial plexus palsy:* entire arm is paralysed with sensory loss.
- *Facial palsy:* causes facial asymmetry.

Most offered paediatric physiotherapy and followed up by paediatricians. Most resolve within a few weeks. In some care cases injury may not resolve, referred to paediatric neurologist. Nerve or tendon release surgery may be considered. Parents need support and reassurance.

## Bone injuries

- *Clavicle fracture:* occurs in some births from shoulder dystocia. Heals rapidly without treatment.
- *Humerus or femur fractures:* can occur in breech deliveries requires immobilization and heals rapidly.
- Parents need support, reassurance, and advice on care of baby while limb immobilized.

## Related topics

&#x1F4D6; New birth visits, p. 168; &#x1F4D6; New babies, p. 173; &#x1F4D6; Complicated labour, p. 389.

## Further information

The Erb's Palsy Group. Available at: &#x266B; www.erbspalsygroup.co.uk/

# Bone and joint problems

## Variations of normal posture

These are common and most resolve without any treatment, but any that are severe, painful, or asymmetrical are referred for specialist opinion. This includes:

- *Bow legs (genu varum):* bowing of tibiae. Common up to age 3yrs and resolves spontaneously. Other causes include rickets (usually caused by vit. D and calcium deficiency and treatable with oral supplements or injections).
- *Knock knees:* seen in children 2–7yrs, usually resolves spontaneously.
- *Flat feet (pes planum):* all babies and toddlers have flat feet. The arch develops after 2–3yrs of walking. Persistent flat feet may be familial or due to joint laxity. If painful referred for specialist advice.

## Disorders of the hip, knee, and foot

### Development dysplasia of the hip

Previously congenital dislocation of the hip. Describes a spectrum of disorders from dysplasia through to dislocation of the hip. 6–10 per 1000 live births. Detected at routine neonatal and 6-wk screening (📖 Overview of the healthy child programme, p. 146). Most resolve spontaneously. Referred for specialist opinion. Treatment depends on when the condition is diagnosed:

- *Young babies:*
    - Splinting—the hips are held in partial abduction using slings under each thigh attached to a body harness, e.g. von Rosen splint.
    - Usually babies wear a splint for ~3mths.
    - Parents need specific advice on handling and hygiene.
- *Older babies, toddlers:* surgery is required.

**Irritable hip** Most common cause of acute hip pain 2–12yrs. Cause is unknown, usually resolves in 7 days.

### Talipes (clubfoot)

- *Positional talipes:* from intrauterine compression is common and resolves with passive manipulation usually demonstrated by physiotherapists.
- *True talipes:* the foot is inverted, supinated, and forefoot abducted. Referred to orthopaedics. Treatment—physiotherapy, splints +/– surgery at 6–9mths.

## Disorders of the back and spine

- *Back pain:* uncommon pre-adolescent. A young child with back pain should be medically assessed. In adolescents common causes are muscle spasm often from sports related injuries and poor posture.
- *Scolioisis:* lateral curvature of the spine, may lead to pain and limitation of activities, respiratory restriction. Causes can be idiopathic, congenital or secondary to another disorder, e.g. 📖 Cerebral palsy, p. 252. Early onset idiopathic usually resolves. Late onset idiopathic scoliosis (most common 85%) mainly affects girls at pubertal growth

spurt (📖 Growth and nutrition 12–18yrs, p. 221). Treatment of severe scoliois is with spinal braces and sometimes surgery.

- *Torticollis (wry neck):* sudden restriction of head turning due to a mobile nodule in muscle. Resolves in 2–6mths.

## Painful limb

### Growing pains

(Also nocturnal idiopathic pain.) Common in pre-school children. Children with hypermobility in joints often also complain of pain in limbs. Cause unknown. Often wakes child at night and settles with massage and comforting.

### Arthritis

Rare in children. Presents with well-localized joint pains +/– hot, tender, swollen joints. Two types:

- *Septic arthritis:* a serious infection of the joint space that can lead to bone destruction. Most common <2yrs. The child is usually systemically unwell and the joint may be swollen, hot, and tender. Often in the hip and picked up when changing nappies. ❶ Requires urgent medical assessment, admission to hospital, and IV antibiotics.
- *Juvenile idiopathic (chronic) arthritis* (📖 Bone and joint problems, p. 249): group of conditions which last >6wks. Includes Still's disease— acute illness, fever, weight loss, salmon pink rash, pains in joints and muscles. Referred to specialist, requires physiotherapy, pain control, and suppression of inflammation by NSAIDs. Child may be identified as having special needs according to severity and effect (📖 A child or young person in need, p. 150).

## Genetic

### Osteogenesis imperfecta

Autosomal dominant inheritance. A group of disorders of collagen metabolism resulting in fragile bones which fracture easily. Other features include lax joints, thin skin, blue sclerae, hypoplastic teeth and deafness. Severe forms present with fractures at birth (many stillborn). Less severe cases present later and may be mistaken for non-accidental injury. Treatment is supportive with treatment of fractures as occur. Child may be identified as having special needs according to severity and effect.

### Osteopetrosis

Marble bone disease. Rare, bones dense, but brittle. Autosomal dominant presents in childhood with fractures, osteomyelitis +/– facial paralysis. Recessive form is more severe causing bone marrow failure (bone marrow transplantation can be curative) and death.

### Marfan's disease

Autosomal dominant disorder of connective tissue associated with altered body proportions, tall stature, hyper-extensible joints, long thin digits, scicloisis, cardiovascular problems, and dislocation of the eye lenses and severe myopia.

## Related topics
📖 Children with special educational needs, p. 227; 📖 Children with complex health needs and disabilities, p. 225.

## Further information
Brittle Bone Society. Available at: ℘ www.brittlebone.org
Childrens Chronic Arthritis Association. Available at: ℘ www.ccaa.org.uk/
Great Ormond St. Hospital Factsheets. Available at: ℘ www.gosh.nhs.uk/medical-conditions/
Scoliosis Association (UK). ☎ 020 8964 1166. Available at: ℘ www.sauk.org.uk
Steps. Charity for lower limb disorders, e.g. hip dysplasia. Available at: ℘ www.steps-charity.org.uk/

# Cerebral palsy

Cerebral palsy (CP) is the most common cause of physical disability in childhood characterized by impaired movement and posture. Due to non-progressive lesion of the motor pathways in the developing brain. It affects about 2 per 1000 live births, ↑ in premature/small-for-date babies.

## Causes

- *Antenatal (80%):* cerebral malformation, infections, e.g. rubella, cytomegalovirus.
- *Intrapartum (10%):* birth asphyxia/trauma.
- *Postnatal (10%):* head trauma, brain infections, e.g. meningitis, hydrocephalus.

## Associated problems

- Intellectual impairment (60%).
- Epilepsy (40%).
- Visual impairment (20%) and squints (30%).
- Hearing loss (20%).
- Speech and language disorders.

## Classification

Three main types—but mixed forms are common:

- *Spastic CP :* 70–80%. Damage to upper motor neurone pathway. Affects motor function and may → hemiplegia, quadriplediga, or diplegia. Affected limbs underdeveloped and have ↑ tone, weakness, and tendency toward contractures. Scissors gait and toe walking characteristic.
- *Athetoid and dyskinetic syndromes:* 10–20%. Damage is to basal ganglia. Constant involuntary movements, poor postural control, and unsteadiness in walking and sitting.
- *Ataxic CP :* 5–10%. Damage is to the cerebellum. Poor coordination, low muscle tone, poor balance, unsteady gait, tremor, and difficulty with and fine movements.

*Diagnosis* Often abnormalities in tone, reflexes, and posture are noted during routine developmental screening and referred to paediatricians.

## Care management

There is no cure. The aim is to enable children to develop maximum independence and support the family in achieving this. A range of health and social care problems have to be identified and addressed through coordinated care plans in MDT approach, involving physiotherapists, OTs, SLTs, community paediatricians, GPs, HV, social workers, early years care staff and teachers, in liaison with the child and parents.

## Related topics

📖 Children with complex health needs and disabilities, p. 225; 📖 Children with special educational needs, p. 227.

## Further information

SCOPE. ☎ 0808 800 3333. Available at: 🖰 www.scope.org.uk/help-and-information/cerebral-palsy

# Cancer in childhood

Cancer in children are rare: about 1500 cases per year in UK[1]. Most cancers occur as a result of mutations in cellular genes, which may be inherited or sporadic. Emphasis with all cancers is on early diagnosis and treatment, e.g. a maximum of 2wks from GP urgent referral of suspected cancer to first hospital assessment. Most children with cancer in UK are initially treated in regional centres, and then returned to care of local specialists, and primary care, including support from specialist outreach nurses from regional centre or children's community nursing team (📖 Children with complex health needs and disabilities, p. 225). Survival rate for many cancers has increased dramatically. The diagnosis has enormous and long-lasting impact on the whole family. In the early days:

- Parents need opportunities to discuss diagnosis and feelings as well as written information on the disease, implications, and treatments.
- The child and siblings need age-appropriate explanations and opportunities to discuss their feelings.
- Family may need help with practical issues such as transport, accommodation, finance, care of siblings while attends tertiary centre.

Once treatment is established and the disease is under control, families are encouraged to return to as normal life as possible:

- Early return to school is encouraged.
- Child and family should be offered ongoing opportunities to discuss feelings and find ways of coping with unknown long-term outcome.
- Parents should be supported in having time out from caring and focusing on themselves and their own needs (📖 Carers assessment and support, p. 412).

## General overview of treatment and management

### Treatment

May involve chemotherapy, surgery, and radiotherapy. Bone marrow transplantation may be used to treat patients after administering very high doses of chemotherapy and/or radiotherapy that damages normal tissue particularly bone marrow. Side effects of chemotherapy include: immunosuppression, bone marrow suppression, gut mucosal damage, anorexia, nausea and vomiting.

*Long-term follow-up* Monitors residual problems, risks of second tumours, and specific problems as a result of the treatment such as poor growth or sexual dysfunction.

### Palliative care

Despite treatment, some children progress to the terminal stages of their cancers. Specialist palliative care or hospice teams may be involved. General principles of palliative care at home apply (📖 Palliative care in the home, p. 509):

- Address pain relief and symptom control.
- Provide emotional support for child and family.
- Ensure continuity with as few professionals as possible.
- Provide on-going support to family members after the child has died.

## Main types

*Acute leukaemia* Peak presentation age 2–4yrs. 80% acute lymphoblastic leukaemia (310 cases/yr), others acute myeloid or acute non-lymphocytic. Usually presents with a short history (weeks) of pallor, fatigue, irritability, fever, bone pain, and/or bruising/petechiae.

### Lymphomas

Malignancies of the cells of the immune system. Peak presentation is at age 10–14yrs.

- *Hodgkin's disease:* usually presents as painless lymphadenopathy, often in neck. May also have a long history of weight loss, sweating, priutius, fever.
- *Non-Hodgkin's lymphoma:* usually presents with painless lymphadenopathy, often in neck, and/or disease in abdomen. There tends to be a rapid progression of symptoms.

### Brain tumours

280 cases/yr. Almost always primary tumours and present with signs of raised intracranial pressure, e.g. headache (worse when lying down), vomiting, squint, nystagmus, personality, or behaviour change. Tumour identified on computed tomography (CT)/positron emission tomography (PET)-CT or MRI scans. Outcome influenced by position and size. Survivors may have very complex problems.

*Neuroblastoma* Derived from neural crest tissue in adrenal medulla and sympathetic nervous system. Tends to affect children <5yrs. Most present with abdominal mass. Children with extra-abdominal tumours, and those who are <1yr at diagnosis have better prognosis.

*Wilms' tumour (nephroblastoma)* Kidney tumour from embryonal renal tissue. 70 cases/yr. Usually affects children <5yrs old. Presents with fever, weight loss, anaemia, abdominal mass and pain.

*Retinoblastoma* Rare tumour of eye—30 cases/yr Usually affects children <5yrs. Usually detected by a white pupillary reflex found at routine developmental screening, or with squint or inflammation of the eye.

*Rhabdomyosarcoma* Presents with a mass at any age. May be at any site.

*Osteosarcoma (bone tumour)* 10–14yrs. Present with persistent bony pain—most commonly in a limb.

## Reference

[1]Cancer Research UK. Childhood cancer incidence statistics. Available at: ℅ www.cancerresearchuk. org/cancer-info/cancerstats/childhoodcancer/incidence/childhood-cancer-incidence-statistics

## Further information

Cancer and Leukemia in Children (CLIC Sargent). Available at: ℅ www.clicsargent.org.uk/
Macmillan cancer support. Available at: ℅ www.macmillan.org.uk/Home.aspx
National Cancer Action Team (England). Tools and information for primary care professionals. Available at: ℅ ncat.nhs.uk/
Together for short lives (UK charity for all children with life-threatening and life-limiting conditions, families and professionals). Available at: ℅ www.togetherforshortlives.org.uk/☎ 0845 108 2201

# Cleft lip and palate

- Cleft lip is the failure of fusion of frontonasal and maxillary processes.
- Cleft palate is the failure of fusion of palatine processes.
- Affects about 0.8 per 1000 children. Most is inherited, but may be part of a syndrome.

Usually referred to regional specialist cleft lip and palate multidisciplinary team at diagnosis. As with all families and children with special needs, primary care professionals work in conjunction providing their services and long-term support.

## Surgical repair

- *Lip*: surgical repair may be performed in first weeks or first 2–3mths.
- *Palate*: usually repaired by 1yr.

## Feeding

Babies may have difficulty combining reflex actions, creating vacuum, and correctly positioning tongue. Regional team provides specialist advice as does the Cleft Lip and Palate Association (CLAPA[1]). Parents need lots of reassurance as milk and foods may pass into nose and cause sneezing. Babies with cleft lip:

- Can breastfeed (☐ Breastfeeding, p. 176), but may need to try different positions and holding breast differently.
- If bottle fed may need larger hole in soft teat (CLAPA has catalogue of types of soft bottles, teats, and feeding systems).
- May be fed with cup and spoon after repair till heals.

### Babies with cleft palate and lip

- May be given an orthodontic plate to help feeding.
- Many can breastfeed if breast held in area that palate is complete, be well latched-on, with good supply of milk.
- Many can bottle fed with teats with larger holes.
- Some babies may need nasogastric tubes (NGTs) to feed, or be fed by cup and spoon.
- After repair depends on age, but may be asked to use cup and spoon, rather than bottle.

## Other issues

The specialist team will monitor speech development and provide therapy if any difficulties, Hearing is also monitored as middle ear infections common. If the gum is affected by the cleft, then teeth may also be missing, twisted, or be misaligned. Orthodontic referral may be required when adult teeth coming in (☐ Dental health in older children, p. 214).

## Related topic

☐ Children with complex health needs and disabilities, p. 225.

## Reference

[1]CLAPA. Available at: ℬ www.clapa.com

# Congenital heart defects

Congenital heart defects affect ~1 in 145 births. ↑ defects detected at antenatal US. ↑ diagnosed by non-invasive echocardiography. ↑ number of defects can be treated non-invasively. The 8th most common congenital heart lesions:

- Non-cyanotic:
  - *Ventriculoseptal defect (VSD) 32%*—a hole connects the 2 ventricles.
  - *Patent ductus arteriosus (PDA) 12%*—ductus arteriosus fails to close after birth.
  - Pulmonary valve stenosis 8%.
  - *Atrial septal defect (ASD) 6%*—a hole connects the 2 atria.
  - *Coarctation of the aorta 6%*—localized narrowing of the descending aorta.
  - Aortic valve stenoisis 5%.
- Cyanotic:
  - *Tetralogy of Fallot 6%*—large VSD and pulmonary stenosis.
  - *Transposition of the great arteries 5%*—aorta and pulmonary artery.

## Signs and symptoms

- Heart murmur, but only 54% of murmurs heard at neonatal examination are due to cardiac defects, most are innocent.
- Heart failure includes:
  - Breathlessness particularly when crying/feeding.
  - Cyanosis.
  - ↑ respiratory and pulse rates.
  - Failure to thrive or weight ↑ due to fluid retention.
  - Recurrent chest infection.
  - Heart and/or liver enlargement.
  - Cool peripheries.

## Treatment

Refer for specialist paediatric and/or cardiology opinion. Specialist treatment of valve lesions depends on the size. Most congenital cardiac lesions require medical treatment plus surgery. May have oxygen therapy at home (📖 Oxygen therapy in the community, p. 581).

## Care management issues

### Feeding

Slow feeding is a common problem (📖 Breastfeeding, p. 176). Long feeds ↑ tiredness in babies and mothers. Vomiting after feeds often a problem. Encourage ↓ amounts, ↑ frequency. If bottle fed then may need to experiment with teats and bottles to aid feeding, but ↓ wind. Night feeds often need longer than other babies. Weight gain may also be a problem. Usually seen by dietitian in specialist team. May need high-calorie formula feed (in addition if breastfeeding). Introduction of high-calorie weaning food at 4mths often aids weight gain. Some babies at home may have NGT or percutaneous endoscopic gastrostomy (PEG; 📖 Enteral tube feeding, p. 546).

*Immunization*

Usual programme (📖 Childhood immunization, p. 156) plus flu vaccine every year to children with heart conditions (check contraindications flu vaccination) from the age of 6mths–12yrs. Vaccinations against pneumonia and bronchiolitis may also be recommended by cardiologist.

*General*

Most children recover quickly after surgery and are back at nursery, playgroup, school within a month. Exercise tolerance varies and each child is encouraged to find own limits. Antibiotic prophylaxis for dental and surgical procedures given as ↑ risk of developing bacterial endocarditis. Many adolescents and adults require revision of surgery performed in early life, e.g. replacement of artificial valves.

## Related topics

📖 Children with complex health needs and disabilities, p. 225; 📖 Children with special educational needs, p. 227.

## Further information

Children's Heart Federation. ☏ 0808 808 5000. Available at: 🖰 www.childrens-heart-fed.org.uk
British Heart Foundation. Available at: 🖰 www.bhf.org.uk/heart-health/conditions/congenital-heart-disease.aspx

# Congenital impairments

Congenital impairments are present in approximately 2% of live births, more common in pre-term and small for dates babies[1]. Approximately 30% genetic and chromosomal, 10% teratogenic (viral, bacterial, medications, alcohol, drugs), remainder multiple causes or unknown. Individual child and family needs should be identified and addressed accordingly (📖 A child or young person in need, p. 150).

## Congenital adrenal hyperplasia

Congenital adrenal hyperplasia is caused by autosomal recessive disorders in 1 per 5000 births. Cortisol deficiencies causes overproduction of adrenal androgens. Results in:

- Virilization of external genitalia of girls requiring corrective surgery.
- Penis enlargement and precocious puberty (📖 Growth disorders, p. 280) in some boys.
- Adrenal crisis in some male babies within first 3wks requires emergency treatment.

All require long-term glucocorticoid therapy (BNF for children 6.3.2) and monitoring of growth by specialists.

## Congenital infections

- *Cytomegalovirus (CMV)*: affects 4 per 1000 births. 90% of affected children develop normally. The remainder have neurological problems, e.g. cerebral palsy, epilepsy, and developmental delay.
- *Rubella*: usually intrauterine <18wks gestation from infected mother. Preventable (📖 Antenatal care and screening, p. 380). May cause deafness, congenital heart defects and cataracts, and other problems.
- *Toxoplasmosis*: 0.1 per 1000 births. About 10% of affected have problems, usually neurological, e.g. hydrocephalus and retinopathy.

## Urogenital problems

### Babies with ambiguous genitalia

Require full biochemical and sometimes surgical (laparoscopic) investigation prior to assigning sex. Time to correctly assign often causes additional distress to parents, but important as has lifelong social, psychological, medical, and legal consequences. Caused by chromosomal (📖 Genetic problems, p. 276) or adrenal problems. Parents, and later child, need psychological support as well as information at different stages. Surgery may be required at different stages of development as well as long-term glucocorticoid therapy and hormone therapy.

### Male genito-urinary problems

- *Hypdospadias*: urethral opening on the underside of the penis. 1 in 300 boys. Corrected surgically <2yrs.
- *Undescended testes*: occurs in 5% full-term boys. Most descend by 3mths. Those that don't are corrected surgically (orchidopexy) about 2yrs.

*Urological malformations*

Increasingly diagnosed by antenatal ultrasound scan (USS). Horseshoe kidney or double elements in the system common and in themselves are not a problem. However, predispose to reflux and recurrent UTIs (📖 Infections in children, p. 282) and cause renal damage. Often prophylactic antibiotics started at birth to prevent renal damage. USS again within first 6wks, some malformations may have resolved. Prophylactic antibiotics continue if malformation remains. Obstructions such as posterior urethral valve require surgical intervention.

## Related topics

See also other topics of congenital impairments:
📖 Bone and joint problems, p. 249; 📖 Cerebral palsy, p. 252; 📖 Cleft lip and palate, p. 255; 📖 Congenital heart defects, p. 256; 📖 Cystic fibrosis, p. 262; 📖 Endocrine problems, p. 270; 📖 Gastrointestinal problems in children, p. 274; 📖 Neural tube defects, p. 289.

## Reference

[1]National Congenital Anomaly System. Office of National Statistics. Available at: ℬ www.statistics.org.uk

## Further information

Great Ormond St. Hospital Factsheets. Available at: ℬ www.gosh.nhs.uk/medical-conditions/
UK Intersex Association. Available at: ℬ www.ukia.co.uk

# Constipation and encopresis

## Constipation

Constipation is the painful passage of hard, infrequent stools. Affects about 5% children at some time, more ♂ than ♀ (see also ▢ Constipation in adults, p. 460). *Note:* babies show considerable variation in bowel habit according to diet (and if breastfed). Babies can change colour when passing a stool and look as if they are straining even when passing a liquid stool. Changing from breastfeeding to artificial feeds and/or solids results in change of stool colour and consistency (▢ Bottle feeding, p. 178).

### Causes

*Babies*

- May occur from hunger, over-strength feeds, and poor hydration.
- *Rare causes include:* congenital abnormalities, e.g. spinal cord lesions, Hirschsprung's disease.

*Older children*

- Poor or chaotic diet, inadequate fluid intake, and activity.
- Failure to establish toileting routine during toilet training.
- Behavioural or psychological problems.
- Developmental problems (learning disability, autism).
- Fear of toilets, especially school toilets.
- Sedentary lifestyle.
- Vicious cycle created of ignoring sensation, hard stool, anal pain, deferring defecation as long as possible.
- Severe loading, i.e. rectum and colon filled with faeces: may also have faecal incontinence or staining.

### Management of short-lived or mild constipation

- Explanation of reasons for problems is important as is engaging the child and parents in promotion of healthy diet, ↑ fluids, and ↑ exercise.
- Ascertain if afraid of the toilet, suggest ways to make toilet appealing.
- *Advice includes:*
  - Ensure adequate fibre and fluid intake.
  - Allow sufficient time and privacy for morning bowel emptying.
  - Eat breakfast and try 20–30min later.
  - On the toilet sit comfortably with feet supported (footstool if needed).
  - Avoid holding breath and straining.
  - Push using abdominal muscles and relax anus.
  - Consider simple rewards (e.g. star chart).
  - Avoid punishments/reprimands.
  - Always respond to 'urge', do not defer (arrange with teacher).
- Mild bulk-forming laxatives used with caution as last resort. Referred for specialist opinion if not resolving or severe.

*Management of severely constipated child*

These children are referred for medical review. May have painful anal conditions, e.g. anal fissure. May need several months of laxatives as per national guidelines[1] to establish a pattern.

## Encopresis

Most children are continent of faeces by 2½–3yrs. Faecal soiling during daytime after this age usually occurs when:

- Child has bowel control, but passes stool in socially unacceptable places. Cause is often emotional. Consider referral to CAMHS/or via GP as local policies suggest.
- Firm stool passed occasionally in the toilet, but usually in the pants. Try a consistent training programme similar to those used for 📖 Nocturnal enuresis, p. 290.
- Soft stool causes child to soil themselves and smell of faeces. Consider possibility of overflow faecal incontinence due to underlying chronic constipation.

## Related topic

📖 Toilet training, p. 203.

## Reference

[1]NICE (2010). *Constipation in children and young people: diagnosis and management of idiopathic childhood constipation in primary and secondary care (CG 99)*. Available at: 🔗 www.nice.org.uk/guidance/CG99

## Further information

ERIC. Education and resources for Improving childhood continence. ☎ 0845 370 8008 (Monday to Wednesday). Available at: 🔗 www.eric.org.uk

NICE Clinical Knowledge Summaries. Management of constipation in children. Available at: 🔗 cks.nice.org.uk/constipation-in-children

# Cystic fibrosis

Cystic fibrosis (CF) is the most common, serious pulmonary and genetic disease, affecting 1 in 2500 children (UK):

- About 1 in 22 of the UK white population are carriers of a copy of CF gene. Rare in children of African or Asian descent.
- Diagnosed through neonatal screening programme (☐ Child screening tests, p. 152) or antenatal test if thought to be at high risk (☐ Antenatal care and screening, p. 380). Pre-conceptual screening also available.
- Affects movement of salt and water across cell membranes and causes thickened secretions; a multi-system disease characterized by life-threatening pulmonary and GI problems.
- No cure for CF, but life expectancy has improved in recent years.

## Care and management

Children with CF should be linked to a specialist centre with aims of:
- Promoting independence, improve quality of life, and life expectancy.
- Working in partnership with child and family for long-term support.
- Good MDT working, especially with school as grows older.

### Care for lung-associated problems

- Twice daily chest physiotherapy and postural drainage to loosen thick mucus. Parents are taught how to do this by hospital staff and ongoing support from community paediatric nurses. Patients can do this themselves as they become adult.
- Immunizations and flu vaccination (☐ Childhood immunization schedule (UK), p. 158; ☐ Targeted immunizations in adults, p. 347).
- Rapid treatment with antibiotics with any sign of chest infection. IV antibiotic therapy in the community offered in many areas. Some children are prescribed prophylactic antibiotics.
- Some children will have inhalers for asthma and inhaled medication to reduce stickiness of secretions (pulmozyme) as well as corticosteroids.
- Home oxygen to aid breathing and in severe cases candidates for heart lung transplants (☐ Oxygen therapy in the community, p. 581).

### Care for GI-associated problems

- Pancreatic enzymes with each meal to aid digestion (BNF 1.9.4).
- Vitamin supplements especially A and D.
- Medicines to reduce/relieve constipation.
- High protein and high calorie diet.

### Complications and associated issues

- Behavioural and psychological problems arising from having life-threatening disease.
- CF related diabetes (☐ Endocrine problems, p. 270).
- Fertility problems and genetic counselling (☐ Problems with fertility, p. 735).

## Further information

Cystic Fibrosis Trust. Available at: ✆ www.cysticfibrosis.co.uk; ✆ www.cftrust.org.uk
NHS Choices. Available at: ✆ www.nhs.uk/Conditions/cystic-fibrosis

# Deafness in children

**Deafness** The prevalence of confirmed childhood hearing impairment (>40Db HL) in the UK is 1.3 children per 1000 live births at age of 5yrs (UK National Screening Committee[1]).

## Causes

*Prenatal*
- 50% genetic.
- Infections in pregnancy, e.g. cytomegalovirus, measles, toxiplasmosis.
- Ototoxic medications in pregnancy.

*Postnatal*
- Prematurity, sequelae of prematurity, e.g. jaundice.
- Infections, e.g. measles, meningitis, mumps.
- Otoxic medications for other infections.

## Types

*Conductive* Also known as glue ear (□ Infections in children, p. 282). Sound cannot pass through outer and middle ear to cochlea and auditory nerve.

*Sensorineural* Fault in inner ear of auditory nerve.

*Mixed* For example, problem with glue ear and auditory nerve.

## Management

Hearing loss/deafness is identified through screening (□ Child screening tests, p. 152). Children are referred to specialists, including audiology, according to local care pathways and protocols. As in all situations where special needs are identified, the parents and child need support, services and information from a multi-disciplinary team (□ Children with complex health needs and disabilities, p. 225).

Management depends on type, severity of loss and impact.

### Hearing aids

Acoustic aids come in a range of shapes and sizes and may be analogue or digital and some children may use radio transmitter systems to reduce background noise, e.g. in classrooms. When a child gains no benefit from acoustic aids a cochlear implant may be considered, the electrodes are inserted surgically and directly stimulate the auditory nerve.

### Communication

Deaf children, like hearing children, needs lots of attention and interaction to learn and develop communication skills. Special needs teams advise on learning additional communication methods, e.g. oral-auditory systems, e.g. lip reading, sign bilingualism, e.g. British Sign Language, total communication, e.g. multiple methods.

## Reference

[1]NHS Newborn Hearing Screening programme ♪ http://hearing.screening.nhs.uk/

## Further information

National Deaf Children's Society. Available at: ♪ www.ndcs.org.uk/
Deafness Research Factsheets. Available at: ♪ http://www.deafnessresearch.org.uk/

# Depressive behaviours

This includes depressive feelings, depressive behaviour, depressive cognitions or beliefs, as well as depressive disorders. Increase in prevalence as children get older. Girls outnumber boys in diagnosed problems in adolescence, 2:1. Predisposing factors include genetic, temperament, biological factors, chronic life adversity. Factors associated with a high risk of depression include:

- *Psychosocial:* family discord, bullying, all forms of abuse.
- *Other disorders:* including drug and alcohol use, and a history of parental depression.
- *Social problems:* including homelessness, living in institutional settings.
- Single life event losses.

## Presentation

Common to suffer >1 internalizing disorder, e.g. anxiety, social withdrawal, loneliness.

- *Pre-school:*
  - Apathy and food refusal, miserable, irritable, cries, and rocks.
  - Growth failure may occur.
- *5–12yrs:*
  - Children use language of emotional affect.
  - Psychosomatic symptoms.
  - Poor concentration, failure to progress at school.
  - Irritability, social withdrawal, temper outbursts.
  - Usually complain of being bored.
- *Adolescence:*
  - Alike to adulthood depression.
  - Complaints of boredom, sadness, apathy, lacking energy.
  - Appetite and sleep disorders more common.

## Assessment in primary care

From NICE guidance.[1]

- Identify if one of following key symptoms present most days, most of the time >2wks:
  - Persistent sadness or low (irritable) mood.
  - Loss of interests and/or pleasure.
  - Fatigue or low energy.
- If any key symptoms present, ask about associated symptoms:
  - Poor or increased sleep.
  - Poor concentration or indecisiveness.
  - Low self-confidence.
  - Poor or increased appetite.
  - Suicidal thoughts or acts.
  - Self-harm thoughts.
  - Agitation or slowing of movements.
  - Guilt or self-blame.
- Find out about past history of depression, life events, family history, associated disability, school contexts, quality of family and peer relationships, and availability of social support.

*Action on assessment*
- If 4 or fewer of these symptoms, no family history, social support present, not actively suicidal then general advice and watchful waiting. Reiterate advice on good nutrition (📖 Nutrition and healthy eating, p. 304), good sleep patterns and need for exercise. Offer emotional support/active listening (📖 Counselling skills, p. 123) or referral to self-help groups or other forms of support, e.g. Connexions, faith group. Respond to identified adverse events/problems such as action in instances of bullying.
- If 5 or more symptoms, past or family history, low level of social support, associated social disability, child or relative requests, self-neglect then more active primary care intervention and/or referral to CAMHS.
- Urgent referral to CAMHS psychiatrist if active suicidal ideas, psychotic symptoms, severe agitation, severe self neglect.

## Mental health treatments

Depends on severity of depression.
- *Ongoing mild depression beyond 4wks:* non-directive supportive therapy, group cognitive behavioural therapy (CBT) (📖 Talking therapies, p. 429), or guided self-help.
- *Moderate to severe depression:* specific psychological therapy, e.g. individual CBT, interpersonal therapy or shorter-term family therapy. If unresponsive, different and combined therapies considered including the use of medication, e.g. fluoxetine.
- *Exercise therapy:* regular programme of exercise.
- Inpatient care considered when child or young person at significant risk of self-harm.

## Advice for family members
- Encourage child to talk about worries; listen and offer help.
- If suspect more than passing phase contact GP/get professional help.

## Outcomes
- Most children (2 out of 3) improve, but full recovery may take years.
- Liability to further episodes.
- Increased risk of depression in adulthood.

## Related topics

📖 Working with teenagers, p. 219; 📖 People with depression, p. 435.

## Reference

[1]NICE (2005). *Depression in children and young people: Clinical Guideline 28.* Available at: 🔗 www.nice.org.uk/CG28

## Further information

Royal College of Psychiatrists. Available at: 🔗 www.rcpsych.ac.uk/expertadvice/youthinfo.aspx
Understanding Childhood. Available at: 🔗 www.understandingchildhood.net. Leaflets on helping parents and children cope with loss events, e.g. divorce, death
Young Minds (charity for improving children's and young people mental health and wellbeing). ☎ Parents Helpline 0808 802 5544. Available at: 🔗 www.youngminds.org.uk

# Eczema in childhood

Atopic eczema is an inflammatory skin condition characterized by dry, itchy, red, and inflamed skin. A genetically determined disorder with hypersensitivity to certain antigens such as pollen, feathers, house dust, household pets, dairy, wheat, soy products which can lead to eczema, asthma, and hay fever. It affects approximately 15% of the child population usually starts <6mths and 90% are in remission by 15yrs. <10% eczema result of food and inhalant allergies. Can affect self-esteem in children and young people and affect the whole family, e.g. through infant sleep disturbance.

## Symptoms and signs
- Dry skin and itchiness.
- Erythema, papules, vesicles.
- Exudation, crusting, scaling, fissures.
- Hyper- or hypopigmentation on some areas.

In the acute stages the skin is red and inflamed leading to vesicles exudations and crusting. In the chronic stages the skin is dry and thickened from repeated scratching. Food allergies considered if reacting to certain foods and inhalant allergies if seasonal flare-ups.

## Care and support
Eczema in a family can cause an increase of stress for other family members. Explain condition and overall good prognosis. Advise:
- Avoid the use of soaps and detergents on the skin.
- Loose cotton clothing next to the skin.
- Nails kept short to reduce damaging the skin if scratching.
- Avoid and minimize irritants, e.g.
  - Dust mites—damp dusting, vacuuming the room and bed, changing the bedding regularly, wash soft toys frequently.
  - Keep pets away.

## Food allergies and eczema
Breastfeeding should be encouraged in all babies to 6mths (💭 Breastfeeding, p. 176). If bottle feeding extensively then hydrolysed cows' milk formula should be recommended, where parents and/or siblings have atopic conditions. Babies allergic to cows' milk should be referred to specialist allergy services and dietician for specialist testing and advice on dietary manipulation.

## Specific treatment
Treatment aims to replace moisture loss on skin and provide a waterproof barrier to prevent further moisture loss and to protect skin. It aims to ↓ inflammation and relieve the intense itch. A stepped up and down approach is used according to severity of eczema (see 💭 NICE guidelines[1]). Referral to dermatologists if the eczema is not responding to treatment or severe presentations.

*Emollients therapy* **(BNF for children 13.2)**
- Emollients help to repair the broken skin barrier by acting like an artificial fat filling the cracks and allowing water to be retained by the skin cells.
- All soaps and detergents (and shampoo in <12yrs) should be replaced with emollient soap substitute, emollient bath oil. A daily soak for at least 15mins hydrates the skin and provides a good base for the applications of emollients.
- Emollient creams and ointment should be applied 3–4x day even when the skin is clear.

*Topical corticosterioids*
Topical steroids (BNF 13.4) are effective to control inflammation and stop itchiness. Benefits of correct usage outweigh potential harms. A stepped approach to usage in response to severity of the eczema.

*Wet wrapping and paste bandaging*
Wet wrapping used, but little evidence about its effectiveness. Aims to:
- Rehydrate and cool the skin.
- Treat inflammation and promote skin healing.
- ↓ itching and protection against scratching.
- ↑ comfort and ↑ sleep if applied before bed.

The wet wrap technique involves the following: bath the child with emollients added, pat dry then apply generous amounts of emollient ointment, then apply wet layer of tubifast (BNF A8.2.3) garment and then a dry layer. It should not be used if child's skin is infected. The community children's nurse, dermatology nurses, or HVs can teach the parents how to apply the wet wrap garments.

Paste bandages are used at night over steroids for lichenified eczema containing emollient, coal tar, or calamine. Usually prescribed by dermatologists.

*Other treatments*
- *Antihistamines* (BNF for children 3.4.1): to stop the itching and scratching. Short-term use in acute phases only. They are used an hour before bed time, daytime use should be avoided.
- *Antibiotic therapy*: to treat any 2° infection.
- *Complementary therapies*: such as Chinese herbal treatment increasingly used, but little evidence and little regulation of still in experimental stages. Referred to dermatology specialists for advice.
- Dermatologists treating severe eczema may prescribe topical calcineurin inhibitors, phototherapy, and oral steroids.

### Related topic
📖 Eczema/dermatitis, p. 636.

### Reference
[1]NICE (2007). *Management of atopic eczema in children from birth up to the age of 12 years. Clinical guidelines, CG57.* Available at: ℘ guidance.nice.org.uk/CG57

### Further information
National Eczema Society. Information, advice and fact sheets. Available at: ℘ www.eczema.org

# Emotional problems in children

This includes a range of internalizing disorders including fear, anxiety, and phobias. Management and treatment approaches are similar.

## Fear and anxiety

*Fear*  Focuses on a specific object or situation.

*Anxiety*

Diffuse and anticipatory (has developmental variations):

- Both fear and anxiety result in the same physiological manifestations: unhappiness, irritability, tantrums, sleep disruption.
- *Age and sex trends:* no consistent sex differences during infancy and pre-school years. In school years it is suggested that girls have more specific fears than boys.

### Anxiety in infants as part of normal development

- *Stranger anxiety:* by 4–5mths, peaks 12mths.
- *Separation anxiety:* related to stranger anxiety, from 8–24mths, peaks 9–13mths, decreases from 30mths.

### Anxiety in childhood and adolescence

- Separation and stranger anxiety diminish as capacity to anticipate events develops.
- Stranger fear may manifest itself as shyness.
- At school age most common fears are for harm coming to others.
- May start to exhibit anxiety about personal adequacy and achievement, e.g. test anxiety.
- Adolescents may show anxieties relating to social situations, e.g. rejection and may develop phobias or sexual fears.

### Generalized anxiety disorder

Characterized as 'worriers'. ~2% of children.

*Key features*

- Not related to environmental circumstances.
- *Four broad features:*
  - Worries.
  - Restlessness, nervousness, inability to relax.
  - Physical symptoms.
  - Difficulty concentrating; irritability.

### Separation anxiety disorder

Anxiety related to separation from people to whom child is attached. ~3% of children. Onset occurs before adolescence, may continue into early adulthood. May result in school refusal—peak occurs at time of transition, also in adolescence, 5yrs, 11yrs, 14–15yrs are most common (~1%).

## Specific phobias

These are fears that results in avoidance behaviour to the point of interfering with daily functioning. These may involve certain objects, situations. The child may develop anticipatory anxiety for phobic situation. Prevalence is unknown.

### Aetiology

- *Genetic and constitutional:* runs in families.
- Temperament.
- *Parental behaviour:* e.g. over-protection, criticism.
- Specific experiences and life events.
- *Cognitive appraisal of stressful events:* e.g. abuse.
- Social adversity.

### Treatment/management

Referred to local CAMHS as per local guidance.

- *Generalized anxiety:* remove/reduce stresses, enhance coping mechanisms, psychotherapy, medication may help.
- *Separation anxiety:* brief, focused counselling; improve understanding of anxiety, behavioural treatment, e.g. behavioural control skills.
- *Other specific phobias:* behavioural methods.
- *Panic disorder:* behavioural methods, medication may help.
- *Social phobia:* behavioural methods.

### Behavioural methods

Modification of acceptable and unacceptable behaviours. Reinforcement of good/wanted behaviour, ignore/distract from unacceptable/bad behaviour. May use training procedures—rewards (reinforcement) and punishments.

Generally children with anxiety disorders have reasonably good prognosis, but may experience some remissions and some exacerbations throughout childhood and into adulthood.

## Advice for parents

Follow guidance on basics for emotional support (see 🕮 Emotional development in babies and children, p. 199), as well as specifics as provided by CAMHS.

## Further information

Mental Health Foundation. Available at: ℘ www.mentalhealth.org.uk
Young Minds. Available at: ℘ www.youngminds.org.uk
Royal College of Psychiatrists. Available at: ℘ www.rcpsych.ac.uk/expertadvice/youthinfo/parentscarers.aspx
Association for Infant Mental Health. Available at: ℘ www.aimh.org.uk

# Endocrine problems

## Diabetes

See 📖 Diabetes: overview, p. 611; 📖 Insulin therapies, p. 618.

Incidence increasing and now affects 2:1000 children <16yrs. Almost all are insulin dependent (type 1 diabetes) with peak years of presentation at 12–13 with polyuria, polydipsia, and weight loss. Type 2 is rare, but increasing in children and is mostly obesity related (📖 Overweight children and adolescents, p. 291). Symptoms of polydipsia, polyuria, tiredness, and weight loss or looking thinner (❶ currently 1 in 4 diagnosed when in diabetic ketoacidosis). On diagnosis the child is referred to specialist diabetes team. Commenced on insulin by SC injection. Young children usually given insulin bd. Older children and teenagers often have three or four injections a day relating insulin more closely to food and exercise, diet and insulin have to be closely matched. NHS funding for delivery via pumps may be available for those >12yrs if multiple injections is impractical or inappropriate. Parents and children need intensive education and support to cover:

• Nature of diabetes.
• Injecting insulin.
• Diet-regular meals and snacks, reduced refined carbohydrates, healthy diet with no more than 30% fat.
• Sick day rules during illness to prevent ketoacidosis.
• Blood glucose monitoring or in young urine testing.
• Recognition and treatment of hypoglycaemia.
• How to get help and advice 24h/day.
• Emotions and coming to terms with the diagnosis.

Children have special needs (📖 Children with special educational needs, p. 227) and schools need to be included in addressing specific needs through the day, e.g. a snack and what to do if child becomes hypoglycemic.

*Hypoglycaemia* Most complain of hunger, dizziness, wobbly feeling in legs, irritability. Treated with easily absorbed glucose, e.g. glucose tablets, gels. Parents and schools should be provided and taught how to use IM glucagon injection kit for hypoglycaemia if child is not responding.

*Screening offered for complications and associated conditions*
• Coeliac disease at time of diagnosis.
• Thyroid disease at diagnosis and annually until transfer to adult services.
• >12yrs retinopathy, microalbuminuria, and BP.

## Neonatal (congenital) hypothyroidism

~1 per 4000 live births. It is due to congenital absence of the thyroid gland. One of few preventable causes of severe learning difficulties. Normally detected by blood spot/heel prick testing (📖 Child screening tests, p. 152). Child is referred for specialist advice. Treatment is with lifelong thyroxine replacement. In most treated infants development is normal.

## Hyperthyroidism

Usually, the result of Graves' disease—characterized by anxiety, restlessness, weight loss, thyrotoxicosis, and exophthalmos. The child is referred to specialist for drug therapy lasting up to 2yrs and then possible surgery if relapse.

## Inborn errors of metabolism

Many hundreds of enzyme defects have been identified mostly with an autosomal recessive inheritance. Very rare and consequently managed at specialist centres. These include:

- *Phenylketonuria (PKU):* deficiency of the enzyme phenylalaninehydroxylase. 1 in 10,000–20,000 live births, detected by blood spot/heel prick test (⌨ Child screening tests, p. 152). Treated with restriction of dietary phenylaline lifelong and particularly during pregnancy. With treatment, growth, and development are normal.
- *Galactosaemia:* deficiency of galactose-1-phosphate uridyl transferase. Inability to mobilize glucose from galactose resulting in hypoglycaemia. When lactose containing milk feeds (including breast) are introduced results in vomiting, jaundice, hepatic failure. Management is by lactose- and galactose-free diet. Even if treated early, severe learning difficulties are common.

## Related topic

⌨ Growth disorders, p. 280.

## National frameworks

NICE (2004 modified 2011). *Type 1 diabetes: Diagnosis and management of type 1 diabetes in children, young people and adults.* Available at: ℘ publications.nice.org.uk/type-1-diabetes-cg15

NICE (2011). Quality Standards for Diabetes (based on the DH *NSF for diabetes 2001*). Available at: ℘ guidance.nice.org.uk/QS6

National Service Framework for Children, Young People and Maternity Services. *Type 1 diabetes in childhood and adolescence.* London: NHS. Available at: ℘ www.gov.uk/government/publications/diabetes-type-1-in-childhood-national-service-framework-for-children-young-people-and-maternity-services

National Service Framework for Diabetes in Wales. Available at: ℘ www.wales.nhs.uk/sites3/page.cfm?orgid=440&pid=3653

Scottish Diabetes Action Plan (2010). Available at: ℘ www.diabetesinscotland.org.uk/

## Information and resources for parents, children, and professionals

Diabetes UK. Available at: ℘ www.diabetes.org.uk including dedicated website for young people.

Juvenile Diabetes Research Foundation. Available at: ℘ www.jdrf.org.uk/

British Thyroid Foundation. Available at: ℘ www.british-thyroid-association.org

National Society for Phenylketonuria. Available at: ℘ www.nspku.org/

# Febrile convulsions and epilepsy

A seizure or fit is when there is a sudden disturbance of neurological function associated with an abnormal neuronal discharge. Occurs in 3–5% of children. The child is referred for paediatric assessment.

## Febrile convulsions

A febrile convulsion is a seizure associated with fever in the absence of another cause:

- 3–5% of children aged 6mths–5yrs.
- Seizures are usually brief (last <5min) and generalized.
- The risk of subsequent epilepsy is low.

### Management

- Most children do not need hospital admission.
- Parent reassurance and education important. Give practical advice given on how to prevent attacks by reducing fevers, e.g. early use of paracetamol and tepid sponging (📖 The sick baby and child, p. 238).
- Those with recurrent or complex febrile convulsions are referred to paediatrician. They are sometimes treated with rectal diazepam (BNF for children 4.8.3) and parents need teaching when and how to administer.

## Epilepsy

(See 📖 Seizures and epilepsy, p. 693) Epilepsy is recurrent seizures other than febrile convulsions and not due to intracranial infection. 60% of adult epilepsy starts in childhood. It affects in about 5 per 1000 school children. See 📖 Epilepsy, p. 693 for diagnosis, treatment, and management. Surgery is increasingly being used for some types of childhood epilepsy. Every child is reviewed at least annually by specialist paediatric services.

### Support and education for parents and children

Epilepsy is a diagnosis that can cause great alarm and fear. Education is very important. Parents, children, and young people need clear information on:

- What to expect.
- What to do during an attack and how to brief other people, e.g. school staff.
- Avoiding risks, e.g. swimming or cycling alone, but not being over-protective.
- Importance of concordance with medication, particularly teenagers.
- When drug withdrawal may be considered if fit-free.
- Adolescent girls in particular may need specific advice around contraception and pregnancy.

School health staff may have a particular role in helping educate school staff and other children about the condition. Some children with recurring and frequent seizures, usually attending special schools, may require rectal diazepam in particular circumstances as prescribed by the paediatrician. See 📖 Working in schools, p. 38.

## Further information

NICE (2012). *The epilepsies: the diagnosis and management of the epilepsies in adults and children in primary and secondary care.* Available at: ℘ www.nice.org.uk/CG137

Great Ormond Street Information on Febrile Convulsions. Available at: ℘ www.gosh.nhs.uk/medical-conditions/search-for-medical-conditions/febrile-convulsions/

NHS Choices. Febrile seizures. Available at: ℘ www.nhs.uk/conditions/Febrile-convulsions/Pages/Introduction.aspx

Epilepsy Action. Available at: ☎ 0808 800 5050. ℘ www.epilepsy.org.uk

Young Epilepsy. ☎ 01342 831 342 Mon–Fri 09.00-13.00 hours. Available at: ℘ youngepilepsy.org.uk/

### Helplines

NHS 111 (England). ☎ 111. Available at: ℘ http://www.nhs.uk/NHSEngland/AboutNHSservices/Emergencyandurgentcareservices/Pages/NHS-111.aspx

NHS Direct (Wales). ☎ 0845 46 47. Available at: ℘ www.nhsdirect.wales.nhs.uk/24hr helpline

NHS 24 (Scotland) NHS. ☎ 08454 242424. Available at: ℘ www.nhs24.com/24-h helpline Scotland

# Gastrointestinal problems in children

Most children experience GI problems, e.g. vomiting. In most instances the symptoms are mild and transient. Advice is given to parents on nursing a sick child and identifying signs as to when to seek medical advice (📖 The sick baby and child, p. 238).

## Vomiting and diarrhoea

*Posseting and regurgitation* Terms used to describe non-forceful return of milk. It usually resolves with the introduction of solid food and by 1yr.

*Vomiting* The forceful ejection of gastric contents. It may be linked to specific events, e.g. travel sickness or a symptom of an infection.

*Projectile vomiting* is a symptom of pyloric stenosis. Infantile hypertrophic pyloric stenosis usually develops in the first 3–6wks of life (rare after 12wks). Failure of the pyloric sphincter to relax → hypertrophy of the adjacent pyloric muscle. Requires paediatric assessment. Treated with surgery with no long-term effects.

### Vomiting and diarrhoea

Parent information important to determine nature and seriousness of problem, including:
- Nature and duration of symptoms.
- Presence of green bile in vomit.
- Presence of blood in the stool.
- Other accompanying symptoms, e.g. fever.
- Contact with anyone else with similar symptoms.
- History of recent foreign travel.

### Possible causes
- Breastfed babies have loose, often explosive 'mustard grain' stools.
- Toddlers often have intermittent loose stools related to diet. Usually resolves by 5yrs.
- *Gastrointestinal infection:* child may have diarrhoea, vomiting or combination of the two. Usually viral in origin, e.g. Norovirus, and common in winter. Parents advised:
  - To ensure adequate fluids, to prevent dehydration.
  - To eat normally, especially in cases of diarrhoea, or re-introduce as soon as possible and in cases of diarrhoea to avoid giving fruit juice and carbonated drinks until diarrhoea has stopped.
  - On nursing sick infant and when to seek medical help.
  - Actions to prevent spread.
- Malabsorption (see 📖 Coeliac disease, p. 666).
- *Acute abdominal problems* includes:
  - *Intussusception*—the invagination of one part of the bowel into the lumen of the immediately adjoining bowel. 2 per 1000 live births. Usually between 5 and 18mths. Presents with acute pain, vomiting, passage of recurrent jelly like stool. Is a medical emergency treated surgically.
  - Appendicitis. See 📖 Small intestine problems, p. 668.

See 📖 Constipation and encopresis, p. 260.

## Advice on preventing spread of gastrointestinal viruses

From NICE guidelines.[1]

- All household members should wash hands frequently with (preferably liquid) soap in warm running water and dry carefully. In particular after:
  - Going to the toilet or changing nappies.
  - Before preparing, serving, or eating food.
- Individual towels and no sharing towels with infected child towels.
- While child/infant has vomiting or diarrhoea they should not attend any school or childcare facility or return until after 48hrs of last episode.
- Children should not swim in swimming pools for 2wks after the last episode of diarrhoea.

## Reference

[1]NICE (2009). *CG84 Management of acute diarrhoea and vomiting due to gastroenteritis in children under 5.* Available at: ℗ www.nice.org.uk/CG84

## Further information

NHS Choices. Norovirus. Available at: ℗ www.nhs.uk/Conditions/Norovirus/Pages/Introduction.aspx

NHS Direct (England). Available at: ℗ www.nhsdirect.nhs.uk 24hr helpline

NHS Direct (Wales). Available at: ☎ 0845 46 47. ℗ www.nhsdirect.wales.nhs.uk/ 24hr helpline

NHS 24 (Scotland) NHS. ☎ 08454 242424. Available at: ℗ www.nhs24.com/ 24hr helpline Scotland.

# Genetic problems

There are 46 chromosomes: 22 are matching pairs with matching genes (autosomes); the remaining pair are sex chromosomes that may match (XX—♀) or differ (XY—♂). Parents of any child affected by a genetic problem are offered genetic counselling and pre-natal diagnosis, if available, for any subsequent pregnancies. Care, support, and treatment depends on specific problems of each child and family. The 1° health care team, specialist health care services, social services, community paediatric services, education services, and voluntary organizations involved as necessary. Each child and family should be reviewed regularly (📖 Children with complex health needs and disabilities, p. 225).

## Down's syndrome

Trisomy 21 (an extra chromosome number 21). Commonest chromosomal abnormality affecting 1:600 births. Life expectancy is ↓, but ~ half live to 60yrs. Incidence ↑ with maternal age at conception.

### Clinical features

- *Facial abnormalities:* flat occiput, oval face, low-set eyes with prominent epicanthic folds.
- Single palmar crease.
- Hypotonia.
- Developmental delay.
- Congenital heart disease.

See 📖 People with learning disabilities, p. 408.

## Edward's syndrome

Trisomy 18. 1 per 8000 births. Life expectancy is ~10mths (♀ >♂).

### Clinical features

- *Facial abnormalities:* low-set malformed ears, receding chin, protruding eyes, cleft lip or palate.
- A short sternum makes the nipples appear too widely separated. Fingers cannot be extended and the index finger overlaps the 3rd digit.
- Developmental delay.
- Umbilical or inguinal hernias.
- Rocker-bottom feet.
- Rigid baby with flexion of the limbs.

## Patau's syndrome

Trisomy 13. 1 per 7500 births. 50% die <1mth. Usually fatal in the first year. Multiple abnormalities including:

- Small head and eyes.
- Brain malformation.
- Heart malformations.
- Polycystic kidneys.
- Cleft lip/palate.
- Skeletal abnormalities, e.g. flexion contractures of hands +/– polydactyly with narrow fingernails.

# Cri du chat syndrome

Deletion of the short arm of chromosome 5 is the most common deletion syndrome. 1 per 25,000–50,000 births. Life expectancy unpredictable. Presents with:

- Abnormal cry (cat-like).
- Microcephaly.
- Developmental delay.
- Marked epicanthic folds.
- Moon-shaped face.
- Alert expression.

# Sex chromosome abnormalities

**Turner's syndrome**  XO—deletion of 1 X chromosome. 1:2500 live births. Mosaicism may occur (XO, XX). Lifespan is normal.

*Clinical features*
- Female appearance.
- Short stature (<130cm).
- Hyperconvex nails.
- Wide carrying angle (cubitus valgus).
- Inverted nipples.
- Broad chest.
- Ptosis.
- Nystagmus.
- Webbed neck.
- Coarctation of the aorta.
- Left heart defects.
- Lymphoedema of the legs.
- Ovaries are rudimentary or absent.

*Specialist management*
Human growth hormone may be considered for short stature.

**Klinefelter's syndrome**  XXY or XXYY polysomy. 1 per 1000 live births. Life span is normal.

*Clinical features*
- Male appearance.
- Often undetected until presentation with infertility in adult life.
- May present at adolescence with psychopathy, ↓ libido, sparse facial hair, gynaecomastia, and small firm testes.

*Associations*  Hypothyroidism, DM, asthma.

*Specialist management*  Androgens and plastic surgery may be used for gynaecomastia.

# Autosomal dominant inheritance

>1000 diseases are known to be inherited in this way. Individually they are rare and together account for <1% of all disease. Heterozygotes demonstrate the disease. 1:2 pregnancies of an affected individual will be affected, usually ♂ = ♀. Expression of the gene in a given individual may vary. Example—Marfan's syndrome (📖 Bone and joint problems, p. 249).

## Autosomal recessive inheritance

>700 known diseases. Only manifest in the homozygote. Heterozygotes may be asymptomatic or show milder abnormalities. To develop severe disease, the affected gene must be inherited from both parents who must both be heterozygotes. The risk of an affected pregnancy is 1:4, usually $\sigma$ = $\mathcal{Q}$. Affected individuals have unaffected children unless their partner is a heterozygote.

### Glycogen storage diseases

*Incidence*

1:25,000. A group of hereditary disorders caused by lack of ≥1 enzyme involved in glycogen synthesis or breakdown and characterized by deposition of abnormal amounts or types of glycogen in tissues. Inheritance is autosomal recessive for all forms except type VI, which follows an X-linked inheritance. Symptoms and age of onset vary considerably:

- *Predominantly liver involvement* (types I, III, IV, VI) → hepatomegaly, hypoglycaemia, metabolic acidosis.
- *Predominantly muscle involvement* (types V, VII) → weakness, lethargy, poor feeding, heart failure.

Treatment involves frequent small carbohydrate meals; allopurinol (to prevent renal urate stone formation and/or gout) +/– limiting anaerobic exercise. A high-protein diet is also helpful for some patients.

**Other examples** Phenylketonuria (PKU) see 🕮 Endocrine problems, p. 270; 🕮 Sickle cell disorders, p. 292; 🕮 Thalassaemia, p. 294; 🕮 Cystic fibrosis, p. 262.

## Sex-linked disorders

~100 are recognized. Most are recessively inherited from the mother and affect only $\sigma$ offspring.

- A male child of a heterozygote mother has a 1:2 chance of developing the disease.
- A female child of a heterozygote mother has a 1:2 chance of carrying the disease.
- A female child can only be affected by the disease if father has the disease and mother is a carrier when she has a 1:2 chance of being affected and, if not affected, will be a carrier.

### Fragile X syndrome

Affects 1 per 1250 $\sigma$ births and 1 per 2500 $\mathcal{Q}$ births. Genetic abnormality carried on the X-chromosome comprising:

- Low IQ (20–70).
- Large testes.
- High forehead.
- Large jaw.
- Facial asymmetry.
- Long ears.
- Short temper.

Half of carrier females have a normal IQ, half are affected. Fragile X syndrome should be considered in any child with developmental delay of unknown cause.

*Management*
There is some evidence that folic acid supplements ↓ hyperactive and disruptive behaviour tendencies in children with fragile X. Antenatal testing is possible for future pregnancies.

**Other examples**
Haemophilia, Duchenne's muscular dystrophy.

## Polygenic inheritance
Familial trends of disease are commonly seen, but there is often no simple inheritance pattern. Usually due to the combination of genes inherited (polygenic inheritance).

**Other examples** 📖 Neural tube defects, p. 289; 📖 Cleft lip and palate, p. 255; Type 1 diabetes mellitus, 📖 Endocrine problems, p. 270; Pyloric stenosis, 📖 Gastrointestinal problems in children p. 274; Schizophrenia, 📖 People with schizophrenia, p. 443.

## Further information
Association for Glycogen Storage Disease (UK). Available at ℡ www.agsd.org.uk
Contact a Family. ☎ 0808 808 3555. Available at ℡ www.cafamily.org.uk/
Down's Syndrome Association. ☎ 0333 1212 300. Available at ℡ www.downs-syndrome.org.uk
Fragile X Society. ☎ 01371 875 100. Available at ℡ www.fragilex.org.uk
Genetics Alliance UK. Available at ℡ www.geneticalliance.org.uk/
National Society for Phenylketonuria. Available at ℡ www.nspku.org/
Reproduced and updated from 'Genetic problems' ir Simon C, Everitt H and Kendrick T (2005)
    *Oxford Handbook of General Practice* 2nd edition. With permission of Oxford University Press.
Turner's Syndrome Support Society. Available at ℡ www.tss.org.uk

# Growth disorders

Growth starts *in utero* and ends after puberty.

## Measurement

Detail of national policies on weight, height, and head circumference measurement is given in ☐ Overview of healthy child programme, p. 146. Good practice is to also record height and weight if there are concerns about a child either because of chronic ill health or requires prolonged follow-up.

## Interpretation

Interpretation of measurements for stage of puberty, including predicting child adult height and comparison with parental height is done with use of UK-WHO growth charts[1]. Review by GP or community paediatrician indicated if child height centile more than 3 centile spaces below mid-parental centile.

## Short stature

Usually defined as height below second centile. Most of these will be normal, but short. Most short children are well adjusted to their size, however, there may be issues at school with bullying, low self-esteem, disadvantages at sport. Also may be treated inappropriately by others as younger than their age.

### Causes

- *Psychosocial deprivation:* children subjected to physical and emotional deprivation (☐ A child or young person in need, p. 150) may be short, underweight with delayed puberty (☐ Puberty and adolescence, p. 215). Growth catches up if placed in nurturing environment.
- Intrauterine growth disorders (☐ Antenatal care and screening, p. 380).
- Chronic illness associated with nutritional problems, e.g. ☐ Coeliac disease, p. 666; ☐ Cystic fibrosis, p. 262.
- Chromosomal disorders, e.g. Down's syndrome, Turner's syndrome (☐ Genetic problems, p. 276), achondroplasia (short limb or disproportionate short stature previously known as dwarfism).
- *Endocrine problems* (☐ p. 270):
  - Hypothyroidism treated with thyroxine.
  - Growth hormone deficiency referred to specialist centres. Treated with biosynthetic growth hormone by SC injection usually daily.

## Tall stature

Most tall stature is inherited from parents. Some adolescents become concerned about excessive height during pubertal growth spurt. Tall children may be disadvantaged by being treated older than their chronological age. Secondary endocrine causes are rare, e.g. pituitary adenoma (gigantism). Some long-legged tall stature seen in children with chromosome syndromes (☐ Genetic problems, p. 276), e.g. Marfan's and Klinefelter's (XXY) syndromes.

## Abnormal head growth

Most head growth occurs <2yrs and 80% of adult head size achieved by age 5yrs, reflecting brain growth. Posterior fontanelle closes by 8wks, anterior by 12–18mths. Small or large heads may be familial. Children with head circumference <3rd or >97th centile referred for paediatric assessment. Abnormal head growth includes:

* *Skull asymmetry:* may be due to an imbalance in growth, or in pre-terms lying on sides in incubators for a long time, and usually resolves.
* *Craniosynostosis:* premature fusion of skull sutures—referred urgently to specialist.
* *Microcephaly:* circumference <2nd centile. Small head out of proportion with the body. Associated with developmental delay (📖 Children with complex health needs and disabilities, p. 225). Causes—genetic, intrauterine infection (e.g. rubella, CMV), hypoxia.
* *Macrocephaly:* circumference >98th centile. Most are normal children with familial large heads. Rapidly rising head circumference may be due to hydrocephalus, subdural haematoma or brain tumour. Referred urgently to specialist.

## Premature sexual development

Development of secondary sexual characteristics before 8yrs ♀ and 9yrs ♂ is outside the normal range, usually referred to specialist for assessment and investigation.

* *Precocious puberty:* usually familial and organic causes rare, e.g. congenital adrenal hyperplasia, or androgen secreting tumor.
* *Premature breast development only (thelarche):* usually in 6mth–2yrs females and self-limiting.
* *Premature public hair only (adrenarche):* usually self-limiting.

## Delayed puberty

Delayed puberty is the absence of pubertal development by 14yrs ♀ and 15yrs ♂. Common in boys with familial history of delayed puberty. May be a source of problems at school and cause low self-esteem. Often referred for specialist assessment to identify any underlying chronic systemic disorders, e.g. Crohn's disease or hormonal problems. May be treated with weak androgenic anabolic steroids, and testosterone (♂) or oestradiol (♀).

## Related topics

📖 Growth 0–2 years, p. 181; 📖 Growth 2–4 years, p. 195; 📖 Growth and nutrition 5–11 years, p. 210; 📖 Growth and nutrition 12–18 years, p. 221.

## Reference

[1]UK-WHO 0–4 years growth chart resources: charts, training materials, fact sheets. Available at: ℘ www.rcpch.ac.uk/child-health/research-projects/uk-who-growth-charts-early-years/uk-who-0-4-years-growth-charts-initi

## Further information

Child Growth Foundation. Available at: ℘ www.childgrowthfoundation.org/
Great Ormond St. Hospital Medical Conditions Achondroplasia. Available at: ℘ www.gosh.nhs.uk/medical-conditions/
NHS Choices. Restricted Growth. Available at: ℘ www.nhs.uk/Conditions/Restricted-growth/Pages/Introduction.aspx
Short Stature Scotland. Available at: ℘ www.shortstaturescotland.co.uk/

# Infections in children

Viral infections are very common in childhood. Advice to parents on caring for a sick child and when to seek medical advice is important (see 📖 The sick baby and child, p. 238).

## Respiratory tract infections

Most are viral in origin and will resolve spontaneously. Evidence suggests there should be no or delayed antibiotic prescribing for self-limiting respiratory tract infections unless systemically unwell, have symptoms suggestive of serious illness at high risk of serious complications because of co-morbidity, e.g. cystic fibrous (📖 p. 262), young children born prematurely and children <2yrs with bilateral acute otitis media and children with otorrhoea who have acute otitis media (see NICE CG69[1]).

- *URTIs:* are extremely common and usually viral in origin. URTIs include the *common cold* (coryza), presents with discharging or blocked nose, malaise, cough, and sometimes mild pyrexia. Resolves in a few days with paracetamol suspension and fluids. May cause exacerbation of asthma and in infants, difficulty in feeding and febrile convulsions. Purulent sputum indicates infection and may require antibiotics.
- *Acute otitis media:* infection (could be bacterial or viral) of the middle ear. 20% of <4yrs experience at least 1/yr. Average total illness length = 4 days. Presents with pain and fever. On visual inspection with auroscope, red bulging drum. Many resolve spontaneously within 24hrs; >80% resolve in <3 days without treatment. Many local policies advocate conservative approaches to prescribing antibiotics, e.g. manage with paracetamol and fluids, antibiotics reserved for unresolved infections after 3 days. Recurrent ear infections can lead to *chronic secretory otitis media* (known as glue ear), most common cause of conductive hearing loss. May be referred for paediatric assessment and insertion of grommets into tympanic membrane. Current debates on effectiveness of this procedure.
- *Sore throat/tonsillitis:* is pharyngitis (infection of throat, usually viral) with intense inflammation of tonsils, often with purulent exudates. May be treated with antibiotics. Children with recurrent infections of tonsils and adenoids referred for paediatric assessment. May have adenotonsillectomy if interfering with development, schooling or has abscess.
- *Bronchiolitis:* serious respiratory infection, usually viral, in <1yr characterized by cold symptoms, followed by dry cough and increasing breathlessness. Requires medical assessment and often hospital admission for humidified oxygen.
- *Croup:* a viral URTI characterized by a barking cough and inspiratory stridor. Steam may help. Requires medical review and may be admitted to hospital in acute phase.
- *Pneumonia:* may be viral or bacterial. Child has fever, malaise, cough, often purulent sputum. Requires medical review and may need hospital admission.

## Urinary tract infections

8% girls and 2% boys experience UTIs, most <1yr. Most caused by normal bowel flora. UTIs may be more common in children with renal abnormalities. Consequences can include renal scarring. Infants and toddlers may present with non-specific symptoms, e.g. fever, vomiting. Older children may present with dysuria, frequency, abdominal pain, enuresis. Diagnosis by MC&S of clean catch urine sample. Treated with antibiotics as per local guidelines for UTI diagnosis. Referred to paediatrician if <3mths and UTI suspected or if recurrent infections as may have renal abnormality.

## Other common infections

See 📖 Infectious diseases in childhood, p. 283.

### Conjunctivitis

Infection (bacterial or viral) of the conjunctiva. Young children are very susceptible to repeated episodes and severe forms. Presents with red eye(s), swollen eyelid(s), discharge often sticks lids together. 64% resolve in 5 days without treatment.

- Treatment with antibiotics eye drops or ointment (BNF for children 11.1 and 11.3.1.).
- Up to 25% physical transmission in household so advise to avoid sharing towels, etc. No need for exclusion from day care or school (see HPA[2]).
- If presenting with these symptoms <1mth (different from new born sticky eye see 📖 New babies, p. 173) swabbed for MS&C. Possibly contracted STI through the birth canal (ophthalmia neonatorum, a notifiable disease).

### Impetigo   See 📖 Bacterial skin infections, p. 632.

## References

[1]NICE (2008). *CG69 Prescribing of antibiotics for self-limiting respiratory tract infections in adults and children in primary care.* Available at: ℘ www.nice.org.uk/CG069
[2]Health Protection Agency. Available at: ℘ www.hpa.org.uk

## Further information

NICE (2007). *CG54 Urinary tract infection: diagnosis, treatment and long-term management of urinary tract infection in children.* Available at: ℘ www.nice.org.uk/CG054
NICE Clinical Knowledge Summaries. Available at: ℘ cks.nice.org.uk/#azTab
NHS Choices. Available at: ℘ www.nhs.uk/Conditions

## Infectious diseases in childhood

Primary immunization (📖 Childhood immunization general, p. 156) has virtually eliminated all traditional childhood diseases with the exception of chickenpox. Key aspects of these diseases are summarized in Table 7.1. Parents should be advised on caring for a sick child and reminded of key indicators when to seek medical advice (see 📖 The sick baby and child, p. 238).

See Table 7.2 for infectious disease exclusion times.

**Table 7.1** Infectious disease in childhood

| Disease | Transmission/ incubation | Presentation | Treatment | Complications | Infectious |
|---|---|---|---|---|---|
| Chickenpox | Physical contact, droplet, airborne. 11–20 days | Rash +/- fever. Spots progress from macule → papule → vesicle. Crops appear for 5–7 days. Vesicles dry out and scab over (usually in <14 days) | Supportive: paracetamol, fluids, topical calamine lotion to lesions | Eczema herpeticum, encephalitis, pneumonia | Until 5 days after skin eruption |
| Diphtheria (very rare in UK) | Droplet 2–5 days | Inflammatory exudate that forms a greyish membrane in respiratory tract | Hospital admission for antitoxin and antibiotics | Respiratory obstruction | |
| Haemophilus influenzae (very rare in UK) | Respiratory droplet. Nasal secretions | Meningitis: 60% | Antibiotics | Permanent neurological sequelae; mortality—5% | Until antibiotic treatment for 24hrs |
| Erthema infectiosum (5th disease) | Respiratory droplet. 4–7 days | Erthematous maculo-papular rash starting on face, then lacy rash on trunk and limbs. Mild disease | Tepid sponging, paracetamol and fluids | | Probably only during prodome. Important for pregnant ♀ to report contact to GP |
| Measles | Respiratory droplet. 10–14 days | Early: fever, conjunctivitis, cough, cold. Later: Koplik's spots (white spots on bright red background inside mouth) red maculopapular rash appears after 4 days Last ≈ 10 days | Tepid sponging, paracetamol and fluids | Bronchopneumonia, otitis media, gastroenteritis, encephalitis | Highly contagious for up to 18 days to non-immune |

| | Transmission / Incubation | Symptoms | Treatment | Complications | Infectious period |
|---|---|---|---|---|---|
| Mumps | Respiratory droplet. 16–21 days | Fever, malaise, tender enlargement of 1 or both parotids +/– submandibular glands | Tepid sponging, paracetamol and fluids | Aseptic meningitis; epididymo-orchitis; pancreatitis | Up to 29 days |
| Pertussis (whooping cough) | Respiratory droplet. 7 days | Catarrhal stage as URTI, coughing stage paroxysmal cough with spasms of coughing followed by a 'whoop' lasts 4–6wks | Antibiotics in catarrhal stage | Pneumonia, bronchiectasis, convulsions | Up to 5 days after start of antibiotics |
| Poliomyelitis (rare in UK) | Droplet or faeco-oral. 7 days | Flu-like prodrome then fever, tachycardia, headache, vomiting, neck stiffness and unilateral tremor, paralysis | Hospital admission | Permanent disability may result. <10% of those developing paralysis die | |
| Rubella (German measles) | Respiratory droplet. 14–21 days | Pink maculopapular rash for 3 days, mild fever | Paracetamol and fluids | Birth defects if infected in pregnancy, arthritis (adolescents); thrombocytopoenia (rare) | 15–23 days |
| Roseola infantum (<2yrs) | Oral secretions. 4–7 days | High fever, sore throat, macular rash appears after 3–4 days as fever drops | Tepid sponging, paracetamol and fluids | | 5–15 days |
| Scarlet fever | Respiratory droplet. 2–4 days | Fever, malaise, headache, tonsillitis, rash, 'scarlet' facial flushing | Penicillin | Rheumatic fever | Not known |

**Table 7.2** Infectious diseases exclusion times

| Disease | Exclusion period from early years care/schools |
|---|---|
| Chickenpox (varicella) | 5 days from start of skin eruption |
| Conjunctivitis | None |
| Gastroenteritis | Usually 48hrs after last episode of diarrhoea or vomiting |
| Glandular fever | None |
| Head lice | None |
| Hepatitis A | 7 days after onset of jaundice |
| Hepatitis B, C, HIV/AIDs | None |
| Herpes simplex | None |
| Impetigo | Until lesions healed/crusted or 48hrs from starting antibiotics |
| Infectious mononucleosis | None |
| Influenza | Until recovered |
| Measles | 4 days from onset of rash |
| Meningococcal disease | Bacterial—duration of illness. Viral—none |
| Mumps | 5 days from onset of swelling |
| Pertussis | 5 days from starting antibiotics otherwise >3wks |
| Rubella | 6 days from onset of rash |
| Scabies | Return after first treated |
| Scarlet fever | 24hrs from start of antibiotic treatment |
| Shingles | Only if rash weeping and can't be covered |
| Tinea (ring worm) | None |
| Threadworms | None |
| Tuberculosis | Smear positive: 2wks after starting treatment |
| Typhoid and paratyphoid | 24hrs after last episode of diarrhoea |
| Warts and verrucas | None |

*Source:* Health Protection Agency (2010). *Guidance on Infection Control in Schools and other Child Care settings.* Available at: ℻ www.hpa.org.uk/Topics/InfectiousDiseases/InfectionsAZ/SchoolsGuidanceOnInfectionControl/

## Further information

Health Protection Agency Topics Infections A–Z. Available at ℻ www.hpa.org.uk/Topics/InfectiousDiseases/
NHS Choices. Available at: ℻ www.nhs.uk/Conditions

# Insects and infestations

## Insect bites and stings

Response depends on the insect involved and the individual's response to the bite. The response ranges from blisters through papules to urticarial wheals. Stings should be removed if still embedded.

- Itching resulting from bites from fleas, flies, and mosquitoes can be treated with topical antihistamine (BNF for children 13.3), although greater allergic reactions may need oral anti-histamines.
- Anaphylactic reactions (see 📖 Anaphylaxis, p. 751).

Prevention includes:

- Animal flea infestation in homes needs treatment of animals and carpets. Sprays available OTC, severe infestations may need widespread spraying by a commercial company or local environmental health department (📖 Environmental health services, p. 23).
- Use of mosquito deterrent (see 📖 Travel health care, p. 350).

## Head lice (*Pediculus capitis*)

These are wingless insects. Most commonly found on children age 4–16yrs ($♀ > ♂$), but can infest anyone. Spread by lice walking from head to head. Eggs are known as 'nits' and laid at base of hair shaft, hatch within 7–10 days. Empty white shells remain 'glued' to hair. Nymph stage is 7–10 days to adult and then able to reproduce. Lice pierce the scalp to feed on blood.

### Prevention

No evidence of effectiveness of prophylactic treatment or use of herbal based lotions. Health promotion schemes with children and parents (e.g. Bug Busters[1]), particularly in early years facilities and schools, encourages:

- Hair management strategies.
- Early detection by weekly combing wet, conditioner covered, hair with light coloured, bevel edged, louse detection comb (fine-tooth).
- Early treatment to prevent spread.

### Symptoms

Itchy scalp and scratching. Detection of a moving louse, not old egg shells, confirms infestation. It is difficult to detect moving louse on dry or damp hair unless very severe infestation. Experts continue to debate effectiveness of wet combing and insecticides.

### Treatment by mechanical removal (wet combing)

- After washing hair, apply conditioner and systematically comb all hair with fine-tooth, detector comb (available from local pharmacies). Rinse comb after each stroke to remove trapped lice and not comb back into hair.
- Repeat on days 5, 9, 13 to remove nymphs. Detailed instruction on sites such as NHS Choices and Bug busters. Bug Buster™ kit can be prescribed on NHS (BNF for children 13.10.4).

*Chemical treatments with insecticides*
• Available OTC and on NHS prescription.
• Malathion, phenothrin, permethrin, and carbaryl mostly effective against lice. To overcome the development of resistance, a mosaic strategy is used rotating to different insecticide if treatment fails (BNF 13.10.4).
• Application as per instructions for contact time of 12hrs, repeated 7d later. Aqueous formulations preferred for small children and those with severe eczema, or asthma. Shampoos are not effective—use lotions or liquids.
• Note: some community concerns about using pesticides including organophosphates on children (see Pesticide Action Network[2]).

*Other treatments*
*Herbal therapies* For example, tea tree oil, herbal treatments. No evidence of effectiveness.

*All close contacts* For example, family, school friends should check their heads and be treated as necessary.

**Scabies** (*Sarcoptes scabie*) The scabies mite is ~½mm long and spread by direct physical contact.

*Symptoms* Appear 4–6wks after infection. Red burrows, tracking in irregular lines, commonly between fingers and toes. Intense itching. Scratching results in excoriations.

*Treatment*
Treated with permethrin 5% aqueous preparation over whole body and washed off after 8–12h (BNF 13.10.4). All close contacts need treatment. All worn clothing and bedding should be washed. Itching may persist for some time after elimination often alleviated by topical antihistamines.

## Threadworm (*Enterobulus vermicularis*)

Threadworm is common among children. Worm lives about 6wks. Causes anal itch as it leaves the bowel to lay eggs on the perineum. Often seen as silvery thread-like worms in stools or at the anus. Scratching transfers eggs to nails and hands, then ingested. Child >2yrs and household members treated with mebendazole. Piperazine for children <6mths. OTC (BNF for children 5.5.1). Prevention includes promoting good hand washing before meals and after going to the toilet, ensuring short and clean nails.

## References

[1]Bug Busting. Available at: ℅ www.chc.org
[2]Pesticide Action Network. Available at: ℅ www.pan-uk.org

## Further information

NICE Clinical Knowledge Summaries. Available at: ℅ cks.nice.org.uk/#azTab
NHS Choices How to treat nits. Available at: ℅ http://www.nhs.uk/Livewell/childhealth6-15/Pages/Nits.aspx

# Neural tube defects

The neural tube fuses in first 28 days after conception. Incomplete fusion leads to 4 types of malformation. Prevention is through folic acid supplements in ♀ planning pregnancy and in first 12wks (☐ Pre-conceptual care, p. 376). Most defects are detected antenatally (☐ Antenatal care and screening, p. 380). Incidence is now about 0.15/1000 births. Mothers who have had one fetus with a neural tube defect have a very high risk of second and should take high-dose folic acid preconceptually and for first 12wks.

## Malformations

- *Anencephaly:* absence of most of cranium and skull. Stillborn or die shortly after birth. Antenatal termination offered if detected.
- *Encephalocoele:* midline skull defect and brain and meninges herniated through. Corrected by surgery, but may be underlying malformations.
- *Spina bifida occulta:* failure of fusion of the vertebral arch. May be associated with skin lesion or tuft of hair. Usually asymptomatic.
- *Spina bifida.* Two types:
  - Meniges only protrude (meningocoele) and repaired surgically with a good prognosis.
  - Myelomeningocoele (meniges and spinal cord) protrude. 80% of spina bifida cases. Surgically treated soon after birth. Problems can include hydrocephalus, scoliosis, paralysis of legs, sensory loss, neuropathic bladder and bowel. Hydrocephalus may be treated by endoscopic surgery or introduction of ventricular shunt to drain cerebrospinal fluid (CSF).

## Long-term care for the parents and child with spina bifida

These children will be treated and managed by specialist multi-disciplinary paediatric teams with long-term follow-up as needs change with age and they become adults. Primary care professionals provide long-term support and primary care services as with all children with special needs (☐ Children with complex health needs and disabilities, p. 225). Need for emotional support as well as physical care and information important for parents and child. Particular issues primary care professionals may need to be aware of include:

- *Prevention of renal problems:* many parents are taught intermittent catheterization when child very young to ensure bladder emptying. More require support at school.
- *Recognition of shunt blockage or infection problems:* onset may be gradual including headaches, irritability, vomiting, general malaise. Schools and other child carers need to be informed of signs. Needs assessment and attention at specialist centre not local hospitals.

## Further information

Scottish Spina Bifida Association. Available at ✍ www.ssba.org.uk/
Spina bifida – Hydrocephalus – Information – Networking – Equality (SHINE). ☎ 01733 555 988.
  Available at: ✍ www.shinecharity.org.uk/

# Nocturnal enuresis

About 30% of children aged 4yrs have nocturnal enuresis (bedwetting), reduces to about 15% at 5yrs, 10% at 7yrs, 5% at 10yrs. More ♂ than ♀. It has a major impact on self-esteem. The causes are unclear, but may be associated with bladder dysfunction, sleep arousal difficulties, polyuria, and also runs in families.

## Principles of care

- Ensure child, young person, and family understands it is not their fault and punitive measures will not help.
- Involve child (irrespective of age) in discussions and planning.
- Discuss with parents if they need additional support in coping.

### Assessment

Includes history, current symptoms, toileting patterns, fluid intake, assess for triggers (e.g. constipation, UTI), developmental problems, neurological or congenital conditions, soiling (double incontinence suggests neurological causes or developmental delay), sleeping arrangements, family dynamics, possible maltreatment. Urinalysis not required unless recent start or other indications of ill-health. Invasive tests and examination not usually indicated initially.

### Management

- Engage child and family.
- Support for the child and family.
  - May be distressed or unconcerned.
  - May be causing strife (or result of it).
- <5yrs advice only as usually resolves spontaneously. See also 📖 Toilet training, p. 203.
- >5yrs more actively managed in stepwise fashion:
  - Review fluid and diet intake. Fluid intake should be: 4–8yrs: 1000–1400mL/day, 9–13yrs: ♀1200–2100 mL/day, ♂1400–2300 mL/day, 14–18yrs: ♀1400–2500 mL/day, ♂2100–3200 mL/day.
  - Advise on reward system (e.g. star chart for dry nights).
  - Enuresis alarms offered (often via school health service run enuresis clinics), may take 4wks for response, used until 2wks of dry nights,
  - Desmopressin nasal spray offered if no response to advice and alarm after 3mths.
- Incontinence nappies/pants may be needed for neurogenic incontinence and if laundry is causing an intolerable burden.

## Further information

NICE (2010). *Nocturnal enuresis - the management of bedwetting in children and young people (CG111)*. Available at: 🖰 www.nice.org.uk/guidance/CG111

ERIC Education and resources for Improving childhood continence. ☎ 0845 370 8008 (Monday to Wednesday). Available at: 🖰 www.eric.org.uk

# Overweight children and adolescents

Obesity in children is major public health concern (📖 Public health in the NHS, p. 10).

## Measurement and interpretation

- Detail of national policies on weight, height, and head circumference measurement is given in 📖 Overview of healthy child, p. 146.
- Interpretation of weight and height measurements are done with use of UK-WHO growth and BMI charts.[1]
- A child whose weight is average for their height will have a BMI between the 25th and 75th centiles, whatever their height centile.
- BMI >91st centile suggests overweight and advice/actions according to local guidelines.
- Review by GP or community paediatrician indicated if >98th centile is clinically obese.

## Advice for overweight children and families

- Children are growing, so the child needs to maintain their current weight (not lose weight) while they continue to grow in height.
- Eat well as a family including, healthy meals (📖 Nutrition and healthy eating, p. 304) eaten together.
- Get active as a family (📖 Exercise, p. 313) including
  - *Increase amounts of physical activity*—<5yrs at least 180min every day, >18yrs at least 60min every day.
  - Decrease sedentary time, e.g. at screens.
- Parents need to help build self-esteem of overweigh children so postive encouragement for all attempts/small steps of the earlier listed points.
- Engage school support through joining in activities, supporting healthy eating opportunities, e.g. healthy lunch boxes.

## Weight management programmes for children

A number of programmes are available tailored to children and young people of different ages and may be available through the NHS according to local guidelines and offer training to local staff in delivering them to children, young people, and families.

## Key reading and resources

[1]UK-WHO 2–18 years growth chart resources: charts, training materials, fact sheets. Available at: 🖱 www.rcpch.ac.uk/

## Further information

NHS Change4life Eat well, Move more, Live longer programme. Available at: 🖱 www.nhs.uk/change4life/Pages/change-for-life.aspx

# Sickle cell disorders

Haemoglobinopathies refers to a range of genetically inherited disorders of red blood cell haemoglobin (Hb). Sickle cell disorders refer to an inherited sickle Hb disorders including sickle cell anaemia. Sickle cell anaemia (Hb SS) is an autosomal recessive genetic condition inheriting two Hb S genes from both parents. Hb S refers to haemoglobin that is deformed, rigid, and 'sickle' shaped, unable to transport oxygen effectively. Sickle cells have a reduced life span, and block small capillaries, reducing oxygen transportation and resulting in thrombosis and ischaemia. This is made worse by factors such as dehydration and cold or situations of reduced oxygen availability, e.g. anaesthesia, high altitudes. About 300 children a year in the UK are born with sickle cell anaemia (NHS Sickle cell screening programme[1]). Mainly affects people of African or Caribbean descent, but also affects people from Asia, the Middle East, and the eastern Mediterranean. The UK has antenatal (&#x1F4D6; Antenatal care and screening, p. 380) and new born screening programmes (&#x1F4D6; Child screening tests, p. 152).

Those with one *HbA* gene and one *HbS* gene have sickle cell trait and are carriers of sickle cell anaemia. They have enough normal HbA to not experience the problems of those with sickle cell anaemia.

Children identified with HbSS are referred to a named paediatrician. Children (and adults) with sickle cell anaemia will vary in the severity of symptoms and problems. Symptoms include:
- Anaemia.
- *Pain as a result of vaso-occlusive crises:* can vary in frequency and severity. Can occur anywhere in the body, but often occurs in the limbs, back, and abdomen. Also presents as dactylitis—hand/foot syndrome is a painful swelling of the hands, feet, or both and affects children <3yrs old. Often the pain is excruciating. Boys can also experience priapism. Types of vaso-occlusive crisis that may require blood transfusions include:
  - *Sequestration crisis*—a sudden ↓ haemoglobin concentration due to pooling of a large volume of blood in the spleen, liver, or lungs, painful swelling of the organ with worsening anaemia. Can affect children within the first 5yrs, and in rare instances, can result in death from circulatory collapse, anaemia, and hypovolaemic shock.
  - *Haemolytic crisis*—when events such as infections cause a serious ↓ in the number of red blood cells.
  - *Aplastic crisis*—occurs at any age as a result of a ↓ of bone marrow activity. May be life threatening.
  - *Megaloblastic changes/crisis*—this is rare due to folic acid deficiency.
- Infections, due to splenic dysfunction causing increased susceptibility.
- Jaundice due to chronic haemolysis.

Long-term problems may include cardiac problems from chronic anaemia, and gall stones due to chronic haemolysis of red blood cells, CVA, ulcerated legs.

## Advice and management

There is no cure or specific treatment for sickle cell disease. Prevention of illnesses includes prophylactic antibiotics and full 📖 Child immunization schedule, p. 158 plus annual influenza vaccination.

### Key areas of advice

- As normal lifestyle as possible, but act early in any illness.
- Ensure a healthy lifestyle and good nutrition (including folic acid).
- Avoid triggers to crisis, e.g. dehydration, cold, strenuous exercise in damp or wet conditions.
- Seek medical advice early for any infections.
- *Travel advice:* ensure adequate malaria prophylaxis—sickle cell disease offers no protection. *Note:* crisis can be precipitated by antimalarials.
- Recommend wearing a medic alert bracelet.

The Sickle Cell Society suggests CBT (📖 Talking therapies, p. 429) can help young people and adults.

Important to ensure child care and school staff understand the condition and support the active management to avoid triggers, e.g. drinking lots of fluids, avoiding cold.

### Management of crises

Minor ones are managed at home with support of GP and primary care team. Key management elements are analgesia, ↑ fluid intake, and warmth. Pain can be helped by:

- Careful assessment, child diaries useful insight into patient's pain experience and coping strategies.
- Warmth, massaging and rubbing, and by heat, e.g. hot water bottles.
- Bandaging to support the painful region.
- Resting the body. Deep breathing exercises and distraction techniques.

*Pain relief prescribed according to severity (see BNF for Children)*

- Paracetamol, tds (30–60mg 1–3mths, 60–120mg 3–12mths, 120–250mg 1–5yrs, 250–500mg 6–12yrs, 500mg 12–18yrs).
- Codeine phosphate, qds, at 3mg/kg daily in divided doses.
- Stronger analgesic non-steroidal anti-inflammatory agent, such as diclofenac, which is tds, of 1mg for every kg of body weight.

Children with more severe crisis will be admitted to hospital, e.g. severe pain, high fever, or other symptoms such as dyspnoea or neurological signs.

### Related topic

📖 Children with complex health needs and disabilities, p. 225.

### Reference

[1] NHS Sickle Cell and Thalassaemia screening programme. Available at: ℘ sct.screening.nhs.uk/

### Further information

The Sickle Cell Society. Available at: ℘ www.sicklecellsociety.org
NHS Choices Sickle Cell Anemia. Available at: ℘ www.nhs.uk/conditions/sickle-cell-anaemia/
    pages/introduction.aspx

# Thalassaemia

Thalassaemia is a less common haemoglobinopathy than sickle cell in the UK. Estimated to be about 700 people having the most severe form thalassaemia (UK Thalassaemia screening programme[1]). Highest prevalence in Cypriot, Italian, Greek, Indian, Pakistani, Bangladeshi, Chinese, and South Asian populations. Also (less common) Northern European population. The UK has antenatal (📖 Antenatal care and screening, p. 380) and new born screening programmes (📖 Child screening tests, p. 152). Any child identified with thalassaemia is referred to a named paediatrican.

## B thalassaemia major

Children (and adults) with this condition are unable to produce haemoglobin resulting in life-threatening anaemia and jaundice from about 6mths. They require regular blood transfusions for life accompanied by regular chelation therapy to prevent iron deposition. Even with treatment, these children often have complex problems including growth and sexual development problems, enlarged spleen, diabetes, and heart problems. Life expectancy is of 2 or 3 decades. A bone marrow transplant can offer a cure.

Thalassaemia intermedia is another less severe form and may require less frequent transfusions.

## Management of care

- These children and their families are primarily supported by specialist services.
- Families and children need continual support and recognition of problems being faced over a lifetime.

## Related topics

📖 Children with complex health needs and disabilities, p. 225.

## Reference

[1]NHS Sickle Cell and Thalassaemia Screening Programme. Available at: ℜ sct.screening.nhs.uk/

## Further information

UK Thalassaemia Society. Available at: ℜ www.ukts.org

# Sudden death of an infant

Sudden infant death syndrome (SIDS) is the sudden, unexpected death of an apparently well baby (also known as cot death). It affects >300 babies in UK each year. Most are <1yr, but the majority <3mths and more ♂ than ♀. Since 1991 the number has decreased in incidence by 75%.

## Risk factors

Are thought to include: prematurity, low birth weight, laying baby face down to sleep (📖 Babies and sleeping, p. 189), parental smoking, smoke, and overheating. The Lullaby Trust[1] produce parent leaflets on reducing risk.

## Protocols

There are joint interagency protocols for SIDS agreed with coroner as part of local child protection procedures (📖 Child protection, p. 230). All sudden, unexpected deaths are under the jurisdiction of the coroner and post mortems have to be carried out. The police investigate if there is any suspicion it may have been unnatural. Protocols likely to include:

• Ambulance staff will attempt resuscitation and always take to ED.
• Immediate notification to coroner's office, GP, police team, and named paediatrician.
• Home visit by paediatrician and police within 24h to talk with parents and inspect the scene.
• Paediatrician collates all medical records and asks social services to check child protection register, keeping in close contact with police and coroner.
• Post-mortem carried out and findings reported to parents as soon as possible by pathologist, paediatrician, and/or GP.
• Case discussion, as per agreed guidelines, usually within 6wks involving all professional involved with family to scrutinize all aspects of death and contributory factors, to plan ongoing support for family at that point, and when they plan another pregnancy. Paediatrician and/or GP and/or HV meet with parents to share conclusions and offer ongoing support.
• Child Death Overview Panel under local child protection reviews the case subsequently to identify any actions to prevent future child deaths.

## Best practice guidance for HVs and primary care nurses

- If first to visit home when SIDS discovered:
  - Check that an ambulance has been called.
  - If in doubt, resuscitation should always be attempted.
  - Ensure parents and siblings have support from friends and family.
  - Spend time listening to the parents. Mention baby by name and don't be afraid to express sorrow.
- If learn later that a baby has died, HV team should liaise with GP to avoid duplication and visit as close to death as possible to offer:
  - Condolences, an opportunity for the parents to talk.
  - Information and support though post-mortem, coroner procedures, funeral, and 🕮 Bereavement, p. 528.
  - If the mother was breastfeeding, discuss methods of suppression of lactation.
  - Ensure the parents have information from The Lullaby Trust and its befriender scheme.
  - Ensure parents have been given, and content discussed, leaflets on post mortems of a baby or child ordered by a coroner (consent not required) and retention of human tissue (consent required).
- Check the following agencies have been informed of the baby's death:
  - Medical records departments of maternity/children's hospitals to avoid follow-up appointments being sent.
  - Child Health records department to avoid letters being sent about immunizations and development checks.
  - The school, if there are school-age children in the family.
- Later revisit following funeral and then follow-up to case discussion to:
  - Offer further time to talk.
  - Information about local bereavement services.
- Remember to talk about the deceased baby by name, at anniversaries, and during any subsequent pregnancies and births.
- Offer information about local Care of Next Infant Scheme (CONI).

## Care of next infant

CONI is a programme set up in many areas of the UK where a local coordinator supports parents and professionals through subsequent pregnancies and first year of child's life. Programme includes additional visits from a HV, symptom diary, loan of apnoea monitors, room thermometer, and additional advice.

## Reference

[1]Lullaby Trust (formerly Foundation for the Study of Infant Deaths (FSID) provides a comprehensive booklet, as well as information, support, befriending scheme for parents and guidelines and information for professionals. Helpline ☎ 0808 802. Available at: 🖰 www.lullabytrust.org.uk/0

## Further information

Child Death Helpline ☎ 0800 282 986. Available at: 🖰 www.childdeathhelpline.org.uk/

# Chapter 8

# Adult health promotion

# Models and approaches to health promotion

Health promotion aims to enable people to increase control over and to improve their health. It involves a wide range of individual, social, and environmental interventions. The Ottawa Charter[1] incorporates three strategies: to enable, mediate, and advocate:

- Build healthy public policy.
- Create supportive environments.
- Strengthen community actions.
- Develop personal skills.
- Reorient health services.

There is no universally accepted model of health promotion. There are three main types of approaches: individual focused, group focused, community focused. Table 8.1 summarizes the main theories and key concepts within these approaches.

## Individual focused approaches

Can involve:

- *Medical/nursing input:* acting to ensure that the individual does not develop a disease or is protected from an agent that might cause a disease, e.g. immunization against disease and screening for disease.
- *Educational input:* giving individuals information, or helping them to interpret evidence, so that they can make informed life choices. Lectures and leaflets by themselves have limited impact.
- *Behavioural input:* giving people information and support to help them cope, or move on with making lifestyle changes, e.g. stopping smoking.

## Group focused approaches

Normally a combination of educational and behavioural change approaches, although can also be community development focused. Requires an understanding of group dynamics.

## Community focused approaches to health promotion

Involves one or a combination of the following:

- *Epidemiological focused approaches:* based on information on prevalence and/or incidence of condition in geographical area. Use standardized statistical information to initiate health promotion initiatives, e.g. TB prevention.
- *Social/societal change:* initiating or lobbying for change involving policy or legislation change or innovation. Often based on epidemiological evidence, but may be initiated by expressed need of community or policy initiative, e.g. physical activity promotion.
- *Community development:* interventions are identified by community. It may involve health and other professionals working with communities to empower them to identify their own health promotion and health improvement needs. These may differ radically from agenda of health and social care professionals.

**Table 8.1** Summary of theories: focus and key concepts of health promotion

| Theory | Focus | Key concepts |
|---|---|---|
| Stages of change model | Individual's readiness to change or attempt to change toward healthy behaviours | • Pre-contemplation<br>• Contemplation<br>• Decision/determination<br>• Action<br>• Maintenance |
| Health belief model | Person's perception of the threat of a health problem and the appraisal of recommended behaviour(s) for preventing or managing the problem | • Perceived susceptibility<br>• Perceived severity<br>• Perceived benefits of action<br>• Cues to actions<br>• Self-efficacy |
| Social learning theory | Behaviour explained via a 3-way, reciprocal theory = personal factors, environmental influences, and behaviour continually interact | • Behaviour capability<br>• Reciprocal determinism<br>• Expectations self-efficacy<br>• Observational learning<br>• Reinforcement |
| Community organization theories | Emphasizes active participation and development of communities that can better evaluate and solve health and social problems | • Empowerment<br>• Community competence<br>• Participation and relevance<br>• Issue selection<br>• Critical consciousness |
| Organizational change theory | Strategies for ↑ chances that healthy policies and programmes will be adopted and maintained in formal organizations, e.g. NHS | • Problem definition (awareness stage)<br>• Initiation of action (adoption stage)<br>• Implementation of change<br>• Institutionalization of change |
| Diffusion of innovation theory | How new ideas, products & social practices spread within a society or from one society to another | • Relative advantage<br>• Compatibility<br>• Complexity<br>• Trialability<br>• Observability |

## Reference

[1]WHO Ottawa Charter for Health Promotion (1986). Available at: ℘ http://www.who.int/healthpromotion/conferences/previous/ottawa/en/

## Further information

Health Scotland. Available at: ℘ www.healthscotlanc.com
Public Health Agency NI. Available at: ℘ www.publichealth.hsci.net/
Public Health England. Available at: ℘ www.gov.uk/government/organisations/public-health-england
World Health Organization. Healthy Settings. Available at: ℘ http://www.who.int/healthy_settings/en/

# Group health promotion

Group work is an effective method of health promotion. HVs and other public health nurses are often more involved in group health promotion work than other nurses in primary care, but all nurses are encouraged to use these techniques. Involvement in group work can mean:

- Teaching health topics as a formal lecture or one-off talk, e.g. antenatal education classes, to a school class.
- Using principles of participatory adult learning in community group situations, e.g. session on contraception in youth group.
- Forming and/or supporting groups for self-help, mutual support, and health information, e.g. carers support group.
- Becoming part of a group, made up of local people/professionals to influence policy and/or services, e.g. estate action group or campaigning group on housing problems.

Each of these types of group work requires different skills and knowledge, some of which may have been part of formal education or undertaken as a part of ongoing professional development.

## Principles of participatory learning in small groups

### Beforehand

- Plan how to use the time together.
- Plan how environment will help group work, e.g. seats in circles, crèche for small children separately.
- Plan to use materials appropriate to group.

### In the session

- Involve everyone from beginning by getting them to introduce themselves and saying what they'd like to get out of session (consider icebreaking activities that encourage each member to speak briefly).
- Establish any ground rules the group think necessary, e.g. listen to each other, discussion confidential to group.
- Activities that include active participation and sharing by the members. Techniques include:
  - *Brainstorming*—e.g. what are the different types of contraception?
  - *Problem solving*—e.g. 3-year-old John has full-blown temper tantrum at supermarket checkout. What would you advise mum to do?
- Break up time and change activities using additional inputs/health promotion materials.
- Summarize activity at end of session, offer time for participants to summarize/raise any issues and offer written materials, e.g. leaflets to back up or provide detailed information, e.g. local directory of services aimed at carers.

## Principles for helping to establish and run a group

- Identify need and partners to help, check there is not already a similar local group that you could support, be clear about its purposes, e.g. support/social opportunity for carers with 'sitting' facilities for person cared for.
- Consider any finance required and possible local sources.
- Find a suitable local venue for the purpose of the group. Consider issues such as access, acoustics, comfort, refreshment opportunities, insurance cover for purpose intended, separate space if need to split into 2, e.g. for crèche.
- Personal invitations to target members plus wider local publicity.
- Plan first meeting and tasks for facilitators, such as arranging space, greeting people, starting and ending the meeting.
- Consider how to involve others in group roles to share workload and increase commitment.
- Consider how group could become self-sustaining.
- Recognize that many groups have their own life cycle, and ending a group or watching it change into something completely different is often appropriate and healthy.

## Further information

Scriven A. (2010). *Promoting Health a Practical Guide*, 6th edn. (Chapter 13: Working with groups, pp. 177–90.) Edinburgh: Baillière Tindall Elsevier.

# Community approaches to health

Three inter-linked concepts relate to community approaches to health.

## Social cohesion and social capital

Social cohesion refers to the shared values of communities that enable them to operate in an integrated manner. Social capital describes the connections and networks among people in a social group or community. Different socio-economic groups are more or less able to act collectively and this contributes to unequal access to the resources necessary for health or unequal exposure to health risks. The ↑ interaction between people, the ↑ sense of being part of a community. Main aspects include:

• Trust and reciprocity.
• Informal and social networks.
• Civic engagement.

Higher levels of social capital and social cohesion in a community → better health, ↑ educational achievement, better employment outcomes, and ↓ crime rates. *Note:* also has the potential to exclude others.

## Partnership approaches

Increasingly, health and care systems are expected to work together to improve the health and wellbeing of their local population and reduce health inequalities. In England, this includes the setting up of Health and Wellbeing boards that have community participation and representation working alongside health and social care. Their remit is to:

• Ensure stronger democratic legitimacy and involvement.
• Strengthen working relationships between health and social care.
• Encourage development of more integrated commissioning of services.

Primary care nurses are encouraged to participate in these partnerships, as well as network with local statutory, voluntary, and self-help organizations to improve service response to local need and develop innovative approaches to locally identified need.

## Community development approaches

Community development work aims to bring about social change and address inequalities by working with communities (defined geographically and/or by specific interests). The community members themselves:

• Identify their needs and acceptable ways to address them.
• Plan and take action.
• Evaluate impact and identifies what else needs to change.

HVs and SNs often take these types of approaches and in some areas, may not have a caseload of individual families or schools so they can focus on these types of community development approaches to health.

## Further information

Community Development Foundation. Available at: ℘ www.cdf.org.uk/
Daily J, Barr A. (2008). Understanding a Community-led Approach to Health Improvement. Available at: ℘ www.scdc.org.uk
Public Health England. Available at: ℘ www.gov.uk/government/organisations/public-health-england

# Expert patients

Expert patients are people living with a long-term health condition, who are able to take more control over their health by understanding and managing their conditions, leading to an improved quality of life.

## Benefits of becoming an expert patient

- Confidence and control of their lives.
- Manage their condition in partnership with health care professionals.
- Communicate effectively with professionals and are willing to share responsibility on treatment.
- Are realistic about impact of their disease on themselves and family.
- Use their skills and knowledge to lead full lives.

## The expert patients programme

The expert patients programme (EPP) is an NHS initiative launched in 2002 to help patients with chronic conditions to develop new skills to self-manage their condition better day-to-day and take control of their lives. It recognizes that people with all kinds of long-term conditions are dealing with similar issues on a daily basis, often including pain, stress, and low self-esteem. It is a training course that teaches people how to manage their conditions by using five core skills:

- Problem-solving.
- Decision-making.
- Making the best use of resources.
- Developing effective partnerships with health care providers.
- Taking appropriate action.

### EPP training courses

A free self-management course provides tools and techniques to have the confidence, skills, and knowledge to manage any chronic health condition. The majority of EPP courses are delivered by trained tutors who have personal experience of living with a long-term health problem. Courses usually run over 6 weekly sessions and include topics such as dealing with pain, extreme tiredness, coping with feelings of depression, relaxation techniques, exercise, healthy eating, communicating with family, friends, and health care professionals, and planning for the future.

### Joining an EPP course

Course contact details are available from the Expert Patients Programme Community Interest Company. This is not currently available in Scotland or Northern Ireland, but patient self-help material is available online.

## Further information

Expert Patients Programme Community Interest Company. Available at: ℘ http://www.expert-patients.co.uk/

Details of >1500 UK patient support organizations, self help groups, health and disease information providers can be found at: ℘ www.patient.co.uk/selfhelp.asp

# Nutrition and healthy eating

Energy is needed to stay alive, grow, keep warm, and be active. Carbohydrates, proteins, and fat provide energy. Estimated average requirements (EAR) for energy:
• *Men age 19–59yrs:* 74kg, 2550kcal/day.
• *Women age 19–59yrs:* 61–63kg 1940kcal/day.

Energy requirements ↓ gradually >50yrs in women and 60yrs in men as typically activity levels ↓. To maintain body weight, it is necessary to expend as much energy as is derived from food; to lose weight, energy must exceed intake.

## Body mass index

BMI is a tool for judging weight. BMI = weight/height$^2$ (see 📖 Adult body mass index chart, p. 306. Not applicable to children, pregnant women, or athletes). Normal BMI = 18.5–24.9; <18.5 underweight; 25–30 overweight; >30 obese; >40 severely obese (📖 Weight management: overweight, obesity, p. 307).

## Waist circumference

Also used to assess obesity and associated health risk. It is measured mid-point between lowest rib and top of right iliac crest. ♂ >102cm (40 inches) and ♀ >88cm (35 inches) associated with ↑ visceral fat mass and co-morbidities. ❶ Increased risk for people of Asian origin at ≥90cm for ♂ and ≥80cm for ♀.

## Nutritional requirements

All diets require the following:
• *Carbohydrate:* recommended as 47–50% of daily intake, a source of energy. Complex (plant derived) or simple (sugars) types. Complex, e.g. bread, potatoes, rice are slower to breakdown and release energy.
• *Protein:* recommended as 15% of daily intake, needed for growth and repair, and energy, e.g. fish, meat, legumes.
• *Fibre:* recommended average 18g/day for an adult, keeps gut healthy and helps prevent constipation, e.g. fruit and vegetables.
• *Fats:* total recommended as up to 33% of daily intake. Made up mostly of unsaturated fats, e.g. nuts, oily fish, vegetable oils, rather than saturated fats, e.g. meat products, hard cheese, butter. Required for absorption of vitamins, energy, and essential fatty acids omega-3 and omega-6.
• *Vitamins (government recommended daily allowance) includes:*
  • *A*—for growth, development, and eyesight.
  • *B group*—help body use energy; *B12:* for blood cells and nerve function.
  • *C*—for skin and tissue growth, also absorption of iron.
  • *D*—for bone metabolism and calcium absorption.

- *Minerals (government recommended daily allowance) includes:*
  - *Calcium*—most adults should aim to eat 700mg calcium each day, post-menopausal women 12000mg for development and maintenance of bones.
  - *Iron*—for red blood cells.
  - *Phytonutrients*—plant compounds that acts as antioxidants against free radicals (substances implicated in cancer, heart disease).
- Intakes of 1.5–2L of fluids/day recommended in temperate climates.
- Protein requirements ↓ for ♂ >50yrs, but increase slightly for ♀.
- After menopause, women's requirement for iron is reduced to same level as that for men.
- >65yrs ↑ vitamin D to 10 micrograms/day.

## A healthy balanced diet

Encourage a diverse diet from the five food groups, eating more from groups 1 and 2 than 3 or 4:

- *Group 1—fruit and vegetables:* five or more portions a day. Portion = 80g, e.g. 1 medium apple, a bowl of salad, 3 heaped tablespoons of peas. Fruit juice, smoothies, beans, and pulses only count as 1 portion per day.
- *Group 2—bread, other cereals, and potatoes:* one-third of total food intake. At least one food from this group at each meal.
- *Group 3—milk and dairy foods:* 2–3 servings a day. A serving = milk 200mL glass, yogurt small pot (150g), cheese 30g (matchbox size).
- *Group 4—meat, fish, and alternatives:* moderate amounts recommended, as well as 2 portions of fish (2 oily fish) each week. Vegetarians and vegans should ensure adequate protein, iron, selenium, and vitamin B12 (especially vegans) in diet.
- *Group 5—foods containing fat and foods containing sugar:* sparingly, e.g. butter and spreads or not eaten too often, e.g. sweets and crisps.

The amounts that should be consumed will vary depending on energy needs (based on age, sex, and physical activity levels) and appetite. See Box 8.1 for healthy eating guidelines

### Box 8.1 Eight guidelines for healthy eating

- Base your meals on starchy foods.
- Eat lots of fruit and vegetables.
- Eat more fish.
- Cut down on saturated fat and sugar.
- Try to eat less salt—no more than 6g a day.
- Get active and try to be a healthy weight.
- Drink plenty of water.
- Don't skip breakfast.

## Further information

British Nutrition Foundation. Available at: ℘ www.nutrition.org.uk
Food Standards Agency pages on nutrition. Available at: ℘ www.food.gov.uk/
NHS Choices Good food. Available at: ℘ www.nhs.uk/LiveWell/Goodfood/Pages/
Eatwell plate. Available at: ℘ www.nhs.uk/Livewell/Goodfood/Documents/Eatwellplate.pdf

# Adult body mass index chart

*Note:* assessing growth and BMI of children and young people is undertaken differently, see 📖 Growth 0–2 years, p. 181; 📖 Growth 2–4 years, p. 195; 📖 Growth and nutrition 5–11yrs, p. 210; 📖 Growth and nutrition 12–18yrs, p. 221. Adult BMI charts (Fig. 8.1) are not accurate for pregnant women, athletes, or older people.

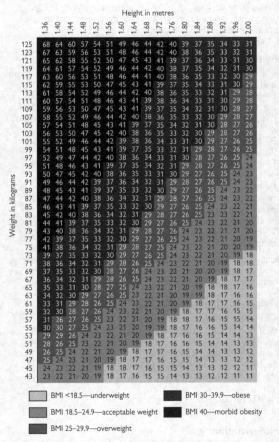

**Fig. 8.1** BMI ready reckoner.

# Weight management: overweight, obesity

All opportunities in primary care should be taken for promoting the principles of good nutrition and healthy eating (📖 Nutrition and healthy eating, p. 304) and exercise (📖 Exercise, p. 313). Particularly important to teach children and young people these principles, as eating patterns continue into adulthood. In 2008, nearly a quarter of adults (over 16yrs of age) in England were obese. Amongst children (2–15yrs of age), one in six boys and one in seven girls in England were obese. The number of overweight children was also around one in seven.

## Overweight

People who take in more energy than they require, store the energy as excess fat and become overweight, and if this continues will become obese. The main contributory factors are sedentary lifestyle and increased energy intake. Obesity is directly linked to increased risks of morbidity, e.g. DM, CHD, hypertension. Classification of BMI:

- 18.5–24.9 healthy weight.
- 25–29.9 overweight.
- 30–34.9 obese Class I.
- 35–39.9 obese Class II.
- >40 morbid obesity.

*Note:* people of Asian origins at ↑ risk of morbidity at lower BMI levels.

## Obesity

*Obesity* is a major public health issue. Many factors interact to cause weight gain, e.g. behavioural, genetic predisposition, lifestyle. Weight gain increases with age, women gain weight more easily, there is ↑ risk in lower socio-economic groups, higher prevalence in some minority ethnic groups, e.g. women of Caribbean and Pakistani origin. 80% of ex-smokers increase weight, but benefits of cessation outweigh not stopping.

People who are obese have a shorter life expectancy, ↑ risk of developing CHD and type 2 diabetes as well as ↑ risk of other problems, e.g. respiratory, musculoskeletal, stress incontinence.

## Raising the issue

Assess willingness to change. Overweight and obesity is an issue that needs to be raised in an open, empathetic manner that acknowledges the complexity of the person's experiences, the causes, and their feelings. Listening to the patient's experience and views establishes their perception of the problem and their willingness to address it. For those not interested in weight reduction at this point, it is important to let them know they can come back or give them information where else to go if they choose to address the issue later.

### Supporting those interested in weight reduction

For those willing to address the issue:

- In general aim to promote good nutrition and healthy eating (📖 Nutrition and healthy eating, p. 304), ↑ physical activity (📖 Exercise, p. 313) and ↓ sedentary behaviour, ↑ self-awareness about day-to-day behaviours.
- Make time to clarify patient expectations and ability to engage. Discuss the options on how to support weight reduction. This may be in or outside of the NHS, e.g. WeightWatchers or the community dieticians, GP practice may have a weight management protocol, or weight management clinic, or HVs may have a weight management group.

### Supporting weight reduction in primary care

The aim is for a realistic, modest weight loss over no more than 12wks. Some local areas are supported by community dietician programmes and protocols. Protocols usually include:

- Agreement between person and professional on goals and means of achieving them.
- Structured assessment, recording and regular follow-up.
- Specific dietary advice and menu sheets for weight loss:
  - ↓ calorific intake by about 600kcal/day to total of 1200–1600kcal will usually achieve target weight loss.
  - ↓ fat intake with accompanying increase in fruit and vegetables.
- Advice supported with weight management leaflets, activity and eating diaries, information on local organizations, increasing exercise.
- Group activities, e.g. WeightWatchers, have higher success rates in reducing and maintaining weight loss than one-on-one consultations

Obese people with attendant health problems and difficulties in losing weight may be considered by GPs for drug therapies or as a last resort surgical intervention.

### Further information

Food Standards Agency pages on nutrition. Available at: ℠ www.food.gov.uk/
National Obesity Forum. Available at: ℠ www.nationalobesityforum.org.uk/
NHS Choices Obesity. Available at: ℠ www.nhs.uk/Conditions/Obesity/
NICE (2006) Obesity: Guidance on the prevention, identification, assessment and management of overweight and obesity in adults and children, CG43. Available at: ℠ www.nice.org.uk/CG43

# Weight management: malnutrition

See also 📖 People with eating disorders, p. 431.

Many factors can lead to under-nutrition and/or dietary deficiencies. Factors include socio-economic (e.g. social isolation), disabilities (e.g. osteoarthritis), physical (e.g. swallowing problems, dental problems), pathological (e.g. dementia), psychological (e.g. depression). Some conditions have specific nutritional consequences (e.g. cancer). Poor nutrition leads to muscle wasting, problems with the immune system, apathy, depression, poor wound healing, and altered drug metabolism. Older people > 85yrs are particularly at risk. Unexplained weight loss may be an early indication of cancer and should be referred for medical assessment.

~1 in 4 people admitted to a UK hospital are malnourished. High-risk groups include:
- Older people >65yrs, including those in long-term care (care home).
- People with long-term conditions, such as diabetes or kidney disease.
- People with cancer.
- People who abuse drugs and/or alcohol.
- People on low incomes.

## Assessment

The most common symptom of malnutrition is unplanned weight loss. Assessment of nutritional status should include:
- All medical, physical, psychological, and social factors.
- Dietary intake over a few days/week.
- BMI repeated over time or evidence of weight loss over time. BMI <18.5 chronic protein–energy under-nutrition probable.

Nutritional risk factor scoring systems use BMI, plus evidence of unintentional weight loss over time, e.g. over last 3mths plus dietary intake in last 5 days. If weight and measurement are not possible then assessment is by checking factors, such as clothes and rings becoming too loose. Height can be estimated from length of ulna. Other symptoms include:
- Lack of strength or energy to undertake routine activities, or poor physical performance.
- Lack of energy and breathlessness (due to anaemia).
- Changes to skin and nails.

In children consider:
- Inability to concentrate or unusually irritable.
- Failure to grow to their expected adult height (stunted growth).

## Management

- Address any problems identified in assessment, e.g. ill-fitting dentures or need for help in preparing food, e.g. Meals on Wheels, difficulty with utensils or to eat in company, e.g. luncheon clubs.
- Difficulty in swallowing should always be referred for medical assessment.
- Advise people with low BMIs and/or malnourishment:
  - On the components of good nutrition and healthy eating.
  - To fortify diet with more high energy/high protein foods, e.g. milk, cheese, butter, and eat small high energy/high protein snacks and drinks in between meals, e.g. whole milk coffee, whole milk yoghurt, peanut butter sandwiches.
  - On simple measures, such as fresh air and exercise increase appetite.
- Monitor and refer to GP or dietician as appropriate.
- Nutritional supplements (e.g. sip feeds) should only be considered if fortifying diet has had no effect after about 4wks.
  - Likely to benefit people with BMI <20.
  - Should be chosen with consideration of nutritional profile and patient preference.
  - Typically 300–400kcal (1–2 cartons) a day can be of benefit. Care should be taken in using supplements not to further depress appetite. Constipation can be a problem.
  - Re-assessment should occur 4–6wks after prescription. They should not be used for longer than 4–6wks without a dietician assessment (or as per local policies).
- Nutritional supplements can only be prescribed within NHS in accordance with Advisory Committee on Borderline Substances (see BNF, Appendix 7) for conditions such as short bowel syndrome, intractable malabsorption, IBD, dysphagia, total gastrectomy, disease-related malnutrition.

## Related topic

📖 Enteral tube feeds, p. 546.

## Further information

NHS Choices Malnutrition. Available at: 🖰 www.nhs.uk/Conditions/Malnutrition/

# Home food safety and hygiene

There were over 80,000 cases of food poisoning in England and Wales in 2010, about 32,000 formally notifiable (see 📖 Infectious disease notifications, p. 103). While the number of cases decreased from 2000 to 2005, they are now rising. All UK countries have food-borne disease reduction strategies.

## Key principles for food safety and hygiene

- *Hand washing:* before starting, after touching any meat or raw fish, after going to the toilet, or touching pets.
- *Cleaning up:* wash all chopping boards and surfaces before and after cooking. Wash and replace tea towels, cloths, sponges frequently.
- *Separate raw meat:* contains harmful bacteria. Store in fridge at the bottom so it cannot drip on ready-to-eat food. Avoid cross-contamination with other ready-to-eat foods by using different cutting boards, cleaning surfaces, cleaning utensils after using on raw meat. Do not place raw meat next to cooked foods, e.g. on barbeques. Always wash hands after handling.
- *Raw fish:* may contain microbes that can cause food poisoning. To prevent this store fish in fridge. Treat raw fish as raw meat above. Elderly or sick people, young children, and pregnant women should not eat raw, or partially-cooked fish and shellfish.
- *Fruit and vegetables:* always wash before use to remove any bacteria. Scrap or peel skin off to remove earth not removed by washing on root vegetables.
- *Cook through:* ensure items are cooked all the way through, i.e. piping hot so steam is rising from centre if pierced with knife or skewer of dish. Fully cook (i.e. no pink flesh) poultry, rolled meat joints, kebabs, burgers, and chicken nuggets to ensure all harmful bacteria are killed.
- *Leftovers:* should be cooled and placed in fridge within 90min and used within 2 days. This includes rice and grains because if they are cooked and then left at room temperature longer than 90min, spores germinate, which produce toxins that cause vomiting and diarrhoea. These toxins are not killed by reheating.
- *Reheating food:* foods should only be reheated once and cooked through.
- *Eggs:* some eggs contain *Salmonella* bacteria. Eating raw eggs, or eggs with runny yolks, or any food containing these, can cause food poisoning. Care is required in preparation not to spread bacteria on work surfaces, utensils, etc. Advise to cook eggs until the yolk and the white is solid especially for the very young (i.e. babies to toddlers) and those who are older, pregnant, or unwell.
- *Freezing at home:* cooked foods should be cooled quickly, placed in clean containers/bags, labelled and stored according to freezer or cookery guide. Uncooked and chilled foods should be frozen and used according to the instructions on retailers' labels.
- *Defrosting foods:* foods that require defrosting throughout should be left at a temperature (e.g. in the fridge) that will not allow bacteria or toxins to multiple during process. Cook within 24hrs. Do not re-freeze.

## Key principles on hygiene elsewhere in the home

### Laundry

- Reduce risk of spread of infection via laundry by washing:
  - *High-risk items*—e.g. those visibly soiled or in contact with areas of the body (bed linen, underwear) that might excrete pathogens at 30–40°C with an oxygen bleach-based laundry product.
  - *Low-risk items*—i.e. not in contact with body or in low risk areas of soiling, e.g. shirts, socks trousers at 40°C or less with non-bleach based products.
- Treat health care workers uniforms as high-risk items.

### Hygienic cleaning

- Hand-to-hand contact surfaces and food contact surfaces can be hygienically cleaned with soapy water, then rinsed.
- Where a surface cannot be adequately rinsed (e.g. large food surfaces, handles, toilet seats), which are likely to leave behind pathogens, then a disinfectant should be used.

## Further information

Food Standards Agency. Available at: ℛ www.food.gov.uk/
Community Infection Control Nurses Network Prevention of infection in the home A training resource for carers and their trainers. Available at: ℛ http://www.nhs.uk/Livewell/homehygiene/Documents/ICNA-TRAINING-RESOURCE-BOOKLET[1].pdf
International Scientific Forum on Home Hygiene. Available at: ℛ www.ifh-homehygiene.org/
NHS Choices, Live Well pages on home hygiene and food hygiene. Available at: ℛ http://www.nhs.uk/livewell/homehygiene/Pages/Homehygienehub.aspx

# Exercise

Physical activity ↓ the risk of morbidity and improves many conditions, e.g. CHD, hypertension, DM, COPD, ↓ risk of some cancers (colon, breast, prostate), prevents osteoporosis (and thus risk of fractures). It also improves mental health and helps in weight management. It is a government priority to encourage the population to become more active and less sedentary. The National Healthy Schools Standard requires all pupils to be offered a minimum of 2hrs physical activity a week. Physical activity levels:

- Decline dramatically with age.
- Vary between people of different social class, gender, and ethnicity, e.g. levels of activity lower for black or minority ethnic groups except African-Caribbean and Irish populations and ♂ from manual classes are more active overall—this is reversed for leisure and sporting activities.

## Definitions

- *Aerobic fitness:* ability of cardiovascular system to supply oxygen to muscles. Achieved through:
  - *Moderate intensity activity*—causes breathing and heart rate to ↑ brisk walking, cycling.
  - *Vigorous intensity activity*—causes rapid breathing and heart rate, e.g. running, climbing stairs.
- *Muscular strength:* maximum force a muscle can exert. ↑ with exercise such as lifting.
- *Muscular endurance:* ability of muscles to work for longer before feeling fatigued. Weak muscles need to ↑ strength before endurance.
- *Flexibility:* maximum range of movement in a joint.
- *Motor fitness:* speed, reaction time, balance, coordination.

## Recommended physical activity levels

### 19–64yrs

Moderate intensity activity for 150min or vigorous activity for 75min over a week. Activities to improve muscle strength undertaken on at least 2 days/wk. Minimize time spent being sedentary.

### 65yrs+

Moderate intensity activity for 150min or, if already active, vigorous activity for 75min over a week. Activities to improve muscle strength on at least 2 days (e.g. chair exercises). If at risk of falls, incorporate activities to improve balance and coordination on at least 2 days (e.g. tai chi, yoga). Minimize time spent being sedentary.

### People with specific health problems

For example, COPD. Require specific advice tailored to them from qualified health or fitness professionals.

**Evidence-based interventions for promoting exercise**

No one health discipline or model has been shown to be more effective than others in delivering exercise promotion. Advise only strategies to ↑ exercise result in ↑ exercise, but it is not sustained for longer than a year. Low intensity exercise incorporated into daily routine is more successfully sustained than commitments to new high intensity exercise, e.g. going to a gym. There is some evidence that activity/exercise in groups is more successfully sustained than exercise on an individual basis and support from family, peers, community and health care professionals is beneficial.

Community/environmental strategies and partners for PHCT include:
• Walking and cycling to work in partnership with employers.
• Preserving and encouraging use of playing fields and open spaces in partnership with LAs.
• Local walking groups including Health Walks run by many PCOs.

Individual exercise promotion strategies should include
• Identification of patient/client's current daily/weekly activity levels as opportunities present, e.g. consultation for contraception or assessment home visit.
• Routine advice given in primary care, including written materials, on recommended levels of physical exercise and how to ↑ levels of physical activity in daily routines, e.g. use stairs, cut down on watching TV/screen time, walk faster, do household chores/garden more energetically and on most days.
• Use of client-centred, individualized, action plans, based on agreed, targeted behaviour change.
• Use of exercise referral schemes to LA exercise groups (sometimes known as prescription for exercise schemes).

*Older people—special considerations*
• For frailer older people, strength should be built up before progressing to dynamic exercise, e.g. through chair-based exercises, which some community nurses now provide following training.
• Moderate physical activity results in physical and emotional health improvements as well as modifies risks/impacts of falls (📖 Falls prevention, p. 327).
  • Training specifically in balance, strength, coordination, and reaction time leads to reduction of injurious falls (📖 Falls prevention, p. 327).
  • Weight-bearing exercise, plus the earlier mentioned points, leads to decrease in fractures (see also 📖 Osteoporosis, p. 558).

**Further information**

NICE (2006). Public Health Intervention Guidance No 2. Four commonly used methods to increase physical activity. Available at: ℗ www.nice.org.uk/PH2
Department of Health (2011). UK physical activity guidelines. Available at: ℗ www.gov.uk/government/publications/uk-physical-activity-guidelines

# Smoking cessation

Smoking is the leading cause of preventable disease and death in the UK. Cigarette smoke contains 50 known carcinogens and metabolic poisons, as well as nicotine. Half of all regular smokers will die as a result of smoking. Rates are higher in people in lower social class groups, in younger people, and in vulnerable groups, e.g. those with mental health problems. Nicotine is addictive, and has psychological and physiological effects. The majority of smoking-related deaths in UK from lung cancer, COPD, CHD.

*Passive smoking* associated with increased risk of CHD and lung cancer. In children, increased risk of cot death, bronchitis, and otitis media sudden unexpected death in infancy (SIDS; 📖 Sudden infant death syndrome, p. 295). Health promotion for young people is aimed at preventing them starting smoking.

## Helping people stop smoking

It is an NHS priority to help smokers quit. Ceasing smoking at any age brings health benefits. About 4 million smokers try each year but only 3–6% succeed. There are smoking status recording standards for general practice in the QOF (📖 Quality and outcomes framework, p. 66). National No Smoking Day is always the second Wednesday in March in the UK.

### Brief smoking-cessation advice

In primary care should include:
- Asking about smoking status at each contact, recording it (at least annually in general practice), including intention to quit.
- Giving advice about the benefits of stopping, particularly if a link can be made to the person's ill health or the effects on children, fetus, etc., and provide leaflets.
- Assessing motivation to stop, e.g. are you ready to give up for good?
  - If person is not ready to quit then provide information for future, e.g. quit smoking helpline.
  - If person is ready to quit then refer to local smoking cessation service, and/or offer nicotine replacement therapy (NRT) prescription and stop smoking support, as follows. *Note:* most cessation services offer specific stop smoking training for primary care professionals.

### Supporting a smoker to quit

- Help smoker set a date to quit and advise seeking support of friends and family.
- Identify triggers to smoking, e.g. alcohol, coffee, and advise on plan to reduce these during the first days.
- Encourage smokers to persist as it can take 3–4 attempts to stop.
  - Explain about nicotine withdrawal symptoms (includes irritability, dizziness, increased appetite) and craving. Symptoms are most intense within 24–48hrs after cessation and decline over 2–4wks.

- Explain about availability of NRT and bupropion and encouraging those smoking >10/day to consider it.
- Identify if person is likely to experience high levels of withdrawal symptoms, e.g. from previous experience, smokes within 30min of waking, smokes >15/day and advise NRT.
- Offer review, follow-up, and motivational support.

## Aids to smoking cessation

OTC nicotine gum, patches, inhalers, etc., are available (BNF 4.10). Complementary therapies are unproven, but some evidence for hypnotherapy. NICE guidance indicates:

### Smoking cessation medication

- Prescribe only for smokers who commit to target stop date.
- Prescription to last initially only for 2wks after target stop date.

NICE[1]: further prescriptions should only be issued if the patient has abstained and remains committed. NHS does not fund prescriptions again within 6mths, if the attempt was unsuccessful.

### Nicotine replacement therapy

↑ cessation rate by 1.5×. Contraindications for those with severe cardiovascular disease and recent CVA. NRT available as tablets, gum, patches, sprays, etc. (BNF 4.10). Some preparations are licensed in pregnancy. Treatment is continued for about 3mths provided the patient is abstaining. The dosage is only reduced after 3mths treatment, reducing every 3–4wks.

### Bupropion (Zyban®)

Smokers >18yrs (contraindicated if history of seizures, risk factors for seizures, eating disorders, experiencing acute symptoms of alcohol or benzodiazepine withdrawal, central nervous system tumour, bipolar disorders, pregnancy, breastfeeding). BP is measured before and during treatment Started 1–2wks before target quit date (BNF 4.10), increased dose after 6 days (not older people) to a max. of 7–9wks.

### Varenicline

Smokers >18yrs, take tablets 1wk before target quit day. 0.5mg od for cessation 3 days, 0.5mg bd for 4 days then 1mg bd for 11wks. Cessation rate increased by 2× if patients has stopped smoking after 12wks, consider further 12wks of treatment to avoid relapse (contraindications caution in psychiatric illness).

## Reference

[1]NICE. Guidance on NRT and smoking Intervention guidance (2006). Available at: ℰ www.nice.org.uk/

## Further information

ASH Action on Smoking and Health. Available at: ℰ www.ash.org.uk/
NHS Smoking Helpline ☎ 0800 022 43320
NHS Choices Smoking. Available at: ℰ www.nhs.uk/livewell/smoking/

# Managing stress

Stress is the feeling of being under too much mental or emotional pressure. A normal body response to stress is ↑ the production of adrenaline and cortisol, which ↑ heart rate, BP, metabolism to improve performance. People react differently to stress. Some respond by ↑ behaviours likely to cause other health problems, e.g. ↑ smoking, ↑ eating comfort food, ↑ drinking alcohol. Continued exposure to stress can lead to mental and physical symptoms, e.g. mood swings, anxiety, depression (🕮 People with depression, p. 435), sleep disturbances, indigestion, diarrhoea. Chronic stress contributes to depression (🕮 People with depression, p. 435), mental health problems and can ↑ risk of CHD (🕮 Coronary heart disease, p. 584). Common sources of stress-related ill health include:

- Relationship problems.
- Work problems.
- Financial problems (🕮 Benefits and support, p. 789).
- Bereavements (🕮 Bereavement, grief and coping with loss, p. 528).
- Exams.
- Change or loss of work.
- Being an informal carer (🕮 Key facts on carers and caring, p. 410).

Early recognitions of signs and symptoms of stress can help reduce their impact. Stress can affect feelings, behaviour, and physical health.

Individuals may notice ↑ irritability, anxiety, pessimism, racing thoughts, low self-esteem, or mood. May experience, headaches, muscle tension, sweating, dry mouth, loss of libido.

Many people benefit from simple advice and support (🕮 Social support, p. 24), while others find one of the talking therapies (🕮 Talking therapies, p. 429) beneficial.

Health promotion advice on managing stress includes:
- *Managing mind set:*
  - Setting realistic goals, thinking about achievements as success, not belittling them or talking them down.
  - Thinking of a stressful event as something to be managed and planned, not as an overwhelming event that leaves patient powerless.
- Make use of people around patient in coping, delegate tasks to others and talk to others about how feelings.
- Actively relax.
- Learn to express anger in an assertive not aggressive way, e.g. speaking in strong, steady voice not shouting.
- Have enough uninterrupted sleep. Actively address sleep problems, e.g. create a bedtime routine that helps relax, cut out late night alcohol, make bedroom as dark as possible, don't read in bed.
- Do things you enjoy, have fun, plan treats—escape to a world of movies, books, music, etc.
- Create time for regular exercise. Exercise helps release physical tension, can be sociable, and releases mood-enhancing endorphins in brain. Smiling and laughter also release endorphins.

*Simple relaxation technique*

Can be practised on own or in groups with one person talking through the steps. (*Note:* used by some nurses in group health promotion (📖 Group health promotion, p. 300).) Steps for simple relaxation:

• Find a quiet place where you won't be interrupted.
• Make yourself comfortable, lying or sitting, with eyes closed. Breathe slowly, deeply, effortlessly.
• Working from your feet to head, tense, then relax each part of body:
  • Starting with feet, tense them, for a count of 5, then release muscles and count to 5.
  • Repeat with small areas of body, including face, until every part of body has been tensed and released.
• Finally, tense all parts of body, count 5, release, then remain in that position, breathe slowly and deeply for at least 5–20min.

There are many different types of guided relaxation exercises. Self-help tapes and books are available at most book stores.

**Related topic**

📖 Counselling skills, p. 123.

**Further information**

Health and Safety Executive Information on workplace stress. Available at: ℔ www.hse.gov.uk/stress/
Mental Health Foundation. Available at: ℔ www.mentalhealth.org.uk
NHS Choices Stress. Available at: ℔ www.nhs.uk/conditions/stress/pages/

# Alcohol

Alcohol misuse is a significant public health concern. Most health-related harm is caused by non-dependent drinkers. Sensible drinking limits are defined as:
- <21U of alcohol a week for ♂, spread over the week and no more than 3–4/day.
- <14U of alcohol a week for ♀, spread over the week and no more than 2–3/day.
- Plus 2 alcohol-free days a week.

1 unit of alcohol:
- ½ pint of ordinary strength beer, lager, or cider.
- ¼ pint of extra strength beer, lager, or cider.
- 1 small glass of white (8 or 9% ABV (alcohol by volume)) wine.
- ⅔ small glass of red (11 or 12% ABV) wine.
- 1 single measure of spirits (30mL).

Alcohol should be avoided in pregnancy, before driving, operating machinery, swimming, working at heights, or using electrical equipment.

Harmful/hazardous drinking is associated with physical problems, e.g. hypertension, cirrhosis of the liver, injuries and accidents, e.g. falls/fights, mental health problems, e.g. depression, social problems, e.g. loss of work, family breakup, homelessness, and offending behaviours, e.g. violence to others.

## Promoting sensible drinking

Nurses in primary care have a wide range of opportunities to promote sensible drinking, e.g.:
- As part of other clinic/surgery consultations, e.g. for travel advice (⬚ Travel health, p. 350), review consultation for LTC.
- As part of specific health promoting care, e.g. pre-conceptual (⬚ Pre-conceptual care, p. 376) or antenatal care.
- In group health promotion, e.g. PSHE in schools (health promotion in schools, ⬚ Health promotion in schools, p. 217), parenting groups.

NICE guidance recommends alcohol use disorders identification test (AUDIT) to help to identify individuals with harmful and hazardous patterns of alcohol consumption. Scores provide guidance on level of intervention from alcohol education to referral for specialist[1].

## Harmful/hazardous drinking

Harmful/hazardous drinking is defined as:
- >28 units of alcohol a week for ♂.
- >21 units of alcohol a week for ♀.

Signs and symptoms of harmful/hazardous drinking include:
- Feeling depressed.
- Feeling nervous or on edge.
- Having difficulty in sleeping.
- Physical symptoms, e.g. gastritis.
- History of accidents or injuries due to alcohol.

- Poor concentration or memory.
- Neglecting themselves, e.g. poor hygiene.

### Interventions and management
Aim to help people reduce drinking at harmful levels. Strategies include:

- Give information on sensible drinking levels and risks of harmful drinking and encourage the person to consider ways of reducing this.
- Encourage patient/client to keep a drinking diary and feed back to patient/client on the number of units of alcohol s/he drinks a week.
- Discuss how and why patient/client believes s/he benefits from drinking and consider willingness to change.
- Discuss how much drinking costs patient/client each week.
- Discuss how to avoid situations where patient/client feels need to drink, e.g. social situations, stressful events.
- Discuss strategies for ↓ intake, e.g. low-alcohol beer, water to quench thirst, and in between drinks, drink with food, switch to half-pints, avoid buying rounds, and avoid friends who drink heavily.
- Discuss benefits of ↓ alcohol intake, e.g. sleep better, ↑ energy, ↓ lose weight, ↑ money.

*Dependent drinking* is when three of the following are present:

- Patient/client has difficulty in controlling drinking.
- There is a very strong urge to drink.
- Patient/client can drink large amounts of alcohol without feeling intoxicated.
- Drinking continues despite harm it causes.
- Day-to-day activities are neglected due to alcohol use.
- If drinking is stopped, withdrawal symptoms, e.g. tremors, anxiety, and sweating occur.

Patients who are drinking at high levels and are dependent drinkers need longer and more detailed interventions, determined by whether patient/client wish to change their drinking behaviour. These patients need to be referred to GP and/or NHS specialist alcohol services.

### Related topic
📖 Substance misuse, p. 433.

### Reference
[1] NICE (2011) CG115 Alcohol-use disorders. Availalbe at: http://guidance.nice.org.uk/CG115

### Further information
Al-anon UK is for anyone affected by another person's alcohol misuse. Available at: ℘ www. al-anonuk.org.uk/index.asp

Alcohol Concern tips for reducing alcohol intake. Available at: ℘ www.howsyourdrink.org.uk/ home.php

### Helplines
ADFAM Support for families. ☎ 0207 7553 7640. Available at: ℘ www.adfam.org.uk
Alcoholics Anonymous. ☎ 0845 769 7555

# UK screening programmes

There are internationally agreed criteria for appraising the viability, effectiveness, and appropriateness of screening before a condition screening programme is initiated. These include:
- The condition is an important health problem.
- Its natural history is well understood.
- It is recognizable at an early stage.
- Treatment is better at an early stage.
- A suitable test exists.
- An acceptable test exists.
- Adequate facilities exist to cope with abnormalities detected.
- Screening is done at repeated intervals when the onset is insidious.
- The chance of harm is less than the chance of benefit.
- The cost is balanced against benefit.

Each country has a committee that appraises the evidence and advises the central health department on implementation of screening programmes. It also lists conditions, which are not recommended for screening because insufficient evidence exists or evidence that screening does more harm than good (and provides links to reasons for decisions). Examples of conditions not recommended for routine screening are diabetes, depression, prostate cancer, domestic violence, speech, and language delay in children.

## Current national screening programmes

See Fig. 8.2.
- Antenatal (📖 Antenatal care and screening, p. 380) and newborn (📖 Child screening tests, p. 152).
- Child health (📖 Child screening tests, p. 152).
- Young person and adult :
  - Abdominal aortic aneurysm (📖 Abdominal aortic aneurysm screening, p. 344).
  - Bowel cancer (📖 Bowel cancer screening, p. 334).
  - Breast cancer (📖 Breast awareness and screening, p. 335).
  - Cervical cancer (📖 Cervical cancer screening, p. 337).
  - Diabetic retinopathy (📖 Diabetes, p. 611).
- Sexually transmitted diseases: *Chlamydia* (📖 Sexually transmitted infections, p. 715).

## Further information

Public Health England. UK NHS cancer screening programmes. Available at: 🕭 www.cancerscreening.nhs.uk/index.html

UK National Screening Committee. Available at: 🕭 www.screening.nhs.uk/uknsc

UKNSC. Policy database. Conditions which should not be screened for. Available at: 🕭 www.screening.nhs.uk/policydb.php

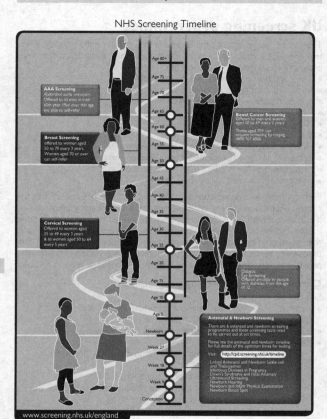

**Fig. 8.2** UK Screening Committee (England) NHS Screening Timeline 2012v3.
Reproduced with kind permission of UK Screening Committee (England).

# Menopause

The cessation of menstruation, usually occurs between 45 and 55yrs. Peri-menopause is the time from when the ovaries start to fail, ↓ oestrogen production and symptoms experienced, until 12mths after the last period. Women experience menopause in many different ways. Most experience peri-menopause over 4–5yrs, some experienced abrupt cessation. Contraception advised for 2yrs after last period if <50yrs and 1yr if >50yrs.

## *Premature menopause*

Cessation of menstruation <45yrs. Occurs in some syndromes, e.g. Turner's, and as a result of some gynaecological surgery or radiotherapy. Lack of oestrogen is associated with ↑ risk osteoporosis and cardiovascular disease. Premature menopause may be treated with HRT.

## Signs and symptoms

- *Menstruation changes:* cycle may shorten or lengthen to many months. Often increases in menstrual loss.
- *Hot flushes and night sweats:* experienced by about 80% of women.
- Thinning of the skin, brittle nails, hair loss, headaches, and generalized aches and pains.
- *Urinary symptoms:* 🕮 Stress urinary incontinence, p. 451; recurrent lower UTIs common.
- *Vaginal discomfort and dryness:* leading to dyspareunia (🕮 Sexual problems, p. 718).

In addition, some women may experience a range of emotional changes, but mostly related to other life events and not a sequelae of menopause. Some mood changes such as irritability and difficulties in concentration may be a result of disturbed sleep through night sweats. Loss of libido may occur, but non-hormonal factors, such as inadequate stimulation, depression, life stresses are usually main contributors.

## Consequences of the menopause

- Many women experience the end of menstruation as very liberating.
- Reduction in oestrogen causes ↑ risk of osteoporosis, urogenital atrophy, cardiovascular disease, and CVA. Increase weight, at or around menopause, to central abdomen area is an additional risk factor for cardiovascular disease.

## General advice

- Osteoporosis prevention (🕮 Falls prevention, p. 327).
- ↓ cardiovascular risk through exercise (🕮 Exercise, p. 313), nutrition and healthy eating (🕮 Nutrition and healthy eating, p. 304), weight management (🕮 Weight management: overweight, obesity, p. 307), smoking cessation (🕮 Smoking cessation, p. 315).
- Pelvic floor exercises (🕮 Urinary incontinence in women, p. 448).
- Stress management through ↑ exercise and relaxation techniques (🕮 Managing stress, p. 317).

## Managing symptoms

Many women experience very mild symptoms and manage them easily. About 40% experience symptoms that are distressing at some point.

### Hot flushes and night sweats

- May be helped by ↑ exercise, ↓ stress, avoiding triggers, such as caffeine, smoking, alcohol.
- Managed through lighter clothing, wearing layers, sleeping in cooler room, etc.
- Hormone replacement therapy.
- Herbal therapies, e.g. red clover, black cohosh, isoflavines, soya products used by many women to some benefit but research evidence is inconclusive (see British Menopause Society Fact Sheet).

**Urinary symptoms** (📖 Urinary incontinence in women, p. 448) HRT may also help with recurrent UTI.

**Vaginal dryness** Helped with lubricants. Short-term topical oestrogens (BNF 7.2.1) may be required. Use limited to 3–6mth. *Note:* some damage condoms and diaphragms (📖 Barrier contraceptive methods, p. 370).

## Hormone replacement therapy

HRT provides oestrogen (and progesterone in women with a uterus or premature menopause). HRT gives a small ↑ risk of DVT, breast, ovarian and endometrial cancer, stroke and CHD (for those starting >10yrs after menopause[1]. Contraindications include history of breast cancer, DVT). HRT is used short term (may be 2–3yrs) for alleviating symptoms or up to age 50 for those with premature menopause or hysterectomy before menopause. Choice of HRT preparation is according to symptoms, medical history, and preferences (BNF 6.4.1.1).

### Key principles in use of HRT

HRT is started with lowest dosage, reviewed after 3mths for side effects and improvements. Side effects may be oestrogen-related, e.g. headaches, fluid retention, or progesterone-related, e.g. bloating, headache, depression. Side effects may be alleviated by change of preparation. Bleeding may be erratic for first 1–2mths and spotting may occur up to 12mths with combined preparations. Reviewed every 12mths including BP.

### Stopping HRT

Can be withdrawn once menopause symptoms are no longer a problem. Trial withdrawals after 1–2yrs of use. Warn women symptoms may reappear.

## Reference

[1]NICE Clinical Knowledge Summaries (CKS) Menopause guidance. Available at: 🖰 http://cks.nice.org.uk/menopause

## Further information

British Menopause Society. Available at: 🖰 www.thebms.org.uk/
Menopause Matters. Available at: 🖰 www.menopausematters.co.uk/

# Healthy ageing

17% people in the UK are >65yrs in the UK with estimates that by 2035, 23% of the population will be >65yrs[1]. However, older people are not homogeneous. Health means different things to different people and may include the ability to lead an active life, ability to get out, independence, financial security. It is important to recognize that:

- Infirmity is *not* inevitable, but disability, dependency, accidents, death, and mental health problems are more common with older people.
- Chronic disease and disability in older people related to social class. Life expectancy at 65yrs is 3.5yrs greater in lower managerial and professional classes than routine occupations[1]. Chronological age is ∴ less appropriate than class as an indicator of potential illness and disability.

## Work and retirement

The traditional view of retirement as 'non-work' is challenged by the concept of the 'third age' as one of productivity, creativity, and contribution to community. Changes in occupational and pension schemes mean people are working in paid employment at older ages. Many employers organize pre-retirement courses, including information on financial management, getting the best from the NHS, skills training/retraining, and how to cope with change.

## Health promotion

Many potential problems which can accompany ageing are amenable to a preventive approach (e.g. falls, grief and loss, depression see 📖 p. 264). *Note:* ageism in public services may mean that older people are not offered access to screening or health promotion. Health promotion interventions should be addressed at individual and community/environmental levels (📖 Models and approaches to health promotion, p. 298).

*Community/environmental interventions* Important as healthy lifestyles information is insufficient if issues such as access to local healthy food, transport, housing, carer support, tackling crime, and improving the environment (e.g. street lighting, pavements) are not addressed.

### Specific topics for health promotion

- *Smoking:* older people and health professionals tend to take a fatalistic approach, but smoking cessation (📖 Smoking cessation, p. 315) is effective for all ages.
- *Diet and nutrition:* older people are at risk of poor nutrition (📖 Nutrition and healthy eating, p. 304) due to disease, drugs, social circumstances, income, and cognitive impairment. Healthy eating programmes and lunch clubs also provide social interaction. Alcohol (📖 Alcohol, p. 319) is related to depression and suicide. Safe drinking levels should be emphasized.
- *Activity:* inactivity is strongly associated with falls. Falls prevention programmes (📖 Falls prevention, p. 327) and exercise referral schemes (📖 Exercise, p. 313) are beneficial.

- *Social engagement:* isolated older people are more prone to poor health. Interest groups (gardening, dance, music) may be helpful. See also 🕮 Social support, p. 24.

**Life course issues related to age** This can mean older people are more vulnerable, and would benefit from statutory and informal services to support them through times of adjustment. Health professionals should be aware of particular issues including:

- *Emotional and mental health:*
  - *Grief and loss*—older people may experience multiple losses including spouse/partner, family, friends, also loss of independence and autonomy, mobility, social connections, dignity, privacy, confidence and self-esteem (🕮 Bereavement, and coping with loss grief, p. 528).
  - *Depressive illness*—depression is commonest mental health problem of old age, often due to bereavement and changing life events, e.g. retirement (🕮 People with depression, p. 435).
- *Physical health:*
  - *Hearing*—about 1 in 3 people >65yrs have a hearing impairment (🕮 Deafness, p. 649).
  - *Vision*—presbyopia (blurring of close vision) is feature of ageing experienced by 90% of >65yrs (🕮 Blindness and partial sight, p. 699).
  - *Respiratory function*—physiological deterioration in lungs due to the ageing process (🕮 Asthma, p. 566; 🕮 Chronic obstructive pulmonary disease, p. 574).
  - Cardiovascular disease and hypertension problems are more likely (🕮 Hypertension, p. 589).
  - *Musculoskeletal system*—reduced bone density may lead to Osteoporosis (🕮 Osteoporosis, p. 558) while wear and tear on large weight-bearing joints may lead to osteoarthritis (🕮 Osteoarthritis, p. 553).

SPICE[2] is a mnemonic for remembering the five aspects of older people's health that can be addressed but are often overlooked. It is particularly useful in general practice or clinic consultations:

- Senses (hearing and vision).
- Physical activity.
- Incontinence.
- Cognition.
- Emotions.

## Related topic
🕮 Individual health needs assessment, p. 110.

## References
### Health professionals and the public
[1]Office for National Statistics. Available at: ℬ www.ons.gov.uk
[2]Iliffe S, Lenihan P, Orrell M, *et al.* (2004). A short instrument to identify common unmet needs in older people in general practice. *Br J Gen Pract* **54**: 914–18.

## Further information
Age UK (2011). Healthy ageing evidence review. Available at: ℬ www.ageuk.org.uk/professional-resources-home/knowledge-hub-evidence-statistics/evidence-reviews/
Age UK Fit as a fiddle programme. Available at: ℬ www.ageuk.org.uk/health-wellbeing/fit-as-a-fiddle/

# Falls prevention

A fall is an unintentional event that results in a person coming to rest on the ground or another lower level. While accident prevention is a public health issue for all ages, falls and their sequelae are a particular issue for older people. Over 30% people >65yrs have a fall in any one year. Falls are a major cause of disability and the leading cause of mortality due to injury in people 75yrs+ in UK[1]. 75% of falls related deaths occur in the home. Falls are under-reported to health professionals.

## Consequences

Falls ↑ the likelihood of osteoporotic hip fracture, thought to be responsible for up to 14,000 deaths year in the UK, accounting for about £1.8 billion NHS spending. Other consequences include other fractures (e.g. Colles), loss of confidence, and restriction of activities. The inability to get up after a fall can result in hypothermia, pneumonia, dehydration, and pressure sores.

## Risk factors

Risk factors can be divided into physical, environmental, iatrogenic. *Note:* there is often no one clear cause.
- *Physical:*
  - Age >75yrs, ♀.
  - Orthostatic hypotension.
  - Cognitive impairment, depression.
  - Parkinson's disease, CVA, balance disorders, acute illness, visual impairment.
  - Urinary urgency.
  - Inability to rise from chair of knee height without use of arms.
  - ↓ mobility, lower limb weakness, foot problems.
  - History of fall in previous year/fear of falling.
- *Environmental factors:*
  - In the home, e.g. bed or chair too low, poor lighting, loose rugs.
  - Outside the home, e.g. ice on pavement, uneven pavements.
- *Iatrogenic:*
  - 4+ medications/day.
  - Antihypertensives, sedatives, diuretics.

## Key policy interventions

Public health strategies to identify, assess, and prevent those at risk of falling exist in each PCO. Strategies also link to activity promotion (📖 Exercise, p. 313). Most PCOs have developed an integrated falls services (see 📖 Falls prevention, p. 327). Most PCOs use clinical guidelines on assessment and prevention of falls, case/risk identification, risk assessment, and interventions (e.g. NICE guidelines[1]). Many have a falls prevention service.

## Falls prevention services

Usually has a named falls prevention coordinator (e.g. clinical nurse specialist) who coordinates information systems, involvement of older people and carers, education for health professionals, and inter-disciplinary and interagency collaborative programmes. A Falls Prevention Service promotes:

- The identification of people at risk through:
  - The promotion of asking older people whether they have experienced falls at each contact with health and, social services, ambulance services, independent sector or voluntary groups.
  - Promoting the comprehensive assessment of people, who report falling, against the risks reported above (also see NICE guidelines[1]).
- Multi factorial interventions of:
  - Strength and balance retraining programmes by trained professional (📖 Exercise, p. 313).
  - Home hazard assessment and modification programmes.
  - Personal, body-worn alarm systems.
  - Optician assessment of vision and correction of visual impairment.
  - Medication review.
  - Education and information provision.

## Related topic

📖 Osteoporosis, p. 558.

## Reference

[1] NICE (2013). Falls assessment and prevention of falls in older people, CG161. Available at: ℘ http://www.nice.org.uk/nicemedia/live/14181/64166/64166.pdf

## Further information

Age UK (2010) Preventing falls: strength and balance exercises for healthy ageing. Available at: ℘ www.ageuk.org.uk/Documents/EN-GB/strength_and_balance_training_PDF.pdf?epslanguage=en-GB?dtrk=true

Gillespie, WJ, Robertson, LD, Gillespie, MC, et al. (2010). Interventions for preventing falls in older people living in the community. *Cochrane Library*. Available at: ℘ http://onlinelibrary.wiley.com/doi/10.1002/14651858.CD007146.pub2/pdf

# Weather extremes

## Heat waves

Even during relatively mild heat waves death rates are significantly, but avoidably raised in the UK. In extreme hot weather there is a risk of developing dehydration leading to *heat exhaustion*:

- Symptoms include headaches, dizziness, nausea and vomiting, muscle weakness or cramps, pallor, high temperature.
- Treatment includes moving somewhere cooler, cool down in water or shower, or sponge down, rest and drink lots of water.

### Untreated heat exhaustion leads to heatstroke

Symptoms include intense headaches, nausea, intense thirst, sleepiness, hot, red, and dry skin, sudden rise in temperature, confusion, aggression, convulsions, and loss of consciousness. Requires urgent medical attention. Can result in organ failure, brain damage, or death.

### Groups at particular risk

- Those >over 75yrs old and/or living on their own, or in a care home.
- People suffering from mental ill health or with dementia.
- People who are bed bound.
- People with serious chronic heart, respiratory conditions, or medications that affect their ability to sweat.
- Babies and young children, especially <4yrs.

Each PCO has to plan with social services to identify individuals vulnerable to heatstroke, especially >75yrs, and actions to support them if a heat wave alert is issued by central government Each country has a heat watch system.

### The Met Office warning system

- *Level one minimum alert:* people should be aware of what to do if alert level is raised. In place from June 1 until September 15.
- *Level two alert:* ↑ chance of heat wave within the next few days.
- *Level three alert:* when a heat wave is happening.
- *Level four alert:* when a heat wave is severe.

### Prevention advice if a heat wave is forecast

- Keep out of the heat:
  - Especially in the hottest part of the day 11am–1pm.
  - If have to go out stay in the shade, wear a hat, carry water.
- *Keep cool:*
  - Stay inside in coolest room as much as possible.
  - Close curtains in rooms that get sun, keep windows closed while room is cooler than outside, open windows when temperature rises above outside and at night.
  - Take frequent cool baths, showers, or splash water over face, neck.
- *Drink regular fluids:* water or fruit juice best, avoid tea coffee, alcohol, eat cool foods.
- Be alert to signs of heat exhaustion and act as above, seek help if concerned.

## Cold weather

Every winter in the UK, 25,000–30,000 deaths are linked to the cold weather. ~4 million households in the UK are in fuel poverty. This is when a household spends more than 10% of its income to keep warm.

*Hypothermia* (📖 Hypothermia, p. 768) occurs when body temperature is <35°C (95°F). It is caused by exposure to cold environment and an inability to maintain body temperature. Those at risk include:
- Babies who cannot regulate their body temperature.
- People exposed to extreme weather conditions or cold water.
- Older people, especially if they are not very active, or have other illnesses.
- People with dementias may not be able to tell when they are cold.
- People with reduced mobility or health conditions that change body's ability to respond to temperature changes.

*Prevention advice*
- Maintain body warmth through activity, eating well, including warm food and drinks, dressing in layers to trap heat and covering head.
- Keeping home heated, or at least one room, and use that for all activities. Use thermometer to check room is between 16°C and 20°C. Government support for heating costs for people on low incomes, disabled and older people (📖 Benefits for people with a low income, p. 791). See also 📖 Homes and housing, p. 21.
- The Warm Front Scheme offers grants for heating and insulation improvements.

All PCOs and social services have to collaborate on identifying individuals vulnerable to hypothermia in cold weather and plan to ensure support is given, particularly for extreme weather conditions.

## Further information

NHS Choices warm and cold weather pages. Available at: 🔗 www.nhs.uk/livewell/weather/Pages/weather.aspx

Met Office Weather forecast and any high temperature health warnings. Available at: 🔗 www.metoffice.gov.uk

Department of Health (2010). Heatwave. Looking after yourself and others. Available at: 🔗 www.dh.gov.uk

Gov.UK. The Warm Front Scheme. Available at: 🔗 www.gov.uk/warm-front-scheme/overview

# Skin cancer prevention

Skin cancer, including non-melanoma skin cancer (NMSC) and malignant melanoma (MM), is the most commonly diagnosed cancer in the UK. Around 80% of MM are $2°$ to exposure to sunlight or artificial ultraviolet (UV) light. UV rays from the sun classified into: UVA and UVB. Majority of UV radiation is UVA. UV light is natural in sunlight or artificial, e.g. sunbeds. UV penetrates cloud, water, and UVA penetrates glass, sand, snow, concrete.

❶ The majority of skin cancers are preventable.

## Risk factors

- UV radiation is most intense between 11.00–15.00 hours British Summer Time (BST) or 10.00–14.00 hours Greenwich Mean Time (GMT).
- Burning from over exposure to UV light, doubles the risk of MM.
- Repeated intense exposure to UV light ↑ risk of development of MM.
- UV damage to skin in the first 15yrs linked to risk of MM in later life.
- Those with naturally fair skin are at ↑ risk of DNA damage.
- Those with fair skin which burns and freckles easily and light eye colour, red or fair hair.
- Large number of moles, >50.
- Family history of skin cancer.
- Previous melanoma and some other cancers, e.g. breast, non-Hodgkin lymphoma, renal cell, prostate, thyroid, and leukaemia.
- Other medical conditions and treatments, e.g. organ transplant possibly through the use of immunosuppressant drugs.

## Prevention

### Sunbeds or sunlamps

Sunbeds and lamps should not be used, can be more dangerous than natural sunlight because they use a concentrated source of UV radiation. ❶ It is illegal for people <18yrs to use a sunbed or be in an area that is allocated for sun bed users.

### Sunscreen

Should be applied around 15min before going into the sun and reapplied every 2hrs. Take extra care to protect babies and children. Buy sunscreen suitable for skin type and blocks both UVA and UVB radiation. Sunscreens with a SPF of 15+ filters out 93% of UVB. ❶ Sunscreens should not be used to ↑ time in the sun. No sunscreen has 100% protection.

Choice of sunscreen should include:
- With a minimum SPF of 15, the higher the better. Broad spectrum'— to protect against UVA and UVB.
- Water resistant, to prevent being washed or sweated off.
- With a valid 'use by' date. Most sunscreens have a shelf life of 2–3yrs. Expensive sunscreens are not more effective than cheaper ones.
- Sun **Smart** code (Cancer Research UK):
  - **S**tay in the shade 11.00–15.00 hours.
  - **M**ake sure you never burn.
  - **A**lways cover up—↑ protection by dark-coloured, close woven, dry (wet fabrics allow more UV through), wide brim wide hats, wrap-around sunglasses (British Standard 2427, or marked with CE mark or a UV 400 label protect vulnerable eyes).
  - **R**emember to take extra care of children.
  - **T**hen use factor 15+ sunscreen.
- Also report mole changes or unusual skin growths promptly to GP.

*The Solar UV index*
Indicates the strength of UV. It is shown in weather reports as a number in a triangle. The level of danger depends on skin type i.e. fair burns, fair tans, brown, black). UV Index 10 means high levels of UV and advice for people of all skin types is to try to stay in the shade. Daily UV ratings are on UK Government Meterological Office website.

## Signs of skin cancer

Advise people to know what their skin normally looks like by looking regularly in a full-length mirror. ❶ The following abnormalities and changes should be referred to the GP for further investigation:
- *Changes of non-melanoma skin cancer:* occurs mainly in older people, often on head, neck, and/or hands:
  - A new growth or sore that does not heal within 4wks.
  - A spot or sore that continues to itch, hurt, crust, scab, or bleed.
  - Persistent skin ulcers that are not explained by other causes.
- *Signs of abnormality of malignant melanoma:*
  - Moles which are asymmetrical or have blurred or jagged edges.
  - Moles that have changed colour, or with multiple colours in them.
  - Moles which are new, growing, or bigger than other moles.
  - Moles which are raised and/or have an uneven surface.
  - Moles which are bleeding, oozing, crusting, itchy, or painful.

## Related topic
📖 Burns and scalds, p. 756.

## References
Cancer Research UK SunSmart. Available at: ℘ www.cancerresearchuk.org/sunsmart/
NHS Choices pages on skin cancer protection and use of suncreen. Available at: ℘ http://www.nhs.uk/Livewell/travelhealth/Pages/SunsafetyQA.aspx
UK Meteorological Office UV information. Available at: ℘ www.metoffice.com

# Early signs of cancer

One person in three is diagnosed with cancer at some time in their life. Cancer usually affects older people, but it can occur at any age. Key advice for prevention against cancer:

* Do not smoke or smoke in the presence of non-smokers (⬚ Smoking cessation, p. 315).
* Avoid obesity (⬚ Weight management: overweight, obesity, p. 307).
* Undertake brisk physical activity each day (⬚ Exercise, p. 313).
* ↑ daily intake and variety of fruit and vegetables to at least five portions daily and ↓ foods containing animal fats (⬚ Nutrition and healthy eating, p. 304).
* Moderate alcohol consumption (⬚ Alcohol, p. 319).
* Avoid excessive exposure to sunlight especially children, adolescents, and those with tendency to burn (⬚ Skin cancer prevention, p. 331).
* Adhere to safety regulations about exposure to known carcinogens.

## Early signs of cancer

Cancer is not just one disease, but at least 200 different types, with a wide range of possible symptoms, not always symptoms of cancer. Early detection aided by knowing what is normal for your body and acting on changes. Signs and symptoms to consult a medical professional about:

* *Ongoing chest or throat problems:* coughing or hoarseness that lasts >3wks, haemoptysis.
* *Changes in bowel function:* unexplained changes, such as chronic constipation, diarrhoea, or a change in the size of the stool, which last for >6wks. Blood in the stool, melaena, occult blood, frank blood.
* *Changes in bladder function:* dysuria, haematuria, or unexplained changes in micturition.
* *Unexplained intermenstrual bleeding or discharge.*
* *Skin changes:* skin changes can occur in internal cancers as well skin cancers. These can include: hyperpigmentation, erythema, pruritus, hirsutism, and ulceration.
* *Changes in skin moles:* in colour, shape or sensation, i.e. pain or itching; bleeding or crusting; moles that have multiple colours, moles with irregular edges, uneven surfaces, raised; moles that are new or growing (⬚ Skin cancer, p. 634).
* Lumps, or thickening that does not go away.
* Ongoing indigestion or swallowing problems.
* Unexplained fatigue.
* Unexplained pain.
* Unexplained weight loss.

## Related topic

⬚ UK screening programmes, p. 321; ⬚ Skin cancer prevention, p. 331.

## Further information

NHS Cancer Screening Programmes website for more information on national cancer screening programmes. Available at: ↗ www.cancerscreening.nhs.uk

Macmillan Cancer Relief. Available at: ↗ www.macmillan.org.uk

NHS Choices. Preventing cancer. Available at: ↗ www.nhs.uk/Livewell/preventing-cancer

# Bowel cancer screening

Bowel cancer is the third commonest cancer in the UK and second largest of cancer deaths. Regular screening for faecal occult blood in older adults avoids 1 in 6 colorectal cancer deaths. The NHS Bowel Cancer Screening Programme invites men and women in their sixties to be screened for bowel cancer every 2yrs. People aged 70yrs and over can request a kit. The faecal occult blood test kit is sent to complete at home and return to a laboratory. Anyone with a positive result is referred for a colonoscopy and any necessary treatment.

## Advice for patients on screening
- The kit includes:
  - Instruction leaflet and a prepaid return envelope.
  - An orange and white cardboard test kit, and six cardboard sticks.
- The kit lasts months, but once opened, all samples must be taken so it is sent and received within 14 days.
- Samples need to be collected from three different bowel motions.
- Write the date of the motion on each flap.
- Collect the stool before it goes in the toilet (e.g. in toilet paper, in plastic bag over hand).
- Uses two sticks to take a small bit from two areas of stool and wipe each thinly over one of the two windows in that flap. Close flap and tuck it under orange part to secure. *Note:* sticks should be wiped and put in rubbish not down toilet.
- Store the kit in a cool place and out of sunlight.
- Repeat for samples 2 and 3.
- Return so the kit arrives within 14 days of opening.
- The instruction leaflet provides confidential helpline numbers.

## Related topic
📖 UK Screening programmes, p. 321; 📖 Early signs of cancer, p. 333.

## Further information
Cancer Research UK. Cancer statistics. Available at: ℘ www.cancerresearchuk.org/cancerstats
Cochrane Database of Systematic Reviews (2006). Screening for colorectal cancer using the fae-
    cal occult blood test: an update. Available at: ℘ http://summaries.cochrane.org/CD001216/
    screening-for-colorectal-cancer-using-the-faecal-occult-blood-test-hemoccult
NHS Bowel Cancer Screening Programme. Available at: ℘ www.cancerscreening.nhs.uk/bowel/
    index.html

# Breast cancer awareness

Breast cancer is the most common cancer to affect women in the UK.
❶ Over 200 men diagnosed with breast cancer a year. Early detection
of changes is encouraged through 'breast awareness'. 2° prevention is
by breast screening by mammography and clinical breast examination.
Rationale for the promotion of breast awareness:

- Approximately 90% of breast cancers are detected by women
  themselves or their partners.
- Early detection of cancer equates to increased chances of survival.

## Teaching breast awareness

The most effective methods of promoting breast awareness are: provision
of verbal and written information; demonstration and return demonstration on the woman's own breast; and feedback to the woman regarding
her own ability.

Women should practise breast awareness from the age of 18yrs onwards
as part of overall bodily awareness. The NHS Breast Screening Programme
Breast Awareness Five Point plan:

- *Point 1—know what is normal for you:*
  - *During activities*—e.g. bathing, showering, and dressing become
    aware of the normal state of the breasts.
  - *Breasts are glandular sensitive to the presence of oestrogen
    and progesterone*—in pre-menopausal ♀, and ♀ taking HRT,
    normal breasts feel different at different times of the month.
    Post-menopausal women's breasts may become softer, and
    less lumpy.
- *Point 2—look and feel:*
  - *Look*—stand in front of the mirror, undressed to the waist, and
    raise arms above head and drop them to sides. Then place hands
    on hips and clench chest muscles.
  - Look at the outline and rise and fall of each breast.
  - *Feel with the finger tips*—breast is pear-shaped and extends into
    armpit, richly supplied by lymph nodes so ensure whole breast and
    surrounding area is felt, including into armpit, nipple, clavicle, and
    sternum.
- *Point 3—know what changes to look for:*
  - Appearance change in the outline or shape of the breast, especially
    those caused by arm movements or lifting the breasts.
  - Skin puckering or dimpling of the skin
  - *Nipple change*—direction, rash, position, shape, discharge, bleeding.
  - Lumps or thickening in breast or armpit or seems different than the
    other breast.
  - Pain or discomfort especially if new and persistent.
- *Point 4*—report any changes to the GP without delay.
- *Point 5*—attend for breast screening if aged 50yrs or over.

## Mammography screening

Mammography is part of the UK screening programme (📖 UK screening programme, p. 321) offered every 3yrs for ♀ aged 50–70yrs (extending to late 40s and early 70s). ♀ >70yrs can make own appointments. It detects ~85% of breast cancers in women aged >50yrs (60% of which are impalpable). Women have a good prognosis in 70–80% of cancers detected by screening. Screening more regularly does not improve outcomes and ↑ exposure to radiation. Most women find having a mammogram uncomfortable and sometimes painful, but it is only for a few seconds.

## Related topics

📖 Menopause, p. 323; 📖 Breast problems, p. 722; 📖 Breast cancer, p. 723.

## Further information

NHS Choices. Breast Cancer Awareness. Available at: ℬ http://www.nhs.uk/Livewell/Breastcancer/Pages/Breastcancersymptoms.aspx

NHS Breast Cancer Screening Programme. Breast Awareness. Available at: ℬ http://www.cancer-screening.nhs.uk/breastscreen/breastawareness.html

NHS Breast Cancer Screening Programme. Breast Screening. Available at: ℬ www.cancerscreening.nhs.uk/breastscreen/about-breast-screening.html

# Cervical cancer screening

Cervical cancer mortality and incidence is ↓ in the UK. In 2008, there were about 2800 diagnoses and 960 deaths[1], about 1% of all cancers. Risk factors are persistent infection with oncogenic HPV types and cigarette smoking. Screening aims to detect cell abnormalities on cervix, which might lead to cancer if untreated.

## Cervical screening programme

Cervical screening is an additional service in the GMS contract (📖 General practice, p. 13) and has specified points in the QOF (📖 Quality and outcomes framework, p. 66).

### Invitation to screening

Local call and recall agency invites ♀ for screening to GP practice, contraceptive and sexual health clinics.

- *In England women aged 25–64yrs:*
  - 3-yearly between 25–49yrs.
  - 5-yearly 50–64yrs.
- At 65+ only those are screened who have not been screened since age 50yrs or have had recent abnormal tests. ♀ 65+yrs who have had 3 consecutive negative smears are taken out of the call–recall system.
- Every 3yrs from 20 to 64yrs in Wales and 20–60yrs in Scotland.

***Cervical cell sampling*** Cervical samples taken by liquid-based cytology (LBC) (📖 Cervical samples, p. 339).

### Results

- ♀ Must receive results within 14 days, sent by local call and recall agency. Some contraceptive and sexual health clinics still send results by letter.
- 90% have normal result and are recalled in 3–5yrs depending on age.
- Types of results and actions: see Table 8.2.
- Abnormal results referred for colposcopy, examination with a low-powered light microscope. May also include biopsies or treatment (usually large loop excision of the transformation zone (LLETZ)) with local anaesthetic.

### Quality assurance

The NHS Cervical Screening Programme has a regional system of quality assurance, in which a regional team reviews the performance of the local cervical screening programmes 3-yearly against national quality standards.

## Human papilloma virus testing

HPV testing introduced in England in 2012. There are two new tests:
- HPV triage offered to all ♀ with either borderline changes or mild dyskarysosis:
  - If oncogenic HPV is detected the ♀ referred immediately to colposcopy.
  - If oncogenic HPV is not detected, ♀ returns to normal recall 3 or 5yrs. Need for ongoing surveillance will be removed.

- HPV test of cure offered to all ♀ who have been treated for cervical intraepithelial neoplasia (CIN), and who have either a normal or low grade abnormality 6mths post-treatment.
  - If oncogenic HPV is not detected, ♀ is returned to normal recall—3yrs for all age groups. Removes approximately 80% of treated ♀ from the current 10-yr surveillance programme.
  - If oncogenic HPV is detected the ♀ remains under care of colposcopy service.

❶ Women with glandular abnormalities (CGIN) do not come under this new protocol.

**Table 8.2** Cervical cancer screening results and action

| Result | Action |
|---|---|
| Inadequate (2–3%; test cannot be interpreted) | Repeat smear at or after 3mths<br>If 3 in a row inadequate referred for colposcopy |
| Negative (90%; no abnormalities detected) | Routine recall as per national programme |
| Borderline changes in squamous or endocervical cells (cellular appearance neither normal or abnormal). Low grade abnormality | HPV test carried out. If HPV +ve refer to colposcopy |
| Mild dyskaryosis (outer third epithelium abnormal consistent with CIN1). Low grade abnormality (6%) | HPV test carried out. If HPV +ve refer to colposcopy (within 8wks) |
| Moderate dyskaryosis (half to two-thirds epithelium abnormal consistent with CIN2). High grade abnormality (0.5%) | Referred for colposcopy within 4wks |
| Severe dyskaryosis (full-thickness epithelium abnormal consistent with CIN3). High grade abnormality(0.5%) | Referred for colposcopy within 4wks<br>Urgent referral for colposcopy (within 2wks) |
| Suspected invasive cancer | |

### Related topics

📖 Sexual health: general issues, p. 711; 📖 Sexually transmitted infections, p. 715; 📖 Gynaecological cancers, p. 726.

### Patient information

Leaflets are available from the NHS Cancer Screening website,[2] including those for women with learning disabilities and other languages.

### References

[1]Cancer Research UK. Cancer statistics. Available at: ℬ www.cancerresearchuk.org/cancerstats
[2]National Cervical Cancer Screening Programme. Available at: ℬ www.cancerscreening.nhs.uk/cervical

# Cervical sample taking

See also 📖 Cervical cancer screening, p. 337.

LBC is used for taking cervical samples in the UK. The sample is obtained using a Cervex-Brush® and immediately placed into a vial of preservative liquid.

**Timing** The sample can be taken at any time during the month except when the woman is menstruating. Mid-cycle remains the optimum time, but is not essential. Appointment times should be available outside normal working hours to encourage attendance.

## Patient comfort and understanding

Aim to minimize embarrassment, anxiety, and discomfort. A sensitive approach is required to ensure women continue in the programme for subsequent tests.
- Ensure understanding of purpose of screening.
- Explain the procedure before and during test.
- Obtain informed consent (📖 Consent, p. 77), for sample and for possibility of HPV test (if in England).
- Offer opportunity to empty bladder before.
- Offer a chaperone (📖 Chaperones, p. 79).
- Ensure privacy in examination room.
- Use modesty paper sheet while on couch.
- Offer tissues and hand-washing after procedure.
- Offer an opportunity to ask questions after and ensure results procedure is explained clearly.

## Protection against infection

Vaginal speculae used to access the cervix *must* be either single-use items or sterilized via a central sterile supplies department. Brushes and vials for the test must be kept in a clean environment.

## Taking a history and forms

- A history should be taken using the request form as a template. Accurate and complete details are essential including:
  - Screening history.
  - Any contraceptive method and HRT.
  - Any abnormal bleeding or discharge symptoms (consider whether referral to other service, e.g. gynaecology is required).
- Forms can be:
  - National, e.g. HMR101 (England).
  - Open Exeter form, pre-populated with the ♀ details and history.
  - An electronic requesting method used for all types of samples.

## Sample taking

The sample must be taken from the squamocolumnar junction (SCJ). This is usually around the cervical os. It is essential to obtain squamous cells and desirable to obtain some endocervical cells from the SCJ.
- Use an appropriately sized, warm speculum to keep vaginal walls apart and visualize cervical os.

- Do not use any lubrication if possible; it may affect analysis of sample.
- If cervix is posterior, woman may need to tilt pelvis by clenching fists under her sacrum. A Winterton speculum may be helpful when cervix is very posterior. Coughing can also help bring cervix into view.
- Insert Cervex-Brush® into endocervical canal, turning 360° × 5 in a clockwise direction. Firm pressure is needed to obtain sufficient cells. See Fig. 8.3.
- If an ectropian/ectopy/eversion is present take care to sample SCJ fully. If a wide ectropian is present two Cervex-Brushes® may be needed.
- If intrauterine device (IUD)/intrauterine system (IUS) *in situ*, 360° sweep × 5 starts and ends at thread position, gently moving it aside.
- Place sample in vial immediately:
  - With ThinPrep®, agitate the Cervex-Brush® in vial to release cells.
  - With SurePath™, place thumb against brush pad and release brush head into vial.
  - Label the vial.
- Record clinical observations of the cervix, such as contact bleeding, polyps on the request form.
- Vial sealed in bag with request form and sent to the laboratory on next available transport.
- Take additional bacterial and viral swabs *only* if indicated clinically.

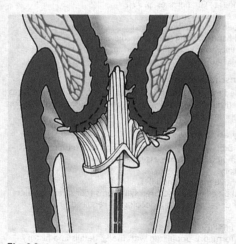

**Fig. 8.3** Cervex-Brush® in the cervical os.
Reproduced with kind permission of Rovers® Cervex-Brush®.

## Further information

Jo's Trust. Information and support on cervical screening, abnormal results and cervical cancer. Available at: ℘ www.jostrust.org.uk/
UK National Cervical Cancer Screening Programme. Available at: ℘ www.cancerscreening.nhs. uk/cervical

# Testicular self-examination

The aim of testicular self-examination (TSE) is the early detection of any changes from normal that may indicate testicular cancer. TSE is method of 2° prevention. The majority of testicular cancers are first detected by men themselves. Testicular cancer responds extremely well to treatment with a cure rate of 97% for testicular cancer, which is detected early. Most of the testicular cancer deaths in UK occur in males aged 30–50yrs of age[1].

## Known risk factors for testicular cancer

- Age 20–49.
- More common in white men.
- Previous testicular cancer.
- Risk ↑ in men with cryptorchidism (undescended testis, risk is ↓ if testicle is repositioned by age of 10yrs), inguinal hernia, subfertility.

## TSE guidelines

Barriers to performing TSE are embarrassment, ignorance, and lack of confidence in their ability to do TSE. The easiest time for men to self-examine is after a bath or a shower, when the scrotal skin is relaxed. Advise self-examination once a month.

- *Know what is normal:*
  - Hold scrotum in palms of hands, and feel testicles' size and weight. It is usual for one testicle to be larger than other, or one that hangs lower.
  - Feel each testicle and gently roll it between thumb and finger. It should feel smooth. Soft, tender tube toward back of each testicle is normal (i.e. epididymis).
- *Know what changes to look for:*
  - Lump or swelling in part of testicle—*Note:* most are not cancer. Lump may be small and hard (pea-sized), although it may be much larger.
  - A dull ache in the testicle and/or lower abdomen. *Note:* there may be no pain.
  - A heavy feeling in the scrotum.
- Report any changes without delay to a GP.

## Reference

[1]Cancer Research UK. Testicular cancer statistics. Available at: ℘ http://www.cancerresearchuk. org/cancer-help/type/testicular-cancer/about/finding-testicular-cancer-early

## Further information

Cancer Research UK. TSE. Available at: ℘ www: cancerhelp.cancerresearchuk.org/type/ testicular-cancer/about/testicular-selfexamination

NHS Choices. Testicular cancer prevention. Available at: ℘ http://www.nhs.uk/conditions/ cancer-of-the-testicle/pages/prevention.aspx

# New patient health check

GP practices offer all new patients registering with the practice a health check as part of the registration process. Each practice decides its own protocols. It provides the practice with the opportunity to get to know the new patient, whilst ensuring their medical information is correct and up-to-date. The aim is to understand new patient's health needs, reduce the incidence of preventable conditions, encourage good health in the practice population, and record any relevant QOF (📖 Quality and outcomes framework, p. 66) indicators.

Note: practices should offer a routine NHS Health Check to all patients aged 40–75yrs every 5yrs. Good practice: all patients >75yrs who have not been seen in the last year should be offered a routine heath check.

## Suggested elements of the new patient health check

- Review current and past illnesses and operations.
- Identify family history (FH) of illnesses with particular reference to diabetes, CHD, stroke, hypertension, cancers, and other significant problems.
- Check and record current medications, OTC medications, and allergies. Refer to GP or non-medical prescriber regarding medication.
- Check screening tests (📖 UK screening programmes, p. 321) are up-to-date, e.g. cervical smear, bowel cancer, and advise as appropriate.
- Check immunization status and offer as appropriate (📖 Targeted immunization in adults, p. 347).
- Check and record smoking status and offer smoking cessation (📖 Smoking cessation, p. 315) advice.
- Measure weight and height for BMI calculation, and waist circumference. Offer as appropriate weight management (📖 Weight management: overweight, obesity, p. 307), exercise advice (📖 Exercise, p. 313).
- Review alcohol units/wk, offer advice or intervention if required (📖 Alcohol, p. 319).
- Undertake urinalysis for proteinuria, glycosuria, haematuria.
- Measure BP: adults should have their BP measured at least every 5yrs (📖 Quality and outcomes framework, p. 66). BP should be <150/90; normotensive = <140/90.[1]

- *Measuring BP:*
  - In both arms, arm with the highest value should be used.
  - Use appropriate size cuff, i.e. bladder encircles at least 80% upper arm and arm must be supported at heart level.
  - Korotkoff phase I and phase V sounds used for systolic BP and diastolic BP, respectively.
  - Take 3 measurements 1–2min apart and record lowest reading.

*Note:* hypertension is sustained BP >140/90 on 3 or more occasions (&#x1F4D5; Hypertension, p. 589). Provide lifestyle advice for reducing BP and reassess yearly.

- Offer other healthy lifestyle advice, e.g. nutrition and healthy eating (&#x1F4D5; Nutrition and healthy eating, p. 304) exercise as appropriate.
- Arrange appointments with appropriate health-care professional if additional intervention necessary.

## Reference

[1]NICE (2011). Hypertension (CG127). Available at: &#x1F56E; www.nice.org.uk/guidance/CG127

# Abdominal aortic aneurysm screening

Aneurysms are weaknesses causing bulges in blood vessels. Abdominal aortic aneurysms (AAA) cause about 6000 deaths/yr in England and Wales. Those most at risk are men >65yrs who smoke, have high BP, or with close family history of AAA. Screening introduced across England in 2013.

All men aged 65yrs are invited in the year of their birthday (those older can contact the local programme for an appointment). Invitation leaflets explain the reasons, procedure, and possible outcomes. The screening is by abdominal ultrasound (takes about 10min), and results are given at the time and in writing.

## Possible results of screening

- *Normal:* i.e. no AAA detected. No further invitations.
- *Small aneurysm:* i.e. aorta is wider than normal and repeat invitations for regular checks will be issued.
- *Large aneurysm found:* i.e. aorta much wider than normal (only 1 in 100 men). Referral to specialist service for further tests and possible treatment, usually surgery.

## Further information

Circulation Foundation (UK Vascular disease charity). Available at: ℘ www.circulationfoundation. org.uk/

NHS Abdominal Aortic Aneurysm Screening. Available at: ℘ http://aaa.screening.nhs.uk/aaainfo

NHS Choices. Abdominal Aortic Aneurysm. Available at: ℘ http://www.nhs.uk/Conditions/ repairofabdominalaneurysm

# Immunization administration

The UK national immunization programme is detailed in the 'Green Book' (Department of Health 2006)[1] and updated on-line to reflect real-time policy decisions and recommendations of the Joint Committee on Vaccination and Immunization. The 1° purpose of vaccination is to protect the individual, who in turn is less likely to be a source of infection to others. High percentages of vaccinated individuals provide 'population' or 'herd' immunity, which benefits those who cannot be vaccinated.

## Key aspects of immunization provision

- The provision of information about the benefits and risks of each vaccination so that informed consent can be given (🕮 Consent, p. 77).
- One individual (and a deputy ) in each clinic or surgery responsible for ordering, receipt, and proper storage of vaccines including:
  - No more than 2–4wks supply stored and used by expiry date.
  - Refrigerate immediately in specialized vaccine fridge.
  - Stored at between +2°C to +8°C as monitored and recorded at least once each working day.
  - As vaccines are POMs, the fridge should lock or be in lockable room.
- Cold chain must be preserved in transportation, storage at manufacturers recommended temperature to point of administration.
- Transporting vaccines to other clinics, care homes, etc., should only be in validated cool boxes with maximum–minimum thermometers.
- All individuals advising and administrating vaccines should be trained and updated in immunization (see 🕮 Immunization, p. 345), and recognizing and treating anaphylaxis (🕮 Anaphylaxis, p. 751).
- Anaphylaxis packs with adrenaline (epinephrine) and protocols must be immediately available at the time of vaccine administration.

## Administration of vaccines

- Ensure suitability and no contraindications to individual vaccines.
- Ensure informed consent.
- Ensure the patient or carer is aware of possible adverse reactions and how to treat them.
- Most vaccines given IM except:
  - BCG given intradermally.
  - Green Cross Japanese encephalitis and varicella vaccines given SC.
  - Cholera vaccine given orally.
- Deltoid area of the upper arm or anterolateral aspect of the thigh are the preferred sites for IM and SC immunization.
- A 23-gauge (blue) or 25-gauge (orange) needle is recommended for IM administration of most vaccines.
- If two or more injections are administered at same time, they should be given at separate sites, preferably in different limb.
- Patient should be given a record of vaccination.

- The nursing/medical records should include:
  - The date of administration.
  - Vaccine and product name, batch number, and expiry date.
  - Dose administered and the site(s) used.
  - Name and signature of vaccinator.

## Reference

[1]Department of Health (England) (2006). *Immunisation against infectious disease.* '*The Green Book*', 3rd edn, and its electronically updated chapters for the UK on Gov.UK. Available at: ℜ www.gov.uk/government/organisations/public-health-england/series/immunisation-against-infectious-disease-the-green-book

## Further information

Health Protection Agency Minimum Standards for Immunisation Training (2005). Available at: ℜ http://www.hpa.org.uk/EventsProfessionalTraining/HealthProtectionAcademy/AdditionalOpportunitiesAndInformation/ImmunisationTrainingResources/

Immunization for professionals. Available at: ℜ www.immunization.org.uk

# Targeted adult immunization

Five doses of diphtheria, tetanus, and polio vaccines in childhood ensure long-term protection through adulthood. Those with <5 doses should be offered the rest. Those with unclear history should be offered all 5. Adults at greater risk are offered targeted immunization.

❶ The 'Green Book' (Department of Health, 2006)[1] is essential reading for immunizations.

## Seasonal flu

The vaccine is prepared each year to WHO recommendations on likely virus strains. Immunization in Sept–early Nov gives 70–80% protection and lasts 1yr. Available for a fee in high street pharmacies. NHS provides free immunization for those 'at risk'. General practice identifies patients and invites them to attend. The DN service vaccinates the housebound. It is an enhanced service under non-GMS contract (☐ General practice, p. 13). Annual guidance should be checked, but in general at-risk groups include:
- All patients 65yrs and over.
- Pregnant women (in all trimesters).
- Patients aged 6mths and over in a clinical risk group(s):
  - Chronic lung (including drug treatment for asthma in last 3yrs), heart, diabetes, liver, kidney, or neurological disease.
  - Immunosuppressed, e.g. chemotherapy (consider also household members).
- In addition programmes usually include:
  - Residents of long-stay care facilities.
  - Frontline health and social care workers.
  - Main carer for an older or disabled person.
  - Those in close contact with poultry (for H1N1).

### Dosage
- *Children and adults >13yrs:* single injection 0.5mL.
- *<13yrs:* unless specified otherwise a single injection of 0.5mL, repeated 4–6wks later if receiving influenza vaccine for first time.

## Meningitis C

Recommended for adults at ↑ risk meningococcal disease:
- Adults 18–25yrs if no prior immunization. Single vaccination.
- Those with asplenia or splenic dysfunction. Single vaccination followed by booster dose >2mths.

See ☐ Childhood immunization, p. 156.

## Pneumococcal

Recommended for adults where infection is more common or serious:

- All patients 65yrs and over and clinical risk groups:
  - Asplenia or splenic dysfunction.
  - Chronic respiratory disease, heart, renal, or liver disease, diabetes.
  - Immunosuppression.
  - Individuals with cochlear implants.
  - Individuals with potential for CSF leaks.

Single dose of 23-valent polysaccharide vaccine. Repeated 5-yearly for patients who are asplenic, splenic dysfunction, or chronic renal failure.

## Hepatitis A

Recommended for:

- Patients with severe liver disease of whatever cause.
- Haemophiliacs receiving plasma derived clotting factors. ❶ Need SC injection.
- Men who have sex with men (MSM) injecting drug users.
- Adults at occupational risk.
- Consider for those with chronic hepatitis B or C, or milder liver disease.

Booster dose 6–12mths after initial dose, further booster every 10yrs.

## Hepatitis B

Recommended for:

- Injecting drug users, their sexual partners and children.
- MSM, male and female commercial sex workers.
- Individuals receiving regular blood or blood products, and their carers.
- Chronic liver disease.
- Adopters and fosterers of children from countries ↑ prevalence hepatitis B.
- Chronic renal failure. ❶ Adult require ↑ dose (40 micrograms).
- Inmates of custodial institutions.
- People with learning difficulties in residential accommodation.
- Workers at occupational risk.
- Travellers to ↑ risk areas (▢ Travel vaccinations, p. 356).

Generally immunization schedule is for 3 doses with or without a fourth booster dose. Check BNF/manufacturers instructions for spacing.

Individuals at continued risk should have a single booster at ~5yrs.

## BCG

Recommended for:
- Previously unvaccinated tuberculin −ve contacts of respiratory TB.
- Unvaccinated tuberculin −ve individuals <35yrs in occupational groups likely to have contact with person(s) with TB:
  - Workers in care homes for the elderly.
  - Laboratory workers.
  - Veterinary and abattoir workers.
  - Prison staff.
  - Workers in hostels for homeless, refugees, asylum seekers.

See ⏛ Childhood immunization, p. 156; ⏛ Tuberculosis, p. 680.

## Reference

### Professionals and the public

[1]Department of Health (England) (2006). *Immunisation against infectious disease*. 'The Green Book', and its electronically updated chapters. Available at: ℘ www.gov.uk/government/organisations/public-health-england/series/immunisation-against-infectious-disease-the-green-book

## Further information

Immunization for professionals. Available at: ℘ www.immunization.org.uk
NHS Choices. Vaccinations. Available at: ℘ www.nhs.uk/Planners/vaccinations/Pages/Adultshub.aspx

# Travel health care

Every year UK residents make >50 million journeys aboard. Primary care services provide a key role in travel health. Patients are encouraged to consult their general practice 8wks prior to planned travel.

## Pre-travel assessment

Key elements that are modified in the light of planned travel details (e.g. country, travel mode, stopovers, purpose, length of stay, etc.) are:
- *Assessment of fitness to travel including:*
  - *General health*—most serious illness abroad is due to pre-existing cardiovascular or pulmonary disease, not tropical disease.
  - *Medical history relevant to vaccination*—anti-malarials, contraception/pregnancy, mental health.
- *Requirements for vaccination, based on:*
  - Current vaccination status (☐ Targeted adult immunization, p. 347).
  - Current NHS advice on need for vaccination according to area of travel (☐ Travel vaccinations, p. 356).
- Need for malaria prophylaxis (☐ Malaria prevention, p. 354).
- Need for health promotion advice.

## Travel health care plan

This includes:
- Health promotion advice (☐ Travel health promotion, p. 352).
- Vaccination as required (☐ Travel vaccinations, p. 356).
- Anti-malarial prophylaxis as required (☐ Malaria prevention, p. 354).
- Advice on medicines for people on long-term medication, including:
  - Adequate prescribed medicine to cover trip.
  - Availability in other countries.
  - Restrictions on taking medicines into other countries (see NaTHNaC website[1]).

## Post-travel care

Consider the presence of imported diseases, as well as usual UK health problems, in travellers consulting for up to 1yr (particularly in first 3mths) on return. Assessment should include details of dates, place, animal contact, swimming in inland waters, sexual contact with people, previous vaccinations, and health of others in travel party.
- *Fever in travellers:* suspect imported disease, including malaria as first priority, typhoid, and paratyphoid. Investigations include full blood screen, including thick and thin films for malaria.
- *Diarrhoea in travellers:* suspect imported disease, such as giardisis, amoebic dysentery, and cholera. Investigations include MC&S of fresh stool sample.

## Useful reading
Chiodini J, Boyne L, Stillwell A, Grieve S. (2012). *Travel Health Nursing: Career and Competence Development, RCN guidance.* London: RCN.
Chiodini JH, Anderson E, Driver C, et al. (2012). Recommendations for the practice of travel medicine. *Travel Med Infect Dis* **10**(3): 109–28.

## Reference
[1]National Travel Health Network and Centre (NaTHNaC). Available at: ℘ www.nathnac.org. See website for details of telephone helpline for professionals.

## Further information
NHS Choices. Available at: ℘ Travel health www.nhs.uk/livewell/travelhealth/pages/travelhealth-home.aspx
Office for National Statistics. *Travel Trends* 2010 Edition (published 28 July 2011)

# Travel health promotion

This may form part of a pre-travel assessment or be offered opportunistically during other consultations. The emphasis is on prevention for a wide range of issues tailored according to travel plans, age, type of activity planned on travel, length of stay.

## Key areas

### On the journey

- *DVT prevention advice for any travel involving sitting for long periods:* avoid alcohol, drink ↑ water, foot, and leg exercises.
- Remind women using combined oral contraception (COC; &#x1F4D6; Combined hormonal methods, p. 361) and travelling across time zones to keep track of the hours, not day of the week, for the next pill.

### Out and about

- *Accidents and injuries:* main cause of death in travellers aged <40yrs, often alcohol related.
  - Advise on using same level of preventive measures as in UK, e.g. crash helmets with mopeds, not diving into shallow water.
  - Need for first aid kit.
  - Need for adequate travel health insurance cover.
- *Safe sex:* supply condoms if appropriate (&#x1F4D6; Sexual health: general issues, p. 711).
- *Blood-borne infections:* use of sterile medical kit (obtainable from chemists, outdoor retailers, online travel equipment shops) and avoidance of blood transfusion.
- Sun protection (&#x1F4D6; Skin cancer prevention, p. 331).
- Danger of altitude sickness if travel to altitudes >2500m.
- No-go areas because of risk of violence (contact Foreign Office help line[1]).
- *Avoid insect bites, advise:*
  - The use of insect repellents, cover up, especially between dusk and dawn (see &#x1F4D6; Malaria prevention, p. 354).
  - Travellers to areas at risk of tick-borne encephalitis to wear long trousers tucked into socks and to spray clothes with insect repellant.
- *Avoid animal bites:* rabies occurs in animals in Europe and North America, as well as less-developed countries. Advise not to touch any wild or seemingly tame animals. Wound management is essential after any potential exposure. WHO guidance advises washing wound with soap and running water for 15min, then apply povidone iodine or alcohol to help kill rabies virus and seek medical help immediately (see Travax[2]).

## Food and drink

Traveller's diarrhoea is common, ~50% travellers (📖 Food-borne disease, p. 682).
- *Remind people of basic hygiene:* e.g. hand cleaning after toilet.
- Avoid foods kept warm or likely to be touched by flies.
- *Advise on oral rehydration:* e.g. 1tsp sugar, pinch salt to 250mL boiled or bottled water, or use commercially available preparation
- *Anti-motility medicines:* available OTC in UK for adults and some older children (patient to be advised by pharmacist).
- Antibiotics could be considered for those with serious pre-existing medical conditions.
- In areas with ↑ risk of cholera, typhoid, hepatitis A, advise people to avoid tap water, salads, seafood, and ice cubes, drink bottled or boiled water, peel fruit.

## Travel health insurance
- Required for foreign travel in case of needing access to health services. Always inform company of any pre-existing medical problems.
- In Europe a European Health Insurance Card provides evidence of eligibility for health services under reciprocal EAA agreements. advise to check it is still in date before travel

## References

[1]Foreign and Commonwealth Office Advice to travellers. Passports, travel, and living abroad. Available at: ℘ www.fco.gov.uk/travel
[2]TRAVAX from Health Protection Scotland (password protected). Available at: ℘ http://www.travax.nhs.uk/ See TRAVAX website for details of telephone helpline for professional TRAVAX users.

## Further information

European Health insurance Card. Available at: ℘ www.applyehic.org/
Fit for travel provided by Health Protection Scotland. Available at: ℘ www.fitfortravel.nhs.uk
MASTA Advice and network of travel health clinics. Available at: ℘ http://www.masta-travel-health.com/
NaTHNaC – Medications – transportation by travellers. February 2010. Available at: ℘ http://www.nathnac.org/pro/factsheets/medications.htm
National Travel Health Network and Centre (NaTHNaC). Available at: ℘ www.nathnac.org. See website for details of telephone helpline for professionals
NHS Choices. Available at: ℘ www.nhs.uk. Found in Live Well and also in the Health A–Z sections.

# Malaria prevention

Malaria is a parasitic disease spread by the bites of infected mosquitoes. Over 1500 cases are imported to the UK each year. Over 70% are the potentially fatal *Plasmodium falciparum* strain, in which death can occur, sometimes within 24hrs of developing symptoms of the disease.

## Key principles

Malaria prevention advice centres on four essential principles:
- A-Awareness of risk.
- B-Bite prevention.
- C-Chemoprophylaxis.
- D-Prompt diagnosis and treatment.

Anti-malarial prophylaxis is required according to the area of travel, as per recommendations from an authoritative source. Patients visiting countries with endemic malaria where they have previously lived should be warned that any earlier immunity is likely to be lost, and that children born in this country have no immunity. Travel to malarial areas should be avoided in pregnancy (📖 Antenatal care and screening, p. 380). Breastfed infants require antimalarials.

## Antimalarial medication

Antimalarial medications are <100% effective against malaria, but appropriately chosen, still give very good protection. Choice of antimalarials depends on:
- Presence of chloroquine-resistant malaria in the travel area.
- Patient's medical history.

Commonly recommended antimalarials include: chloroquine, proguanil, mefloquine, doxycycline, proguanil/atovaquone.
- Specific advice on dosages for children are available at the BNF website (📖 Useful websites, p. 800).
- Specialist advice is addressed in the UK Malaria Guidelines for long-term prophylaxis[1].
- Tablets must be taken in accordance with instructions:
  - All are started pre-travel (varying from 1 to 2 days up to 2½ wks before travel, depending on the malaria chemoprophylaxis selected).
  - All are continued on return to UK for 4wks, except atovaquone/proguanil, which is taken for 1wk on return.
  - Anti-malarials are best taken after meals to ↓ side effects.
- Malaria prophylaxis is not prescribed from NHS so requires a private prescription. Some are available OTC.

## Anti-malarial precautions to avoid being bitten

- Cover arms and legs with appropriate clothing from dusk to dawn.
- Use effective anti-mosquito repellent: most effective ones contain DEET (up to 50% content), including children over 2mths of age and pregnant women. Reapply regularly.
- Sleep with windows closed, use a permethrin-impregnated mosquito net, spray room with knockdown spray, burn a mosquito coil overnight, air conditioning is an effective deterrent. Note: electronic buzzers are not effective.

## Reference

[1]Chiodini P. (2007). Guidelines for malaria prevention in travellers from the UK. London, Health Protection Agency, January 2007. Available at: ℘ www.malaria-reference.co.uk

## Further information

Health Protection Agency. Available at: ℘ www.hpa.org.uk and www.malaria-reference.co.uk for specific advice via the fax helpline

National Travel Health Network and Centre (NaTHNaC). See website for details of telephone helpline for professionals and country specific information. Available at: ℘ http://www.nathnac. org/ds/map_world.aspx

Health Protection Report (2011). Malaria imported into the United Kingdom in 2010: implications for those advising travellers. *Hlth Protect Rep* **5**(17). Available at: ℘ www.hpa.org.uk/hpr/ archives/2011/hpr1711.pdf

# Travel vaccinations

All travellers should be up to date with routinely recommended vaccinations according to the national schedule (⌨ Childhood immunization, p. 156).

## Children

Routine child immunization given earlier if travelling to high-risk areas if for prolonged stay or travel is likely to delay the routine programme.

## Live vaccines

Special considerations for pregnant women, people with a suppressed immune response, people treated with chemotherapy or radiotherapy (see Department of Health 2006). If two live vaccines are required they should be given simultaneously at different sites or 4wks apart.

## Immunization advice by country

❶ Authoritative up-to-date information on requirements for area and countries of travel should be consulted.

Table 8.3 lists vaccine information against each disease.

## Prescribing and administration of vaccines

Prescribing and administration of vaccine should follow legal and good practice guidelines, as well as relevant protective procedures against blood-borne viruses and sharps injuries (⌨ Sharps injuries, p. 107). Only travel vaccines available under the NHS can be administered under patient group direction in NHS setting. Vaccines administered privately in NHS GP setting must be administered under a patient specific direction, or by prescription prior to administration (⌨ Prescribing, p. 130).

## Payment and availability of vaccines

Travel vaccination can be supplied at commercial travel clinics and in general practice (see Table 8.3). Protection against the diseases cholera, hepatitis A, polio, and typhoid (and any combination vaccine containing any of these diseases) is free of charge to NHS patients in an NHS GP surgery. Other vaccines can be charged for privately. Yellow fever vaccination and the international certificate of vaccination or prophylaxis (required for entry to some countries) are available only at designated centres (see NaTHNaC[1] and TRAVAX[2] for more details).

# References

[1]NaTHNaC National Travel Health Network and Centre. Available at: ℘ www.nathnac.org/index. htm. Advice line for professionals ☎ 020 7380 9234

[2]Travax is a NHS UK-wide resource. Available at: ℘ www.travax.scot.nhs.uk

# Further information

Department of Health. *Immunisation against infectious disease* (3rd Edition) London: TSO, 2006. Available at: ℘ http://immunisation.dh.gov.uk/category/the-green-book/ ❶ Use online resource only.

Field VF, Ford L, Hill DR. (eds) (2010). *Health Information for Overseas Travel*. London: National Travel Health Network and Centre. Available at: ℘ www.nathnac.org/yellow_book/YBmainpage. htm

For professionals. Available at: ℘ http://immunisation.dh.gov.uk/ and www.medicines.org.uk for the Summary of Product Characteristics of travel vaccines and malaria chemoprophylaxis

For vaccinations for the public. Available at: ℘ http://www.nhs.uk/Planners/vaccinations/Pages/Aboutvaccinationhub.aspx

**Table 8.3** Travel vaccination

| Disease | Vaccination schedule | Comments |
|---|---|---|
| Cholera | Oral; 2 doses separated by 1wk; complete 1wk before travel | May be advised for humanitarian aid workers and travellers with remote itineraries in areas of cholera outbreaks |
| Typhoid | IM: single dose; or oral: 3 doses | Reinforcing dose of IM typhoid vaccine at 3 years if at continued risk. Oral vaccine requires annual booster of 3 doses. Not all recipients of typhoid vaccine will be protected—(see Department of Health 2006) |
| Hepatitis A | IM; 2 doses; interval 6–12mths | Can be given in combination with typhoid vaccine or hepatitis B vaccine |
| Hepatitis B | IM; 3 doses; interval 0, 1, 6mths (4 doses if using accelerated schedule) | Accelerated regimens can be used if time is short (see Department of Health 2006). Booster 5yrs if continued risk |
| Tetanus, diphtheria, polio | 5-dose course usually given in national schedule | Boosters at 10yrs if travelling ↑ risk area |
| Meningitis ACW$_{135}$Y | IM; single dose | Required for those making pilgrimage to Hajj and Umrah, Saudi Arabia |
| Rabies | IM; 3 doses 0,7, and 28, or 21 days if less time | Booster not advised if at intermittent risk (see Travax) |
| Japanese B encephalitis | IM; 2 doses 0 and 28 days with booster at 12–24 or at 12mths if at continuous risk<br><br>Currently no data on further booster doses | Licensed vaccine available for adults, Unlicensed vaccine only available for children (see Department of Health 2006) |
| Yellow fever | Deep SC, single dose | Protection lasts 10yrs. ❶ As per all live vaccines. Caution in use in those over 60yrs (Department of Health 2006) |
| Tick-borne encephalitis | IM, 3 doses, intervals 0, 1–3, and 5–12mths | Booster every 3yrs if at continued risk |

❶ Always seek current advice on recommendations, e.g. NaTHNaC (www.nathnac.org) or TRAVAX (www.travax.nhs.uk – password protected)

# Contraception: general

Fertility control is important for the health of ♀, families, and societies. Contraceptive services are available in NHS clinics, some sexual health clinics, young people's clinics, general practice, and not-for-profit organizations, e.g. Marie Stopes and Brook Advisory Service (under 25yrs). Contraception is free if provided in NHS clinics, prescribed in general practices, or commissioned by a PCO. Barrier methods, and fertility monitoring and the emergency contraceptive, Levonelle®, can be bought OTC.

## Choice of method

Informed by:

- Patient preference and accurate knowledge of methods, effectiveness (see Table 8.4), benefits, and risks.
- Patient age, medical history, immediate family medical history, gynaecological history.
- Past contraceptive history and experience.

## All consultations are an opportunity for health promotion

Includes:

- 📖 Smoking cessation, p. 315.
- 📖 Weight management, p. 307.
- 📖 Exercise, p. 313.
- 📖 Breast cancer awareness, p. 335; self-examination, and mammography programme for >50yrs
- 📖 Cervical cancer screening, p. 337.
- Safer sex practices, STI assessment, and screening.
- 📖 Pre-conceptual care, p. 376.
- 📖 Menopausal symptom management (📖 Menopause, p. 323) and 📖 Osteoporosis, p. 558 prevention.
- 📖 Emergency contraception, p. 374 provision.

## Under 16s and contraception

### Sexual and reproductive health advice and treatment

Fraser Guidelines (a House of Lords ruling) should be applied when assessing anyone under the age of 16yrs. This states that a health professional is able to provide contraception, sexual and reproductive health advice and treatment, without parental knowledge or consent provided:

- The young person understands health professional's advice.
- The health professional cannot persuade the young person to inform his or her parents or allow health professional doctor to inform parents that s/he is seeking contraceptive advice.
- The young person is very likely to begin or continue having intercourse with or without contraceptive treatment.
- Unless he or she receives contraceptive advice or treatment, the young person's physical or mental health or both are likely to suffer.
- The young person's best interests require health professional to give contraceptive advice, treatment, or both without parental consent.

See also 📖 Consent, p. 77; 📖 Confidentiality, p. 86.

## Menopausal women and contraception

- ♀ <50yrs contraception required 2yrs after last period.
- ♀ >50yrs contraception required 1yr after last period.

**Table 8.4** Effectiveness of all contraceptive methods

| Method | Effectiveness |
|---|---|
| Male condom | 98%* |
| Female condom | 95%* |
| Diaphragm, cervical cap, and spermicide | 92–96%* |
| Fertility awareness methods | 98%* |
| Combined hormone contraception: oral, patch, or ring | >99%* |
| Progestogen-only pill (POP) | 99%* |
| Progestogen subdermal implant | >99% |
| Progestogen injection | >99% |
| IUS | 99% |
| IUD | >99% |
| Sterilization: male and female | >99% |

* If used according to instructions.

## Key reference texts

Clinical Effectiveness Unit (2009) United Kingdom Medical Eligibility Criteria For Contraceptive Use. Faculty of Sexual and Reproductive Health care. Available at: ℜ http://www.fsrh.org/pages/Clinical_Guidance_1.asp

Faculty of Sexual and Reproductive Health care. Clinical Effectiveness Guidance Publications. Available at: ℜ http://www.fsrh.org/pages/clinical_guidance.asp

Guillebaud J. (2009). *Contraception: Your Questions Answered*, 5th edn. Philadelphia: Churchill Livingstone.

## Further information

Family Planning Association UK Helpline ☎ 0845 122 8690; FPA Northern Ireland ☎ 0845 122 8687. Available at: ℜ www.fpa.org.uk

Brook Advisory Centre's for under 25yrs. Available at: ℜ www.askbrook.org.uk ☎ 0808 802 1234 or text – Ask Brook on 07717989023

# Combined hormonal methods

## Combined oral contraceptive pill

COC is an oral drug containing synthetic oestrogen and progestogen. It prevents pregnancy by suppressing ovulation, thickening cervical mucus, thinning endometrium. 1 pill x 21 days at same time each day then 7 days pill free (unless everyday preparation). 24hr window to take the next pill before efficacy ↓. See Box 8.2 for absolute contraindications

### Advantages

↓ bleeding, ↓ dysmenorrhoea, ↓ pre-menstrual symptoms, protects against uterine and ovarian cancer, ↓ ovarian cysts, ↓ PID.

### Risks in taking COC

Venous and arterial thrombosis (resulting in MI, CVA, PE, DVT), breast cancer—risk returns to normal within 10yrs.

---

**Box 8.2  Absolute contraindications for taking COC**

- Smokers >35yrs.
- BMI >35kg/m$^2$.
- Unexplained vaginal bleeding.
- Focal migraines.
- Pregnancy, breastfeeding.
- First-degree relative with arterial or venous disease diagnosed <45yrs.
- Oestrogen-dependent neoplasm.
- Active liver disease, heart disease, lipid disorders, conditions affected by sex steroids.
- Past venous thrombolytic embolism (VTE), arterial thrombosis, CVA, TIA.
- 4wks before and 2wks after major or leg surgery.

---

### Conditions that are relative contraindications

Sickle cell disease, severe depression, systemic lupus erythematosus (SLE), Crohn's, splenectomy, diseases with high-density lipoprotein (HDL), DM, diseases with drug treatments that interact, e.g. epilepsy, TB, BMI >30kg/m$^2$.

### Choice of COC

- First choice COC is low in progestogen and low in oestrogen, 2nd-generation pill (e.g. Levest®, Microgynon 30®).
- COC with gestodene and desogestrel (e.g. Femodene®, Femodene ED®, Femodette®, Marvelon®, Mercilon®, Minulet®, Triadene®, and Tri-Minulet®), known as '3rd-generation' pills associated with a slight ↑ VTE risk than 2nd-generation pills.

*Starting routines*

For immediate efficacy (otherwise additional contraception required for 7 days) are one of the following:

- Day 1 menstruation.
- Day 21 post-partum and not lactating.
- Same day as miscarriage/termination of pregnancy (TOP).
- Instant switch to higher dose COC.
- Switch to lower dose COC after 7-day break.
- Day 1 of menstruation in a switch to POP.

*Advice on starting COC*

- Seek medical attention if chest pain, pain and swelling in calf, shortness of breath, ↑ headaches, or with speech or visual disturbances, jaundice, severe stomach pain, BP >160mmHg systolic, 100mmHg diastolic.
- Situations of ↓ effectiveness. Additional contraception, e.g. condoms required if:
  - Severe vomiting and/or diarrhoea >24hrs.
  - Taking interacting drugs, e.g. enzyme-inducing drugs, such as anticonvulsants, antitubercule, St John's wort herbal preparation. Need to change to another method of contraception whilst taking them and for 4wks after stopping enzyme-inducing drugs.
- Missed pill rules (see 📖 Contraception: missed combined oral contraceptive rules, p. 364).
- How to obtain emergency contraception (EC) if required.
- Follow-up 3mths after starting or changing COC (earlier if problems) and then 6mths (or 1yr according to local protocols).

At each consultation review/check the following:
- Age, BP, weight and BMI, smoking habits, change in health or family health status.
- Any minor side effects.
- Date and any problems with last menstrual period.
- Problems with missed pills or missed pill rules.
- Any questions or concerns.
- Medications and allergies.

*Minor short-term side effects*

- *Breakthrough bleeding:* not unusual in first months, but check pill routine/missed pills/diarrhoea and vomiting/drug interactions/disease of cervix, screen for STIs. If persistent may need higher dose pill.
- *Nausea, bloating, weight gain, breast tenderness, loss of libido, depression:* may need change of pill.

## Contraceptive patch

A transdermal patch, releasing oestrogen and progestogen, stuck on skin for 7 days x3 then patch-free 7 days. As for COC for advantages, risks, contraindications, starting regimens, follow-up and minor short-term effects. If patch falls off:

• <24hrs apply new patch immediately, no additional contraception needed.
• >24hrs apply new patch immediately, then use condoms for next 7 days.
• >48hrs after usual start day, apply new patch immediately, then use condoms for next 7 days.

## NuvaRing®

The vaginal ring, releases oestrogen and progestogen, and stays *in situ* for 3wks then ring-free 7 days. As for COC for advantages, risks, contraindications, starting regimens, follow-up, and minor short-term effects. If ring falls out:

• <3hrs rinse ring with cool water and re-insert, no additional contraception needed.
• >3hrs rinse ring with cool water and re-insert, then use additional methods for next 7 days.
• If out>3hrs in 3rd wk then either insert a new ring and begin next 3wk cycle or wait for period and insert new ring no later than 7 days from when last ring slipped out. See further information, 📖 Contraception: general, p. 359.

## Key reference texts

Faculty of Sexual and Reproductive Health care. Clinical Effectiveness Guidance Publications. Available at: ✍ http://www.fsrh.org/pages/clinical_guidance.asp

Guillebaud J. (2009). Contraception: Your Questions Answered, 5th edn. Philadelphia: Churchill Livingstone.

## Further information

Family Planning Association UK Helpline ☎ 0845 122 8690; FPA Northern Ireland ☎ 0845 122 8687. Available at: ✍ http://www.fpa.org.uk/

Brook Advisory Centre's for under 25yrs. Available at: ✍ http://www.askbrook.org.uk/ ☎ 0808 802 1234 or text – Ask Brook on 07717989023

# Contraception: missed combined oral contraceptive rules

The basic principles (see Fig. 8.4) are:
- Whenever a woman realizes she has missed COC pills she should take a pill as soon as possible, then resume her usual pill-taking schedule.
- Also, if missed COC pills are in week 3, she should omit pill-free interval.
- Also, a back-up method (usually condoms) or abstinence should be used for 7 days if two or more pills are missed:

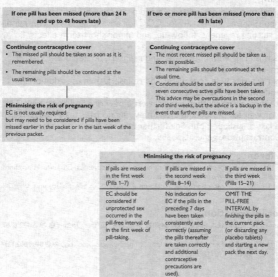

**MISSED COMBINED ORAL CONTRACEPTIVE PILLS (COCs): CEU ADVICE FOR HEALTH PROFESSIONALS**

| If one pill has been missed (more than 24 h and up to 48 hours late) | If two or more pill has been missed (more than 48 h late) |
|---|---|
| **Continuing contraceptive cover**<br>• The missed pill should be taken as soon as it is remembered.<br>• The remaining pills should be continued at the usual time. | **Continuing contraceptive cover**<br>• The most recent missed pill should be taken as soon as possible.<br>• The remaining pills should be continued at the usual time.<br>• Condoms should be used or sex avoided until seven consecutive active pills have been taken. This advice may be overcautious in the second and third weeks, but the advice is a backup in the event that further pills are missed. |
| **Minimising the risk of pregnancy**<br>EC is not usually required<br>but may need to be considered if pills have been missed earlier in the packet or in the last week of the previous packet. | |

| Minimising the risk of pregnancy | | |
|---|---|---|
| If pills are missed in the first week (Pills 1–7) | If pills are missed in the second week (Pills 8–14) | If pills are missed in the third week (Pills 15–21) |
| EC should be considered if unprotected sex occurred in the pill-free interval of in the first week of pill-taking. | No indication for EC if the pills in the preceding 7 days have been taken consistently and correctly (assuming the pills thereafter are taken correctly and additional contraceptive precautions are used). | OMIT THE PILL-FREE INTERVAL by finishing the pills in the current pack (or discarding any placebo tablets) and starting a new pack the next day. |

**Fig. 8.4** Missed combined oral contraceptive pills (COCS): CEU advice for health professionals.

Faculty of Sexual & Reproductive Healthcare 'CEU Statement (May 2011) Missed Pill Recommendations'. London. Reproduced with kind permission of the Faculty for Sexual and Reproductive Health.

## Key references

Faculty of Sexual and Reproductive Healthcare Clinical guidelines. Available at: ℘ www.fsrhc. org.uk

BNF section 7.3.1. Available at: ℘ www.bnf.org/bnf/

## Further information

FPA UK Helpline ☎ 0845 122 8690; FPA Northern Ireland ☎ 0845 122 8687. Available at: ℘ www. fpa.org.uk

# Progestogen-only methods

## Progestogen-only pill (also known as mini-pill)

POP is an oral method. Prevents pregnancy by thickening cervical mucus, in some cycles suppresses ovulation, makes endometrium unreceptive and ↓ fallopian tube function. Efficacy: see ▢ Contraception: general, p. 359.

### Advantages

Alternative to COC when oestrogens are contraindicated (▢ Combined hormonal methods, p. 361), e.g. ♀ >35yrs and smokes, focal migraines, breastfeeding. It may ↓ dysmenorrhoea and pre-menstrual symptoms. It can continue to be taken prior to surgery.

### Initial consultation

Opportunity for health promotion topics (▢ Contraception: general, p. 359), discussion of POP method, benefits, and side effects —particularly alteration of menstrual pattern.

*Risks* ↑ Ovarian cysts; if became pregnant ↑ risk of ectopic, small ↑ risk breast cancer, but returns to normal within 10yrs.

### Contraindications to POP

Pregnancy, previous ectopic pregnancy, past or present severe arterial disease, severe lipid abnormalities, liver disease or liver cancer, recent trophoblastic disease, concurrent enzyme-inducing drugs, e.g. anti-epileptics (▢ Seizures and epilepsy, p. 693).

### Choice of POP

Cerazette®, as this inhibits ovulation and has greater ↑ effficacy than other POPs; also has larger window to take the pill—12h compared with 3h with other POPs.

### Starting POP

- *Day 1 of menstruation:* offers immediate protection. Additional contraceptive measures if started day 2 for 2 days.
- *Changing from a COC:* immediate protection if POP from day 21 of COC pill, i.e. omitting the 7-day break.
- Post-partum to start on day 21 otherwise additional contraceptive measures for the first 2 days.

### Taking the pill

Daily pill with no pill-free breaks, taken at the same time each day within 12h for Cerazette® and 3h for all other POP's. ♀ >70kg should be prescribed Cerazette® or 2 pills/day for all other POPs (unlicensed use see ▢ Prescribing, p. 130).

*Missed pills*

If a pill is later than 12h for Cerazette® and later than 3h for all other POPs continue taking POP at usual time and use additional precautions for 2 days. Ensure ♀ knows about EC (📖 Emergency contraception, p. 374).

- *Severe diarrhoea or vomiting within 2h of taking pill:* continue taking POP, but assume pills 'missed' and additional precautions for 2 days.
- *Enzyme-inducing drugs:* such as rifampicin and griseofulvin reduce efficacy need to use additional precautions or different method required whilst taking these and for 4wks after stopping them.

*Review*

3mths after starting POP, earlier if problems, then 6mthly (or yearly according to local protocols). Check age, BP, weight, change in health or family health status, minor side effects, any problems with menstruation or missed pills, any questions.

*Side effects*

- *Menstrual irregularities:* duration, volume, and flow may alter. ♀ may experience inter-menstrual episodes, may experience amenorrhoea. This is the commonest reason for stopping method. STIs need to be excluded, and pregnancy test if amenorrhoea. Consider changing type of progestogen i.e. to a different POP.
- *Others:* breast discomfort, bloatedness, depression, weight changes, nausea, skin problems (e.g. acne or chloasma), changes in libido. Consider changing progestogen, i.e. to a different POP.

# Progestogen injectables

Progestogen injectables have a main preventative action through suppression of ovulation. Efficacy see 📖 Contraception: general, p. 359.

*Advantages* As for POP, lasts 8–12wks.

*Disadvantages*

Irregular bleeding, amenorrhoea, fertility may take up to 1yr to return, may ↑ weight, may ↓ mood, cannot be withdrawn. Long-term use has a possible link ↓ oestrogen levels and requires medical reassessment and review of risk factors for osteoporosis after 2yrs use.

*Contraindications:* as POP.

*Initial consultation:* as POP.

*Preparations*

- *Depo-Provera® (DMPA):* 150mg IM injection lasts 12wks. Licensed for long-term use.
- *Noristerat® (NET-EN):* 200mg IM lasts 8wks. For short-term use only.

Contraceptive effect immediate if 1st injection is given:
- Within 5 days of onset of menstruation.
- <5 days post-partum if not breastfeeding or 6wks if breastfeeding.
- 1–5 days after miscarriage or TOP.

Otherwise advise ♀ to use additional contraception for 7 days after the 1st injection.

*Repeat injections*

Effective immediately if given <12wks + 5 days after previous injection (<8wks for Noristerat®) If not, exclude pregnancy before repeat injection and use additional contraception for 7d. Consider EC >14wks and 1 day (DMPA), >10wks and 1 day (NET-EN) (📖 Emergency contraception, p. 374).

## Progestogen subdermal implants (e.g. Nexplanon®)

Small (40mm), thin rod inserted and removed by specially trained doctor or nurse into upper arm. Lasts for 3yrs with no check-ups required.

*Action* As for injectables. Contraindications and side effects as POP above. Effect rapidly reversible.

## Further information

Faculty of Sexual and Reproductive Health care (2008). Clinical Effectiveness Unit. Progestogen only injectables. Available at: 🔗 http://www.fsrh.org/pages/Clinical_Guidance_4.asp

Faculty of Sexual and Reproductive Health care (2012). Clinical Effectiveness Unit. Drug Interactions with Hormonal Contraception. Available at: 🔗 www.fsrh.org.uk

# Intrauterine devices and systems

### Intrauterine devices

IUDs are inserted via the cervical canal into the uterus. It is a small plastic device often incorporating copper, with threads hanging into vagina and tucked around the cervix. IUDs prevents pregnancy by impeding sperm transport, altering gametes, and blocking fertilization.

*Disadvantages* Heavier and more painful periods, ↑ risk of ectopic if pregnant, ↑ risk of pelvic inflammatory disease, rare risk of perforation of the uterus during insertion, risk of expulsion.

*Advantages* Effective immediately (☐ Contraception: general, p. 359), not reliant on user for efficacy, safe. Easily removable.

### Contraindications

Previous ectopic pregnancy, abnormalities of uterus, allergy to copper, at risk of STI, e.g. multiple partners or short-term partners. History of fibroids and endometriosis, dysmenorrhoea, menorrhagia need careful individual assessment.

### Pre-insertion

- Health promotion (☐ Contraception: general, p. 359).
- Counsel on advantages/disadvantages particularly menstrual impact.
- STI screening (☐ Sexually-transmitted infections, p. 715).
- Ensure effective method of contraception until insertion or abstinence from day 1 of period in that cycle. If changing IUD, no sex for 7 days before in case new IUD cannot be inserted and sperm survive.
- Information about insertion procedure, and likelihood of cramping pains that day.

### Insertion

- Performed by specially trained doctors and nurses.
- Optimum time for insertion:
  - End of main menstrual flow to days 14–28 of cycle.
  - 4–6wks post-partum (6–8wks post-Caesarean section).
- Mefenamic acid 500mg orally pre-insertion ↓ pain post-insertion.

Emergency equipment should be available in case of vasovagal attack or anaphylaxis (☐ Anaphylaxis, p. 751). Insertions usually performed with two professionals for reassurance and in case of emergency.

### Post-insertion

- ♀ encouraged to rest, then get up slowly.
- Use sanitary towels not tampons until next period.
- Advised on feeling threads monthly and to return if cannot.
- Abstain from sex for 3 days or use condoms as insertion interferes with protective mechanism of cervix.
- Advised to seek medical attention if pelvic pain and/or vaginal discharge.
- Give patient a record of date of insertion and type of IUD.

*Review and follow-up*
- Review 4–6wks post-insertion. Ask about periods, pelvic pain, vaginal discharge, discomfort to partner, frequency of thread checks. Threads should be checked visually (through speculum) also felt, as well as cervix moved gently side-to-side to detect partial expulsion of device.
- Subsequent reviews according to local protocols. Many now state only required if woman has a problem or cannot feel threads.

*Life span of IUDs*
- Check BNF 7.3.4 by brand. Modern copper devices, e.g. T-safe® Cu 380 A is effective for 10yrs: older types for 3–5yrs.
- ♀≥40yrs: most IUDs effective until the menopause.

*Removal*
- Any time if considering pregnancy.
- 7 days after alternative method of contraception established.
- 1yr after menopause (📖 Contraception: general, p. 359).

*Actinomycete-like organisms (ALOs)*
See 📖 Cervical cancer screening, p. 337.

## Intrauterine systems (IUSs)

IUSs have a slow-release progestogen (levonorgestorol) reservoir around the vertical stem. Mirena® is the only IUS in UK and licensed for 5yrs use.

*Advantages*
As IUDs plus:
- ↓ heavy periods.
- ↓ dysmenorrhoea.
- Protects against ectopic pregnancy.
- Suitable for women with history of PID.

*Disadvantages*
- Associated with irregular bleeding, may be constant spotting over first few months, although this settles down.
- Amenorrhoea after first few months.
- More expensive than IUDs, so it is important ♀ fully understands disadvantages.
- Expulsion and possible increased risk of ectopic pregnancy.

*Pre-insertion, insertion, post-insertion, and removal* As IUDs.

## Key reference texts

Faculty of Family Planning and Reproductive Health (2004) *Copper IUD and IUS systems*. Available at: 🖰 www.ffprhc.org.uk
NICE (2005). *Long Acting Reversible Contraception Clinical Guidelines*. Available at: 🖰 www.nice.nhs.uk

## Further information

FPA UK Helpline: ☎ 0845 122 8690; FPA Northern Ireland: ☎ 0845 122 8687. Available at: 🖰 www.fpa.org.uk

# Barrier contraceptive methods

## Male condoms

A male condom is a single-use latex sheath. It is applied to the erect penis before contact with vulva. The closed end is squeezed to expel air before unrolling down the length of the penis. After ejaculation the penis is removed, holding condom firmly in place. Efficacy, see 📖 Contraception: general, p. 359.

*Advantages* Protection against STIs, no systemic effects, easily available OTC.

*Disadvantages* Perceived as an interruption to sex, loss of sensitivity. Plain-ended and thin condoms ↑ sensitivity.

*Contraindications* Erectile problems.

*Allergy problems* Hypoallergenic brands available if allergic to latex. ❶ Should only be used with water-based lubricants, e.g. KY jelly®. Oil-based products, e.g. baby oil, Vaseline®, damage latex and ↓ effectiveness.

## Female condoms

A female condom is a lubricated polyurethane tube with inner and outer ring, inserted into vagina. Inner ring aids insertion. Outer ring at open end, sits flat against vulva. Femidom® is the only female condom licensed in UK.

*Advantages* As for male condom. It can be used with oil-based products.

*Disadvantages* Can be perceived as noisy during sex.

## Vaginal diaphragms and caps

A diaphragm is a latex rubber dome used with spermicide and inserted into vagina to cover the cervix (see Fig. 8.5).

*Advantages* Non-systemic, can be used during menstruation.

*Disadvantages* Requires motivation, may be perceived as messy.

*Contraindications* Poor vaginal tone or prolapse, allergy to rubber or spermicide, recurrent UTI, past history of toxic shock syndrome.

*Type of diaphragm* Flat spring type is suitable for ♀ with anterior or mid-plane cervix. Coiled spring type is suitable for those who find flat spring uncomfortable. Arcing spring type is suitable for ♀ with posterior cervix.

### Fitting

Must be performed by a doctor or nurse trained to fit diaphragms. The woman then practises in the clinic room:
• Insertion (see Fig. 8.5).
• Checking the diaphragm covers cervix.
• Removal.

Then ♀ has a trial period for >1wk in which she uses the diaphragm while using another form of contraception. Any problems of insertion, fit, removal, and comfort are addressed at a follow-up appointment, and size and fit checked before prescribing the diaphragm for contraceptive use.

*Advice on correct use*
- Diaphragm used with 2-cm strips of spermicide on both sides. Spermicide effective for 3hrs. If intercourse takes place ≥3hrs later, more spermicide is needed.
- Insert diaphragm before intercourse and leave in place ≥6hrs afterwards but no longer than 24–48hrs, depending on the brand.
- ❶ Caps can be damaged by some oil-based products, e.g. Vaseline®, baby oil, and vaginal medications, e.g. Nystan® cream (full list in leaflet in box).
- After use, wash diaphragm in warm soapy water, dry, and store in box.

*Follow-up*
Fit and comfort checked after ~1wk. Advice on use and care discussed. Advised to return for check of fit if problems, or weight changes by 5kg or more, or after pregnancy. New diaphragm prescribed annually, or if develops hole, or after treatment of a vaginal infection.

## Spermicides
Used in combination with barrier methods and are not protective on their own (see BNF 7.3.3).

*Different forms* Cream—Gygel®.

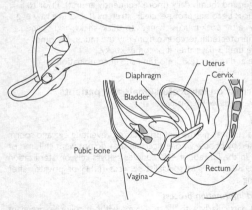

**Fig. 8.5** Inserting a diaphragm.
Reproduced from Szarewski A, Guillebaud J. (2000). *Contraception.* Oxford: OUP. By permission of Oxford University Press.

## Key reference texts
Faculty of Sexual and Reproductive Healthcare. Clinical Effectiveness Guidance Publications. Available at: ℛ www.ffprhc.org.uk/
Guillebaud, J. (2009). *Contraception: Your Questions Answered,* 5th edn. Philadelphia: Churchill Livingstone.

## Further information
FPA UK Helpline: ☎ 0845 122 8690; FPA Northern Ireland: ☎ 0845 122 8687. Available at: ℛ www.fpa.org.uk

# Natural family planning and sterilization

Natural family planning involves fertility awareness through observation of changes that indicates ovulation (usually between 12–16 days before menstruation). From this information the couple will either decide to abstain or use additional contraception (or have sex for a pregnancy).

## Methods of estimating ovulation

- A hand-held computerized system for testing early morning urine for hormone changes. Commercial system (Persona®) available to buy plus additional urine dip sticks. Not suitable if menstrual cycle <23 or >35 days, or menopausal, or breastfeeding, or has kidney or liver disease, or using hormonal treatment.
- *Temperature:* taken orally in morning prior to drinking or getting up (ovulation thermometer available on FP10). Charted from 1st day of period. An ↑ of 0.2–0.4°C indicates progesterone release from corpus luteum. Once temperature has ↑ and been maintained for 3 days then intercourse can be unprotected until next period.
- *Mucus texture (Billing's method):* texture of vaginal secretions is felt between finger and thumb daily (more frequently at first). Prior to ovulation mucus becomes profuse, clear, stretchy (looks like raw egg white). 4 days after peak mucus changes to thick, sticky, and opaque. Advise no unprotected intercourse from day the mucus becomes more profuse until 3 days after it becomes sticky.
- Temperature and mucus texture often used in combination as a double check method.

## Further information for professionals and patients

Fertility UK. Available at: ♪ www.fertilityuk.org/

## Sterilization

Sterilization is a surgical, permanent procedure preventing egg and sperm meeting. It is used by people who are certain they do not want children or more children. In the UK about 45% couples >40yrs rely on sterilization of one partner. Referral is to specialist services (NHS or private) after initial counselling.

### Counselling and information process

Very important particularly with those <25yrs, without children, pregnant women, those in reaction to a loss of relationship, or those who may be at risk of coercion by their partner or others. Prior sanction by a high court judge sought in all cases where there is doubt over an individual's mental capacity to consent (📖 Mental capacity, p. 424). Key information should include:

Alternative long-term contraceptive methods:
- Sterilization should be thought of as permanent, reversal is <50% successful.
- Post-procedure pregnancy rate: 1:200 ♀ (plus ↑ ectopic risk); 1:2000 ♂.
- *Procedures:*
  - ♀—laparoscopic tubal occlusion with clips or rings. Usually done under general anaesthetic (GA) as a day case.
  - ♂: vasectomy, usually done under local anaesthetic as a day case.
- Risk of operative complications.
- *Need for contraception before and after operation:*
  - ♀ other contraception until 1st post-procedure menstruation.
  - ♂ other contraception until two consecutive, but 2–4wks apart semen analyses (>8wks post-vasectomy) shows sperm free.

**Key reference text**

Guillebaud J. (2009). *Contraception: Your Questions Answered*, 5th edn. Philadelphia: Churchill Livingstone.

**Further information**

FPA UK Helpline: ☎ 0845 122 8690; FPA Northern Ireland: ☎ 0845 122 8687. Available at: 🖰 www.fpa.org.uk

# Emergency contraception

Three time-limited forms of EC are available to prevent pregnancy post-unprotected sexual intercourse (UPSI):

- Levonorgestrel tablets.
- Ulipristal acetate tablets.
- Insertion of copper IUD.

Choice depends on time from earliest UPSI in that cycle, and medical, contraceptive, and menstrual history.

## Levonorgestrel (Levonelle®)

May be used <72hrs after UPSI. Given as a single oral dose of 1.5mg. Most effective closest to UPSI in time. Acts to prevent ovulation or blocking implantation of egg. If pregnant ↑ risk of ectopic. If given from 27 to 120hrs after UPSI is as unlicensed use (BNF 7.3.5).

*Contraindications* Porphyria.

*Cautions* Efficacy reduced with liver disease, enzyme-inducing drugs (may need double dose to 3mg—unlicensed use), severe malabsorption syndromes, active trophoblastic disease.

*Side effects* Nausea and vomiting, menstrual irregularities, breast tenderness.

*Advice to ♀*

- Take tablet immediately.
- Not 100% effective and if pregnant may ↑ risk of ectopic.
- If vomit within 2hrs of taking tablet to return for replacement dose.
- Levonorgestrel deals with UPSI in last 72hrs not future: so use a barrier method until next period.
- To seek medical attention if lower abdominal pain.
- To re-consult if period unusual or >5 days late.
- Discuss future contraceptive needs (📖 Contraception general, p. 359):
  - If starting oral hormonal contraception should start on day 1 of normal period or may be quick started and commenced the next day after Levonelle®, with extra precautions for the COC for 7 days or for Qlaira® 9 days, or for the POP 2 days and a pregnancy test should be done in 3wks.
  - *Injectables:* implants, and IUS should commenced with next normal period and advised to have no sexual intercourse from day 1 of cycle prior to starting.
- Advise STI screening in 14 days if appropriate.

## Ulipristal acetate (EllaOne®)

This may be used up to 120h after UPSI. Given as a single oral dose of 30mg (BNF 7.3.5).

*Contraindications* Hepatic impairment, breastfeeding, severe asthma.

*Cautions* EllaOne® reduces the efficacy of combined and progestogen-only methods. Enzyme-inducing drugs the efficacy, advice is to give 3mg of Levonelle® (unlicensed use) or if suitable fit IUD,

*Side effects* Nausea and vomiting, menstrual irregularities, breast tenderness, and headaches.

*Advice to* ♀
- Take tablet immediately.
- Not 100% effective and if pregnant may ↑ risk of ectopic.
- If vomit within 3h of taking tablet to return for replacement dose.
- To seek medical attention if lower abdominal pain.
- To re-consult if period unusual or >5 days late.
- Discuss future contraceptive needs (📖 Contraception general, p. 359).
  - If starting oral hormonal contraception should start on day 1 of normal period or maybe quick started and commenced the next day after EllaOne®, with extra precautions for the COC for 14 days or for Qlaira® 16 days, or for the POP 9 days and a pregnancy test should be done in 3wks.
  - *Injectables*—implants, and IUS should commence with next normal period and advised to have no sexual intercourse from day 1 of cycle prior to starting,
- Advise STI screening in 14 days if appropriate.

## Insertion of copper IUD

Acts as a post-coital method by preventing implantation and may also block fertilization (100% effective). May be inserted up to 5 days after single UPSI or if several UPSI in that cycle up to 5 days after the earliest calculated date of ovulation (usually 12–16 days before next menstrual period).

*Pre-insertion counselling, insertion, post insertion care, and removal* as IUD (📖 Intrauterine devices and systems, p. 368). As the pre-insertion *Chlamydia* results will not be available prophylactic antibiotics are given.

## Rape and sexual assault See 📖 Victims of crime, p. 404.

## Key reference texts

Faculty of Sexual and Reproductive Healthcare (2012) Emergency contraception. Available at: ℘ http://www.fsrh.org/pages/Clinical_Guidance_2.asp

Faculty of Sexual and Reproductive Healthcare (2010) Quick starting contraception. Available at: ℘ http://www.fsrh.org/pdfs/CEUGuidanceQuickStartingContraception.pdf

## Further information

FPA UK Helpline: 📞 0845 122 8690; FPA Northern Ireland: 📞 0845 122 8687. Available at: ℘ www.fpa.org.uk

*Young people advice and information*

Brook Advisory Centre's for under 25yrs. 📞 0808 802 1234 or text – Ask Brook on 07717989023. Available at: ℘ www.askbrook.org.uk

# Pre-conceptual care

Pre-conceptual care and advice can be offered as part of other consultations as well as those for contraception, cervical screening checks, etc. It may be given opportunistically or as part of a planned consultation. The aims are to:

- ↓ problems in pregnancy.
- ↑ chances of conceiving in an optimum state of health.

## Key areas to discuss

### Rubella

Rubella infection in early pregnancy results in a high risk of fetal abnormalities, including deafness and blindness. Rubella status should be checked. If not immune, should be immunized with MMR (exclude pregnancy beforehand) and advised to avoid pregnancy for 1mth.

### Screening

♀ Should be encouraged to ensure any screening is up to date, e.g. cervical cancer screening (📖 Cervical cancer screening, p. 337) or undertaken if at risk, e.g. STI, HIV.

### Genetic screening and counselling

Genetic screening and counselling is aimed at detecting carriers, identifying levels of risk, and then couples having informed choices about pregnancy. Sometimes direct access to services, e.g. some haemoglobinopathy centres or offered through referral from GP to couples who:

- Have personal or family history of genetic abnormality.
- Have had a previous pregnancy, baby with genetic abnormality.
- Have an ethnic background in which high risk of carrier status, e.g.
  - *South East Asia and Southern China*—thalassaemias.
  - *Mediterranean, parts of North and West Africa, Middle East and Indian subcontinent*—thalassaemias and sickling disorders (📖 Sickle cell disorders, p. 292).
  - *Black African and Caribbean*—sickling disorders (📖 Sickle cell disorders, p. 292).
  - *Ashkenazi Jewish*—Tays–Sachs, Gaucher's disease, and cystic fibrosis.

### Diet

- Encourage healthy diet and BMI in normal range (📖 Nutrition and health eating, p. 304) plus:
  - *Folate-rich foods*—e.g. breakfast cereals, leafy green foods; prior to pregnancy and in the first 12wks.
  - *Avoid high levels of vitamin A*—e.g. in liver.
  - *Avoid unpasteurized dairy products*—e.g. brie and camembert cheeses; uncooked eggs, undercooked meat, pâtés, pre-prepared salads to prevent infection (e.g. listeriosis, salmonella) during pregnancy as associated with ↑ risk of stillbirth and miscarriage.

- *Start folic acid supplementation:* OTC or prescribed, which ↓ risk of neural tube defect by 72%.
  - All ♀ should take 0.4mg daily when pregnancy is being planned and for 12wks after conception.
  - ♀ At higher risk of pregnancy with neural tube defect take 5mg daily until 12wks after conception. This group includes women who have had a previous affected pregnancy, one of the couple has a neural tube defect, ♀ has coeliac disease, or takes anti-epilepsy medication, or has sickle cell disease.

## Smoking

Encourage cessation (☐ Smoking cessation, p. 315) in both partners because:
- In ♀ it affects ovulation.
- In ♂ it ↓ the sperm count and sperm motility.
- In pregnancy, smoking increases the miscarriage rate (×2), increases the risk of pre-term delivery, and is associated with a low birth weight.

## Alcohol

Opportunity for brief intervention on reduction of alcohol consumption. Current advice is to avoid alcohol in pregnancy, but if alcohol is taken it should be a maximum of 1U/day. Heavy drinking is associated with increased risk of miscarriage. Fetal alcohol syndrome (brain damage, growth retardation, facial malformations) occurs to ~1/3rd of ♀ drinking >18U/day (see also ☐ Alcohol, p. 319).

***OTC medicines*** Few have been established as safe in pregnancy so avoid use while trying to conceive.

***Toxoplasmosis*** Parasitic infection causing fetal brain damage and blindness. Avoid raw meat, cat faeces, sheep and goat milk.

***Fertility awareness*** Review knowledge of fertile period and optimum days in menstrual cycle to have sex for conception. Ovulation usually 12–16 days before period.

**♀ with pre-existing medical conditions** Should consult their GP for review and advice, particularly on suitability of medication in pregnancy.

**♀ with previous problems in pregnancies** Should consult their GP for review, advice, and possible early referral to specialist.

## Related topic

☐ Antenatal care and screening, p. 380.

## Further information

Family Planning Association. FPA UK Helpline: ☎ 0845 122 8690; FPA Northern Ireland: ☎ 0845 122 8687. Available at: ⬥ www.fpa.org.uk

# Pregnancy

Pregnancy is a continuous process of growth and development from the time of conception to the birth of the baby. The early signs and symptoms include missed period (or very light spotting), sickness and/or nausea, breast tenderness and enlargement, tiredness, frequency of urine, constipation. Urine dipstick pregnancy tests can detect hormone human chorionic gonadotrophin at about 14 days (see instructions on different brands) after conception. OTC pregnancy testing kits are available.

Normal pregnancy varies from 37 to 42wks. The date of the last menstrual period (LMP) is used for calculating the length of a pregnancy, using 280 days as the length of pregnancy, and EDD. Length of gestation (and thus EDD) confirmed with USS, which is accurate to within 3–5 days.

### The first trimester

- During first 12–14wks of pregnancy, baby develops from an early embryo into fetus with all organs and systems in place. Placental circulation also becomes established.
- If a woman is going to experience a miscarriage, it is more likely to happen in first trimester, most likely due to developmental problems with either fetus or placenta, or genetic defects.
- Antenatal screening for fetal abnormality takes place towards end of first trimester.

### The second trimester

- From 14–30wks, mother experiences a growing sense of wellbeing as early symptoms, like nausea, diminish.
- Baby continues to grow and develop with nervous system maturing progressively so fetal movements become more pronounced.
- He/she is also able to experience sensations like warmth and can taste amniotic fluid swallowed. Some even develop hiccups from time to time. A baby born late in this trimester would be unable to sustain independent life, and would require respiratory *and* nutritional support.

### The third trimester

- From 30wks to birth is a time of continued growth and maturation.
- Baby doubles in weight between 34 and 40wks. Every week spent in mother's uterus is significant in respect of maturity of respiratory and digestive system.
- Baby also develops a layer of SC fat, which helps to protect it from hypothermia and hypoglycaemia in neonatal period, so it is essential that mother maintains adequate healthy diet throughout pregnancy.

### Further information

Midirs Informed Choice Information Leaflets for professionals and expectant parents. Available at: ℘ www.infochoice.org/

National Childbirth Trust. ☏ Pregnancy and Birth Line 0300 330 0772. Available at: ℘ www.nct. org.com

NHS Choices pregnancy and baby. Available at: ℘ www.nhs.uk/conditions/pregnancy-and-baby/pages/pregnancy-and-baby-care.aspx

# Antenatal education and preparation for parenthood

Antenatal education can take place during any encounter a pregnant woman may have with a health professional, e.g. during antenatal visits to a midwife.

## Parent education classes

Women are also invited to locally held, free NHS parent education classes. Some localities offer a range of different preparation to suit local needs for instance, Aquanatal classes that take place in a swimming pool under the direction of a midwife or other specially trained instructor. In many areas, HVs work with midwives to provide community antenatal classes. Other organizations, e.g. NCT, also offer parent education, but will charge a fee for attendance at their classes.

## Aims of classes

The aim of antenatal education is to build confidence to enable parents to take control over their labour and the birth of their child. Antenatal classes provide a place to discuss fears and worries, and exchange views with other parents-to-be. Parents attending classes find meeting new friends who will be going through the same experiences beneficial, particularly if first-time parents. The needs of parents attending antenatal classes are broadly:

- To obtain balanced realistic information so they know what to expect.
- To learn skills that will help them to cope during labour.
- To learn about emotional and social aspects of birth and parenthood.
- To learn about life after birth and caring for their new baby.

The content of a series of classes might include:

- Development and growth of the baby and what mother might expect during pregnancy.
- Common screening tests/blood tests.
- Healthy eating for pregnancy.
- Going into hospital to give birth and what to take.
- Recognizing when labour has started and when to seek advice. Coping skills for labour. What happens if help is needed to give birth (assisted birth, Caesarean section, etc.).
- Common types of pain relief available during labour.
- Breastfeeding and caring for new baby.
- Life at home with new baby/how partners can help.
- Common problems in the postnatal period.

Most sessions would probably include practising labour coping skills, such as relaxation and breathing techniques.

## Further information

Midirs Informed Choice Information Leaflets for professionals and expectant parents. Available at: ℘ www.infochoice.org/

National Childbirth Trust. ✆ Central course information 0300 330 0017. Available at: ℘ www. nct.org.com

# Antenatal care and screening

Pregnancy is a time of tremendous physical, psychological, social, and emotional change.
- Professional care and advice at an early stage of pregnancy allows identification and management of any initial problems.
- Most women seek advice from their GP as a first point of contact. The GP makes early referral to either a midwife or an obstetrician according to need. Midwives are employed by a NHS Trust, working in community teams (3–6), or in hospital, or both.
- Women who are at risk of experiencing problems in their pregnancies may also be referred to an early pregnancy assessment unit or a high-risk day care unit.

## The pattern of antenatal care

It is best delivered at a venue easy to reach for the mother and provided by same midwife or team for continuity of care. Mothers hold their own pregnancy record so that continuity is maintained. The aim of antenatal appointments is to check on the mother's and baby's progress, and provide information, explanations about care, and health promotion advice. The pattern varies according to need and is regularly reviewed.

### Antenatal care appointments

All women should have appointments and screening (as per Fig. 8.6):
- *First appointment before 12wks:* full assessment is undertaken. This may be a lengthy appointment. Blood tests include:
  - *Routine*—full blood count (FBC), blood group and Rhesus factor, Venereal Disease Research Laboratory test (VDRL), rubella antibodies.
  - *Recommended, but optional*—HIV, hepatitis B.
- *Around 14wks:* perform US for dating/fetal anomaly/nuchal fold measurement and serum Down's risk screening.
- *16wks:* review results of scan and screening tests. If a congenital abnormality is detected the woman and her family will need to choose whether or not to continue with pregnancy. Genetic counselling available for all women in this situation.
- *18–20wks:* if mother requests a fetal anomaly scan.
- *28wks:* to offer prophylactic anti-D to women who are Rhesus negative (2nd dose at 34wks) and obtain FBC to monitor mother's Hb level.
- *34, 36 (presentation of baby checked), and 38wks:* to monitor mother and baby.
- *All women not delivered by 41wks:* a further visit to arrange induction of labour.

Nulliparous women have another three appointments to a total of 12 visits.

*Monitoring*
- BP and urinalysis for proteinuria at each visit.
- Measurement of symphysis fundal height at each visit from 25wks.
- Pregnant ♀ are also offered the opportunity to disclose domestic violence (💷 Domestic violence, p. 402).
- If, at any time, a complication arises, the woman should be referred to obstetrician for advice.

*Women whose pregnancies are assessed as medium or high risk*
Extra antenatal visits if long-term condition, e.g. diabetes, previous problems in pregnancies, age >40yrs or <18yrs, BMI >35 or <18, mental health problems, or problematic social circumstances.

## Key reference texts
National Institute of Clinical Excellence/National Collaborating Centre for Womens' and Child Health (2008). *Antenatal Care: Routine care for the Healthy Pregnant Woman.* (CG62). Available at: ℱ http://guidance.nice.org.uk/CG62

NICE Public Health Guidance Maternal and child nutrition. Available at: ℱ http://publications.nice.org.uk/maternal-and-child-nutrition-ph11

Policies and frameworks for maternity services in all countries are available on central health departments' websites (💷 Useful websites, p. 800).

## Further information
National Childbirth Trust. ● Pregnancy and Birth Line 0300 330 0772. Available at: ℱ www.nct.org.com

NHS Choices pregnancy and baby. Available at: ℱ www.nhs.uk/conditions/pregnancy-and-baby/pages/pregnancy-and-baby-care.aspx

Pregnancy Book 2010 (published by Health Departments in England and Wales). Available at: ℱ http://webarchive.nationalarchives.gov.uk/20130107105354/http://www.dh.gov.uk/en/Publicationsandstatistics/Publications/PublicationsPolicyAndGuidance/DH_107302

Public Information version of *Antenatal Care: Routine care for the healthy pregnant woman.* Available at: ℱ www.nice.org.uk

Ready Steady Baby (Scotland). Available at: ℱ http://www.readysteadybaby.org.uk/

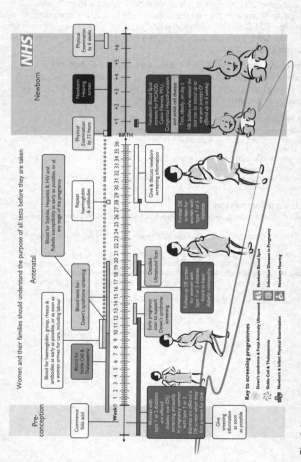

**Fig. 8.6** Antenatal and newborn screening time line (2012).
Reproduced with kind permission of the UK National Screening Committee, English Programmes.

# Maternity rights and benefits

Pregnant women and new mothers in employment are protected by a number of regulations specific to their welfare and wellbeing while at work, and protected against discrimination on the basis of pregnancy.

Employers of pregnant women must:
- Carry out a risk assessment.
- If aspects of job pose risk to health of woman, adjust working conditions, working hours, or offer another job.
- Provide a rest area, preferably smoke free.
- After returning to work, provide a private room for breastfeeding mothers to express and store their milk.

Pregnant women in employment have:
- Paid time off to attend antenatal care.
- Normal sick pay rights for pregnancy-related illness.
- Accrual of contracted holiday entitlement while on maternity leave.
- A right to return to the same job.

## Maternity leave

All employed women are entitled to 26wks ordinary maternity leave and 26wks additional maternity leave, irrespective of whether they are entitled to maternity benefits (see 📖 Benefits for mothers and those responsible for children, p. 793).

### Key regulations
- They must inform the employer, preferably in writing with a medical certificate (MATB1), by the end of the 15th wk before baby is due, when they wish to commence maternity leave. MATB1 is signed by midwife or GP to verify pregnancy and EDD at 20wks before EDD.
- The leave can start any time after 11wks before EDD.
- Maternity leave starts automatically if a woman is sick with a pregnancy-related illness during the 4wks before EDD.
- A woman may not return to work within 2wks of birth (4wks if they work in a factory).
- Maternity leave rights remain if baby is stillborn after 24wks or born earlier than EDD.

## Maternity benefits
### Statutory maternity pay (SMP)
- A weekly payment made by employers to employees or former employees if they meet the qualifying conditions:
  - Employed for 26wks continuously by the 15th week.
  - Earning at least an average of £107/wk before tax.
- An entitlement whether or not they intend to return to work for that employer.
- Paid for a maximum of 39wks, can start 11wks before EDD.
- The first 6wks of SMP are 90% of weekly earnings (with no upper limit). Then 33wks of £135.45 or 90% of earnings.

## Maternity allowance

- Available to some employed and self-employed women who don't qualify for SMP, but meet criteria on weeks of continuous employment and earning on average £30/wk.
- Paid by Department of Works and Pensions (DWP) and claimed on form MA1 from Jobcentre Plus.
- Paid for 39wks at rate of £135.45 or 90% of weekly earnings.
- Reduces amount received from other state benefits.

## Paternity leave and pay

Fathers are entitled to statutory paternity leave of 1 or 2wks at time of birth if they have been employed continuously for 26wks at the 15th week before EDD. They have to inform employer in writing. A self-certification form is available at DWP website (see 📖 Useful websites, p. 800). This leave is paid if they are earning enough to pay National Insurance, otherwise the father may be able to claim income support (📖 Benefits for people with a low income, p. 791).

## Sure Start maternity grants

- Available to parents on low incomes receiving Jobseeker's Allowance, Income Support, Pension Credit, Child Tax Credit at a rate higher than family element, or Working Tax Credit where a disabled worker is included in the assessment. This grant is only available if there are no other children under 16 years of age in the family.
- A payment of £500, which does not have to be paid back (see also 📖 Benefits for people with a low income, p. 791).
- Claimed on SF100 Sure Start form from local Jobcentre Plus office, Social Security office.

## Other benefits

Pregnant women and up to 12mths after birth are entitled to:
- Free prescriptions on production of exemption card (MATEX) from prescription pricing authority on completion of form FW8 (obtainable from GP or midwife).
- Free NHS dentistry.
- Healthy Start tokens for milk, fruit or vegetables if receiving low income benefits, from 10wks of pregnancy by claiming on form available at 🖰 www.healthystart.nhs.uk countersigned by GP or midwife (☎ Helpline 0845 607 6823).

## Related topic

📖 Benefits for people with a low income, p. 791.

## Further information

GOV.UK. Time off work section for full advice on maternity and paternity employment rights and benefits. Available at: 🖰 www.gov.uk/browse/working/time-off

Local Citizens Advice Bureau and online guide. Available at: 🖰 www.adviceguide.org.uk/

# Common problems in pregnancy

During pregnancy a woman may experience a range of problems for which she can be given timely advice, making these easier to manage and improving her wellbeing. Problems include nausea, constipation, indigestion, varicosities, backache, and frequency of micturition. These so-called minor disorders of pregnancy are a series of commonly experienced symptoms related to effects of pregnancy hormones and consequences of enlargement of the uterus as the fetus grows.

## Nausea

- Nausea and vomiting are common, with about 50% of pregnant women suffering anything from mild nausea on awakening, to nausea throughout day with some vomiting, during first half of pregnancy.
- For many women symptoms subside after 12th–14th week of pregnancy coinciding with ability of placenta to take over support of growing embryo.
- Advice includes maintaining good fluid intake, eating little and often throughout day, and avoiding alcohol, caffeine, spicy, and fatty foods.
- Doctor should be consulted if woman is vomiting more than 4 times a day, if she is losing weight, or fluids are not being kept down.

## Indigestion

- Caused when progesterone relaxes smooth muscle in cardiac sphincter, leading to reflux of acid into oesophagus.
- Taking fluids separately to meal times, and sleeping with more than 2 pillows so chest is raised slightly higher than abdomen can ease the symptoms.
- Woman can be prescribed a suitable antacid if this advice doesn't work and she needs additional help to manage symptoms.

## Constipation

- Caused by progesterone relaxing the smooth muscle in bowels.
- The woman can be advised to take extra fluids, increase amount of fruit and vegetables consumed, and that exercise such as walking may help (☐ Nutrition and healthy eating, p. 304).
- If constipation is very difficult to manage, a gentle laxative may be prescribed by midwife or doctor dependent on stage of pregnancy.

## Varicosities

- They are caused when weight of growing uterus creates back pressure in veins of lower body, overcoming normal flow of blood.
- Accompanied by smooth muscle relaxation in vessel walls due to influence of progesterone.
- Can occur in legs, vulva, or anal canal (haemorrhoids).
- Support tights, and close fitting supportive underwear will minimize leg and vulval varicose veins. If legs are aching, resting with them elevated will ease symptoms.
- Haemorrhoids can be treated by avoiding constipation (see ☐ Constipation in adults, p. 457). A soothing haemorrhoidal preparation (BNF 1.7.1) may be prescribed in cream or suppository form.

## Backache

- Complaint is common, both during and after pregnancy.
- Ligaments supporting lower spine and pelvis become softer and stretch more readily during pregnancy. Poor posture exacerbates this, leading to backache.
- Advice includes not standing or sitting for long periods. Pay attention to posture, particularly if woman uses keyboard or computer at work. Using a chair with good lumbar support at work and at home, and regular gentle exercise, such as walking can all be beneficial.

## Frequency of micturition

- Usually apparent during early pregnancy when uterus is still a pelvic organ, and later in pregnancy when fetal head enters maternal pelvis.
- Both situations create pressure on bladder, reducing amount of space available; hence, the need to pass urine more often.
- This does not normally inconvenience woman, but she should be asked about other symptoms, such as burning, stinging, or discomfort during micturition to rule out UTI.

## Further information

National Childbirth Trust. ☎ Helpline 0300 330 0700. Available at: ℘ www.nct.org.uk/

National Institute of Clinical Excellence/National Collaborating Centre for Womens' and Child Health (2008). *Antenatal Care: Routine care for the Healthy Pregnant Woman.* (CG62). Available at: ℘ www.nice.org.uk/CG62

NHS Choices pregnancy and baby. Available at: ℘ www.nhs.uk/conditions/pregnancy-and-baby/pages/pregnancy-and-baby-care.aspx

Ready Steady Baby (Scotland). Available at: ℘ http://www.readysteadybaby.org.uk/

# Birth options and labour

For most mothers-to-be, planning the birth of the baby is an exciting prospect. Previous experience can, however, make this a daunting prospect. The midwife usually discusses options with the mother and her family once a risk assessment (includes medical history, pregnancy, and previous complications) is completed, as it may limit the woman's choices.

## Place

A mother may give birth at home, in a birth centre, or midwife-led unit, or in a hospital consultant-led unit. Healthy, low-risk mothers whose pregnancies are progressing normally can deliver with their midwife at home or in a midwife-led setting. Arrangements may change if complications occur in pregnancy and mother is referred to a consultant obstetrician. A mother may have a preference for a particular type of care, e.g. epidural pain relief, which requires she is cared for in hospital.

## Care in labour

During labour, the mother will be cared for on a one-to-one basis by either her named midwife, if she is low risk, or another midwife from the same team. Mothers with high-risk pregnancies are cared for by a midwife from a high-risk team, working alongside the consultant obstetrician. In a hospital setting, also available if required, are an obstetrician, anaesthetist, paediatrician, and operating department staff. It is very rare that mothers being cared for at home will require any assistance other than that of the midwife; however, the midwife can call to her aid any other clinicians should the situation warrant this. A decision to transfer into hospital is made if there is any deviation from normal during the labour or birth.

## Pain relief

Usually, a discussion about such choices will have taken place during pregnancy and any preferences included in the birth plan. During labour in any setting a mother also has choices about how she will be cared for. She may wish to be upright and mobile, and give birth in a standing, kneeling, squatting, all fours, or seated position. A range of pain relief is available including epidural analgesia (not in home deliveries), opiates, nitrous oxide, and oxygen. A range of complementary therapies may be available if the mother wishes to use these.

During pregnancy the uterus contracts painlessly and passively to assist circulation of blood to the uterine muscles and placenta. These are called Braxton Hicks contractions. At the end of pregnancy, hormone changes result in the uterus becoming more sensitive to oxytocin and so these formerly passive contractions become more active.

## The process of labour

### Initiation of labour

The cervix has to become softer and stretchier to allow it to dilate during labour. In a first-time mother, these changes start to occur from 36wks gestation. Prostaglandins are responsible for these changes and some mothers might experience a blood-stained mucous discharge as the cervix alters. This is because the protective plug sealing the cervix is disturbed as the cervix alters its shape and size.

### First stage

- *Effacement of the cervix*: i.e. cervix gradually becomes shorter (3cm long to almost flat) as early labour contractions pull cervical tissues up into lower part of uterus. These contractions can stop and start again several times before labour establishes.
- Cervix then gradually dilates until completely open in response to contractions and pressure from baby's head.
- Meanwhile, membranes containing amniotic fluid in front of baby's head start to bulge through opening cervix. This 'bag' of water does not normally break until cervix is fully open.
- First stage of labour can last anything up to 12–18h.

### Second stage

- Characterized by contractions becoming more expulsive in nature, creating an almost uncontrollable urge to push as descending baby's head is pressed against rectum.
- Mother will push during contractions and gradually this stretches perineum allowing baby's head to be born. The next contraction delivers baby's body.
- Second stage of labour can last from 30min to 1h or more, depending on type of analgesia used. Use of epidural analgesia lengthens this stage as mother does not experience bearing down sensations.

### Third stage

Uterus continues to contract until placenta and membranes deliver. Most women are offered an injection of syntocinon to prevent excessive bleeding during this stage, which lasts 5–15min.

## Further information

Royal College of Midwife guidelines and position statements. Available at: ℜ www.rcm.org.uk/college/policy-practice/guidelines/

Midirs Informed Choice Information Leaflets for professionals and expectant parents. Available at: ℜ www.infochoice.org/

National Childbirth Trust. ☎ Pregnancy and Birth Line 0300 330 0772. Available at: ℜ www.nct.org.com

Ready Steady Baby (Scotland). Available at: ℜ http://www.readysteadybaby.org.uk/

NHS Choices pregnancy and baby. Available at: ℜ www.nhs.uk/conditions/pregnancy-and-baby/pages/pregnancy-and-baby-care.aspx

# Complicated labour

## Induction of labour

Labour may be induced with the mother's consent if the mother is 10 days overdue, or if there are any concerns about maternal or fetal wellbeing at any other point during late pregnancy.

### Key points

- Induction methods aim to mimic normal labour so synthetic prostaglandin gel or pessaries are used to soften cervix, followed by IV oxytocin, which causes regular contractions to become established.
- Process of labour then continues as normal. Because contractions are artificially induced they may be more painful, especially if rupture of membranes is also performed.

## Caesarean section

This operation is performed with the mother's consent if it is anticipated that a vaginal birth poses unacceptable risks to the mother and/or the baby. This can be planned in advance if a problem is identified before labour or be carried out in an emergency should a problem develop unexpectedly either during pregnancy or during labour.

### Key points

- Common for this operation to be performed under epidural anaesthetic as this leads to reduced post-operative complications.
- Caesarean section on demand is discouraged as it is statistically more likely for a woman to die as a result of a Caesarean than a vaginal birth.
- Postnatal recovery can be delayed due to giving birth by Caesarean section.
- Complications such as infection, urinary problems, haemorrhage, and thrombo-embolic disorders are managed by administering prophylactic antibiotics, and low molecular weight heparin.
- Before surgery an in-dwelling urinary catheter is inserted to prevent urinary complications.
- Analgesia is usually required for a number of days/weeks after birth. The mother stays in hospital 3–4 days afterwards.
- Caesarean section can sometimes lead to delay in lactation, so extra support is required by breastfeeding mothers (⬚ Breastfeeding, p. 176).
- There are also some risks to baby of being delivered by this method. These include difficulties establishing respiration, transient tachyapnoea of newborn, which requires admission to special care baby unit (if delivered before 39wks gestation) scalpel cuts to head, face, or neck area.

## Forceps/ventouse

These instruments are used in 12% of births when either the mother or baby become tired or distressed, or the second stage of labour is considered too slow. Having an epidural increases the risk of needing an instrumental delivery. After use of ventouse, oedema on baby's head can take up to 2wks to resolve (⬚ New babies, p. 173).

## Episiotomy

This is a cut made by the midwife or doctor into the perineum under local or epidural anaesthetic. Its purpose is to enlarge the vaginal opening and assist birth. It can be performed if the baby is in distress and needs to be born quickly, or during an instrumental delivery to protect the vaginal wall, or to assist a slow birth. 12% of births are aided by episiotomy. An episiotomy is repaired with dissolvable stitches (as are tears). It heals in about 2wks. Mothers are advised by midwife on perineal hygiene, pain relief, and other remedies, e.g. ice packs, warm baths that may ease discomfort.

## Further information

Midirs Informed Choice Information Leaflets for professionals and expectant parents. Available at: ℘ www.infochoice.org/

National Childbirth Trust. ☏ Pregnancy and Birth Line 0300 330 0772. Available at: ℘ www.nct. org.com

NICE Clinical guideline (2011). *Caesarean Section*: (CG132). Available at: ℘ www.nice.org.uk/cg132

Royal College of Midwife guidelines and position statements. Available at: ℘ www.rcm.org.uk/college/policy-practice/guidelines/

# Postnatal care

The postnatal period is the time when the mother recovers from the birth, her reproductive and other organs regain their normal function, and lactation is established if she is breastfeeding. She adjusts to motherhood and becomes confident in the care of her baby receiving advice and support initially from the midwife and, subsequently, from the HV. The midwife visits according to the needs of the mother and baby up to 28 days (although may be involved up to 6wks. *Note:* there is variation according to national and local frameworks), visiting frequently in the first 10 days. The midwife liaises with the HV and in most instances the HV makes contact from day 10 (📖 New birth visits, p. 168).

Most of the physical changes take place in the first 6wks after the birth. Social, psychological, and emotional adjustment can take considerably longer even up to a year after the birth. The rate at which a woman recovers will depend on several factors:
- Her health during pregnancy.
- The length of labour.
- Whether birth was complicated or uncomplicated.
- Whether baby is healthy and makes normal progress.
- Whether there were any problems for mother or baby in immediate postnatal period.
- Level of support she receives as she recovers.

## Maternal health

At first postnatal contact the mother will be offered information on the physiological process of recovery after birth and that some health problems are common. The midwife will advise the mother about the signs and symptoms of potentially life-threatening conditions, and to contact a health care professional immediately if any of the following occur:
- Sudden and profuse loss of blood or persistent increased blood loss.
- Signs and symptoms of infection.
- Headache in first 72h accompanied by visual disturbances, vomiting, or feeling faint.
- Signs and symptoms of thrombo-embolism.
- If the mother has not passed urine within 6h of birth.

During the 1st week after birth the mother is given guidance and advice on the following:
- Tiredness, a normal consequence of new parenthood.
- Perineal hygiene or care of Caesarian wound.
- Involuntary leakage of small amounts of urine, commonly experienced after birth.
- Haemorrhoids, common in postnatal period.
- Importance of appropriate diet and fluid intake.
- Contact details for expert contraceptive advice.
- *Intercourse:* may be uncomfortable at first and contraception (📖 Contraception: general, p. 359) should be used by 21 days post-birth.
- Normal patterns of emotional changes.

The mother is advised to contact a midwife, GP, or HV if:
- Any changes in mood outside of normal pattern.
- Itching or bleeding around anus.
- Faecal urgency or frank faecal incontinence.

Between 2 and 6wks, the mother is advised to contact a midwife, GP, or HV if:
- Still bleeding after 6wks.
- Sex still painful.
- Severe, long-lasting backache is preventing normal daily activities.

Midwife and HV remain alert to signs of domestic violence during this period (📖 Domestic violence, p. 402).

### Infant feeding

Infant feeding information and advice is given during the first week. The midwife will support each mother in her feeding method of choice (📖 Breastfeeding, p. 176; 📖 Bottle feeding, p. 178) and knows to contact midwife or GP urgently if signs of mastitis (flu-like symptoms, red and painful breasts).

### Infant health

At each postnatal contact the parents are offered information and advice to help them to assess their baby's general condition, identify warning signs to look for if their baby is unwell, and how to contact a health care professional or emergency service if required.

The midwife will assess the physical wellbeing of the baby during each postnatal contact, as well as advising the parents on:
- Parenting and attachment, social capabilities of baby.
- *Neonatal screening:* obtaining neonatal blood spot screen.
- *Health promotion and well baby care:* including skin, thrush infection, nappy rash, constipation, diarrhoea, colic, fever, jaundice, vitamin K, and care of umbilicus before and after cord separation.
- Each visit is an opportunity to evaluate relevant safety issues, safety equipment, and reinforce the recommendations about sudden infant death and co-sleeping.
- Midwife will be alert to risk factors, and signs of child abuse and children in need.

Either the midwife or HV will give the parents PHCHR and a NHS-produced child health promotion information according to local protocols.

### Further information

National Childbirth Trust. ☎ Postnatal Line 0300 330 0773. Available at: ℘ www.nct.org.com
Net Mums. Available at: ℘ www.netmums.com
NICE (2006 reviewed 2012). *Postnatal Care: routine postnatal care of women and their babies (CG37)* Professional and public versions. Available at: ℘ www.nice.org.uk/CG037
NHS Choices pregnancy and baby. Available at: ℘ www.nhs.uk/conditions/pregnancy-and-baby/pages/pregnancy-and-baby-care.aspx
Ready Steady Baby (Scotland). Available at: ℘ www.readysteadybaby.org.uk/

# Postnatal depression

## Definition

A depressive illness that occurs following childbirth during the first 12mths and lasts for several weeks/months. It appears more long-lasting and debilitating than depression at other times. It occurs in 10–15% of women. It is distinguishable from postnatal 'blues' (i.e. brief low mood felt at some point by many women in first 2wks postnatally) by greater severity and longer duration. It is also distinguishable from more severe post-partum psychosis (symptoms include loss of contact with reality, hallucinations, severe thought disturbance), which only occurs in 2:2000 births, and requires immediate medical assessment and treatment.

## Causes

- Unknown, probably no single reason.
- In some cases, is result of hormonal changes.
- Stress of looking after a young baby, having sleep disrupted may also help to bring on illness in susceptible people.

## Risk factors

- Main risk factor is a previous history of depression.
- *Others include:*
  - *Stressful life events*—especially during pregnancy (negative life events, previous miscarriage/stillbirth).
  - *Family and marital difficulties*—poor marital relationship, conflict between woman and parents.
  - Inadequate levels of social support.
  - *Personality factors, attitudes*—perfectionism, low self-esteem, negative maternal attitudes towards child rearing.
  - Mood during pregnancy.
  - FH of depression.
  - Infant temperament and mother–infant difficulties.
  - *Early experiences*—poor relationship with own mother, history of sexual abuse.
  - Unrealistic expectations of motherhood.

## Symptoms

- Variable, but persist most of the time.
- Low mood, tearfulness/crying, anxiety/panic attacks, self-blame/guilt, undue health worries, lethargy/tiredness, irritability, ↓ appetite, inadequacy, emotionally labile, loss of interest in activities.

## Onset

- Usually develops within first 3mths following childbirth.
- Second peak at 6–8mths post-partum.

## Assessment and management

### Assessment

- Should be through, simple, brief self-report on symptoms of depression (📖 People with depression, p. 435), at minimum on antenatal booking and postnatally at 4–6wks and 3–4mths.
- Edinburgh Postnatal Depression Scale (EPDS) is *not* a screening tool and is not ratified by UK National Screening Committee (see 📖 UK screening programmes, p. 321). However, NICE clinical guidance[1] suggests it can aid in assessment of mood when used by trained professionals. Local protocols apply in management and referral to GP and mental health services of women identified at different levels of risk.
- *Primary prevention:* focuses on raising awareness antenatally, and provision of extra support and prevention of social isolation, e.g. through schemes, such as Sure Start (see 📖 Working with parents, p. 164; 📖 Support for parents, p. 166). Additional 'listening visits' may be offered by HVs to women identified as at 'at risk' of depression.
- Management of women diagnosed with postnatal depression is as for any depression (see 📖 People with depression, p. 435). It may include 'listening visits' by HVs, non-directive counselling, dynamic psychotherapy, CBT (see 📖 Talking therapies, p. 429), and antidepressants. Occasionally hospital admission to a mother and baby unit is necessary. Additional support may be required to aid the mother and child relationship (see 📖 Working with parents, p. 164; and 📖 Support for parents, p. 166), and prevent social isolation.
- Women diagnosed with puerperal psychosis are managed in the same way as any psychotic illness (see 📖 People with schizophrenia, p. 443) and may be admitted to mother and baby unit.

### Potential long-term effects

- Woman's mental health may predispose for future postnatal depression.
- *Mother–infant relationship:* may have a negative influence on this relationship and future child development.
- It may have a negative effect on partner/marital relationship.

## Reference

[1]NICE (2006). *Postnatal Care: routine postnatal care of women and their babies.* Professional and public versions. Available at: ℜ www.nice.org.uk

## Further information

Association for Postnatal Illness. Available at: ℜ www.apni.org

Health Care Improvement Scotland and Scottish Intercollegiate Guidelines Network IGN Guideline 127 (2012). Management of perinatal mood disorders. Available at: ℜ http://sign.ac.uk/patients/publications/127/index.html

National Childbirth Trust. Available at: ℜ www.nct.org.com ☏ Postnatal Line 0300 330 0773

NICE. Antenatal and postnatal mental health: clinical management and service guidance (CG45). Available at: ℜ www.nice.org.uk/CG45

# Chapter 9

# Adults with extra needs

# Asylum seekers and refugees

The UK is a signatory to the 1951 UN Convention relating to the Status of Refugees. Most refugees and asylum seekers in the UK are from areas of conflict and are single men <40yrs. In 2012 193,510 with accepted status as refugees, 15,170 pending asylum cases, and 205 people stateless in the UK[1]. In the UK:

- *Asylum seeker:* person that has lodged an asylum claim with Government (Home Office) and is waiting for a decision on their claim.
- *Refugee:* person is recognized as *refugee* only when application for asylum has been accepted by Home Office.

## People seeking asylum

People claiming asylum from persecution make their application at a UK Border Agency centre in South London. Asylum seekers are not allowed to work after they make an application and have to comply with restrictions and stay in contact with their case worker. Those without personal means of support and are classed as destitute (homeless or without means to buy food), receive some cash support at fixed rates and are placed in temporary accommodation (outside of London). People making an application have the right to NHS care and education for children. Secure detentions centres are used to accommodate people and children who are considered to have failed to comply with restrictions or have no right to remain and will be removed. Failed applicants are expected to leave the UK voluntarily or their removal is enforced. If asylum claim is unsuccessful, support stops 21 days after the decision (unless appealed against).

## People recognized as refugees

People recognized as refugees by the UK Border Agency are given a residence permit for 5yrs in the first instance, at which point their case will be reviewed again and they may have to return to their own country or be given indefinite leave to remain. Those not recognized as refugees, within the terms of the Refugee Convention, but can demonstrate a need for international protection, may be granted Humanitarian Protection or Discretionary Leave.

## Unaccompanied children

See 📖 Children in special circumstances, p. 160.

## Health issues
The health problems of asylum seekers and refugees are dependent on:
- The communicable diseases, disease patterns, and availability of health services to them in their home country.
- The events that led them to flee their country, e.g. civil war, persecution, imprisonment, and torture.
- The events that have happened to them while travelling to the country of asylum and since their arrival in the UK (40% of ♀ have experienced sexual assault in the UK).

Refugees and asylum seekers are not homogeneous. Health care needs have to be assessed individually. While all refugees and asylum seekers have experienced loss, they also demonstrate great resilience and courage in facing enormous challenges and losses. Key issues for health care professionals:
- Ensuring good communication (📖 Adults and children with additional communication needs, p. 119) using interpreters and advocates.
- A recognition of different cultural attitudes to norms in health and expectations of health care services.
- Recognizing that asylum status may make accessing health care services problematic, e.g. in temporary accommodation, may be moved on at short notice, if in hostel accommodation may have to be present at meal times or may not eat.

## Key reference texts
Burnett A, Fassil Y. (originally 2002, updated online). *Meeting the health needs of refugees and asylum seekers in the UK.* Available at: ℘ www.migranthealthse.co.uk/dhnhs-specialist-support

Wilson R, Sanders M, Dumper H. Sexual health, asylum seekers and refugees: a handbook for people working with refugees and asylum seekers in England. Available at: ℘ www.fpa.org.uk/professionals/publicationsandresources/healthprofessionals/sexualhealthasylumseekersandrefugees

## Reference
[1]UNCHR 2012 Asylum Trends Report. Available at: ℘ http://unhcr.org/asylumtrends/UNHCR%20ASYLUM%20TRENDS%202012_WEB.pdf

## Further information
UK Border Agency. Available at: ℘ www.ukba.homeoffice.gov.uk/asylum/

Refugee Council. Available at: ℘ www.refugeecouncil.org.uk/

Medical Foundation for the care of victims of torture. Available at: ℘ www.freedomfromtorture.org/

ROSE Information and advice for health care professionals who are refugees in the UK. Available at: ℘ www.rose.nhs.uk/

# Homeless people

The UK has legal definitions of homelessness (📖 Homes and housing, p. 21). LAs have a legal duty to provide advice to all those who meet the criteria and duty to provide emergency accommodation to groups legally eligible for assistance, e.g. pregnant women, those with dependent children (see 📖 Homes and housing, p. 21). In 2012 >34,000 households with children accepted as homeless and numbers ↑.

## Single and hidden homeless

Numbers are difficult to estimate, but thought to be >350,000 single homeless people in the UK. One-quarter of these live in hostels or bed and breakfast accommodation, or are facing imminent threat of eviction through debt. Three-quarters live in what are known as concealed households, with friends or family, often in unsatisfactory accommodation. Estimates of 6000 people sleeping rough in London in 2010/11. The average life expectancy of a rough sleeper is 42yrs.

Rough sleepers will access primary care health services provided that they are provided in an appropriate and sensitive way.

## Causes of homelessness

Complex, interrelated, and different for different age groups:
• Mental health needs.
• Family breakdown.
• Abuse or violence in the home.
• Alcohol, drug, and substance misuse.
• Debt and unemployment.
• Leaving armed forces, prison, or residential care (e.g. looked-after children).

Policy in all countries of UK is to address complex problems of single homeless and ensure minimal numbers of rough sleepers.

## Health needs

In addition to health needs that have contributed to homelessness people are vulnerable to a wide range of health problems:

Homeless people are about 40 times more likely not to register with a GP than members of the general population.

• 30–50% of homeless people have mental health problems, including depression.
• 70% misuse drugs (📖 Substance misuse, p. 433).
• TB (📖 Tuberculosis, p. 680) and respiratory problems.
• Hepatitis (📖 Viral hepatitis, p. 676).

- Skin problems (📖 Bacterial skin conditions, p. 632; 📖 Eczema/dermatitis, p. 636; 📖 Fungal infections, p. 638).
- Malnutrition.
- Antenatal and postnatal complications.

*Needs of homeless children:* see 📖 Children in special circumstances, p. 160.

## Access to health care

Policy expectations are that:
- Health organizations and LA have local plans for improving access to health care of families in temporary accommodation and homeless people, particularly in areas of known health need.
- Close liaison between mental health service providers, charitable providers, and primary health care.
- In urban areas where there are higher numbers of homelessness more likely to be specialist providers/teams and GPs offering enhanced services (📖 General practice, p. 13).

*Access to help with housing*
- Local CABs and Housing Action Centres are key resources for advice and help on housing issues.
- Emergency accommodation found through Shelter national helpline ☎ 0808 800 4444, and local councils, e.g.:
  - *Night shelters*—free, often found in redundant public buildings, e.g. old churches and halls. One night's accommodation.
  - *Hostels*—provide a few nights to a few months, require payment, and may need to book ahead. Some have entry criteria, e.g. age, no substance abuse, religious and cultural background.
  - *Nightstop*—for young 16–25-yr-olds single homeless for one night only, provided by people with spare rooms.
  - *Foyers*—for young people, provide accommodation up to 9mths, support to acquire new skills, and long-term housing.
- *Support and advice for other forms of accommodation:* e.g. bed and breakfast (subject to eligibility), housing association, council housing, and private rental can be accessed through local council, homeless outreach teams (charitable or council based) and main homeless charities, e.g. Shelter, Crisis.

## Related topics

📖 Asylum seekers and refugees, p. 396; 📖 Alcohol, p. 319; 📖 People with depression, p. 435; 📖 Substance misuse, p. 433; 📖 Homes and housing, p. 21.

## Further information

Shelter advice for homeless people. Available at: ℘ www.shelter.org.uk
Crisis Homeless Charity. Available at: ℘ www.crisis.org
Nightstop services for young homeless people. Available at: ℘ www.depaulnightstopuk.org/
Homeless UK. Search for advice services, day centres and hostels. Available at: ℘ www.homelessuk.org

# Gypsies and travellers

## Definition of terms

'Traveller' is overarching term covering various groups, estimated 100,000 nomadic and 200,000 in housing:

- *Romany gypsies and Irish travellers*—recognized minority ethnic groups, ~300,000 in UK.
- *New travellers*—not a recognized ethnic group).
- Also covers *Scottish travellers, European Roma, show people* (fairground and circus people), and *bargees* (occupational boat dwellers).

## Gypsies and travellers in the UK

- Legally covered under terms of the Race Relations (Amendment) Act (2000).
- One of most marginalized ethnic minorities in the UK; subject to widespread prejudice.

### Accommodation

Trailers (caravans) on privately-owned or rented sites, or on unauthorized encampments (due to limited site availability). Cultural importance of close proximity to extended family for support and wellbeing. Possibly half the population lives in houses. House dwelling is associated with long-term illness, poorer health state, and anxiety.

### Health profile

Gypsies and travellers have significantly worse health than the general population. ↑ respiratory problems, anxiety and depression, excess prevalence of stillbirths, neonatal deaths, and premature death of older offspring. Possibly the highest maternal death rate among all minority ethnic groups. Research in Leeds and Ireland shows ↓ life expectancy and ↑ mortality rates for all causes, than the general population.

### Access to services

There is an inverse relationship between their health needs and use of health and related services. Contributory factors:

- Reluctance of GPs to register travellers or visit sites.
- Practical problems of access.
- Mismatch of expectations between travellers and health staff, accompanied by travellers' defensive expectation of racist attitudes from health staff.
- Attitudinal barriers and cultural inappropriateness of service delivery.
- Lack of readily available health records for continuity of care.
- Low literacy levels and poor knowledge of services amongst travellers.

## Good practice guidance

- Never make assumptions about cultural practices—ask!
- Use client-held and PHCHR health records (📖 Client- and patient-held records, p. 87).
- Seek advice and support from specialist health workers for gypsies and travellers.

- Maximize opportunistic health promotion and protection, e.g. 📖 Child immunization, p. 156.
- Consider provision of services to sites if no specialist health workers are already doing so.

At an organizational level:

- Involve gypsies and travellers in cultural competence training of health service staff.
- Use specialist health workers in partnership with gypsy and traveller communities and agencies to address wider determinants of health through community development and capacity development (📖 Community approaches to health, p. 302).
- Include in NHS ethnic monitoring to address 'invisibility' in public health terms.

### Related topics

📖 Anti-discriminatory health care, p. 76; 📖 Professional conduct, p. 74.

### Key reference texts

Derbyshire Gypsy Liaison Group. *A Better Road: An Information Booklet for Health Care and Other Professionals.* c/o Ernest Bailey Community Centre, Office 3, New Street, Matlock DE4 3FE. Tel: 01629 732 744.

Francis G. (2009) Traveller Voices FAQs on the Cultural Identity and Health Needs of Gypsy Travellers. Available at: ✎ www.qni.org.uk/docs/MSA%20Traveller%20booklet.pdf

### Further information

Friends, Families and Travellers. Available at: ✎ www.gypsy-traveller.org
Gypsy & Traveller Law Reform Coalition. Available at: ✎ www.travellerslaw.org.uk
Irish Traveller Movement. Available at: ✎ www.itmtrav.ie
Irish Travellers organization in Dublin. Available at: ✎ www.paveepoint.ie
The Gypsy Council. Available at: ✎ www.gypsy-association.co.uk

# Domestic violence

Any incident or pattern of incidents of controlling, coercive or threatening behaviour, violence or abuse between those aged 16 or over who are or have been intimate partners or family members regardless of gender or sexuality. This can encompass, but is not limited to, the following types of abuse: psychological, physical, sexual, financial, emotional.[1]

Describes a continuum of behaviour ranging from verbal, physical, emotional, and sexual abuse, to rape and murder (including so-called 'honour killings').

### In the UK
- Majority of victims (>90%) are women.
- Affects about 1 in 4 ♀, 1 in 6 ♀ in lifetime.
- 2 ♀ murdered every week by partners, 40% after separation.
- Estimated that ♀ suffer at least 35 assaults before contacting police.
- Violence starts in 30% cases during pregnancy.
- >52% of reported ♀ rapes committed by current or former partner.
- Estimated over 30,000 children affected each year.
- In 50% cases where mother abused, children also abused.
- >50% child protection cases involve domestic violence.

There is an impact not just on ♀ health, but also on children. Both women and are children likely to have long-term emotional and mental consequences. ♀ stay in abusive relationships for many reasons, including self-blame, shame, loss of confidence, fear of losing children, financial dependency, fear that no one will believe them.

### Potential indicators of domestic violence
Include:
- Multiple injuries at various stages of healing to areas such as breast, genitals, and abdomen.
- Explanations vague or inconsistent with injuries.
- Partner insists on being present at all appointments, speaks for ♀.
- ♀ appears depressed, or overly anxious.
- ♀ fails to attend for medical appointments, comply with treatment.

Women are particularly at risk during pregnancy and following separation from a violent partner.

### Key principles in the role of health professionals
- Create a supportive environment that allows ♀ to talk.
- Ask ♀ (only if alone) direct questions about domestic violence.
- Have information on local agencies that can help readily available and in a format that ♀ can easily conceal.
- Keep the ♀'s safety in mind and that of any children.
- Know how to refer ♀ to local support agencies if that is what she chooses. Respect their decisions.
- Document all discussions and assessments accurately.
- Never try to mediate between partners, ensure own and colleagues' safety.

*Selective enquiry* Ask the ♀ (when alone) directly if she is experiencing violence or fear of violence from another adult in the home when there are indicators suggesting it might be a possibility.

*Routine enquiry* Ask all women, but particularly pregnant women about domestic violence as part of usual care. Introduced in many areas as part of government initiatives to reduce domestic violence. Routine enquiry includes being clear on the limits of confidentiality (📖 Confidentiality, p. 86).

## On disclosure of domestic violence

- Reassure, support, give national helpline[2] and local specialist domestic violence services contact details, e.g. women's refuge, police domestic violence unit.
- Undertake a risk assessment with ♀ to determine extent of danger.
- High risk includes children present, pregnancy, previous violence, alcohol and/or drug misuse, weapons present, stalking, separation, suicide threat.

❶ If immediate risk, e.g. partner acting aggressively in the same building, call police.

❶ If there are children in the household, follow local child protection procedures (📖 Child protection, p. 230).

❶ If high risk, seek senior clinician/manager support to follow multi-agency guidelines.

- If low risk of danger then help ♀ think through need for a safety plan if still living with perpetrator (e.g. think about escape routes, calling 999 if violence starts, keep money and keys easy to grab) and if now living separately (e.g. changing locks, think about escape routes).
- Document fully in records all observations, actions, and events.

## Related topics

📖 Vulnerable adults and abuse, p. 406.

## Key reference texts

DoH (England) (2005). *Responding to Domestic Abuse: A Handbook for Health Professionals* London: DoH. Note: all countries have guidance. Available at: 🔗 www.domesticviolencelondon. nhs.uk/uploads/downloads/DH_4126619.pdf

## References

[1]Home Office (2013) Information for Local Areas on the change to the Definition of Domestic Violence and Abuse. Available at: 🔗 www.gov.uk/government/publications/definition-of-domestic-violence-and-abuse-guide-for-local-areas

[2]UK National Domestic Violence. 24-h Helpline Freephone ☎ 0808 2000 247

## Further information and sources of help

Broken Rainbow (for lesbian, gay, bisexual and transgender people). 0300 999 5428. Available at: 🔗 www.broken-rainbow.org.uk

Refuge. Available at: 🔗 www.refuge.org.uk (includes links to UK wide domestic violence services and information)

Womens' Aid. Available at: 🔗 www.womensaid.org.uk/ and their resource for children. Available at: 🔗 www.thehideout.org.uk

## Victims of crime

UK public perceive levels of crime and anti-social behaviour as higher than surveys and reporting suggest:

- <80% of all crimes are reported to the police. Common assault and sexual assault least likely to be reported.
- Young men aged 16–24yrs most at risk of being a victim of violent crime and people with mental health problems at higher risk of being a victim of any crime.
- Eight metropolitan areas account for >40% of all recorded crimes in England and Wales, 40% of all UK reported robberies occur in London. No geographical variation in reported domestic violence (📖 Domestic violence, p. 402).
- Distraction burglaries (i.e. bogus callers) target older people.
- About 15% of victims of violent crime require medical attention.
- No injuries in >70% mugging, >50% assaults by acquaintances or strangers, <30% domestic violence (📖 Domestic violence, p. 402).
- Sexual offences account for 5% of recorded crime. 93% of victims of reported rapes ♀.

Source: Office for National Statistics Crime Summaries. Available at: ℘ www.ons.gov.uk/ons/taxonomy/index.html?nscl=Crime

### Crime reduction

- LAs with others work in partnerships with the police, health organizations, community organizations and businesses in developing local strategies for tackling crime and disorder, e.g. Neighbourhood Watch.
- All police forces have crime prevention officers to give public and victims of crime advice on personal and property security.
- LAs usually have a lead contact for addressing anti-social behaviour (includes problem neighbours, vandalism, fly-tipping, graffiti).
- Anti-Social Behaviour Orders (ASBO) are court orders to protect public from behaviour likely to cause distress, alarm, or harassment.

### Reporting crimes

Important in order to catch criminals and prevent further crime. For some types of crime also require a police crime number to claim compensation through insurance or to claim criminal injuries compensation.

- *Emergencies:* dial 999.
- *Non-emergency crimes:* call 101 to contact police or local police station or reported to the police online ℘ www.police.uk
- *Anonymously:* via Crimestoppers, an independent charity for reporting information about crime and criminals and passes on to police. ☎ 0800 555 111. ℘ www.crimestoppers-uk.org

## Post-assault consultations with health professionals

Victims may need physical and psychological care, as well as considering the need to collect forensic evidence.

### Assault

Any professional consulted should document carefully the extent of injuries as this may be required for legal purposes. Measurements and photos if possible of injuries should be taken. Encourage the victim to report the incident to the police.

### Rape or sexual assault

If the victim is willing to report the assault then they should not be examined except by a specialist trained in collecting forensic evidence. Most areas now have sexual assault referral centres, i.e. one stop shop offering medical care, counselling, collection of forensic evidence, and police investigation into the alleged offences.

Victims unwilling to access such services should be offered medical examination, assessed for need for EC, STI screening, offered prophylactic antibiotics, assessed for need for HIV prophylaxis, etc. Also offer counselling and information on support organizations.

## Victims of crime

Many people experience a range of emotions, including anger, fear, anxiety, and sorrow after a crime, depending on the type and consequences. Counselling and the opportunities to talk through the experience may help many victims. Some assault victims and many sexual assault victims develop post-traumatic stress disorder (PTSD), with symptoms such as flashbacks, leading to insomnia, depression etc. Referral to either counselling services or psychology services as appropriate.

### Victim Support

A national charity that works with police, in some areas receives referrals, and provides free and confidential support for victims of crime and witness support. Available at: ℘ www.victimsupport.org.

### Criminal Injuries Compensation Scheme

This aims to provide blameless victims with material recognition of their pain and suffering, and to allow society to express its regret to them. The level of compensation is set in a tariff determined by Parliament. Individual applies directly. England, Wales, and Scotland available at: ℘ www.cica. gov.uk; and Northern Ireland available at: ℘ www.compensationni.gov.uk/

## Further information

UK government information on reporting crimes and getting compensation. Available at: ℘ www. gov.uk/browse/justice/reporting-crimes-compensation

UK Police Services. Available at: ℘ www.police.uk

Victim Support UK. ☎ 0845 30 30 900. Available at: ℘ www.victimsupport.org

Rape Crisis Centres for advice, support, and counselling. Available at: ℘ www.rapecrisis.org.uk/

Rape and Sexual Assault Referral Centres locations in England and Wales. Available at: ℘ http:// www.nhs.uk/Service-Search/Rape%20and%20sexual%20assault%20referral%20centres/ LocationSearch/364

# Vulnerable adults and abuse

*A vulnerable adult* One who is unable to take care of themselves and/or unable to protect him or herself against significant harm or exploitation through mental or other disability, illness, and/or age.

*Abuse* A violation of human and/or civil rights and may be one off or repeated acts of physical, psychological, sexual, financial (includes theft as well as intimidation about wills), discriminatory (includes hate crime) abuses, or acts of omission or neglect. Most abuse is a criminal offence and the police lead the investigations.

*Patterns of abuse* May take different dynamics, e.g. may be opportunistic, or involve repeated acts by person in position of power over another, or long-term slow increase in violations (e.g. grooming). Perpetrators may be household members, carers, neighbours, professionals, or multiple staff members in institutions where neglect, acts of omission, use of punishment e.g. withholding medication, have become a cultural norm.

*Predisposing factors* May include vulnerable adults living with financially dependent family members, vulnerable person isolated, personal or family history of violence, abuse, alcohol, or drug misuse, carer stress.

## Acting on concerns

Often when anxieties or concerns are raised about possible abuse of a vulnerable adult, it is not clear the extent or nature of the harm.

All primary care staff receiving allegations or having concerns about harm or possible harm to vulnerable adults (either by unpaid carers/family/neighbours or professional/carer) should discuss this with their line manager or named senior clinician, and follow local agreed multi-agency procedures for safeguarding or protection of vulnerable adults.

All areas should have agreed multi-agency procedures, often follows the model of those for child protection, Social services has the key coordinating role. Every health organization should ensure that copies or internet access to the policies are available to all primary care staff.

### Concerns for vulnerable adults at home

Should be referred to social services as per local guidance. Many areas have a facility for a pre-referral consultation with the social service designated or safeguarding officer. The procedures usually involving in-depth assessment of the level and impact of the abuse, the individual's safety, rights, and views. This may lead to police involvements and decision to offer an immediate place of safety or the designated officer may convene a multi-agency case conference to establish the facts, and plan to prevent further abuse.

*Key principles*
- Active empowerment of the individual through the services provided.
- Supports the rights of the individual to lead an independent life.
- Recognizes the right to self-determination involves risk.
- Active interagency collaboration.
- Ensures the individual receives the full protection of the law.

*Concerns about a care service*
Everyone has a duty to report any allegations or suspicions of abuse or potential abuse of a vulnerable adult either to their immediate line manager or to discuss their initial concerns with the social services agency, the regulatory authorities, or the police. Local agreed procedures should be followed. Suspected abuse by staff of a regulated service, e.g. care agency, care home, should also be reported to the relevant regulatory bodies.

*Whistle blowing* Individual staff members should also be aware of policies supporting 'whistle blowing' (📖 Whistle blowing, p. 80).

*Situations of immediate danger or need for emergency treatment* Primary care staff should call for police or ambulance without referring to a senior staff member.

## Disclosure of abuse
- Listen carefully and allow them to tell as much as they want to at that point, don't press for details.
- Be sympathetic, non-judgemental, reassure them it is not their fault.
- Explain this has to be shared to get them the help they require.
- Discuss with senior staff member and refer to social services/police as per local guidelines.
- Document in detail the disclosure conversation as soon as possible.

## Related topics
📖 Domestic violence, p. 402; 📖 People with learning disabilities, p. 408; 📖 Child Protection, p. 230; 📖 Key facts on carers and caring, p. 410; 📖 Mental capacity, p. 424.

## Further information
Action on Elder Abuse. ☎ Helpline: 080 8808 8141. Available at: 🔗 www.elderabuse.org.uk
DoH (England) (2011). Statement on government policy on adult. Available at: 🔗 www.gov.uk/government/publications/adult-safeguarding-statement-of-government-policy
Practitioner Alliance for Safeguarding Adults. Available at: 🔗 www.pasauk.org.uk/home

# People with learning disabilities

Learning disability (LD) is a reduced intellectual ability and difficulty with everyday activities. All types of LD are lifelong, and occur <18yrs. People with profound and multiple LDs require significant help, while those with mild/moderate LD will usually be able to live independently with support. Approximately 1.5 million people in the UK have a LD. Government policies for people with learning disabilities have key principles of: rights, independence, choice, and inclusion at the heart of strategy for the 21st century.

## Health profile

Children and adults with learning disabilities have significantly worse health in comparison to the general population, in particular, respiratory problems, diabetes, GI problems, heart disease, epilepsy, depression, schizophrenia, hypothyroidism, and sensory impairments. Mortality rates are ↑ for all causes compared with the general population.

### Access to health services

There is an inverse relationship between the high level of health needs and the low use of health services. Contributory factors:

- Attitudinal barriers by professionals.
- Communication difficulties.
- Diagnostic overshadowing (i.e. the disability masks the illness).
- Lack of accessible information.
- Confusion about law regarding consent to treatment (📖 Consent, p. 77; 📖 Mental capacity, p. 424).

## Good practice guidance

- Never make assumptions.
- Speak clearly and not too fast.
- Avoid medical jargon—use simple everyday language.
- Photographs and objects to accompany information may help.
- Use concrete terms.
- Try to avoid negative words such as don't.
- Use key events in the person's life, such as Christmas, birthdays, to help recall.
- Use open-ended questions.
- Use active language, e.g. Jane will give you a blood test.
- Use health action plans or personal hand-held records.
- Use Makaton or British sign language when required.

## Specialist support for children and adults

*General health care* is provided through primary care services.

*Multi-professional specialist teams* are, in most areas, providing specialist support to children and adults with learning disabilities.

*For children* these services may be located at Child Development Centres (📖 Children with complex needs and disabilities, p. 225), some areas may have specialists staff working in mainstream services such as CAMHs.

*For adults*

These services are usually called Community Teams for Learning Disabilities (CLDT). These are made up of staff from health and social care professionals, such as LD nurses, social workers, physiotherapists, OTs, psychologists, speech and language therapists and psychiatrists. CLDT have an open referral system.

These services can help with finding a home, benefits, occupation, education, leisure, bereavement, respite care, relationships, health access, communication, mobility, aids, appliances, and dealing with behavioural difficulties.

*Adolescence to adulthood* This is a vital transitional point, and it's crucial that services work in partnership with the young person to ensure that they are actively involved in the choices, and decisions about their future.

*Growing older* Adults with learning disabilities are living longer and require service supports to be robust, as they often do not have close family support. Bereavement and palliative care needs often overlooked.

*Family carer*

Play a critical role, often providing lifelong support to their relative. They need access to information, training and support, and can also make valuable contributions to staff and service development services need to work sensitively, and help families plan for the future.

*Challenging behaviour*

This is a term used to describe a wide range of behaviours that puts themselves or others at risk of harm. Much behaviour can be attributable to environmental stresses, and lack of occupation and opportunities. Physical complaints should always be considered as a cause of change in behaviour, and then a psychiatric assessment to exclude a mental health disorder.

*Adult protection* People with learning disabilities are often at risk of abuse, this may be physical, verbal, or psychological. Local adult protection guidance should be available. See 🛈 Vulnerable adults and abuse, p. 406.

**Related topic**

🛈 Sexual health and adults with a learning disability, p. 720

**Further information**

Breaking Bad News. Available at: ✆ http://www.breakingbadnews.org/
Challenging Behaviour Foundation. Available at: ✆ www.challengingbehaviour.org.uk
Foundation for People with Learning Disabilities. Available at: ✆ www.learningdisabilities.org.uk
Intellectual Disability Health Information. Available at: ✆ www.intellectualdisability.info
Mencap. Available at: ✆ www.mencap.org.uk
Scottish consortium for learning disability. Available at: ✆ www.scld.org.uk/
Turner's Syndrome Support Society UK. Available at: ✆ www.tss.org.uk

# Key facts on carers and caring

A carer is someone who provides care on an unpaid basis and provides that care either in association with paid carers (e.g. care workers, nurses, and social workers) or instead of paid carers. GPs both through QOF and direct-enhanced services (DES; Scotland) should record care, status, and provision of services for carer. Estimated to be >7 million carers in the UK who are key to the support of dependent family members and friends in the community of carers, believed to save the economy £119 billion pa.

## Contribution

- Many carers derive high levels of personal satisfaction in their role, but this does not mean they do not need support and regular review.
- 1.9 million carers provide 20hrs or more care/wk. Caring is often provided in conjunction with other work/family responsibilities. Majority of carers look after older people and may themselves be old with health needs.
- Carers may provide:
  - Personal care.
  - Physical help with daily activities.
  - Practical support, e.g. help with medication and shopping.
- Women more likely to be carers (58%). Peak age for caring 50–59yrs. 1 in 4 of ♀ in this age group provide care.

## Impact of caring

- There are significant financial consequences from being a carer and the majority of carers worry about finances.
- Caring is often detrimental to health, carers providing high levels of care are 2½× more likely to experience mental health problems.
- Spouse carers and mothers of disabled children have increased likelihood of psychological distress.
- Carers may benefit from respite from their caring responsibilities. For those who are already depressed, respite care alone is unlikely to be sufficient.

*Note*: carers are not a homogenous group. The quality of the relationship between the carer and the dependent person prior to a person taking on a caring role, directly affects emotional health and caring relationships.

Carers need their role and knowledge acknowledged and respected by health and social care professionals. Primary care nurses are well placed to offer ongoing support, advice, and help with direct care.

❶ Health professionals that are in contact with carers should ensure that the carer's needs are considered *independently* of the dependent person.

It is important that:
- Individual has made an informed choice about being a carer and does not feel coerced into the role through guilt or expectations of others.
- Carers have access to proper assessment of their needs and are aware that they are entitled to a carer's assessment from social services (☐ Carers assessment and support, p. 412).

- Carers are fully consulted on decisions that affect them.
- Receive information about benefits services (📖 Benefits and support, p. 789) and sources of peer and voluntary/charity-based support.
- That services are coordinated between health, social care, housing, and, when relevant, education.
- Services are *not* withheld because a carer is present.
- Risks of being socially excluded are addressed. Carers often cannot take up paid employment because of need for flexible working or give up holidays and ↓ leisure activities because of low incomes and costs.
- Black and ethnic minority carers are not overlooked by mainstream services.
- Practice complies with the Carers (Equal Opportunities) Act 2004.
- *Note*: confidentiality is an issue when involving carers in discussion about patient care. Consider 'carer contract': patient gives written consent for information to be shared with carer. GPs through QOF and Direct Enhanced Services (Scotland) should record carer status and services received.

**Young carers** (see also 📖 Children in special circumstances, p. 160). A minority of young carers are being identified or assessed for support though national census figures show steady increase. Defined as anyone <18yrs whose life is in some way restricted because of the need to take responsibility for someone who is:
- Ill (physically or mentally).
- Has a disability, ongoing mental health problems, or is affected by substance misuse.
- Caring responsibilities can have adverse effects on:
  - Schooling: learning and attendance.
  - Relationships with peers.
  - Relationships within the family.
- Health professionals should consider:
  - The need to be proactive in identifying children who may be carers.
  - Term 'young carer' is important and differentiates from a child of someone who has a disability or needs extra help.
  - That young carers value support groups that affirm their contribution and prefer individual non-intrusive support to statutory service provision.
  - Carers Act 1995 and Framework for Assessment of Children in need should be a starting point in assessment a young carer's needs.

**Related topics**

📖 Carers assessment and support, p. 412; 📖 Children with complex health needs and disabilities, p. 225; 📖 Social support, p. 24; 📖 Assistive technology, p. 776.

**Further information**

Age UK. Available at: ℘ www.ageuk.org.uk/home-and-care/advice-for-carers
Carers Trust: host interactive online resource for young carers. Available at: ℘ www.carers.org
Carers UK. ☎ 0808 808 7777. Available at: ℘ www.carersuk.org/
SCIE. Social care Institute for Excellence Research briefing 11:The health and wellbeing of young carers. Available at: ℘ www.scie.org.uk/publications/briefings/briefing11

# Carers assessment and support

Carers (Equal Opportunities) Act 2004 gives carers rights to information and places a duty on LAs to inform carers of their right to a carers assessment. This gives LAs powers to enlist the help of housing, health, education, and other LAs in providing carer support.

## Carers assessment

Anyone who is a carer or who is contemplating becoming a carer has the right to an assessment by social services. They can request an assessment directly or ask the GP or nurse to do so on their behalf. The assessment does not assume that the individual should take on the caring role. The purpose is to:

- Discuss with social services, help needed to support caring role.
- Explore how an individual feels about being a carer.
- Provide information about benefits.
- Discuss how to balance caring responsibilities with other responsibilities and interests.
- Plan and consider how caring responsibilities might change.
- If caring is likely to continue for foreseeable future then review date should be set.

*Assessment includes a review of:*

- Housing: possible needs for aids and adaptations.
- Health and likely health needs of the carer.
- Work: if there is a need to ↓ working hours because of caring role, desire to return to work, challenges of balancing demands.
- Other interests: e.g. leisure access to lifelong learning.
- Time spent on caring: where support is needed and opportunities for respite/care breaks.
- Relationships, feelings, and emotional consequences of caring.
- The contingency plans in place for emergencies or situations where it is not possible to carry on caring.

## Types of help and support that should be available to carers and their dependents

*Note*: there is considerable local variation.

- *Help at home:* means-tested support from social services is available to carers in need of support.
- *Carers Allowance:* for people>16yrs who spend at least 35h/wk caring for someone who is in receipt of Disability Living Allowance or Attendance allowance. Carer must not be in full-time education of earning above a specified amount per week. Currently, £58.45/wk. *Note*: person being cared for benefits may be affected. People in receipt of a state pension are not eligible (may be eligible for underlying entitlement) iCare4 website (⌘ www.icare4.co.uk/moneymap_2.php) provides money map for carers to see financial support options
- *Caring with confidence:* DH-backed knowledge and skills-based learning for carers through a self-study programme.
- *Voluntary organizations:* e.g. crossroads can offer sitting services.

- Involvement of district nursing service to provide support and relevant specialist nursing support, e.g. Admiral nurses, MS CNS.
- *Day care:* social services will have a list of centres providing day care for older people and children
- *Respite care:* care homes and specialist residential settings can provide short-term care to provide carer with planned breaks. Social services may provide support with costs.
- Involvement of district nursing services.
- Aids and equipment (📖 Assistive technology, p. 776).
- *Adapting the home environment:* the person being looked after may be eligible for a home improvement grant.
- *Carer specific support services:* local carer support groups, carer services offered by social services, e.g. help with taxi fares for hospital visits.
- *Pharmacy support:* e.g. delivery of repeat prescriptions.
- *Continuing care:* since 2007 national service framework for assessing eligibility for NHS continuing care for people with ongoing needs outside hospital

LAs are required to set out how they make decisions arising from the needs identified according to their eligibility criteria. If carers are dissatisfied with the support they have been offered then carers' organizations provide support and advice about how to appeal and what it is reasonable to expect.

### Related topics
📖 Key facts on carers and caring, p. 410; 📖 Benefits for illness, disability and carers, p. 795; 📖 Children with complex health needs and disabilities, p. 225; 📖 Social support, p. 24; 📖 Assistive technology and equipment for home nursing, p. 778.

### Further information
AgeUK. Available at: ℘ www.ageuk.org.uk
Carers Trust. Available at: ℘ www.carers.org
Carers UK. Available at: ℘ www.carersuk.org/
NHS Choices Caring with confidence online learning. Available at: ℘ www.nhs.uk/carers-learning-online

# Principles of rehabilitation following stroke

## Definition

- *Stroke:* a focal or global neurological deficit due to local disturbance in blood supply to brain; may have abrupt onset, but lasts longer than 24hrs.
- *FAST test:* if there is a yes to any one of these questions then get emergency help:
  - *F*acial weakness—can person smile? Has their mouth drooped?
  - *A*rm weakness—can the person raise both arms?
  - *S*peech problems—can person speak clearly and understand others?
  - *T*ime to call 999.

## Prevalence

Stroke is a major health problem in the UK. Most people survive a first stroke, but often have significant morbidity. More than 900,000 people in England live with the effects of stroke. Incidence ↑ with age; 80% are >65yrs and ♂:♀ equal. > 30% have ongoing disability post-stroke. Recovery can take years.

## Risk factors

↑ BP, smoking, DM, heart disease, peripheral vascular disease (PVD), past TIA, raised lipid levels, obesity, lack of exercise, MI, atrial fibrillation (AF), excessive alcohol intake.

## Effects of stroke

- *Motor deficits:* speech difficulties (e.g. dysarthria, dysphasia), hemiplegia and hemiparesis, facial paralysis → difficulties in swallowing.
- *Sensory deficits:* visual deficits, poor response to heat and cold, perceptual deficits (e.g. environment), lack of awareness of disabled part of body.
- *Altered consciousness:* memory loss, short attention span.
- *Emotional deficits:* personality change, loss of self-control, confusion, depression.
- *Bladder and bowel dysfunction:* incontinence, frequency, urgency.
- Altered sexual function.
- Impact on family

## Secondary prevention

Control risk factors, if an embolic stroke aspirin or warfarin (Ⅲ Patients on anticoagulant therapy, p. 600) may be prescribed by GP/hospital consultant. Management of hypertension (Ⅲ Hypertension, p. 589) and hyperlipidaemia (Ⅲ Hyperlipidaemia, p. 593). All patients with history of CVD should be treated with a statin.

*Principles*

Patients and carers should have active involvement in the rehabilitation process, agree care plans that have realistic goals, and be offered information, e.g. voluntary stroke services, benefits such as disability living allowance and attendance allowance (📖 Benefits for illness, disability and carers, p. 795). Return to work issues should be identified as soon as possible and the physical, cognitive, communication, and psychological demands of the job identifying any impairments on work performance (e.g. physical limitations, anxiety, fatigue) and measures that may support a gradual return to work.

## Rehabilitation

An active process in which people with a disability work together with MDT, relatives, and members of the wider community to achieve optimum wellbeing. Should have a systematic approach to assessment (📖 Integrated assessment process, p. 114) that considers the physical deficits arising from stroke, emotional consequences, immediate physical needs, e.g. adjustments to clothing, equipment aids, and housing, ability to be independent in and outside the home, and range of social support networks. Key elements:

- People with residual disability after stroke should receive rehabilitation in a dedicated stroke in-patient rehabilitation unit and, subsequently, from a specialist stroke team within the community.
- Assessment should consider previous functional status, current limitations including emotional functioning and pain, environmental factors (social, physical, and cultural).
- Early mobilization exercises (passive, assisted, or active) and weight-bearing and mobilization should be encouraged.
- Based on the pattern of recovery. Recovery of leg function occurs before arm function, and arm function prior to hand function.
- Prevention of deformity and damage based on maintaining correct position, which opposes direction of flexion. Avoid over-using unaffected side.
- In collaboration with physiotherapist, repetitive task training after stroke on a range of tasks can help to improve upper limb weakness (such as reaching, grasping, pointing, moving and manipulating objects in functional tasks) and lower limb weakness (such as sit to stand transfers, walking, and using stairs).
- *Visual problems/visual neglect:* focus on relevant functional tasks taking account of impairment. e.g. encourage people to scan to neglected side, use brightly coloured lines or highlighter at edge of page.
- Swallowing problems should be regularly reviewed in collaboration with SLT.
- Repetitive task performance, such as dressing.
- Assess cognitive, attention span and memory function, and suggest aids such as diaries and prompts, etc.
- Monitor progress through use of valid tools, e.g. Barthel Index (📖 Standardized assessment tools for adults, p. 116)

- *Psychological rehabilitation:* e.g. engaging patient in conversation, encouraging participation in social activities.
- MDT: patient, family/carers, nurses, GP, physiotherapy, OT, SLT, and social services. Specialist referral where necessary.
- *Carer support:* stroke often called the family illness.
- Provision of stroke family care workers/nurses where they exist.
- *Driving after a stroke:* patients with a stroke who make a satisfactory recovery should not drive for at least 1mth after their stroke.
- Patients with residual disability at 1mth must inform DVLA and can only resume driving after formal assessment by GP or other professional.

## Related topics

📖 Assistive technology and equipment for home nursing, p. 778; 📖 Carers assessment and support, p. 412; 📖 People with depression, p. 435; 📖 Coronary heart disease, p. 584.

## Further information

NHS Choices Standards for stroke care includes links to National stroke strategy. 10-point plan and forthcoming revised NICE guidance on rehabilitation. Available at: ℘ www.nhs.uk/NHSEngland/NSF/Pages/Nationalstrokestrategy.aspx

NICE (2008). Clinical Guidance CG68. Diagnosis and initial management of acute stroke and transient ischaemic attack. Available at: ℘ www.nice.org.uk/CG68

Stroke Association. Available at: ℘ www.stroke.org.uk

# Principles of working with someone with dementia

For definitions, prevalence, risk factors and signs, symptoms, and assessment see 📖 People with dementias, p. 438.

People living through the early stages of dementia often adopt strategies to hide symptoms. It is important to recognize that dementia presents as an interplay of factors that all influence an individual's experience.

• Neurological impairment.
• Personality (temperament, psychological defences, coping style).
• Biography and recent life events.
• Physical health and sensory awareness.
• Individual's existing relationships with individuals and groups.

❶ Health professionals and carers can rob people with dementia of their self-esteem, confidence, and sense of personhood by their actions, e.g. being patronizing and infantalizing them, using deception to gain compliance, not acknowledging feelings and subjective reality, ignoring their presence, denying them choices, blaming them.

Focus on abilities and function that are retained. Emphasize maintaining a healthy lifestyle. Very unhelpful to characterize dementia as a condition of relentless decline where patients and carers have no control, process of normalization as individuals family and carers adjust to living with the disease.

National policy commitment to improve diagnosis and care of people with dementia and related initiatives to promote dementia friendly environments, e.g. Dementia Friends.[1]

## Needs of people with dementia

• *Comfort:* feeling of security, people with dementia experience ongoing loss and bereavement.
• Inclusion and feeling of connectedness.
• Occupation.
• *Identity:* continuity with individual's past.

## Communication with someone with dementia

• Speak clearly and use short sentences.
• Make eye contact before speaking.
• Give time for person to respond; avoid creating feeling of pressure to answer.
• Do not interrupt, talk for the person or over them.
• Avoid asking multiple questions.
• Pay careful attention to body language (including how your own body language could be misinterpreted) and how someone communicates distress.
• *Use visual aids:* e.g. object linked to conversation, a photo that can be left in patient's home as reminder of who you are. Consider how the environment can help act as a cue for conversations, e.g. talking about eating in the kitchen.

- If unsure what has been said, ask them to repeat or check accuracy of what you think they have said.
- Highly patterned clothing may be visually disturbing and very dark clothes may affect how the person sees you. Consider wearing block colours that are bright.

## Management information and advice

See also NICE Dementia Quality Standard and supporting resources.[2]

- Refer to memory services; also specialist services as needed, e.g. consultant, old age psychiatrist, geriatrician, neurologist, community mental health team, social services.
- Encourage person with dementia to live as full life as possible and make full use of remaining abilities; promote choice.
- Monitor safety in daily activities and assess safety in home, e.g. cooking (see Alzheimer's Society factsheets).
- It is important to work with carers and family, sharing information, and providing ongoing support.
- Understand person's story and what is important to them, e.g. encouraging recall of early memories of childhood, school, family, work, etc.
- Encourage full use of remaining abilities, interests and hobbies by, e.g. writing things down, making lists. Suggest person carries a Helpcard with key information and phone numbers. Checklist by the door can prompt appropriate clothing and taking keys, etc.
- Encourage maintenance of physical health and fitness through good diet, exercise, and swift treatment of physical illness.
- Suggest membership of a support group or organization, which may help caring, though some find these distressing in short term.
- Financial and legal matters need to be discussed, consider organizing bills using direct debit, review eligibility for benefits and establish power of attorney (📖 Mental capacity, p. 424).
- 'Behaviours that challenge (sometimes called behavioural and psychological symptoms of dementia (BPSD)) e.g. screaming, wandering, shouting, may be attempts to communicate or expressions of pain, hunger, etc. Careful listening and affirmation of what is being expressed important.
- Ensure carers to receive advice on help with caring, accommodation, financial advice, benefits, and support groups, e.g. Alzheimer's Society.
- Medication and medicines management includes observation for effects and side effects:
  - Antipsychotics are usually contraindicated if used should be reviewed regularly and used on a short-term basis.
  - Avoid sedative or hypnotic medications if possible.
  - In Alzheimer's disease patients may be referred to primary care for assessment and initiation of anticholinergic drugs, to postpone onset of more severe symptoms.
  - Using medication devices to aid memory may help but should be considered on a person by person basis.

- As dementia and its effects ↑, more intensive care will be required utilizing statutory and voluntary services (📖 Care homes, p. 28; 📖 Mental capacity, p. 424; 📖 Palliative care in the home, p. 509).

*Needs of family caregivers*
- To know someone will provide care when they no longer can.
- Access to telephone support.
- Strategies for dealing with stress.
- Respite.
- Strategies for dealing with feelings of being trapped.

*Admiral nurses*

Not available across whole of UK; check Dementia UK website. Specialist nurses who:
- Work with family carers as their prime focus.
- Provide practical advice, emotional support, information, and skills.
- Deliver education and training in dementia care.
- Provide consultancy to professionals.
- Promote best practice in person-centred dementia care.

Also available in some areas: Dementia care centres and memory clinics.

Palliative care teams will also provide support to people with end stage dementia.

## References

[1]Dementia Friends. Available at: ℗ www.dementiafriends.org.uk
[2]NICE. Dementia Quality Standard. Available at: ℗ http://guidance.nice.org.uk/QS1

## Further information

AgeUK. Available at: ℗ www.ageuk.org.uk
Alzheimer's Society. Advice for all types of dementia not just Alzheimer's disease. Available at: ℗ www.alzheimers.org.uk
DementiaUK. Admiral Nursing service. ☎ 0845 257 9406. Available at: ℗ www.dementiauk.org
NHS Choices. Living well with dementia. Available at: ℗ www.nhs.uk/Conditions/dementia-guide/Pages/living-well-with-dementia.aspx
NICE. Supporting People to live well with dementia (QS30) issued 2013. Available at: ℗ www.nice.org.uk

# Principles of working with someone with compromised immunity

Healthy people fight infections through the immune system, mainly the lymphatic system. This can be compromised by age, infection, burns, neoplasms, metabolic disorders, irradiation, foreign bodies, cytotoxic drugs, steroids. Causes include:

- *Immunodeficiency:*
  - 1° causes.
  - 2°, e.g. lymphoma, myeloma, malnutrition, chemotherapy, HIV, post-organ transplant.
- *Hypersensitivity:* i.e. excessive immune response, e.g. asthma, hay fever, eczema, anaphylactic shock.
- *Autoimmune diseases:* e.g. pernicious anaemia, rheumatoid arthritis, systemic lupus erythematosus, myasthenia gravis.
- Graft rejection and transplantation.

## Principles of care

Most people with compromised immunity live independently. Care is related to the severity and type of symptoms. Many of the associated disorders have support groups and organizations providing information.

## Principles of care for people with immunodeficiency disorders

- Lack of awareness about antibody defects → considerable under-diagnosis. Be alert to patients with multiple infections per year (ear, sinus, chest, skin), failure of an infant to gain weight, or when family history of immune deficiency.
- Aim to prevent infections and complications and to enable a normal working capability and life expectancy.
- Educate patient in self-care and disease management.
- Involve MDT, medical, and other specialists.
- Smoking should be discouraged.

### Prevention of infection

*Note:* adhere to principles of infection prevention and control.

- Patients exposed to specific infections (e.g. rheumatic fever, TB, meningitis (should receive prophylactic antibiotics)).
- Treat prophylactically patients with HIV and pneumocystis and granulocytopenia for prevention of bacterial infections.
- Immunization against influenza, meningococcal, and pneumococcal infections.
- Hepatitis B immunization given to people who regularly receive blood products.

## Related topic

📖 Principles of working with someone with an infectious disease, p. 421.

## Further information

International Patient Organisation for Primary Immunodeficiencies. Available at: ℞ www.ipopi.org

# Principles of working with someone with an infectious disease

Infectious or communicable diseases are illnesses caused by micro-organisms not normally present in the body. These contrast with those acquired as a result of poor asepsis, antibiotic therapy, immuno-suppressive drugs, or inadequate hand washing (see also 📖 Principles of working with someone with compromised immunity, p. 420).

## Causes

- *Bacteria:* e.g. *Streptococcus*, salmonellosis, meningococcal meningitis.
- *Viruses:* e.g. influenza, hepatitis, chickenpox.
- *Protozoa:* e.g. malaria, toxoplasmosis.
- *Infestation:* e.g. head lice.

Knowledge of the organism important in planning care.

**Transmission** May be by ingestion, inhalation, innoculation (through a cut, skin abrasion or needle stick injury), and direct contact.

## Care principles

- For common infectious diseases (e.g. herpes simplex, chickenpox), only general care is needed with precautions to prevent spread (e.g. hand hygiene (📖 Hand hygiene, p. 94), contact avoidance, washing cutlery, not sharing toiletries).
- *Isolation precautions:* for being nursed at home include wearing gloves and apron when in contact with body fluids or contaminated surfaces is likely, hand washing after removing gloves and before leaving house.
- Carry paper towels and a small container of alcohol hand rub, when visiting premises with inadequate hygiene facilities.
- Advice to patients and relatives: hot, soapy water adequate for dishes and a hot wash (60°C) for clothes.
- Clinical waste: should be disposed of in appropriately coloured bags designated for clinical waste in the community (see also 📖 Managing health care waste, p. 105).
- *Other isolation precautions:* rarely necessary in the home.
- There should be referral to specialist advice if available and indicated (e.g. nurse or HV TB specialists).

## Related topics

📖 Infectious disease notifications, p. 103; 📖 Cleaning, disinfection, and sterilization of equipment, p. 95; 📖 Managing health care waste, p. 105; 📖 Sharps injuries, p. 107; 📖 Bacterial skin infections, p. 632; 📖 Fungal infections, p. 638; 📖 Viral skin infections, p. 643; 📖 Viral infections, p. 672; 📖 Methicillin-resistant *Staphylococcus aureus*, p. 674; 📖 Viral hepatitis, p. 676; 📖 Pandemic influenza, p. 678; 📖 Tuberculosis, p. 680.

## Further information

Public Health England Primary care guidance and useful reference guide. Available at: 🔗 www.hpa.org.uk/Topics/InfectiousDiseases/InfectionsAZ/PrimaryCareGuidance

# Principles of care for people with mental health problems

1 in 4 people in the UK are affected by mental illness. *No Health without Mental Health*[1] sets out six objectives:

- *Objective 1:* more people will have good mental health.
- *Objective 2:* more people with mental health problems will recover.
- *Objective 3:* more people with mental health problems will have good physical health.
- *Objective 4:* more people will have positive experience of care and support.
- *Objective 5:* fewer people will suffer avoidable harm.
- *Objective 6:* fewer people will experience stigma and discrimination

There are ten areas identified as to how these objectives can be achieved:

- *Mental health has 'parity of esteem' with physical health within health and care system:* i.e. commissioning and planning of services reflect mental health needs in all systems and services.
- People with mental health problems, their families and carers, are involved in all aspects of service design and delivery.
- Public services improve equality and tackle inequality.
- More people have access to evidence-based treatments, e.g. all age groups and people from Black Minority Ethnic groups have access to Improving Access to Psychological Therapies (IAPT) programme.
- Public health systems includes mental health and all organizations recognize the value of promoting mental health.
- *Services intervene early:* e.g. services promote mental health from birth.
- Services work together around people's needs and aspirations.
- Health services tackle smoking cessation (☐ Smoking cessation, p. 315), obesity (☐ Weight management: overweight and obesity, p. 307) and co-morbidity for people with mental health problems.
- People with mental health problems have a better experience of employment.
- *Stigma and discrimination faced by people with mental health problems are challenged:* health care staff are trained to understand mental health and principles of recovery.

## Primary care and access to services

Service users who contact their 1° health team with a common mental health problem should:

- Have their mental health needs identified and assessed.
- Be offered effective treatments, including referral to specialist services for further assessment, treatment, and care if they need it.
- Provided with advice, information and sources of self-help and support.

## Effective services for people with serious mental illness

- Individuals receive care that optimizes engagement and anticipates, or prevents a crisis, thereby reducing risk, a care programme approach (CPA).
- Have a copy of their written care plan, which states action to be taken in a crisis by service user, their carer, and care coordinator, and advises GP how they should respond if service user needs additional help.
- Is regularly reviewed by their care coordinator.
- Enables them to access services 24h/day, 365 days/yr.

Service users who are assessed as needing a period of care away from their home should have:
- Timely access to an appropriate hospital bed or place which is:
  - In the least restrictive environment, and consistent with need to protect them and the public.
  - As close to home as possible.
- A copy of a written care plan, agreed on discharge, which sets out their care and rehabilitation, identifies their care coordinator, and specifies the action to be taken in a crisis.

## Caring about carers

All carers or people who provide regular and substantial care for a person on CPA should:
- Have an assessment of their caring, physical, and mental health needs repeated on at least an annual basis ([box] Carers assessment, p. 412).
- Have their own written care plan given to and implemented with them.

## Preventing suicide

Local health and social care services should aim to prevent suicides by:
- Having a local delivery plan based on local need.
- Support local prison staff in preventing suicides among prisoners.
- Ensure staff are competent to assess risk of suicide among individuals.
- Develop a local system for suicide audit, to learn lessons, and take any necessary action.

## Reference

[1] Centre for Mental Health, Department of Health, Mind, NHS Confederation Mental Health Network, Rethink Mental Illness, Turning Point (2012). *No Health Without Mental Health: Implementation Framework*. London: DH. Available at: ℘ www.dh.gov.uk/health/2012/07/mentalhealthframework/

## Further information

MIND. Available at: ℘ www.mind.org.uk
SANE. Available at: ℘ www.sane.org.uk
Rethink. Available at: ℘ www.rethink.orgMIN
NHS Choices. Care Programme Approach. Available at: ℘ www.nhs.uk/CarersDirect/guide/mental-health/Pages/care-programme-approach.aspx
NHS Choices. Mental Health. Available at: ℘ www.nhs.uk/CarersDirect/guide/mental-health/Pages/Mentalhealth.aspx

# Mental capacity

~2 million people in Britain are thought to lack mental capacity, including those that suffer from dementia. Mental capacity is complex, and care must be taken to consider the person's rights and responsibilities. As a basis for assessment the following should always be considered:

- *Everyone* has capacity unless it is established otherwise.
- Person is not to be treated as being unable to make a decision unless all attempts to help them have been tried and been unsuccessful.
- Any assessment should consider who person was and is (especially where sense of self alters or diminishes, as in dementia).
- How to achieve a balance between older person's last-known wishes and current wishes (as expressed through words and behaviour).
- Previously communicated directives or instructions.
- Person's unique responses to their physical and mental health, and how they see their future.
- How capacity is being supported or hindered by others on a day-to-day basis.
- Full and open discussion of multiple perspectives and not simply clinical interests of one or other professional group or family member.
- How capacity has been formally assessed and in what situations it does and does not exist.

Lack of capacity is defined in regard to:

- Inability to make a decision because of impairment of the brain or mind at the material time whether temporary or permanent.
- Inability to make a decision is based on the central tenets of informed consent (📖 Consent, p. 77); i.e. understanding, weighing up, using, and communicating information.

## Mental Capacity Act 2005 (England & Wales)

(Note Scotland has a similar Act called the Adults with Incapacity Act (2008)). Governs decision-making on behalf of adults, where they lose mental capacity at some point in their lives or where the incapacitating condition has been present since birth. The Act covers all decisions made, or actions taken on behalf of people lacking capacity on:

- *Personal welfare:* including day-to-day and major life-related health care.
- *Financial matters:* also provides substitute decision-making by attorneys, court-appointed 'deputies', and clarifies position where no such formal process has been adopted.

Provides guidance on:

- Paying for goods and services.
- Lasting power of attorney and financial issues.
- Court of protection and court appointed deputies.
- Advance decisions to refuse treatment.
- Protection and supervision of those responsible for making decisions or taking actions on behalf of those who lack capacity, and links with mental capacity and finally data protection

*Key principles*
- Need to consider when deciding what's in a person's best interests.
- Do not make assumptions on basis of age, appearance, condition, or behaviour.
- Consider all relevant circumstances.
- Consider whether or when person will have capacity to make decision.
- Support person's participation in any acts or decisions made for them.
- Do not make a decision about life-sustaining treatment 'motivated by a desire to bring about his (or her) death'.
- Consider the person's expressed wishes and feelings, beliefs, and values.
- Take into account views of others with an interest in person's welfare, their carers, and those appointed to act on their behalf. A person must be assumed to have capacity unless it is established that (s)he lacks capacity.
- Person is not to be treated as unable to make a decision merely because they make an unwise decision.
- An act or decision made under this Act or done on behalf of the person who lacks capacity must be in the best interests of the person.
- Before the act or decision, consider if it can be effectively achieved in ways less restrictive of the person's rights and freedom.

*Assessing capacity*
Consider the presence of impairment, its likely consequences, and if the person has been unable to make a decision. Attention is given to minimizing disability. Situational capacity is recognized as is fluctuating capacity. Assessing capacity should be done when the person is at their highest level of functioning. Assessment is to be carried out by the relevant professional. Within health care this is the doctor or the professional proposing treatment.

Multi-disciplinary consultation is recommended. Refusal to consent to capacity assessment must be respected.

**❶** Decision-making regarding capacity is contextual, and varies between persons and within a person over time.

Professionals have a duty to ensure they take reasonable steps to establish consent *first*. So professionals must have assessed a person's lack of capacity prospectively, i.e. before care is given. Where professionals are satisfied advance directives are valid *and* applicable to the proposed treatment they should be followed.

*Lasting powers of attorney*
Powers of attorney can be made at any time when the person making it has the mental capacity to do so. A person can grant a lasting power of attorney (LPA) to another person or people to enable them to make decisions should it become necessary, over their personal welfare property, and financial affairs. There will be a separate legal document in respect of each of these, appointing one or more attorneys. LPA must be registered and a personal welfare LPA will only be effective once the person has lost capacity to make their own decisions.

(An enduring power of attorney (EPA) under the previous law is restricted to decisions over property and financial affairs. An EPA made before 1 October 2007 remains valid.)

### The Court of Protection

The Court of Protection oversees the Mental Capacity Act and deals with all issues, including financial and serious health care matters, concerning people who lack the mental capacity to make their own decisions. It is involved in disputes when the person's carer, and health care or social worker disagree about what's in the person's best interests, or when the views of the attorneys in relation to property and welfare conflict. The Court of Protection can appoint 'deputies' who can also take decisions on health and welfare, as well as in financial matters. They will come into action when the court needs to delegate an ongoing series of decisions, rather than one decision.

### The Public Guardian

The Office of the Public Guardian is to protect anyone who lacks mental capacity to make decisions for themselves. It registers LPA and supervises court-appointed deputies. It works with a range of agencies, such as the police and social services, to investigate concerns.

### The Independent Mental Capacity Advocate service (IMCA)

The independent mental capacity advocate helps people:
• Who do not have mental capacity.
• Who have not given powers of attorney to anyone.
• Who do not have a court-appointed deputy.
• Who have no friends or family to speak on their behalf.

They are involved in decisions about serious medical treatment, such as heart surgery or electro-convulsive therapy (ECT), and long-term accommodation in a hospital or care home.

### Related topics

📖 Consent, p. 77; 📖 People with dementias, p. 438; 📖 End-of-life issues, p. 530.

### Further information

Department for Constitutional Affairs (2005). *A Guide to the Mental Capacity Bill.* Available at: 🔊 www.justice.gov.uk/downloads/protecting-the-vulnerable/mca/mca-code-practice-0509.pdf

Making Decisions Alliance: alliance of national disability and older peoples' organizations. Available at: 🔊 www.mentalhealthalliance.org.uk

# Patients receiving antipsychotic medication

Antipsychotic medication is a common form of treatment for psychotic illnesses, such as schizophrenia. It can be administered either orally or by depot injection. Prescribed to address symptoms, such as hallucinations, delusions, thought disorder, and extreme mood swings, e.g. with bipolar disorder. Choice of administration depends on past history of drug effectiveness, preference, tolerability, and adherence. It is often prescribed alongside psychosocial interventions (📖 Talking therapies, p. 429).

## Monitoring

Antipsychotic medication can cause distressing and disabling side effects. These include extrapyramidal symptoms, i.e.:

- Parkinsonism.
- Dystonia.
- Akathisia.

Need to be monitored to help the patient cope with them, help to ↓ effects and ↑ adherence.

> If a patient is taking antipsychotic medication, any consultation is a good opportunity to assess the patient's general health, monitor for side effects, and liaise with GP or community mental health team (CMHT) key worker/care coordinator if there are problems.

## Assessment tools

Liverpool University Neuroleptic Side Effect Rating Scale (LUNSERS)[1].

### Face/mouth/neck

- Unchanged facial expression (e.g. rigid looking face with little spontaneous movement).
- Increased salivation.
- Involuntary movements of mouth, lips, or tongue.
- Looking sleepy.

### Extremities

- Tremor/involuntary movements of fingers, hands, arms, i.e. pill rolling.
- Restlessness of feet/legs.

### Trunk/posture/gait

- Pelvic gyrations.
- Rigid shuffling gait.
- Reduced arm swinging.
- Slowness and reduced spontaneity.

*General*
- Dizziness.
- Drowsiness.
- Sexual problems (ejaculatory/erectile/libido/menstrual).
- Constipation.
- Urinary problems.
- Skin problems.
- Excessive weight gain.
- Blurred vision.
- Lack of energy.

## Management of side effects and support
Side effects need to be managed in discussion with GP or whoever is prescribing medical treatment; patient's case worker and/or CMHT Commonly achieved by dose titration and/or addition of other pharmacological treatments.

## Some general advice on side effects and strategies
- *Appetite increase:* eat a low-fat, high-fibre diet; avoid sugary or fatty foods; drink low-calorie soft drinks.
- *Constipation:* increase exercise, dietary fibre, and fluid intake (📖 Constipation in adults, p. 460).
- *Dizziness:* get up slowly from lying or sitting; avoid excessively hot showers or baths; avoid alcohol, sedatives or other sedating drugs, e.g. marijuana.
- If possible take medication before bedtime (discuss with GP first).
- *Dry mouth:* ensure regular fluid intake; limit alcohol and caffeine; use sugarless gums, fruit pastilles and lollies; suck on ice cubes.
- *Sensitivity to sunburn:* avoid midday sun; regularly use sunscreen and wear a hat, sunglasses and shirt (📖 Skin cancer protection, p. 331).

Antipsychotic medications are effective in the treatment of the more troublesome symptoms of psychotic illnesses. Other treatments may be added to antipsychotic treatment rather than replacing it. These include CBT (📖 Talking therapies, p. 429), family therapy, psycho-education, and hearing voices groups.

## Related topics
📖 People with bipolar affective disorder, p. 441; 📖 People with schizophrenia, p. 443.

## Reference
[1]Day JC, Wood G, Dewey M, Bentall RP. A self-rating scale for measuring neuroleptic side-effects. Validation in a group of schizophrenic patients. *Br J Psychiatry.* 1995 May;166(5):650–3.

## Further information
Hearing Voices Network. Available at: 🖑 www.hearing-voices.org
NICE (2009). *Schizophrenia (update): core interventions in the treatment and management of schizophrenia in primary and secondary care (CG 82.).* Available at: 🖑 www.nice.org.uk/CG82
Rethink. ☎ General Enquires 0845 456 0455; National Advice Service 0208 974 6814. Available at: 🖑 www.rethink.org

# Talking therapies

Talking therapies provide an opportunity to talk in a way that assists the person to understand themselves better and then work out ways of living in a more positive, constructive way. May be used as part of a staged approach to mental health problems e.g. depression (📖 People with depression, p. 435).

There are a wide variety of talking therapies including:
- Self-help and support groups.
- Individual counselling or therapy.
- Couple or family therapy.
- Group therapy.
- Therapeutic communities.

The most common types in the NHS are counselling, CBT, and psychoanalytic or psychodynamic psychotherapy, usually provided by counsellors, psychologists, psychiatrists, or psychotherapists, but also by nurses and social workers in some services. There may be variation in local NHS availability. Anyone seeking a private therapist should ensure they belong to a recognized professional body, such as the UK Council for Psychotherapy.

## Counselling

Counselling can help with ordinary problems of living and life crises, e.g. bereavement (📖 Bereavement, p. 528), relationship problems, minor depression, disability, or loss. Can help prevent mental health problems. A key element is active and reflective listening to encourage people to think about their own difficulties and feelings and try to find ways to address them. It does not involve giving advice. Usually short term, e.g. 6 sessions of 45–50min. Counsellors may be available in general practice, local mental health services, or sometimes primary care nurses may be involved in offering brief intervention counselling or active listening sessions to particular groups, e.g. women with postnatal depression. Often also available through local voluntary sector, e.g. Cruse (bereavement counselling), Relate (relationship counselling).

## Cognitive behaviour therapy

CBT aims to help people change patterns of thinking or behaviour that are causing problems. The focus is on the thoughts, images, beliefs, and attitudes, and how this relates to the way the person behaves. This also changes how they feel. CBT has been shown to be effective for a variety of mental health problems, including depression, anxiety, panic attacks, phobias, obsessive compulsive disorder, and some eating disorders, especially bulimia. It is also thought to be helpful for people with psychoses as part of treatment. It is a structured approach, with goals for treatment and activities to try out between sessions.

*CBT resources:*
- *Beating the Blues:* for people with mild to moderate depression.
- *MoodGYM:* information, quizzes, games, and skills training to help prevent depression.
- *Living Life to the Full:* free online life skills course for people feeling distressed and their carers.
- *Fear Fighter:* for people with phobias or panic attacks. Free access if prescribed by GP in England and Wales.

## Psychoanalytical and psychodynamic therapies

Psychoanalytic/psychodynamic therapy can help people get to know themselves better, improve their relationships, and get more out of life. The therapist listens to the person's experiences, explores connections between present feelings, actions, and past events. Therapists have different approaches and different styles of working. Psychoanalytic and psychodynamic therapy often continues for a year or more. It can help people with long-term or recurring problems get to the root of their difficulties. Some evidence that it can help depression and some eating disorders (🕮 People with eating disorders, p. 431); however, some people, e.g. those who feel vulnerable or who are experiencing psychosis, can find psychotherapy unhelpful.

## Benefits and risks

- Talking therapies work for some, but not all people.
- Some people find that just knowing a therapist is there and focused on their concerns makes them feel valued.
- Some people can find it disappointing, or feel they did not relate to therapist or the therapist did not seem to understand them.
- A bad experience with a therapist can leave some people feeling worse.
- One of the most important ingredients in effective talking therapies is whether person feels they can make a good relationship with therapist.

## Further information

British Association for Counselling and Psychotherapy provides information on counselling, choosing a counsellor, and lists of private counsellors. Available at: 🔗 www.bacp.co.uk

MoodGym. Available at: 🔗 https://moodgym.anu.edu.au

Beating the Blues. Available at: 🔗 www.beatingtheblues.co.uk

Living Life to the Full. Available at: 🔗 www.llttf.com

MIND produces public information leaflets on all talking treatments. Available at: 🔗 www.mind.org.uk

Department of Health (2007). *Improving access to psychological therapies (IAPT) programme: computerised cognitive behavioural therapy (cCBT) implementation guide.* London: Department of Health.

NICE (2007). CG22: Anxiety: management of anxiety (panic disorder, with or without agoraphobia, and generalised anxiety disorder) in adults in primary, secondary and community care. Available at: 🔗 http://guidance.nice.org.uk/CG22

NICE (2011). CG123: Common mental health disorders: Identification and pathways to care. Available at: 🔗 http://publications.nice.org.uk/common-mental-health-disorders-cg123

# People with eating disorders

**Anorexia nervosa** Anorexia nervosa is a condition where there is a marked distortion of body image, low weight, and weight loss behaviours. 1:10 ratio of ♂:♀ with an equal distribution across social classes, but with mostly upper- and middle-class people seeking treatment.

## Presentation
- *Low body weight:* 15% below expected BMI (📖 Adult body mass index chart, p. 306).
- *Self-induced weight loss:* vomiting, purging, excessive exercise, use of appetite suppressants.
- *Body image distortion:* dread of fatness, imposed low weight threshold.
- *Patients with symptoms of starvation:* sensitivity to cold, bradycardia, low BP, hypothermia, constipation.
- Children with poor growth.
- Amenorrhoea, reduced sexual interest or impotence, small body frame, altered thyroid function.
- *Delayed puberty:* if the onset is prior to puberty.
- *Endocrine disorders:* involves hypothalamus, pituitary, adrenal glands.

## Causes
- *Genetic:* 6–10% of female siblings develop the condition.
- *Life events:* physical or sexual abuse can be risk factors.
- Psychodynamic:
  - *Family relationships*—may be rigid, over protective, weak parental boundaries, lack of conflict resolution.
  - *Individual*—disturbed body image due to dietary problems in early life, parents' preoccupation with food, lack of sense of identity.
  - *Analytical*—regression to childhood, fixation on the oral stage, avoidance of problems in adolescence.

## Related problems and complications

Patients who are pregnant or have diabetes are at particular risk. Everyone involved in their care should be aware of the eating disorder.

- *Mental health problems:* poor memory, irritability, depression, low self-esteem, loss of libido, reduced decision-making.
- *Physical problems:* fatigue, cold, fainting and dizziness, reduced immunity, amenorrhea, hair loss, dry skin.
- Loss of muscle mass, brittle nails.
- Can cause compromised cardiac function.
- Anaemia.
- Calluses on finger joints, eroded tooth enamel.
- Hypotension, bradycardia.
- Atrophy of the breasts.
- Swollen tender abdomen.
- Loss of sensation in extremities.

## Screening questions
- Do you worry excessively about your weight?
- Do you think you have an eating problem?

*Treatment*
- Patients are referred to specialist eating disorder clinic where available. Often treated as an outpatient, with a combined approach including:
  - *Pharmacological*—antidepressants, medication to stimulate appetite.
  - *Psychological*—family therapy (may be effective if early onset). Individual therapy, such as CBT (☐ Talking therapies, p. 429) may improve long-term outcomes.
  - *Education*—nutritional, self-help manuals.
- Hospital admission if there are serious medical problems. Compulsory admission when feeding is regarded as treatment. Ethical issues around a person's right to die, and their right to treatment.
- Offer ongoing support and information to patient and families if no ongoing 2° care. Patients should receive annual physical and mental check-up.
- Poor prognostic factors include chronic illness, late age onset, bulimic features, and anxiety when eating with others, excessive weight loss, poor childhood social adjustment, poor parental relationships, males.

## Bulimia nervosa
- Recurrent episodes of binge eating well in excess of normally accepted amounts of food.
- Inappropriate behaviours to prevent increase in weight, e.g. vomiting, use of laxatives and diuretics, appetite suppressants.
- People with bulimia can be divided into those who purge and those that just use fasting and exercise to control their weight.

*Management*
- Evidence-based self-help programmes.
- Refer to GP for assessment for antidepressants. If unsuccessful referral to eating disorders clinic or CBT for binge eating disorder (CBT-BED),
- Avoid brushing teeth after vomiting, rinse with a non-acid mouthwash.
- Where laxative abuse, advise to gradually reduce intake. *Note:* laxatives do not significantly reduce calories intake.
- Family members, including siblings, should normally be included in treatment of children and adolescents with eating disorders. Interventions may include sharing information, advice on behavioural management and facilitating communication.

## Related topics
☐ Overview of the healthy child programme, p. 146; ☐ The assessment of children, young people, and families, p. 148; ☐ Growth and nutrition 12–18yrs, p. 221; ☐ Child and adolescent mental health services, p. 229.

## Further information
Beat (formerly the Eating Disorders Association) ☎ 0845 634 1414.

NICE Core interventions in the treatments and management of anorexia nervosa bulimia nervosa and related eating disorders. Available at: ✒ http://publications.nice.org.uk/eating-disorders-cg9/implementation-in-the-nhs

# Substance misuse

Substance misuse refers to the harmful use of any substance, such as alcohol (☐ Alcohol, p. 319), street drugs, or misuse of prescribed drugs. 1 in 10 adults report using illicit drugs in the last year, most frequently abused drugs, e.g. cannabis, amphetamine, ecstasy, and cocaine, but the main ones are opioids (e.g. heroin and methadone). Likelihood of substance abuse is influenced by:

- Availability of drugs.
- Peer and social pressure.
- Vulnerable personality.

Individuals may present with inappropriate behaviour, lack of self-care, constricted or dilated pupils, and evidence of injecting, hepatitis, or HIV (☐ Human immunodeficiency virus, p. 686).

## Features of substance misuse disorder

- *Acute intoxication:* pattern of reversible physical and mental abnormalities caused by direct effect of substance, such as disinhibition, ataxia, euphoria, visual, and sensory distortion.
- *At-risk use:* where person is at ↑ risk of harming their physical or mental health. Not dependent on how much taken, but on situations and associated behaviours, e.g. cannabis use while driving.
- *Harmful use:* continuation of substance misuse despite damage to mental health, social, occupational, or familial wellbeing. Damage is denied or minimized.
- *Dependence:* includes both physical and psychological dependence.
- *Withdrawal:* where abstinence leads to features of withdrawal. Different substances have different symptoms; often the opposite of acute effects of substance. Clinically significant withdrawals are recognized in alcohol, opiates, benzodiazepines, amphetamines, and cocaine.
- *Complicated withdrawal:* development of seizures, delirium, or psychotic features.
- *Substance-induced psychotic disorder:* hallucinations and/or delusions occurring as a direct result of substance neurotoxicity. Differentiated from 1° psychotic illness by non-typical symptoms, e.g. late first presentation, prominence of non-auditory hallucinations.
- *Cognitive impairment syndromes:* reversible cognitive deficits occur during intoxication, persist in chronic misuse → dementia. Occurs in alcohol, volatile chemicals, benzodiazepines, and possibly cannabis.
- *Residual disorders:* continuing symptoms exist despite discontinuing substance.
- *Exacerbation of pre-existing disorder:* all other psychiatric illnesses, e.g. anxiety, mood disorders, and psychotic disorders may be associated with co-morbid substance misuse → an exacerbation of the patient's symptoms and a decline in the effectiveness of treatment.

### The Dependence Syndrome

Describes the features of substance dependence:

- *Primacy of drug seeking behaviour*: it is the most important thing in the person's life, taking priority over all activities and interests.
- *Narrowing the drug taking repertoire*: the person takes a single substance in preference to all others.
- *Increased tolerance to the effects of drug*: increased amounts needed for same effect; person explores other routes such as IV.
- *Loss of control of consumption*: inability to restrict consumption.
- Signs of withdrawal on attempted abstinence, and drug taking to avoid withdrawal symptoms.
- Continued drug use despite negative consequences, such as marital break-up, prison sentence, loss of job.
- Rapid reinstatement of previous pattern of drug use after abstinence.

## Aims of care

- Reduce or modify drug abusing behaviour.
- Reduce risk of other health problems. e.g. infections, depression, psychoses, threats to personal safety.
- Reduce social consequences of substance abuse, e.g. family crisis, criminality, financial crisis, and homelessness.

## Care and management

Achieved as part of MDT and should involve community substance misuse teams when available.

- Education, safer routes of administration, risks of overdose, hepatitis immunization for injecting drug users and close contacts, needles exchange.
- Treatment of dependence: provided as part of PHCT, involving community pharmacist and specialist services: work to set realistic goals, reduce dosages, and review regularly.
- Family and carer support liaison with voluntary agencies and support groups.
- Talking therapies, counselling (📖 Counselling skills, p. 123), and possible alternative therapies such as acupuncture.

## Related topics

📖 Homeless people, p. 398; 📖 Alcohol, p. 319.

## Further information

Adfam charity supporting families of drug abusers. Available at: ✍ www.adfam.org.uk

NHS Choices. Live Well: Drugs—includes video clips providing advice for parents. Available at: ✍ www.nhs.uk/livewell/drugs/Pages/Drugshome.aspx

Talk to FRANK: government run information and referral services. ☏ 0800 77 66 00. Available at: ✍ www.talktofrank.com

# Depression

Depression is the most common mental disorder in primary care. One in five people become depressed at some point. Suffering from depression feelings don't go away quickly or become so bad they interfere with their everyday life. Often undetected and often linked to long-term conditions. Characterized by:

- Feelings of unhappiness that interfere with everyday life.
- Everything is a struggle.
- Feelings of hopelessness about the future.
- Unable to see any positives in life.
- Feel apathetic and unable to participate in activities once enjoyed.

Severity of depressive symptoms varies. At its worst, depression → feelings of helplessness and lack of worth that people begin to consider suicide.

## Causes/risk factors

Multidimensional including:

- Biological, genetic.
- Stress, vulnerability.
- Social and physical reasons, e.g. health inequalities.

Patients should be screened who have:

- Past history of depression.
- Significant physical illnesses/events causing disability and other mental health problems (📖 People with dementias, p. 438; 📖 Postnatal depression, p. 393; 📖 Alcohol, p. 319; 📖 Parkinson's disease, p. 628).

## Signs and symptoms

If experiencing four or more signs, for most of the day, nearly every day, for >2 weeks, consider referral to GP or other mental health specialist.

- Tiredness and loss of energy.
- Persistent sadness.
- Loss of self-confidence and self-esteem.
- Difficulty concentrating.
- Not being able to enjoy things.
- Undue feelings of guilt or worthlessness.
- Feelings of helplessness and hopelessness.
- Sleeping problems.
- Avoiding other people, sometimes even your close friends.
- Finding it hard to function at work/college/school.
- Loss of appetite.
- Loss of sex drive and/or sexual problems.
- Physical aches and pains.
- Thinking about suicide and death.
- Self-harm.

### Screening and assessment

See the NICE guidelines for management of depression in 1° and 2° care.[1]

Two initial screening questions recommended with patients:
• During the last month, have you often been bothered by feeling down, depressed, or hopeless?
• During the last month, have you often been bothered by having little interest or pleasure in doing things?'

If patients answer yes to these, further symptoms to assess for are:
• Low energy.
• Changes in appetite, weight, or sleep pattern.
• Poor concentration.
• Feelings of guilt or worthlessness.
• Suicidal ideas.

#### Assessment tools
❶ Risk. Always ask depressed patients about suicidal ideas and intent; a common misconception is to believe asking will introduce suicidal ideas.
• Advise patients and carers to watch out for changes in mood, negativity and hopelessness, and suicidal intent.
• If a patient expresses suicidal ideas refer to GP.
• If a patient is of considerable immediate risk to self or others, refer urgently to specialist mental health service.
• Contact depressed patients not attending follow-up appointments.

❶ Some cultures do not have a term for depression and may present with physical symptoms or use culturally specific phrases like 'sadness in my heart'.

#### Treatment
The stepped care model of the NICE guidelines should be followed.

*Step 1* Recognition and assessment of depression by the GP or nurse.

*Step 2* Treatment of mild depression by primary care team and primary care mental health worker; watchful waiting—if patient does not want treatment or may recover with no intervention ask patient to return within 2wks for further assessment.

#### Sleep and anxiety management
• Encourage regular sleep pattern.
• Avoid caffeine and excess alcohol before bed.
• Advise relaxation methods, encourage structured problem-solving.
• Advise patients to exercise (📖 Exercise, p. 313).
• Consider guided self-help programmes, i.e. booklets or leaflets.
• If available, consider computerized CBT; refer for psychological therapy, e.g. brief CBT and counselling (📖 Talking therapies, p. 429).

Step 3 Treatment of moderate or severe depression by primary care team and primary care mental health worker. Antidepressant medication is usually routinely offered to patients. Key advice for patients:

• They do not cause addiction or craving.
• Patients should not suddenly stop taking their medication.
• Medication takes time to start working—as much as 4wks.
• Patients should take medication exactly as prescribed.
• Continue antidepressants for at least 6mths after remission.

*Monitor for side effects*
• Selective serotonin reuptake inhibitors (SSRIs) may cause nausea, vomiting, abdominal cramps, diarrhoea, anorexia, weight loss, headaches, anxiety, tremor, dizziness, drowsiness, sexual dysfunction.
• Tricyclic antidepressants (TCAs) may cause arrhythmias, drowsiness, dry mouth, constipation, blurred vision, urinary retention, dizziness, syncope, hyponatraemia. If symptoms persist refer to GP.

❶ Monitor risk of suicide frequently. Review patients regularly if an acute risk refer to 2° care.

*Steps 4 and 5* Treatment for patients with treatment-resistant, recurrent, atypical, and psychotic depression or at significant risk. Refer to mental health specialists, crisis teams, and in-patient care.

## Related topics
📖 Risk of suicide and deliberate self-harm, p. 445; 📖 People with dementias, p. 438; 📖 Alcohol, p. 319.

## Reference
¹NICE. Depression pathway including Depression in adults: The treatment and management of depression in adults. Available at: ✍ http://pathways.nice.org.uk/pathways/depression

## Further information
Depression Alliance. ☎ 0207 768 0123. Available at: ✍ www.depressionalliance.org
Geriatric Depression Scale public domain. Available at: ✍ www.patient.co.uk/doctor/geriatric-depression-scale-gds
Patient Health Questionnaire Depression Scale (PHQ-9) The PHQ developed by Robert L. Spitzer, et al. Available at: ✍ www.phqscreeners.com/instructions/instructions.pdf
Samaritans. ☎ 08457 909090. Available at: ✍ www.samaritans.org.uk

# People with dementias

## Dementia

A descriptive term for symptoms affecting the brain = generalized impairment of memory, intellect, and personality. >100 different kinds of dementia. Average lifespan of dementia sufferers 7yrs, but can live for 15yrs.

- Alzheimer's disease most common in people aged 65+ and can occur as early as 30yrs.
- ↑ with advancing age. 1:5 people >80yrs. By 2050 it has been estimated that there will be 1.5 million dementia sufferers in the UK.
- Prevalence ↑ in people with learning disabilities.

## Types

- Alzheimer's disease is characterized by amyloid plaques and neuro-fibrillary tangles in the brain.
- Vascular dementia = 20% of all dementias. Caused by brain damage from cerebrovascular or cardiovascular problems—usually CVA. Can also result from genetic diseases, endocarditis, or amyloid angiopathy.
- *Lewy body dementia*: fluctuating, but persistent dementia, cognitive impairment hallucinations, and Parkinsonianism.

## Signs and symptoms

Patients (carers may also seek help) may describe the following features and may have compensated for these deficiencies for some time before seeking help (also see Table 9.1).

- Steady ↓ in memory for recent events and forgetfulness.
- ↓ mental functioning e.g. getting muddled.
- Difficulty finding words.
- Feeling depressed.
- Steady ↓ in thinking, judgement, orientation, and language.
- Patient appears indifferent or subdued but can appear alert.
- ↓ in daily activities such as washing and dressing.
- Changes in personality or emotional control.
- In some cases, persecutory delusions.

All patients should be referred to Memory services for formal diagnosis, exclusion of treatable causes, ongoing specialist support, and care planning. The transition to becoming a person with dementia is difficult for both patient and carer. Continuity of care and involvement of a key worker identified as very important.

### Assessment tools

See ℜ www.alzheimers.org.uk

- *Clifton Assessment Procedures for the Elderly (CAPE):* assesses both functional ability and cognitive function.
- *Mini Mental State Examination (MMSE):* effective instrument for assessing cognitive function. *Note:* influenced by educational level.
- *Abbreviated Mental Test Score (AMTS):* quick 10-item cognitive function test. **Note: none of these tests are diagnostic.**

- *Carer Strain Index:* use scale to profile the carer, particularly when considering a request for a needs assessment under the Carers (Equal Opportunities) Act (📖 Carers assessment and support, p. 412).

Note: depression and delusional states can be confused with or coexist with dementia.

## Functional capacity

More important than a test score. Assessments of functional impairment can ↑ quality of life and ensure networks of support from social services, voluntary organizations, and specialist medical services are established.

*Points to consider*
- Continence.
- Dressing.
- Self-care.
- Cooking ability and nutrition.
- Shopping/housework.
- Degree of orientation in the home.
- Social contacts.
- Safety in the home.
- Financial capacity.

## Physical problems

Toxic confusional states and other physical disorders can coexist with and/or complicate dementia. Consider referral to the appropriate specialist:
- State of nutrition.
- Drug regimen, if any.
- Hearing.
- Eyesight.
- Mobility.
- Continence.

## Related topics

📖 Principles of working with someone with dementia, p. 417; 📖 People with depression, p. 435.

## Further information

AgeUK. Available at: ℘ www.ageuk.org.uk
Dementia Friends. Available at: ℘ www.dementiafriends.org.uk
Alzheimer's Society. Advice for all types of dementia. Available at: ℘ www.alzheimers.org.uk
DementiaUK. Admiral Nursing service ☎ 0845 257 9406. Available at: ℘ www.dementiauk.org
NHS Choices Living well with dementia. Available at: ℘ www.nhs.uk/Conditions/dementia-guide/Pages/living-well-with-dementia.aspx
NICE. Supporting People to live well with dementia (QS30) issued 2013. Available at: ℘ www.nice.org.uk
NICE. Dementia Quality Standard. Available at: ℘ http://guidance.nice.org.uk/QS1

**Table 9.1** Features of dementia at different points in its path

|  | Early changes | Later changes |
|---|---|---|
| Emotional changes | Shallowness of mood, frustration<br>Lack of emotional responsiveness and consideration of others<br>Depression and/or anxiety | Irritability and hostility<br>Aggression |
| Cognitive changes | Short-term memory deficit with particular difficulty in registration and recall of new information<br>Thinking becomes concrete with a reduced range of concerns<br>Perseveration of thoughts and actions, accompanied by repetitive speech | Language disorder. Both receptive and expressive dysphasia can occur<br>Thought process becomes fragmented, so that speech becomes disordered and fragmented<br>Psychotic features in 30–40%<br>Persecutory ideas and delusions<br>Auditory and visual hallucinations. Not mood congruent |
| Behavioural changes | Social withdrawal<br>Emotional and physical disinhibition<br>Difficulty in carrying out purposeful tasks; domestic tasks, dressing, etc.<br>Socially inappropriate behaviour, self-neglect<br>Disorientation progressively for time, place, and eventually for person | Wandering and restlessness<br>Evening and nocturnal restlessness prominent<br>Turning night into day<br>Aggression and violence |

Adapted with permission from Iliffe S, Drennan V. (2001). *Primary Care and Dementia.* London: Jessica Kingsley Publishers.

# People with bipolar affective disorder

People with bipolar affective disorder can experience recurrent attacks of depression and mania or hypomania, sometimes called manic depression, which is more common in women, with average age of onset at around 21yrs. Children of a parent with bipolar disorder have a 50% chance of developing a mental illness. There is no significant racial difference. Morbidity and mortality rates are high in terms of lost work, productivity, effects on marriage and family. 25–50% of people with bipolar affective disorder attempt suicide and 10% kill themselves.

- *Poor prognosis:* associated with poor employment history, alcohol abuse, psychotic features, and depression in between episodes of mania, being male, and not complying with medication.
- *Good prognosis:* associated with manic episodes of short duration, later age at onset, few thoughts of suicide or symptoms of psychosis, good treatment response and compliance.

The course of the illness is extremely variable. The onset can be hypo-manic, manic, mixed, or depressive; and may be followed by 5 or more years without a further episode. The length of time between episodes may then begin to diminish. People with hypomania share the same symptoms as mania, but to a lesser degree, and the condition may not significantly disrupt work or lead to social rejection.

**Table 9.2** Core features of mania

| | |
|---|---|
| Elevated mood, usually out of keeping with circumstances | |
| Increased energy, which may manifest as: | • Over-activity<br>• Pressured speech (flight of ideas)<br>• Racing thoughts<br>• Reduced need for sleep |
| Increased self-esteem, evident as: | • Over-optimistic ideation<br>• Grandiosity<br>• Reduced social inhibitions<br>• Over familiarity (may be over-amorous)<br>• Facetiousness |
| Reduced attention span or increased distractibility | |
| Tendency to engage in risk behaviour that could have serious consequences | • Preoccupation with extravagant impractical schemes<br>• Spending recklessly<br>• Inappropriate sexual encounters |
| Other behavioural manifestations: | • Excitement<br>• Irritability<br>• Aggressiveness or suspiciousness<br>• Disruption of work, usual social activities, and family life |

Reproduced from Callaghan P, Waldock H. (2006). *Oxford Handbook of Mental Health Nursing*. Oxford: OUP. By permission of Oxford University Press.

## Psychotic symptoms

In severe mania, psychotic symptoms may develop (Table 9.2):

- Grandiose ideas may become delusional with special powers or religious content.
- Suspiciousness may develop into well-formed persecutory delusions.
- Pressured speech may become so great that clear associations are lost and speech becomes incomprehensible.
- Irritability and aggression may lead to violent behaviour.
- Preoccupation with thoughts and schemes may lead to self-neglect, not eating or drinking, and living in dishevelled circumstances.
- Catatonic behaviour, also termed manic stupor.
- Total loss of insight and connection to the outside world.

## Supporting a patient, and their family or carers

It is important to have good multidisciplinary working with GP, the CMHT, and, where appropriate, the care co-ordinator for the patient (England and Wales have implemented a care programme approach (CPA)), which draws on case management to deliver care to people with mental health problems.

- *Acute episodes:* may require hospitalization and if patient is unwilling to be hospitalized may need to be reviewed under the Mental Health Act for compulsory admission.
- *Treatment:* lithium drug of choice. To avoid nephrotoxicity it is important that levels are checked weekly until the dose is constant for 4wks, then every 3mths as long as the dose is constant.
- Plasma creatinine and TFTs should be checked every 6mths.
- Patients may need encouragement to continue with drug therapy.
- Over time, patients can come to recognize situations and events that can trigger episodes of mania or depression. Encourage them to seek help and review of treatment when they think they are at risk.
- Talking therapies (📖 Talking therapies, p. 429) may be helpful. Ensure both patient and family have adequate social support and access to disability benefits (📖 Benefits for illness, disability and carers, p. 795).
- Living with someone with bipolar disorder can be very stressful. Give particular attention to individual needs of family, children, and carers of sufferers (📖 Carers assessment and support, p. 412).
- Patients must inform DVLA.

## Related topics

📖 People with depression, p. 435; 📖 Talking therapies, p. 429; 📖 Alcohol, p. 319.

## Further information

Callaghan P, Waldock H. (2006). *Oxford Handbook of Mental Health*. Oxford: Oxford University Press.
MDF—The bipolar organization. Available at: ℘ www.mdf.org.uk
MIND. Available at: ℘ www.mind.org.uk
NHS Choices. Bipolar Disorder. Available at: ℘ www.nhs.uk/conditions/Bipolar-disorder
NICE. Bipolar disorder: The management of bipolar disorder in adults, children and adolescents, in primary and secondary care CG38. Available at: ℘ http://publications.nice.org.uk/bipolar-disorder-cg38

# People with schizophrenia

Schizophrenia is a highly variable disorder characterized by disordered perception, disordered thoughts (hallucinations and delusions), and withdrawal of the individual's interest from other people and the world.

Schizophrenia is one of the most common serious mental health conditions. About 1 in 100 people will experience schizophrenia in their lifetime, with many continuing to lead normal lives. Schizophrenia is most often diagnosed between the ages of 15 and 35yrs. Men and women are equally affected. There is no single test for schizophrenia. Often diagnosed after an assessment by a psychiatrist. A form of psychosis, it typically develops in the late teens or early twenties, although males tend to have an earlier onset than females.

- *Mortality:* suicide is the most common cause of premature death, accounting for 10–38% of all deaths.
- Genetic factors.
- *Environmental factors:* complications of pregnancy, delivery, and neonatal period; delayed walking and neurodevelopmental difficulties; early social services contact, and disturbed childhood behaviour.

The symptoms of schizophrenia are divided into positive (new symptoms) and negative (loss of a previous function) symptoms (see Box 9.1).

## Box 9.1 Symptoms of schizophrenia

### Positive symptoms
- Delusions
- Hallucinations

### Negative symptoms
- Loss of motivation
- Loss of social awareness
- Flattened mood
- Poor abstract thinking

### Other symptoms
- Thought disorder
- Agitation
- Depression
- Poor sleep
- Cognitive impairment

The following symptoms have a special significance as they occur often in schizophrenia and more rarely in other disorders (sometimes referred to as first-rank symptoms):
- *Auditory hallucinations:*
  - Voices heard arguing.
  - Thought echo.
  - Running commentary on what the person is doing.

- *Delusions or thought interference:*
  - Thought insertion.
  - Thought withdrawal.
  - Thought broadcasting.
- *Delusions of control:*
  - Passivity of affect.
  - Passivity of impulse.
  - Passivity of volitions.
  - Somatic passivity.
- *Delusional perceptions:*
  - A 1° delusion of any context reported by the person as having arisen from a normal perception.

## Prognosis

- Approximately 15–20% of first episodes will not occur again.
- Few people will remain in employment.
- 52% will be without psychotic symptoms in the last 2yrs.
- 52% are without negative symptoms.
- 55% show good/fair social functioning.

## Supporting patients, families, and carers

Patients will be under the care of a psychiatrist and all care should be in liaison with CMHT and, where appropriate, the care coordinator for the patient (England and Wales have implemented a care programme approach which draws on case management to deliver care to people with mental health problems).

- Antipsychotics treatment of choice for sufferers. Many have side effects. Long-acting depot injections often used in maintenance therapy. Administered with Z track technique. There is a reduced risk of relapse if medication is maintained.
- Encourage healthy lifestyle and discourage use of illicit drugs.
- Patients may benefit from CBT and related talking therapies.
- Patients must inform DVLA.
- CMHT regularly review patients, including review of social support available for patients and carers, addressing individual needs of family, children, and carers who are living with and supporting patients.
- Many areas now have crisis intervention teams to provide a rapid community-based response to out-of-hours crisis and prevent hospital admission.

## Related topics

📖 Risk of suicide and deliberate self-harm, p. 445; 📖 Social support, p. 24; 📖 Carers assessment and support, p. 412; 📖 Benefits and support, p. 789; 📖 Talking therapies, p. 429.

## Further information

Callaghan P, Waldock H. (2006). *Oxford Handbook of Mental Health*. Oxford: Oxford University Press.
Rethink (formerly National Schizophrenia Fellowship). Available at: ℘ www.rethink.org

# Risk of suicide and deliberate self-harm

Suicide is the most common cause of death in ♂ <35yrs. Suicide rate can be reduced by early recognition of people at risk

## Aims of risk assessment

- *Establish if there is ongoing suicidal intent:* such as a continuing wish to die, sense of hopelessness, or ambivalence about survival.
- *Establish if there is evidence of mental illness:* e.g. depressive illnesses or alcohol dependence.
- *Establish if there are any non-mental health issues to address:* e.g. emotional problems, family and/or relationship difficulties, school, employment, debt, or legal problems.

## Assessing suicide risk

Consider:
- History.
- Information from relatives and carers.
- Ideation/mental state.
- Intent.
- Planning.
- Person's awareness of risk.
- Benefits and harm from risk.
- Formulation.

### Predictors of suicide risk

- History of self-harm.
- Depression.
- Dual diagnosis.
- Inpatient care.
- Loss of contact with mental health services.
- Within 1wk of discharge from psychiatric in-patient care.
- Member of an ethnic minority.
- Homelessness.

### People at higher risk of suicide

- ♂ >65yrs, ♂ 15–30yrs.
- Separated, widowed, divorced.
- Live alone, socially isolated, or loss of supports.
- Poor physical health.
- Poor mental health.
- Substance misuse.
- Previous episodes of self-harm.
- Suicide by relative.
- Hopelessness, despair, loss of interest.
- Mild learning difficulty.

## Deliberate self-harm

Deliberate non-fatal act committed in the knowledge that it was harmful, e.g. drug overdose, poisoning. Self-harm is often aimed at changing a situation (e.g. where there has been a relationship breakdown), a communication of distress/cry for help or a genuine failed suicide attempt.

Common misconception that asking about suicidal intention can plant the idea into the patient's mind and make it more likely.

### Useful questions if you consider someone to be at risk

- Do you feel you have a future?
- Do you feel that life is no longer worth living?
- Do you ever feel completely hopeless?
- Do you ever feel you would be better off dead?
- Have you ever made any plans to take your life?
- Have you ever attempted to take your life?
- What prevents you doing it?
- Have you made any arrangements for your affairs after your death?

Hopelessness is a good predictor for subsequent and immediate risk of suicide. Any concerns about a patient should be shared with their GP and relevant primary health care team members.

Suicide risk is high when:

- There is direct statement of intent, severe mood change, hopelessness, alcohol or drug dependence, abnormal personality. Refer to GP for admission to ED as psychiatric emergency. May involve using the Mental Health Act for compulsory admission if voluntary admission declined.
- If risk of suicide believed to be lower (decision should be made as part of MDT), then arrange for someone to stay with patient until follow-up and remove all potentially harmful drugs. Community Mental Health Team should be involved.

People who have attempted suicide/self-harmed should be treated with the same care, respect, and privacy as any other patient.

### Support of those bereaved through suicide

Those bereaved following a suicide need extra support to help deal with the death and possible stigma. Self-help groups or counselling may help.

### Related topics

📖 People with depression, p. 435; 📖 Bereavement, grief, and coping with loss, p. 528.

### Further information

Callaghan P, Waldock H. (2006). *Oxford Handbook of Mental Health Nursing.* Oxford: Oxford University Press.

NHS Choices. Suicide. Available at: ℘ http://www.nhs.uk/Livewell/Suicide

NICE. *CG16 Self harm: the short term physical and psychological management and secondary prevention of self harm in primary and secondary care.* Available at: ℘ www.nice.org.uk/CG16

Papyrus Confidential Young Suicide Prevention Advice. ☎ HOPELineUK 0800 068 41 41. SMS: 07786 209697. Email: pat@papyrus-uk.org

Samaritans 24-hr emotional support. ☎ 08457 909 090.

Self injury and related issues. Available at: ℘ www.siari.co.uk

# Chapter 10

# Care provision

# Urinary incontinence in women

Involuntary loss of urine is a common problem with 38% ♀ admitting to having had symptoms of incontinence over a 12mth period. Prevalence of daily incontinence ↑ with age:
- 12.2% in women 60–64yrs.
- 20.9% in women 85yrs+.

## Evidence of a hereditary link

♀ with incontinence often have lower self-esteem and physical and emotional health compared to those who do not have continence problems. Anxiety and depression often linked to continence problems. Types of urinary incontinence experienced by ♀:
- Overactive bladder.
- Stress urinary incontinence (see 🕮 p. 451).
- Mixed urinary incontinence, i.e. leakage associated with urgency and also with exertion, effort, sneezing, or coughing.

## Assessment of problem

- Ask ♀ about severity of incontinence, extent to which it affects everyday life, history, specific symptoms, and her desire for treatment.
- Mobility and access to toilets.
- Consider menopausal status, atrophic vaginal changes.
- General health issues obesity, fitness, smoking.
- Level of fluid intake.
- Consider possibility of constipation.
- Review medication some drugs exacerbate symptoms, e.g. diuretics, antihistamines.
- Pelvic floor assessment (🕮 Stress urinary incontinence, p. 451).
- For people with dementias include any family carers in identifying the problem(s) which may be related to cognition, behavioural, or psychological.

## Investigations

- Test urine for UTI.
- Ask ♀ to complete a frequency and volume chart for 3 days (see ℘ www.bladderandbowelfoundation.org for example of chart).
- Refer to continence specialist service/bladder and bowel care specialist service for bladder ultrasound to ensure voiding to completion and ♀ is not in retention.
- Consider referral to urodynamics service for possibly invasive tests if there is a complex history of previous vaginal surgery, neurological problems, and/or the type of incontinence is uncertain.

## Overactive bladder/urge incontinence

Occurs when bladder contracts unintentionally; cause often unknown. Can occur with MS, dementia, Parkinson's, and local irritation, e.g. infection. Characterized by frequency and an overwhelming desire to void. May experience nocturia (voiding more than once overnight). Symptoms can be antagonized if women smoke or are obese. Evidence is unclear about the negative effects of caffeine and fizzy drinks, but diet drinks and sweeteners should be avoided (see 📖 Stress urinary incontinence, p. 451).

*Care and management*

• Treat UTI (📖 p. 707).
• Advise and address any constipation (📖 Constipation in adults, p. 457).
• Advise on healthy diet and smoking cessation (📖 Smoking cessation, p. 315).
• Advise overweight to reduce weight as this can lead to increases in symptoms especially at night.

Discuss the possible benefits of ↓ diet drinks, sweeteners, caffeine, and fizzy drinks.

• Advise on bladder re-training.
• Suggest/prescribe topical HRT (BNF 7.2.1) for atrophic changes in vagina (📖 Menopause, p. 323).
• Pelvic floor exercises (📖 Stress urinary incontinence, p. 451).
• Consider provision of incontinence pads for those with intractable problems according to local guidance (📖 Continence products, p. 468).
• If symptoms do not respond refer for specialist assessment and treatment, e.g. drug therapy.
• Possibilities of relapse so review and reassess every 3–4mths.

## Related topics

📖 Stress incontinence, p. 451; 📖 Continence products, p. 468; 📖 Menopause, p. 323; 📖 Constipation in adults, p. 460.

### Bladder training programme: advice for patients

Aim to establish a normal pattern of bladder emptying of between 6–8 times a day by increasing the length of time of holding urine so bladder is trained to fill and stay relaxed.

Drink 3–4 pints (2L) of liquid daily—avoiding coffee, tea, cola, hot chocolate, and alcohol.

Based on the recorded frequency of passing urine set a target that lengthens the time before going to the toilet to pass urine and increases the volume passed, e.g.
• Week 1: each time you feel the urge, hold urine and wait before going to the toilet for 5min longer.
• Week 2: hold for 10min.
• Week 3: hold for 15min.
• Week 4: hold for 20min.
• Week 5: hold for 25min.
• Week 6: hold for 30min.

The urge feeling is the first sign that your bladder is filling up, but it will subside. When going to the toilet, do not rush. Sit down on the seat, do not hover over it, and do not push or strain to empty. Strategies that can help control the initial urge to pass urine include:
• Sitting on a hard seat or tightly rolled towel to put pressure on pelvic floor muscles.
• 5 quick squeezes of the pelvic floor muscles can help to manage the feeling of urgency.

### Further information

Alzheimer's Society Fact Sheet. Coping with Incontinence. Available at: ℘ www.alzheimers.org.uk/site/scripts/documents_info.php?documentID=136
Bladder and Bowel Foundation. Confidential Helpline ☎ 0845 3450165. Available at: ℘ www.bladderandbowelfoundation.org
EVIDEM-C. Add on continence assessment tool and information for people with dementia and their carers. Available at: ℘ www.evidem.org.uk
NICE. Guideline Urinary Incontinence: the management of urinary incontinence in women. CG40. Available at: ℘ www.nice.org.uk/cg40

# Stress urinary incontinence

See 📖 Urinary incontinence, p. 448 in women. Loss of urine (often small amounts) upon physical exertion (cough, exercise). Occurs in 30% ♀ and for up to 10% ♀ it is a significant problem limiting activities; rare in ♂ except post-prostatectomy. Caused by incompetent urethral sphincter mechanism (e.g. following childbirth, surgery, pelvic floor weakness, hormone deficiency, ageing).

## Assessment

- Symptoms, history, and patient's desire for treatment.
- Childbirth (number, mode of delivery, birth weight).
- Menopausal status, atrophic vaginal changes.
- Obesity, fitness, smoking.
- Pelvic floor strength, voluntary contraction.

## Investigations

- Test urine for UTI.
- Fluid-volume chart for 3 days.

Invasive tests not indicated unless complex history of previous vaginal surgery.

## Care and management

- Advise on ↓ weight, smoking cessation (📖 Smoking cessation, p. 315), and management of constipation (📖 Constipation in adults, p. 460).
- Pelvic muscle exercises (see Box 10.1). Exercises should achieve optimum results in 3–6mths.
- If simple exercises do not work, consider referral to continence advisor or physiotherapists, specialist bladder and bowel care specialists for biofeedback or electrical stimulation.
- *Vaginal cones:* small graduated weights placed in vagina, intention to use pelvic floor muscles to keep cone in place. Little evidence to support effectiveness, but may help ♀ when doing pelvic floor exercises.
- Local HRT for atrophic changes in vagina.
- If symptoms severe, life-limiting, and do not respond to exercises discuss with patients if they want surgical referral. Surgery may be minimally invasive (e.g. tension free vaginal tape (TVT) or via abdominal incision or laparoscopic (e.g. colposuspension)). Good success rates, but some morbidity (e.g. voiding difficulties).

## Prevention

Management of labour; lifelong pelvic muscle exercises; ↓ obesity and smoking.

## Specialist support

Every area should have a continence advisor/nurse specialist (specialist bladder and bowel care services) practitioners and patients can access for specialist assessment and advice.

## Box 10.1  Pelvic floor exercises

### Exercise 1

- Tighten the muscles around the anus, vagina, and urethra and lift up as if trying to stop passing urine and wind at the same time.
- Hold for as long as possible. Build up to a maximum of 10sec—rest for 4sec repeat to a maximum of 10 contractions.

Advise ♀ to try and isolate their pelvic floor as much as possible by
- Pulling in the abdominal muscles.
- Not squeezing legs together.
- Not holding breath or tightening buttocks.

Practise maximum number of contractions up to 6x a day.

### Exercise 2

- Practise quick steady contractions, drawing in the pelvic floor muscles and holding for 1sec before releasing muscles.
- Aim for strong muscle tightening with each contraction up to maximum of 10x.

Advise to do 1 set of slow contractions (exercise 1) followed by 1 set of quick contractions (exercise 2), 6x each day.

Adapted from Continence Foundation advice.

## Related topics

📖 Urinary incontinence in women, p. 448; 📖 Menopause, p. 323; 📖 Continence products, p. 468; 📖 Constipation in adults, p. 460.

## Further information

Bladder and Bowel Foundation. Confidential Helpline ☎ 0845 3450165. Available at: ℅ www.bladderandbowelfoundation.org

NICE Guideline. Urinary Incontinence: the management of urinary incontinence in women. CG40. Available at: ℅ www.nice.org.uk/cg40

# Urinary incontinence in men

Incontinence is the involuntary loss of urine that is a social or hygienic problem. 1:3 seek help at first sign of problem, 1:3 later, and 1:3 suffer in silence. Opportunistic questioning can reveal problems. Causes:
- Outflow obstruction (enlarged prostate, tumour, neurogenic).
- Under-active detrusor muscle.
- Sphincter damage (e.g. post-prostatectomy).
- Functional incontinence arising from other problems: e.g. toileting difficulties (physical immobility or cognitive impairment/confusion).
- Neurological problems (e.g. stroke, MS, PD, spinal cord injury).
- Constipation/faecal impaction.
- *Note:* some drugs can exacerbate incontinence, e.g. anticholinergics, diuretics, antihistamines, sedatives, and hypnotics.

## Assessment

(See 📖 Urinary incontinence in women, p. 448.)
- Obtain history of symptoms (urgency, urge or stress leakage, nocturia, voiding difficulties, constant dribbling).
- Check urine for infection.
- Discuss with patient their own goals for treatment.
- Ability to self toilet whether any co-existing problems/morbidities.
- Fluid volume chart for 3 days.
- Refer to specialist nurses or community nursing team for bladder ultrasound to assess if having voiding problems or retention.

## Care and management

- Treat reversible causes, e.g. altering pattern of medication, 📖 UTI, p. 707; 📖 Constipation in adults, p. 457.
- Accessible toileting advise on aids.
- For post micturition dribble refer to continence/bladder and bowel care specialists (see 📖 Stress urinary incontinence, p. 451).
- Patients with retention refer to GP for review and referral for flow rate and urological assessment, possibly intermittent catheterization to be taught by specialist services.
- Patients post prostatectomy may need specialist review.
- Patients with an overactive bladder/urge incontinence referral for bladder retraining to continence/specialist bladder and bowel care services (described in 📖 Urinary incontinence in women, p. 448). Anti-muscarinics may also be used.
- Psychological support for distress and embarrassment. *Note:* carer may not be appropriate person to offer support.
- Provide male appliances or absorbent products according to needs and patient's wishes (📖 Continence products, p. 468).

## Key reference text

NICE (2010). *The management of lower urinary tract symptoms in men.* Available at: ℘ www.nice. org.uk/nicemedia/live/12984/48575/48575.pdf

## Further information

Bladder and Bowel Foundation. Confidential Helpline ☏ 0845 3450165. Available at: ℘ www. bladderandbowelfoundation.org

# Urinary catheter care

## Indwelling catheters

Used as a last resort due to complications including trauma, urinary tract infection, stricture formation, encrustation, urethral perforation, and carcinoma of the bladder. Not advised by International Continence Society for people with dementias due to additional risks of trauma and infection due to non-comprehension and trying to remove. See Table 10.1 for types.

### Indications for using catheter

- Urethral obstruction with urinary retention.
- Where it will enhance QoL or independence.
- Occasionally if important to protect healing wounds, e.g. pressure sores.
- Patient is terminally ill and it increases their comfort.
- Intermittent catheterization is an alternative for some, especially patients with neurogenic retention, e.g. MS.

**Table 10.1** Choice of types

|  | Lengths | Gauges | Balloon sizes |
|---|---|---|---|
| ♂ | Standard 40–45cm | 10–22Ch | 10–30mL |
| ♀ | 20–26cm | 10–22Ch | 10–30mL |
| Paediatric | 30–31cm | size 6–10Ch | 3–5mL |

- ❶ Only standard length catheters should be used for male catheterizations.
- Obese or chair-bound females may require standard length catheters.
- ❶ Use smallest size which provides adequate drainage—sizes 12–16Ch usually adequate for adult, seek guidance if considering larger sizes.
- ❶ 30mL balloons only used post urological surgery or when bladder neck damage present (not routinely).

### Catheter materials and coatings

The material and coating determines time it can remain *in situ*.
- Latex or plastic up to 14 days.
- Teflon-coated latex up to 28 days.
- Hydrogel coated up to 12wks.
- All silicone up to 12wks.
- Silicone elastomer-coated up to 12wks.

❶ Consideration should be given to patients sensitive to latex products. Also consider supra-pubic rather than urethral (↑ comfort, non-interference with sexual activity ↓ infection rates).

All catheters and bags available on prescription.

*Inserting an adult indwelling catheter*
- Check local policy regarding catheterization of females by male nurses.
- Check local policy regarding circumstances nurses can undertake male catheterizations, e.g. often prohibited if patient is in acute retention, or history of pelvic trauma, and when haematuria present.
- Offer chaperone (📖 Chaperones, p. 79) and use aseptic technique.

As many female nurses have little experience of male catheterization, procedure is outlined.

Retract foreskin if present, cleanse urethral meatus with soap and water and dry thoroughly.

Instil lubricating gel from single-use container into urethra and massage gel along male urethra. ❶ Caution with local anaesthetic products in patients taking anti arrhythmic medication, patients with cardiac conditions, hepatic insufficiency, and epilepsy.
- Allow 5min to elapse.
- Hold penis vertically and gently introduce catheter into urethra for 15–25cm until urine flows (if resistance is felt at the external sphincter, increase traction on penis slightly and apply steady, gentle pressure on catheter whilst asking patient to gently strain as if passing urine).
- When urine begins to flow, advance catheter almost to its bifurcation.
- Inflate balloon with sterile water or integral air bulb. ❶ Never inflate balloon until catheter is fully inserted into bladder.
- Observe for pain, discomfort, and bleeding.
- Gently withdraw catheter until slight resistance felt and connect catheter to closed drainage system, then secure drainage system.
- Return foreskin to original position.
- Document type of catheter (size, length, material, balloon size, batch, and manufacturer), lubricant instilled, problems negotiated, colour and consistency of urine, and patient's condition following procedure.

## Drainage and support systems
The type of drainage and support system depends on individual assessment.
- *Intermittent drainage:* by catheter valves give greater independence, but are inappropriate with detrusor over activity, poor bladder capacity, ureteric reflux, or renal impairment.
- *Continuous drainage systems:* either body worn systems or suspensory systems and larger capacity, night drainage bags.
  - Care should be taken to prevent infection entering the closed system.
  - Non-ambulant or confined to bed patients can have a sterile, drainable, 2L night bag and emptied as required.
  - Body worn systems should use a non-drainable night bag, discarded in the morning.
  - Drainage bags incorporating a sample port removes the need to break the closed system when obtaining a urine sample.
  - Bags should be changed weekly.

## Blockages

- *Encrustation:* caused by formation of calcium phosphate and magnesium ammonium phosphate salts when the urine becomes alkaline due to urease-forming bacteria.
- Prevention may involve acidification by drinking fluids with citric acid in such as lemonade or systemic agents such as ascorbic acid (vitamin C).

## Management

Advice to patients and carers:

- Advise a fluid intake 1.5–2L a day.
- Avoid constipation (📖 Constipation in adults, p. 457).
- Avoid kinking of tubing and keep catheter bag below bladder.
- *Meatal care:* gentle soap and water bd.
- *Emptying bag:* high risk of contamination and subsequent infection—encourage careful hand hygiene (see NICE[1] guidance on infection control).

If no problems with blockage catheter can be *in situ* 3m.

### Problems

- *People who frequently block their catheters:*↓ risk of blockage—acidify urine by encouraging vitamin C and cranberry juice, regular saline washouts, and planned catheter changes.
- *Infection:* all long-term catheters become infected. Treat symptoms only e.g. fever.
- *Leaking catheters:* try smaller catheter and/or smaller balloon size.
- Bag can be changed every 5–7 days or more often if discoloured, damaged, odourous, or build up of sediment. Also change following catheter change or instilling of maintenance solution.

## Valves

Catheter valve can be used in place of drainage bag:

- Bladder drained intermittently.
- Good for patients who can recognize when bladder is full, can operate a valve and with a minimum bladder capacity of 200mL.
- Catheter valves should be changed every 5–7 days.

> A spigot must never be used in place of a catheter valve.

## Related topics

📖 Urinary incontinence in women, p. 448; 📖 Urinary incontinence in men, p. 453.

## Key reference texts

Dougherty, Lister S. (eds) (2011). *The Royal Marsden Hospital Manual of Clinical Nursing Procedures,* 11th edn. Chichester: Wiley Blackwell.

Getliffe K, Dolman M. (2007). *Promoting continence a clinical and research resource.* London: Elsevier.

Catheter care RCN guidance for nurses (2012). Available at: ℘ www.rcn.org.uk/_data/assets/pdf_file/0018/157/003237.pdf

## Reference

[1]NICE (2012). CG139 Infection control. Available at: ℘ http://guidance.nice.org.uk/CG139

## Further information

Bladder and Bowel Foundation: Confidential Helpline ☎ 0845 3450165.
Available at: ℘ www.bladderandbowelfoundation.org

# Constipation in adults

3 million GP consultations pa; 10% DNs time spent remedying problems; NHS spends £45m pa on laxatives. Myths abound. (See 📖 Faecal incontinence, p. 462.)

## Definition

Constipation <3 stools per week and/or straining, hard stools, or sense of incomplete evacuation at least 25% of the time. Associated symptoms:
- Abdominal discomfort, pain, and bloating.
- Lethargy and malaise.
- 'Spurious diarrhoea'/overflow incontinence in frail impacted patients.

## Prevalence

5–10% population. 50%+ in care homes and neurological patients. More people believe that they are constipated than fit the definition.

## Causes

May co-exist with:
- Slow colonic transit.
- Evacuation difficulty.

Underlying causes include:
- Poor diet (amount, frequency, fibre), low fluid intake, immobility.
- Local anal pathology (e.g. haemorrhoids).
- Neurological disorders affecting sensory or motor function (e.g. spinal cord injury, multiple sclerosis, spina bifida, any neuropathy).
- Pregnancy.
- Endocrine disorders (e.g. hypothyroidism, DM, hypercalcaemia).
- Difficulty with toilet access.
- Drug side effects (e.g. analgesics, especially opioids).
- Idiopathic (may be associated with laxative abuse, anorexia).

## Nursing assessment

Need adequate privacy and time for patient to relax. Bowel diary and symptom questionnaire useful aid. Should include:
- History of the problem and former bowel habit.
- Current symptoms, severity, and frequency.
- Diet (especially fibre) and fluid intake.
- Medication (include laxative history) and other medical conditions.
- Effects of symptoms and limitations to lifestyle.
- Co-existence of faecal incontinence.
- Ability to use the toilet independently.
- Availability and involvement of carers.
- *General observation:* patient's mobility and ability to self-toilet.
- Digital rectal examination for presence and consistency of stool when faecal impaction is suspected.

❶ Consider possibility of serious bowel pathology (rectal bleeding, unexplained change in bowel habit, anaemia, or weight loss) → referral to GP for further investigations.

## Management

Always try non-drug options first.
- Reassurance and patient education.
- Ensure toilet is accessible (supporting feet on footstool may help evacuation).
- Address diet, fluids, mobility as possible.
- Eat regularly and do not skip meals.
- ↑ fibre slowly and mix types.
- Unrefined bran can = bloating, mineral malabsorption, and impaction.
- 1.5L fluids per day (but excessive will not help).
- *Immobile:* passive exercise or abdominal massage may help.
- Regular toileting pattern after breakfast or evening meal (capitalize on the gastro-colic response).
- Change constipating medications if feasible.
- Consider short-term laxatives or evacuants to establish a pattern.
- Refer for specialist investigations if initial management fails.

## Laxatives

Greatly over-used. Most become ↓ effective with continuous use. Abdominal discomfort and bloating may be 2° to laxatives. Re-evaluate regularly. See Fig. 10.1.
- Start with low dose of cheap preparation, discontinue ASAP.
- Evacuation difficulty/hard stool: use softener or rectal preparation.
- Slow transit: use a stimulant.
- If long-term use is likely, find several and rotate.
- Newer prokinetic agents which stimulate the enteric nerves, and thus peristalsis, directly are reported to help with severe constipation in women, but long-term results are awaited.

## Rectal preparations

See 📖 Constipation in adults, enemas and suppositories, and manual evacuation, p. 460.

## Rectal irrigation

Irrigation using tap water is becoming more widely used as equipment to allow patients to self-administer is available on prescription. Evidence for use sparse at present, except in patients after spinal cord injury.

## Related topics

📖 Faecal incontinence, p. 462; 📖 Palliative care in the home, p. 509.

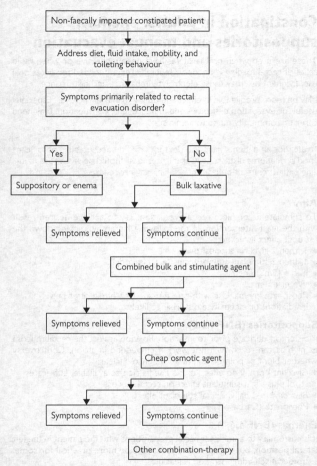

**Fig. 10.1** Decision-making flow chart for use of laxatives.

Reproduced from the Royal College of Physicians (2002). The use and abuse of laxatives. In: Potter J, Norton C, Cottenden A (eds). *Bowel care for older people*. London: RCP. With permission from the Royal College of Physicians, London.

## Further information

Bladder and Bowel Foundation. Confidential Helpline ☎ 0845 3450165. Available at: 🖰 www. bladderandbowelfoundation.org

Müller-Lissner SA, Kamm MA, Scarpignato C, *et al.* (2005). Myths and misconceptions about chronic constipation. *Am J Gastroenterol* **100**(1): 232–42.

NHS Choices Constipation. Available at: 🖰 www.nhs.uk/Conditions/Constipation/Pages/ Introduction.aspx

# Constipation in adults: enemas, suppositories and manual evacuation

These are used when oral laxatives have been ineffective or when rapid relief of rectal loading is needed. Generally recommended for occasional use, frequent use may cause electrolyte imbalance and disturbance.

May be more predictable in effect and timing than oral laxatives. Especially useful for evacuation difficulties and in neurogenic constipation. May need carer or community nurse to administer.

*Note:* not all patients have the dexterity or find acceptable, and/or can find procedures distressing. Careful attention should be given to obtaining patient consent before undertaking any procedure.

## Aim

To stimulate a complete rectal evacuation. Try to achieve desired result with the least intervention, in the following hierarchy, moving down the list until effect achieved:
- 1, then 2 glycerin suppositories.
- 1, then 2 stimulant suppositories (e.g. bisacodyl).
- Micro (5mL) enema.
- Water enema.
- Phosphate enema. Use with care if tissue fragile (e.g. after pelvic irradiation) or electrolyte disturbance likely.

## Suppositories (BNF 1.6.2)

Moisten or lubricate prior to insertion. Position against the rectal mucosa as high as can reach (will not work if embedded in stool). Controversy whether blunt or pointed end first, evidence unclear:
- *Glycerin:* 1 prn. If no effect, use 2. Paediatric size available. Lubricates stool plus slight stimulant effect on rectal mucosa.
- *Bisacodyl:* 1–2 daily. Rectal stimulant effect.
- Phosphate (Carbalax®).

## Enemas (BNF 1.6.4)

It is customary to administer rectal preparations with the patient in the left lateral position, but sitting on the toilet may be more practical for some. Consider if self-administration is feasible.
- *Micro enemas (5mL):* sodium citrate.
- *Tap water enemas:* use 50–200mL warm tap water.
- *Arachis oil (peanut oil) enema:* as softener for hard stool. Do not use in nut allergic patients.
- *Phosphate enemas:* 120mL. Acts osmotically. Also as preparation prior to flexible sigmoidoscopy. Use with care if tissue fragile (e.g. after pelvic irradiation) or electrolyte disturbance likely (hyper-phosphataemia and perforation are RARE, but have been reported).

## Manual evacuation

Some constipated patients find this helpful, especially those with neurological disorders and associated faecal incontinence (e.g. spinal cord injury, spina bifida). Also indicated with faecal impaction and when other bowel emptying techniques have failed.

- Can be a very distressing procedure for patients.
- Check for abnormalities that might contraindicate procedure, e.g. prolapse, anal lesions, haemorrhoids.
- Lubricate the finger with gel, if not a regular procedure consider using lignocaine gel on finger and anus.
- If stool is a solid mass push finger into the centre, split it and remove small sections until none remains.
- Encourage patient to assist with valsalva manoeuvre.
- *Before and during procedure check pulse:* stop if it changes or drops.
- In spinal patients consider risk of autonomic dysreflexia (where BP rises very rapidly) observe for headache, flushing, sweating, hypertension and stop procedure immediately.

## Digital stimulation

Possible to stimulate a defecation reflex voluntarily by stimulation of the anus or anal sphincter in spinal injury patients if lesion above the cauda equine.

## Related topics

&#x1F4D6; Constipation in adults, p. 457; &#x1F4D6; Urinary incontinence in women, p. 448; &#x1F4D6; Urinary incontinence in men, p. 453; &#x1F4D6; Spinal injury, p. 471; &#x1F4D6; Hand hygiene, p. 94; &#x1F4D6; Managing health-care waste, p. 105.

## Further information

Ness W, Hibberts F, Miles S, et al (2008). *Bowel Care, Including Digital Rectal Examination and Manual Removal of Faeces: RCN Guidance for Nurses*. London: RCN.

# Faecal incontinence in adults

## Definition
Faecal incontinence (FI) is the involuntary loss of stool which is a social or hygienic problem. Anal incontinence is used to denote involuntary loss of stool or flatus.

## Prevalence
5% of community-dwelling adults, 1% having a regular and life-limiting problem. >25% in nursing home care. It is experienced as very embarrassing and many are reluctant to report symptoms. ❶ Active case-finding is very important.

## Causes
FI is a symptom not a diagnosis. Results from any combination of:
- Anal sphincter disruption or weakness, e.g. obstetric trauma.
- Iatrogenic injury during anal surgery.
- Impalement injuries.
- Idiopathic anal sphincter degeneration.
- Neurological disorders affecting sensory or motor function (e.g. spinal cord injury, multiple sclerosis, spina bifida, any neuropathy).
- Severe constipation with faecal impaction and 'overflow spurious diarrhoea' (frail and dependent people).
- Local anal pathology (haemorrhoids, prolapse, skin tags).
- Difficulty with toilet access, drug side effects.

## Typical symptoms
- Urgency and urge FI (usually external sphincter disruption).
- Passive faecal soiling (usually internal sphincter disruption).
- Diarrhoea, loose stool or intestinal hurry (inflammation, diet, anxiety, irritable bowel syndrome) (📖 Irritable bowel syndrome, p. 663).

## Nursing assessment
See Box 10.2.

Takes time, need adequate privacy for patient to relax. Bowel diary and symptom questionnaires give added information. Include:
- History of the problem and former bowel habit.
- Current symptoms, severity, and frequency (see Box 10.2).
- Diet (especially fibre) and fluid (especially caffeine) intake.
- Medication and other medical conditions.
- Effects of symptoms and limitations to lifestyle.
- Co-existence of urinary incontinence (about 50%).
- Mobility and ability to use the toilet independently.
- Availability and involvement of carers.

❶ Important to consider possibility of serious bowel pathology (rectal bleeding, unexplained change in bowel habit, anaemia, or weight loss) referral → GP for further investigation.

## Management

- Aim = firm loose stool (e.g. diet, antidiarrhoeals, loperamide 2–16mg daily).
- ↓ caffeine intake.
- Make sure toilet is accessible.
- Pelvic muscle exercises (☐ Stress urinary incontinence, p. 451).
- Bowel retraining for urgency (urge resistance, practice deferment).
- Address constipation if present.
- If initial management fails. Refer to GP for referral for specialist investigations.

---

### Box 10.2  Checklist for faecal incontinence symptom assessment

- Onset of symptoms.
- Usual bowel habit.
- Changes in bowel habit.
- Stool consistency (Bristol stool form scale).
- Amount and frequency of faecal incontinence.
- Urgency or urge faecal incontinence.
- Passive soiling.
- Difficulty wiping clean after toilet.
- Nocturnal bowel symptoms.
- Abdominal pain and bloating.
- Evacuation difficulty:
  - Straining.
  - Incomplete evacuation.
  - Pain.
  - Digitation.
- Control of flatus.
- Rectal bleeding or mucus.
- Products used to manage faecal incontinence.

---

### Related topics

☐ Constipation in adults, p. 457; ☐ Urinary incontinence in men, p. 453; ☐ Urinary incontinence in women, p. 448; ☐ Continence products, p. 468.

### Further information

NICE (2007). Faecal incontinence: the management of faecal incontinence in adults. Available at: ᔐ www.eguidelines.co.uk/eguidelinesmain/guidelines/summaries/gastrointestinal/nice_faecal_incontinence.php

Norton C, Chelvanayagam S. (2004). *Bowel Continence Nursing*. Beaconsfield: Beaconsfield Publishers.

# Toileting problems and incontinence in people with dementia

As dementia progresses, people have difficulties in remaining continent for a number of reasons (*note:* in addition to the effects of other conditions, e.g. arthritis and loss of dexterity to remove clothing):

- Loss of cognition and memory requiring assistance to find, recognize (visual agnosia)/use the toilet and attend to personal hygiene afterwards.
- Expressive and receptive aphasia results in difficulties in communicating needs and understanding others.
- Behavioural and psychological symptoms resulting in depression, apathy (results in making no attempt to find the toilet), loss of inhibition or decisions to urinate or defecate in unusual places, and reluctance/refusal to have aid in going to the toilet.
- Loss of physical function and mobility in the late stage of dementia.

In addition embarrassment or a desire to protect loved ones from socially unacceptable excreta and problems with cognition may lead people with dementia to conceal soiled clothing or items and then forget they have done this. Difficulties with managing constipation and/or post toilet-personal hygiene may lead to faeces on hands, which are then transferred elsewhere, inadvertently or in poorly conceived attempts to remove.

> Family carers report that managing incontinence can be one of the most stressful aspects and it is known to be significant in the decision for the person to move to a care home. Be aware that some family carers strategies may be unintentionally problematic to a person with dementia, e.g. restricting fluids from the afternoon onwards to prevent nocturia.

## Key principles in assessing and addressing problems

- Establish from the person, if possible, and the family carer exactly what the problem is and what needs to be addressed Undertake a usual continence assessment as per local guidelines, but with the manifestations and consequences of dementia to the forefront.
- Remember to exclude tractable causes such as UTI.
- Use of ABC model (A = antecedents, B = behaviours, C = consequences) of understanding behaviours may assist in identifying contributory issues and problem-solving.
- Always establish whether suggested strategies or aids are acceptable to the person with dementia and/or acceptable and feasible for the family carer (📖 Carers assessment and support, p. 412).
- Effective containment of excreta will be of paramount importance and may be the most appropriate aim of care planning through the use of incontinence pads and pants (📖 Continence products, p. 468).

## Aspects to consider and advise on

- *Preventing constipation:* may need considerable thought as to how to ensure adequate fluids, fibre-rich diet, and physical activity.
- Aids to assist in finding, recognizing the toilet, and managing the bathroom, e.g. plug in lights that turn on, on sensing movement, contrasting colour toilet seats, toilet sign on bathroom door, disabling locks or having ones that can be opened from outside.
- Easily undone or removed clothing, e.g. tracksuit bottoms rather than trousers with zips.
- Aids to the toilet or commodes (📖 Assistive technology, p. 776; 📖 Assistive technology and equipment for home nursing, p. 778).
- Family carers and/or paid carers reminding and offering to assist to the toilet (known as prompted voiding, but may be unacceptable to the person with dementia).
- Advising/teaching men, who have mobility or no longer remember how to hold the penis to urinate, to sit to urinate.
- The importance of good communication techniques, attending to and ameliorating anxiety and distress in being assisted to use the toilet, e.g. through verbal reassurance, distraction techniques, use of 'comforters'.
- Out and about:
  - RADAR keys for access to toilets for the disabled ℬ www.radar. org.uk/.
  - Taking extra pads, changes of clothing in case of accidents.
- Design of incontinence pads. Many people with dementia and family carers prefer pull up pants as more like ordinary underwear and easy to use. Different designs and levels of absorbance may be needed at different times of the day or night or if outside the home.
- Consider whether referral needed, e.g. for depression to GP or specialist multi-disciplinary advice, e.g. OTs working in mental health care of older people services.

## Further information

Alzheimer's Society Fact sheets. Available at: ℬ www.alzheimers.org.uk/site/scripts/documents_ info.php?documentID=136

EVIDEM-C applied research to improving evidence based care for people with dementia and toileting problems in primary care. Available at: ℬ www.evidem.org.uk/

Drennan V, Cole L, Iliffe S (2011). A taboo within a stigma? Carers experiences of management of incontinence in people with dementia living at home. *Br Med Council Geriat* **11**: 75.

DuBeau CE, Kuchel GA, Johnson T 2nd, et al. (2010). Fourth International Consultation on Incontinence: Incontinence in the frail elderly: report from the 4th International Consultation on Incontinence. *Neurourol Urodyn* **29**: 165–78.

Promocon: a national service offering product information, advice and practical solutions to both professionals and the general public. Available at: ℬ www.disabledliving.co.uk/PromoCon/ About

# Stoma care

~ 100,000 people with stomas in UK. Majority in people >50yrs. Many will
need an adjustment period after stoma formation. Support for patient and
family crucial.

Three main types of stoma (temporary stomas formed to allow intestinal
healing post surgery):
- *Colostomy (most common). Colonic:* 1–2 formed bowel actions per
  day usual.
- *Ileostomy:* 15,000 in UK. Small bowel content, continuous semi-liquid
  and corrosive. Alternatively, an artificial pouch can be created inside
  the body, which can be regularly emptied when required.
- *Urostomy (ileal conduit):* continuous urine.

## Reasons for needing a stoma
- Inflammatory bowel disease (☐ Inflammatory bowel disease, p. 664).
- Bowel cancer.
- Diverticular disease (appendicitis, diverticulitis, hernias, and intestinal
  obstruction, ☐ Gastro-oesophageal conditions, p. 661).
- Accidental damage to the bowel wall.
- Urostomies rare, → cancer, or pelvic or abdominal surgery, incontinence.

## Nursing assessment and management
*Note:* output from stoma will change in the first 7wks post surgery:
- Discuss with patient, and ask about preferences, concerns, and their
  understanding of how their stoma works.
- Recognize there is a substantial adjustment required to living with a
  stoma and reassure them that they can lead a normal and active life.
- Note size, colour, and position of stoma and surrounding skin check
  for any signs of retraction, prolapse, infection, stenosis excoriation, etc.
- If possible observe how patient manages stoma, check they can see
  stoma and their dexterity with equipment.
- Encourage normal balanced diet, emphasize importance of ↑ fluids (2L
  for patients with ileostomies) some people find sensitivities or flatus
  from some foods. Occasional blocking of small diameter stoma with
  nuts/seeds, mushrooms, sweetcorn.
- Leaking appliances usually caused by poor fit. Stoma may change
  shape, especially post-operatively and if body weight changes. May also
  be poor siting or skin deformities (can build up by using paste/wafers).
- *Sore skin:* true allergy is rare. Often a leaking appliance or inappropriate
  management (changing too often or without due care; use of skin
  products on sensitive skin). Cleanse with water avoid deodorants
  and creams. Check bag fit around stoma. Watch bag, change routine.
  Observe pattern of soreness.
- *Flatus:* chew food carefully and note foods and drinks that cause flatus.
- *Constipation:* ↑ fluid and dietary fibre intake.
- *Pain:* patients with pain associated with the stoma should be referred
  to the GP.
- Patients do not need to wear an appliance when swimming or bathing.
- *Travel:* take adequate supplies and avoid heat when storing pouches.

*Products*
- Very individual.
- Important to find the best product for each patient. Many companies will send samples.
- Two piece—to avoid frequent flange changes.
- Drainable bag for urostomy and ileostomy (with night extension if needed).
- In UK all products are on prescription and patients are exempt from prescription charges.
- Some bags are flushable.

*Stoma care nurses*
Available for home visits or clinic consultations in most areas. Should be contacted when problems with stoma care arise

## Related topics

📖 Faecal incontinence, p. 462; 📖 Constipation in adults, p. 457.

## Further information

British Colostomy Association. Available at: ℘ www.bcass.org.uk and links to products and clothing suppliers
Ileostomy and Internal Pouch Support. Available at: ℘ www.the-ia.org.uk
NHS Choices. Ileostomy. Available at: ℘ www.nhs.uk/conditions/Ileostomy/Pages/Introduction. aspx

# Continence products

Most people with continence problems can achieve a successful resolution without continence products. However, for others the appropriate product gives confidence and an unrestricted quality of life.

Many continence products provided through NHS (local policies apply) and the range and number of products available may be determined by local policy. Laundry costs are usually the responsibility of individual and carers.

## Points to consider when assessing and choosing a product

- *Lifestyle of the patient:* e.g. level of activity, cosmetic effect.
- *Pattern of incontinence:* e.g. more protection needed at night.
- Visual acuity, cognitive ability, and dexterity for using products.
- If patient is alone or has help with personal care.
- Costs especially if product not provided by NHS.

## Reason for choosing a continence product

- Maintenance of skin integrity.
- Protection of furniture and equipment, e.g. covers and pads.
- Protection of individual and their clothes, e.g. pads and pants.
- Specialist products, e.g. sheaths, alarms, catheters.
- Need an alternative to the toilet because of access problems or urgency, e.g. commode, male or female urinals.

See Bladder and Bowel Foundation and Promocon websites for detailed list of products and prices (available at ℘ www.bladderandbowelfoundation. org). Local continence specialist staff will also produce information.

## Points about bedding protection

- *Mattress covers:* breathable fabrics preferable (PVC covers often hot and uncomfortable only suitable for short-term use).
- 'No launder duvets' can be wiped down, dried, and reused.
- Covers with terry towelling surface preferable for occasional episodes of incontinence at night.
- Reusable bed pads often used in conjunction with personal body protection. Can be difficult to launder at home.

## Points about personal protection from urine and faeces

Wide range of choice to reflect patient preference and type of continence problem. The absorbency of a product depends on the materials used and not its cost, size, or thickness. Barrier creams should not be used with pads as they affect product's ability to absorb urine.

❶ Sanitary towels are inappropriate for urinary incontinence:

- *All in one (pad and pant combined):* disposable or reusable. Suitable for heavy urinary or faecal incontinence especially if confined to wheelchair/bed bound. Hip measurements important to ensure good fit. *Note:* any form of toileting difficult with this product.
- *Insert pads (disposable and reusable):* cater for slight/moderate and heavy urinary incontinence. Held in place by close-fitting underpants (net or stretch pants). If pads do not have waterproof padding then use with waterproof pants or pants with waterproof pouch. For men with light/dribbling incontinence possible to have pouch pad held in place with adhesive strip in tight fitting underpants.
- *Absorbent pants:* disposable and reusable. Suitable for slight urinary leaks or faecal staining. Use hip measurements for women and waist measurements for men and children. Useful when travelling or where laundry difficult. Most like ordinary underwear does not require manual dexterity (i.e. to fit pad, etc.). Can be used over insert pad for extra absorbency. Disadvantage—every pad change=change of underwear.
- *Penile sheaths:* condom urinal, incontinence sheath. Soft rubber sleeve available on prescription, available in one or multiple sizes (some manufacturers provide sizing chart/measuring device). Good for men with physical disabilities, but may not be suitable for:
  - Men with a small or retracted penis.
  - If patient is confused or demented and may pull sheath off.
  - If patient has limited dexterity and needs help to fix it on.
  - Skin sensitivity, e.g. latex intolerance.
- *Self adhesive sheaths:* a strip of double side special adhesive wrapped round the penis and the sheath is rolled up over it. Men with sensitive skin or those who make frequent changes may prefer external fixing around the outside of the sheath—a foam strip with adhesive on one side or a rubber adjustable strap fixed with a button or Velcro. To apply:
  - Make sure foreskin is not pulled back.
  - Keep a gap between tip of penis and outlet of sheath to allow for sudden gushing of urine, but not enough to allow twisting.
  - Avoid pressure on penis and check for soreness/tissue damage.

## Aids for the toilet and toileting

- Range of aids designed to promote continence and independence, e.g. bottom wipers and customized commodes for use in cars, etc. Information from Promocon (available at ✍ www.promocon.co.uk) see aids to independent living (📖 Assistive technology and equipment for home nursing, p. 778).
- Male and female hand-held urinals. Allows people with limited mobility to be continent and independent especially in situations where access to toilets difficult. Useful for carers if moving and handling is difficult. Can be used in bed, seated or standing depending on the users' capabilities.
- Radar Keys or mobile phone app for people who need quick access to public toilets, access to over 9000 toilets across the UK ✍ www.radar.org.uk/.

**Related topics**

📖 Urinary incontinence in women, p. 448; 📖 Urinary incontinence in men, p. 453.

**Further information**

Bladder and Bowel Foundation. Confidential Helpline ☎ 0845 3450165. Available at: 🖰 www.bladderandbowelfoundation.org

Promocon. Promoting continence and product awareness. Available at: 🖰 www.promocon.co.uk

# Spinal cord injury

Approx 700 new spinal injuries pa in the UK, most common in 16–30yrs and >80% ♂. Most common causes falls (41%) and RTA (37%).

Extent of paralysis depends on level of injury.
• C4 injury = complete paralysis below the neck.
• C6 injury = partial paralysis of hands and arms as well as lower body.
• T4 injury = paralysis from chest down.
• L1 injury = paralysis below the waist.

Where there is incomplete injury there is more variation between patients in the amount of movement they have. Patients with acute spinal injury will be managed in neurosurgery and/or spinal unit; majority will go home to adapted living accommodation often with carer support.

Common longer-term problems patients may encounter include:
• Psychological problems including depression.
• Financial hardship.
• Family and relationship stress and breakdown.
• Bladder and bowel dysfunction.
• Autonomic dysreflexia.
• Pressure sores.
• Temperature regulation.
• Cardiovascular and respiratory disorders.
• Risk of DVT and PE.

## Care and management

• Common responses to spinal injury are disbelief, low self-esteem, anger, guilt, and depression. Both patients and their families can take a long time to adjust. Important they receive emotional support from the MDT and voluntary/charitable groups with specialist knowledge of living with a spinal injury.
• People with spinal injury will be eligible for range of disability benefits, e.g. higher rate disability living allowance for mobility—schemes like motobility can provide a car or motorized wheel chair (📖 Benefits for illness, disability and carers, p. 795).
• Citizens Advice Bureau (📖 Useful websites, p. 800) and specialist legal centres can provide advice on employment and welfare rights and access to education and sport and leisure.
• Patients with complete spinal cord injury do not sweat below the level of their injury therefore in environments of high humidity and heat the body temperature rises. The use of wet towels around the neck and water spray to mimic the effect of sweat can help. In cold environments patients may become hypothermic. Important they have access to warmth and warm drinks and clothes.
• *Prevention of UTI and bladder management:* retention or urine with overflow incontinence can put patient at risk of long-term renal damage. Ensure bladder drained by self-catheterization or patient may need a urinary diversion formed.
• *Bowel care:* prevention of constipation and establishing a predictable bowel regime. May require manual evacuation of faeces.

- Autonomic dysreflexia (see 📖 Urinary catheter care, p. 454) in manual removal of faeces in patients with injury above T6, caused by noxious stimulus (e.g. full bladder/bowel, pain) occurring below injury. Monitor symptoms of dramatic ↑ BP, patient appears flushed above level of injury and pale below (due to vasoconstriction), bradycardia, pounding headache, blurred vision, nausea, and profuse sweating. Can lead to cerebral haemorrhage and seizures. ❶ Medical emergency— remove stimulus immediately, give GTN spray 1–2 puffs sublingually or nifedipine 5–10mg capsule sublingual (BNF 2.6).

**Related topics**

📖 Expert patient, p. 303; 📖 Carers assessment and support, p. 412.

**Further information**

Disability law service. Available at: 🔗 www.dls.org.uk

Motobility. Available at: 🔗 www.motobility.co.uk

Spinal Injuries Association: Freephone Advice Line ☎ 0800 980 0501. Available at: 🔗 www.spinal. co.uk

Spinal injuries Scotland. Available at: 🔗 www.sisonline.org

# Pressure ulcers

Pressure ulcers are areas of localized damage to the skin and underlying tissue caused by combination of pressure, shear, and friction. Overall prevalence is 10.3% and 50% of ulcers are hospital acquired. Potential to develop pressure ulcers may be exacerbated by moisture to the skin and certain medications. Pressure ulcers are generally avoidable. Risk factors in individuals include:

• Immobility.
• Sensory impairment (especially with spinal injury).
• Acute illness.
• Impaired consciousness.
• Incontinence.
• >70yrs.
• Vascular disease.
• Chronic or terminal illness.
• History of pressure damage.
• Malnutrition and dehydration.

## Formal risk assessment

Initial assessment should be included within 6hrs of any first contact with patients likely to be at risk. Subsequent assessments as indicated by the patient's condition. Risk assessment tools (e.g. Braden Scale) that give scores are an aide memoir and do not replace clinical judgement. Assessment includes:

• Consideration of individual risk factors and patient and carer's understanding of their at-risk status.
• Document skin inspection (frequency determined individually):
  • Inspect heels, sacrum, ischial tuberosities, shoulders, back of head, toes, parts of the body affected by anti-embolic stockings, equipment and clothing, and parts of the body where pressure, friction, and shear is exerted.
  • Observe for persistent erythema and non-blanching erythema on light skinned patients, purplish/bluish localized patches on dark skinned patients, blisters, localized heat, localized oedema, and localized induration.
  • Encourage patients to inspect own skin (teach mirror use for wheel chair users).
  • Document skin changes.

Wheelchair users should have specific seating assessments, usually by physiotherapists or OTs. Some areas have wheel chair clinics.

## Care plan should include:

### Essentials of care

• Involve patient and carer in decision-making.
• Monitor BMI and advise on nutritional status.
• Effective management of incontinence and skin cleaning.
• Apply moisturizers to dry skin.
• Avoid skin rubbing and massage over bony prominences.

*Ensure correct moving and handling to avoid shearing*

*Pressure redistribution devices*

- Choice based on patient comfort, lifestyle and abilities, critical care needs, and acceptability of proposed equipment to patient and carer.
- Availability, maintenance, cleaning, etc. of devices for home use subject to local policies.
- Patients at 'risk' require low-pressure or overlay mattresses.
- Patients at 'high risk' require alternating pressure mattresses.

**❶** Do not use doughnut type devices, synthetic sheepskins, genuine sheepskins, or water-filled gloves as ineffective and potentially harmful.

*Positioning and seating*

- Frequency of repositioning should be determined on individual basis and aim to minimize prolonged pressure on bony prominences.
- Repositioning to continue even when pressure redistribution devices in use.
- Patients at very high risk should restrict chair sitting to <2hrs.
- Keep bony prominences from direct contact with one another.
- Teach patients and carers to redistribute weight.
- Remove slings and other parts of manual handling equipment from underneath patient after manoeuvring.
- Consider distribution of weight, postural alignment, and support of feet when seating patients.

## Pressure sore grading systems

Many classification systems exist and can be useful. 4 grades are the simplest to use as follows:

- *Grade 1:* non-blanchable erythema of intact skin. Discolouration of the skin, warmth, oedema, induration, or hardness.
- *Grade 2:* partial thickness skin loss involving epidermis, dermis, or both.
- *Grade 3:* full thickness skin loss involving damage to or necrosis of subcutaneous tissue.
- *Grade 4:* extensive destruction, tissue necrosis, or damage to muscle, bone, or supporting structures with or without full thickness skin loss. (adapted from European Pressure Ulcer Advisory Panel 2009. Available at: &#8767; www.epuap.org).

### Key reference text

NICE (2005). Pressure Ulcer Management Pathway which includes guidance on risk assessment, surgery for treatment of pressure ulcers and nutrition in the treatment of pressure ulcers. Available at: &#8767; www.nice.org.uk

### Further information

Braden Scale. Available at &#8767; www.bradenscale.com can be used with permission (no charge).
European Pressure Ulcer Advisory Panel and National Pressure Ulcer Advisory Panel. *Prevention and treatment of pressure ulcers: quick reference. guide.* Washington DC: National Pressure Ulcer Advisory Panel; 2009. Available at &#8767; www.epuap.org
Tissue Viability Society. Available at &#8767; www.tvs.org.uk

# Wound assessment

Accurate assessment is vital to provide correct treatment and evaluate its effectiveness. It must always be part of a wider, holistic approach.

## Aims of wound assessment
- Determine cause/aetiology.
- Identify healing and non-healing wounds.
- Early detection of complications.
- Monitor treatment effect.
- Support clinical decision-making.
- Improve patient concordance.

Practical indications that a wound is responding to treatment include:
- Reduction in exudate production.
- Improvement in condition of the wound bed.
- Reduction in % surface area of the wound.

These parameters are subjective and difficult to measure, particularly in chronic wounds, which do not always follow the expected sequence of healing. Wounds can be objectively assessed in a variety of other ways: wound dimensions, protease levels, and exudates production.

In clinical practice the most commonly assessed objective parameter is wound size.

## Wound dimensions
- Simple length and width measurements overestimate size of larger, irregular wounds.
- More accurate results obtained by tracing the wound circumference using acetate sheets and a pen, *but* is subjective.
- Use of portable digital planimeters ↑ accuracy of wound circumference measurement.
- NICE (2005) guidelines[1] recommend photographing and/or tracing pressure ulcers at initial assessment.

## Wound healing curves
Monitoring wound healing curves particularly within the first 4wks of treatment can determine efficacy of treatment.

Wound healing curves plot the reduction in % area of the wound surface against time on a graph to determine progression towards healing.

This requires 3 key elements:
- *Measurement:* a recording of wound surface area.
- *Time:* a recording made at consistent intervals.
- A consistent approach.

A ↓ of wound area between 20–40% from initial assessment, between 2–4wks of treatment = a reliable indicator of healing. A ↓ in surface area <10% per month is indicative of a non-responding chronic wound. Every 7 to 10 days measure the % reduction of wound surface area.

### Characteristics of wound bed

Identification of tissue type will indicate the depth of the wound, potential complications (e.g. infection) and length of time to healing. Knowledge of anatomy is important as a relatively shallow wound or a finger may involve tendons, and bone. Need to ask what the tissue involvement is, e.g. bone, fascia, muscle, tendon, subcutaneous fat, dermis, epidermis, etc.

### Colour of wound bed

The predominant colour of a wound can be used as a method of classifying wounds to inform treatment.
* *Pink:* epithelial cells—protection.
* *Red:* granulation tissue—protection.
* *Yellow:* loose = slough; adherent= fibrinous tissue—debridement.
* *Black:* necrotic tissue (wet or dry)—debridement.

### Exudate

No standard definitions/methods of assessing exist. What is 'normal' varies depending on wound type, size, and stage of healing. Exudate is described subjectively:
* *Volume:* low, medium, high.
* *Viscosity:* low, medium, high.
* *Colour:* straw coloured (serous), red (blood), creamy off-white (purulent) (LL Infected wounds, p. 483).

### Wound edges and surrounding skin

Wound margin condition provides information for wound status and dressing suitability:
* *Flat migrating sides:* healthy, moist, dividing epithelial cells.
* *Steep non-migrating sides:* unhealthy, dry, epithelial cells.
* *Eschar:* dry wound secretions, dead cells.
* *Induration:* firm swelling with or without redness.
* *Inflammation:* pink/red, warm indicative of inflammatory process.
* *Maceration:* white, soft, wet tissue. Indicates poor exudate control.

### Documentation

The following should be included in wound assessment documentation.
* *Patient details:* gender, age, relevant PMH.
* Previous wound treatment.
* Pressure ulcer risk assessment.
* *General skin condition:* dry, sensitive, eczema, trauma.
* Wound type, duration, e.g. chronicity, location, dimensions.
* Exudate type/amount, wound odour, consistency.
* *Characteristics of wound bed:* colour, tissue type, e.g. slough, necrotic tissue.
* *Condition of wound margin/surrounding skin:* dry escar, macerated, fungal infection.
* *Wound pain/discomfort:* intermittent/continuous, descriptors, e.g. shooting, burning, associated with signs of infection.

## Related topics

📖 Management of chronic wounds, p. 480; 📖 Pressure ulcers prevention, p. 473; 📖 Infected wounds, p. 483; 📖 Leg ulcer assessment and management, p. 496; 📖 Fungating wounds, p. 488; 📖 Wound dressings, p. 492.

## Reference

[1]NICE (2005). The prevention and treatment of pressure ulcers. Available at: ℘ www.nice.org.uk

## Further information

Fette, A. (2006). A clinimetric analysis of wound assessment tools. Available at: ℘ www.world-widewounds.com

Wounds International. Website for specialist information on wound care. Available at: ℘ www.woundsinternational.com

# Post-operative wound care

The aims of post-operative wound care are to promote healing, minimize complications, e.g. surgical site infection, and produce the best cosmetic result possible. Surgical wounds can be closed by primary or secondary intention. Potential wound complications include haematoma, infection, dehiscence, sinus, and fistula formation.

## Wounds healing by primary intention

Wound edges opposed and secured using sutures (absorbable and non-absorbable), staples, tissue adhesives, and adhesive skin tapes. The 3 most common suture lines seen in primary care are continuous sutures (a series of stitches taken with one strand of material, proximal and distal ends knotted), interrupted sutures (a number of strands closing the wound, each knotted and cut after insertion), and subcuticular sutures (continuous sutures placed in the dermis, beneath the epithelial layer, proximal and distal ends knotted or secured with an anchoring device). See Fig. 10.2. A light absorbent dressing is required until haemostasis is achieved and the wound is sealed by a fibrin scab. Post-operative dressings can usually be removed after 24–48hrs. Alternatively a semi occlusive dressing may be applied (e.g. foam or film dressing) and left in place until the wound closure material is removed. Occlusive dressings should not be used with tissue adhesives. Surgical incisions should *only* require cleaning when excessive leakage has occurred. Adhesive skin tapes are left in place until they peel off by themselves and tissue adhesives slough off in 7–10days.

## Removal of sutures or staples

- Establish number of sutures/staples and when to remove, e.g. from discharge letter or referral. Most removed 7–10 days (less if on face and more for high tension areas, e.g. back).
- Examine wound to assess whether suture/staple removal appropriate Encourage patient to wash area prior to procedure.
- Perform procedure using aseptic technique and PPE (📖 Personal protective equipment, p. 98).
- Clean wound with normal saline 0.9%.
- For continuous sutures, lift knot of suture with forceps, snip stitch close to the skin, and gently remove entire suture.
- For interrupted sutures, lift knot of suture with forceps, snip stitch close to the skin, and gently remove individual suture. Repeat on alternating sutures. If wound remains intact remove remaining sutures.
- For subcuticular sutures, lift knot or anchoring device, e.g. bead, snip stitch close to the skin, and gently remove entire suture.
- For staples, hold staple remover device at 90° angle, slip lower jaw under bridge of staple, gently close handles and the staple is automatically released. Repeat on alternating staples. If wound remains intact remove remaining staples. Dispose of staples in sharps box.
- Ensure no sutures/staples have been left in skin unintentionally.
- If wound gapes use adhesive tape to oppose wound edges.
- If wound dehiscence occurs, inform surgeon and lightly pack with absorbent dressings Record condition of wound closure line and surrounding skin.

(a) Interrupted suture

(b) Continuous suture

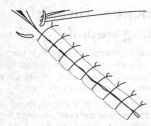
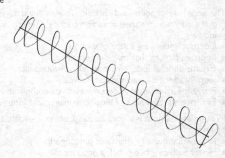

**Fig. 10.2** Sutures.

## Wounds healing by secondary intention

Wound edges come together naturally by means of granulation and contraction (for example, abscess cavities such as peri-anal abscesses). These wounds require a moist healing environment. Dressing materials include alginates, hydrogels, foams, hydrocolloids. Cavity wounds should be lightly filled with an absorbent dressing material. Tight packing can lead to tissue ischaemia and tissue death. Surgical wounds healing by secondary intention often require cleaning. This can be achieved by the patient having a shower and so irrigating the wound with warm water. Infected wounds should be irrigated with normal saline 0.9%. Hydrocolloids and film dressings should be avoided on infected wounds.

### Key reference text

Dougherly L, Lister S. (eds) (2011). *The Royal Marsden Hospital Manual of Clinical Nursing Procedures*, 11th edn. London: Wiley Blackwell.

### Further information

Website for specialist information on wound care. Available at ℅ www.woundsinternational.com

# Management of chronic/ non-healing wounds

In chronic wounds the normal repair process becomes disrupted. Chronic wounds traditionally are classified according to their underlying pathology, e.g. pressure ulcers, venous leg ulcers, etc. The use of the term healing and non-healing wound is more clinically relevant.

Although some chronic wounds heal and respond to conventional therapy, many become unresponsive and need advanced technologies to stimulate healing. It is important to differentiate between a healing chronic wound and a non-healing wound.

The aetiology of acute and chronic wounds are different (Table 10.2) and require different management approaches. General wound management principles:
• Correct underlying cause of wound.
• Improve factors that may delay healing.
• Create optimal local environment at wound site.
• Identify specific treatment objectives.
• Prevent further wound deterioration or complications.
• Evaluate effectiveness of wound management interventions.

Wound assessment is a continuous process. Evaluate the status of healing by asking:
• Is the inflammatory response prolonged?
• How much exudate is being produced?
• Are there any signs of wound infection?
• Are there any signs of tissue ischaemia?
• How much necrotic tissue is present?
• Is the granulation tissue healthy?
• Are there any signs of delayed epithelialization?
• What is the condition of the surrounding skin?

## Specific chronic wound management principles

Wound management decisions rely on assessment, complex decision-making skills, and experience (📖 Wound assessment, p. 475) including wound type, size, and location as well as the patient's psychological response.

## Wound bed preparation

An approach that can remove barriers associated with chronic non-healing and aims at ↓ oedema, ↓ exudate, ↓ bacterial burden and, correct abnormalities contributing to impaired healing. There are 4 components:
• Tissue management.
• Inflammation and infection.
• Moisture balance.
• Epithelial (edge) advancement.

## Tissue management

Chronic wounds have a 'necrotic burden' that consists of devitalized tissue, dead cells, and exudate that delay healing. Following initial debridement a temporary improvement in healing may be observed followed by gradual deterioration. Recommend steady continuous removal of necrotic burden (□ Wound debridement, p. 486).

## Inflammation and infection

↑ bacterial load within chronic wounds can lead to delayed healing. Regardless of the type of organism, substantial impairment of healing occurs, when there is between $10^5$ and $10^6$ organisms per gram in a wound bed. However, the number of organisms in a wound may not necessarily be as critical as the type and pathogenicity of the organism present (□ Infected wounds, p. 483). Removal of bacterial burden at the wound surface ↓ the possibility of infection, but also may ↓ the prolonged inflammation response characteristic of chronic wounds. ↓ the bacterial count, by debridement or slow-release antimicrobials can help.

## Moisture balance

Moisture balance at the wound/dressing interface is agreed to be a key factor responsible for optimizing wound healing. Control of excess wound exudate is important as it increases the risk of:
• Prolonged inflammation.
• Cellular inhibition.
• Wound infection.
• Odour.
• Skin maceration.
• Excoriation.

Exudate can be managed using direct means such as:
• Wound cleansing.
• Absorbent dressings.
• Compression therapy.
• Topical negative pressure.
• Skin protection.

Or indirectly by alleviating underlying cause, e.g. heart failure, diabetes, venous insufficiency, and managing symptoms, e.g. infection, excoriation.

## Epithelial (edge) advancement

Epithelialization = final stage of wound healing needs well-prepared wound bed and a source of healthy epidermal cells, promoted by:
• Well vascularized granulation tissue.
• Absence of infection.
• Optimal moisture levels.
• Hydration of wound margins.
• Minimal dressing trauma.

Healing can be monitored using a series of wound measurements plotted as a graph (□ Wound assessment, p. 475). This allows early detection of complications and prompt intervention.

**Table 10.2** Differences between chronic and acute wounds

|  | Acute wounds | Chronic wounds |
| --- | --- | --- |
| Healing process | Regulated | Haphazard |
| Pathology | None | Underlying |
| Time to healing | Rapid | Slow |
| Inflammatory response | Short | Prolonged |
| Exudate | Reduced after 48hrs | Prolonged |
|  | Promotes cellular proliferation | Inhibits cellular proliferation |
| Bacterial load | Low | High |
| Fibroblast proliferation | Active | Inactive |
| Excoriation/maceration | Infrequent | Frequent |
| Extracellular matrix | Normal remodelling | Defective remodelling |
| Vascular network | Good | Poor |
| Complications | Infrequent | Frequent |
| Progress | Heal | Fail to heal/recur |

Reproduced from Flanagan, M and Fletcher, J (2006). Wound pathologies; causes of acute and chronic wounds in Bale, S and Gray, D (eds). *A pocket guide to Clinical Decision Making in wound management*. Wounds UK Publishing, Aberdeen. By kind permission of Wounds UK Ltd.

### Related topics

📖 Wound assessment, p. 475; 📖 Infected wounds, p. 483; 📖 Leg ulcer assessment and management, p. 496; 📖 Fungating wounds, p. 488; 📖 Wound dressings, p. 492; 📖 Principles of wound management following amputation, p. 490.

### Further information

European Wound Management Association. Available at: 🖱 www.ewma.org
World Union of Wound Healing Societies (WUWHS) (2007). Principles of best practice: Wound exudate and the role of dressings. Available at: 🖱 www.woundsinternational.com.
Wounds International (2008). *Hard-to-heal wounds: a holistic approach*. London: MEP Ltd. Available at: 🖱 www.woundsinternational.com

# Infected wounds

## Wound infection

Defined as the presence of bacteria within a wound with multiplication and an associated host reaction. If a wound contains $10^6$ bacteria per gram of tissue = usually defined as being infected. Wound infection initiates the body's immune response locally, then systemically if untreated will delay healing.

Bacterial colonization is of no clinical significance and should not be confused with wound infection.

## Critical colonization

Is the term used to describe a wound where the bacterial burden is rising due to multiplication of organisms which are beginning to cause a delay in healing. Critical colonization initiates the body's immune response locally, but not systemically.

### Risk factors

- Number of organisms present.
- Bacterial pathogenicity.
- Host resistance—immune-competence.
- Local anoxia.
- Devitalized tissue.
- Haematoma.
- Foreign bodies.

### Surgical wounds

- Presence of an existing chronic infection.
- Nature of invasive procedure—especially bowel.
- Extent of tissue loss and/or trauma to tissues during surgery.
- Adequacy of wound drainage.

### Signs and symptoms

- Raised temperature—shivering, fever.
- Tachycardia.
- Generally feeling unwell.
- Confusion (older people).
- Lymphangitis.
- Neutrophilia.

## Local signs
- Erythema—spreading cellulitis.
- Localized oedema, heat.
- Increased pain/tenderness.
- Increased exudate levels.
- Increased slough/necrosis.
- Pus formation.
- Increased odour.
- Bridging/pocketing at the wound base.
- Fragile granulation (bleeds easily).
- Dark red (cherry) granulation tissue.
- Wound breakdown.
- Non-healing wound.

## Investigations
- *Bloods:* FBC, ESR.
- Swab for C&S if listed signs present.
- *Diabetic foot ulcers:* if listed signs present, X-ray foot to exclude osteomyelitis.

## Care and management
Objectives of treating infected wounds are:
- Identify the infective organism.
- Remove devitalized tissue and excess exudate.
- Eliminate wound infection using appropriate antimicrobial agents.
- Protect the surrounding skin from the effects of maceration.

Select wound dressings for exudating wounds. Assess wounds daily change dressings frequently. Some evidence that topical antimicrobials could be used selectively for:
- Stimulation of previously unresponsive chronic wounds.
- Treatment of infected wounds.
- Eradication of MRSA from contaminated wounds (📖 MRSA, p. 674).

There is limited evidence to support the routine use of silver dressings for infected wounds. Critically colonized wounds may benefit from use of local formulary for topical, sustained, antimicrobial dressings. If no improvement seen in 14 days, treatment should be discontinued.

Reserve systemic antibiotics for diagnosed wound infection.

### Adjunctive measures
- Wound debridement may be necessary (📖 Wound debridement, p. 486).
- Exudate management.
- Skin protection may be necessary.

Spreading infection, i.e. visibly spreading from wound site, requires systemic antibiotics (possibly IV), dressing selection will have little impact on the spreading infection. Seek appropriate medical help immediately.

## Complications

- Delayed/non-healing wounds.
- Wound dehiscence.
- Oesteomyelitis (especially diabetic foot ulcers, sacral pressure ulcers).
- Septicaemia.
- Death.

## Related topics

📖 Wound assessment, p. 475; 📖 Fungating wounds, p. 488; 📖 Wound dressings, p. 492.

## Further information

Storm-Versloot MN, Vos CG, Ubbink DT, *et al.* (2010). Topical silver for preventing wound infection. *Cochrane Database System Rev* Issue 3. Art. No.: CD006478.

Wound Infection in Clinical Practice: an international consensus. (2008). World Union of Wound Healing Societies. Available at ℘ www.woundsinternational.com/clinical-guidelines/wound-infection-in-clinical-practice-an-international-consensus

# Wound debridement

Removal of non-viable tissue is essential (provided there is an adequate blood supply) to promote wound healing and ↓ the risk of local infection. When necrotic tissue collects at the wound surface it may:

- Delay wound apposition and closure.
- Prolong inflammation.
- ↑ wound odour.
- ↑ risk of infection.
- Limits effectiveness of antibiotic therapy.
- Inhibits epithelial cell migration.
- Prevents accurate wound assessment.
- ↑ scarring.

## Methods

The most common methods of debridement include:

- Sharp (surgical or conservative).
- Autolytic.
- Chemical.
- Enzymatic.
- Mechanical.
- Biological.

*Sharp conservative debridement* The removal of dead tissue, with a scalpel, at the bedside above the level of viable tissue is quickest and most cost-effective method. The decision to use a particular method depends upon a number of factors, e.g. wound type, location, extent of tissue damage, amount of exudates. For chronic wounds debridement may take several weeks and require more than one method.

*Sharp surgical debridement:* An extensive procedure performed by surgeons. Debridement using a scalpel must be performed by an experienced, competent clinician. Issues to be considered—training, adequate supervised practice, informed patient consent, need for local anaesthesia, and patient reassurance.

## Contraindications

- Ischaemic wounds.
- Blood clotting disorders/long-term anticoagulant therapy.
- Necrotic tissue close to or involving blood vessels/nerves/tendons.
- Fungating/malignant wounds.
- Patients with reduced sensation.
- Debridement of the feet/hands (excluding the heel).
- Debridement of the face.

## Autolytic debridement

### Autolysis

Commonest method of debridement using moist or occlusive dressings, e.g. hydrogels, hydrocolloids, and medical grade honey dressings. These dressings have a high water content that help to soften devitalized tissue. The speed of debridement will vary between products. Speed of autolysis depends on the wound size and the patient's general physical condition. Rapid debridement may occur within 2–3 days making it safe and effective in the home care setting.

**Chemical debridement** Strong chemical agents, e.g. hypochlorites are rarely used due to adverse side effects and increased availability of less toxic and more effective products. Iodine (either povidone or cadexomer) has a broad-spectrum antibacterial activity and a secondary effect of drying out wet slough to facilitate sharp debridement.

### Enzymatic debridement

They have limited use for wounds with hard, dry eschar. Enzymatic preparations collaginase may be used on chronic wounds as the active ingredient proteases penetrate soft, devitalized tissue. Enzymatic preparations are applied either in solution or in combination with a hydrogel which makes it difficult to separate the enzymatic activity from the autolytic effect. They may also be inactivated by antimicrobial dressings and detergents.

**Mechanical debridement** Is a non-discriminatory method that physically removes debris from the wound and may cause additional tissue damage and patient discomfort. Examples of non-selective mechanical debridement include—wet-to-dry dressings, high pressure wound irrigation, and whirlpool therapy.

### Biological debridement

Larvae only digest necrotic tissue, slough and bacteria, leaving the wound bed clean. Larval therapy can quickly eradicate infection and wound odour, may be effective against MRSA. They can be left in place for up to 3 days, but may require changing sooner in ischaemic wounds. Increased exudate production may occur during early stages of treatment which may be associated with increased odour. Disadvantages of maggot therapy—aesthetic reasons, local discomfort, itching, and application problems. Available on FP10.

### Maintaining debridement

In chronic wounds, difficult to fully remove the necrotic burden as non-viable tissue and exudate continues to accumulate. After initial debridement in chronic wounds, a temporary improvement in healing is often observed followed by gradual deterioration. Initial debridement followed by repeated debridement important whilst the wound is open to maintain steady, continuous removal of necrotic burden.

### Related topics

📖 Wound assessment, p. 475; 📖 Management of chronic wounds, p. 480; 📖 Infected wounds, p. 483; 📖 Fungating wounds, p. 488; 📖 Wound dressings, p. 492.

### Further information

NICE (2001, reviewed 2004). *Guidance on the use of debriding agents and specialist wound care clinics for difficult to heal surgical wounds*. Available at: 🖰 www.nice.org.uk

Wounds International. Website for specialist information on wound care. Available at: 🖰 www. woundsinternational.com

# Fungating wounds

Fungating wounds develop from 1° skin tumours, an underlying tumour, or metastatic disease. Occasionally chronic, non-healing wounds, e.g. leg ulcers may become malignant. Often develop in older patients (>70yrs) with metastatic cancer. Lesions may develop into a 'cauliflower'-shaped nodular growth, or ulcerate into a wound with a crater-like appearance or both. The commonest site of fungating wounds is in the breast, although 25% develop in the head and neck area. Fungating wounds have significant psychological impact, and can be a constant reminder of a condition's progression.

## Assessment

Assessment of fungating wounds should consider the patient's views, psychological state, pain, and local wound factors (📖 Wound assessment, p. 475).

## Factors delaying healing

- Advanced malignancy.
- Immunosuppression—chemotherapy, radiotherapy.
- Malnutrition/dehydration.
- Psychological stress.

The aim of care is symptom control and to promote patient comfort and sense of wellbeing.

## Exudate

Fungating wounds often produce moderate to high levels of exudate. Use dressings that absorb excess exudate, but maintain a moist wound environment to avoid dressing adhesion, trauma, and bleeding. For smaller high exudating wounds, a wound manager/wound drainage pouch can be used. Skin barriers around the wound can be an effective method of ↓ damage associated with exudate's leakage. Alcohol polymer barrier film helps prevent excoriation and gives a surface dressings can adhere to.

### Odour

- *Debridement:* most effective treatment for malodorous wounds. Surgical/sharp debridement, not recommended due to ↑ tendency of wounds to bleed. Autolytic or enzymatic debridement better (📖 Wound debridement, p. 486), monitor to check no ↑ exudate production.
- Antibiotic therapy may be effective if it destroys the bacteria responsible for malodour. ↓ local blood supply can reduce the effectiveness of systemic treatment. Metronidazole (BNF 5.1.11) can be given systemically, but side effects, e.g. nausea, neuropathy can be problematic. Topical preparations of metronidazole gel applied daily for between 5–7 days may help; odour may reoccur once treatment stops.
- Charcoal-based dressings may help in the management of odour.

- Occlusive dressings contain wound malodour, but may not be available in an appropriate size or conform to the wound surface. Meticulous wound hygiene, gentle irrigation with normal saline/water, daily dressing changes and the correct disposal of soiled dressings, can help ↓ odour.

## Pain

Assess to determine type of pain. Specialist advice should be sought regarding management of cancer pain, persistent, and dressing-related wound pain. Anti-cancer therapies, e.g. chemotherapy, radiotherapy, hormone therapy may help to ↓ the wound mass.

## Bleeding

Use low-adherent dressings that maintain a moist environment. Cleanse by irrigation rather than swabbing, →↓ risk of bleeding.

Sucralfate paste or alginate dressings may be applied to the surface of wounds with a small amount of bleeding. *Note:* alginates should be used with care in fragile tumours—may cause bleeding. Loosen alginates by irrigating with normal saline to ensure complete removal.

*Alternative:* haemostatic surgical sponges can be left in place and covered with an appropriate dressing.

Topical adrenaline (epinephrine) can also be applied under medical supervision.
- Wounds should be inspected daily and dressings changed regularly.
- Care is required when removing dressings to avoid further trauma and bleeding.
- Skin barriers may minimize skin excoriation/maceration.
- These patients will be at high risk of pressure damage.

## Related topics

📖 Wound assessment, p. 489; 📖 Infected wounds, p. 483; 📖 Leg ulcer assessment and management, p. 496; 📖 Wound debridement, p. 486; 📖 Wound dressings, p. 492.

## Further information

Macmillan Cancer Support. Fungating cancer wounds. Available at: ℰ http://www.macmillan.org.uk/Cancerinformation/Livingwithandaftercancer/Symptomssideeffects/Othersymptomssideeffects/Fungatingwounds.aspx

NHS Clinical Knowledge Summaries on care of malignant ulcers. Available at: ℰ www.cks.library.nhs.uk

# Principles of wound management following amputation

Amputation has significant social, medical, and economic consequences. Lower limb amputations are the most common. Two-thirds of amputees are ♂. Lower limb amputations are more common in diabetics; 50% of all amputations occur in people with diabetes.

Patients who go on to need an amputation may have had one or more of the following problems/symptoms:
- Cold pale limb.
- Absent or ↓ foot pulses.
- Altered sensation/paraesthesia.
- Paralysis.
- Pain on limb elevation—note that intermittent claudication is not always present in diabetic people with ischaemia.

## Factors delaying stump healing
- Poor health status.
- Level of amputation.
- Need for revision.
- Vascularity of skin flap.
- Position of stump wound.
- Ability to mobilize with prosthesis.

## Complications
Wound complications:
- Oedema (misshapen stump).
- Haematoma.
- Ischaemia.
- Infection.
- Wound dehiscence.

General:
- Delayed prosthetic fitting.
- Delayed independent ambulation.
- Flexion contractures.

## Management of post amputation wounds
Assessment should include pain management, specialist advice should be sought regarding post-operative phantom pain, e.g. referral/consultation to pain clinic.

Use of appropriate dressings allows earlier mobilization of patients with unhealed trans-tibial stumps with promising results. No strong evidence of clinical or cost effectiveness—wound dressings that best match clinical experience, patient preference, and the wound site. Useful dressing types:
- Alginates.
- Foams.
- Hydrofibres.
- Low-adherent contact layers.

## Care of patient with amputation wound

- Wounds should be inspected daily and dressings changed regularly.
- Stump wounds produce ↑ levels of exudate—use absorbent, non-bulky dressings that do not cause skin tension on transfer.
- Skin barriers may minimize stump excoriation/maceration.
- Tight/elasticated bandages should be avoided in vascular amputees.
- Once healing begins the stump can be shaped with a graduated pressure stump sock.
- Care must be taken to protect the contralateral leg from trauma.
- The patient's sacrum and heel will be susceptible to pressure damage.

## Related topics

📖 Wound assessment, p. 491; 📖 Wound debridement, p. 486; 📖 Infected wounds, p. 483; 📖 Leg ulcer assessment and management, p. 496; 📖 Wound dressings, p. 492.

## Further information

Website for specialist information on wound care. Available at: ✍ www.woundsinternational.com

# Wound dressings

Range of dressings available, often very little difference between competing brands. No dressings address all the requirements of an ideal dressing and no one dressing is suitable for all wound types. Choose dressings based upon wound characteristics (see Table 10.3 and refer to local formularies).

## Passive dressings

Products which have no direct effect on the wound. They protect the wound by covering it, e.g. low adherent dressings.

## Interactive dressings

Interact with the wound bed to provide an optimum local environment at the wound/dressing interface.

## Ideal dressing characteristics dressings should be:

- Highly absorbent.
- Comfortable to wear.
- Resistant to external contaminants.
- Low adherent.
- Moisture vapour permeable.
- Cost effective.
- Hypoallergenic.

## Dressing types

This list excludes those not recommended.

### Activated charcoal

*Contraindications:* dry, black necrotic wounds. Anaerobic bacteria causes wound malodour. This can be controlled by using active or antimicrobial dressings. Charcoal deodorizes, but once in contact with exudate, its odour adsorbing properties are ↓ and will require changing. Dressings containing activated charcoal—charcoal sandwiched between 2 fabric layers (BNF A5.2.8).

### Alginates

*Contraindications:* dry wounds, or those covered with dry necrotic tissue. Suitable for use with medium to heavily exuding wounds. Available as a loose 'rope' or packing for cavities, a ribbon for narrow wounds or sinuses, and a flat non-woven pad for larger open wounds. Alginates can be soaked off with saline or water (BNF A5.2.6).

### Anti-microbials

Dressings containing iodine, silver, honey, polyhexamethylene biguanide (PHMB).

*Dressings containing iodine*

A single course of treatment should not exceed 3mths. Contraindications:
• Known or suspected iodine sensitivity.
• Impaired renal function, thyroid disorders.
• Children, pregnant, lactating mothers.
• Iodosorb should not be used on dry wounds.

Suitable for suspected or infected, exuding wounds. *Available as:* polysaccharide paste between 2 fabric layers, polysaccharide paste/ointment. knitted viscose dressing impregnated with povidone iodine (BNF A5.3.2).

*Dressings containing silver*
*Contraindications:* dry wounds.

Powerful antimicrobial capable of killing antibiotic resistant strains of micro-organisms. Ability to kill micro-organisms influenced by:
• Distribution of silver in the dressing.
• The chemical/physical form of the silver.
• Dressing's affinity to moisture.

Dressings with silver concentrated on the surface have ↑ antimicrobial effect. Dressings with sustained silver-ion release effective against MRSA and vancomycin-resistant enterococci (VRE). Dressings containing silver—activated charcoal. Plus foams, hydrocolloid, hydrocolloid fibrous, non-woven fabric dressing (BNF A8.1.4).

### Films

*Contraindications:* highly exudating, deep, cavity or infected wounds. Suitable for lightly exudating, superficial wounds. Permeable to water vapour and oxygen and impermeable to micro-organisms, moist environment promotes epidermal regeneration in superficial wounds. Variety of uses in securing primary dressings and other medical devices, e.g. OpSite® Flexigrid, Tegaderm®. Adhesive films with absorbent pad, e.g. Mepore® Ultra, OpSite® Plus.

### Hydrocolloids

*Contraindications:* highly exudating, or infected wounds. Suitable for light to medium exuding wounds. Need margin of good skin around wound edges to ensure adhesion. Frequent changes with heavily exuding wounds. Thin hydrocolloid without border and fibrous hydrocolloid (BNF A8.1.4).

### Hydrogels

*Contraindications:* highly exudating wounds. As they contain 80% water hydrogels hydrate dry wounds and facilitate autolytic debridement of moist, sloughy, or dry necrotic wounds. Although gels look similar, fluid donating properties vary considerably. Some are able to absorb a limited amount of fluid from exuding wounds. Secondary dressing (film or foam) is required to retain amorphous hydrogels at the wound surface (BNF A8.1.3).

### Low-adherence dressings

*Contraindications:* highly exudating wounds especially if fluid is viscous. Suitable for light to medium exuding wounds, e.g. perforated plastic film faced dressing, cellulose dressings, knitted viscose primary dressing, adhesive bordered dressings, knitted fabric impregnated with silicone (BNF A5.4.2).

### Medical grade honey

*Contraindications:* if localized wound pain occurs discontinue. Suitable for suspected or infected, exuding wounds. Honey has powerful antimicrobial effects capable of killing antibiotic resistant strains of micro-organisms. Medical grade honey. Products containing honey—antibacterial medical wound gel, Mesitran range of products, e.g. hydrogel honey dressing, hydrocolloid honey dressing, polyester net honey dressing and ointments.

### Polyurethane foams

*Contraindications:* dry, necrotic wounds, narrow necked sinus. Suitable for light to medium exudating wounds, are hydrophilic, highly absorbent, and have low adherence. Absorb excess fluid, but maintain a moist wound surface—foam non-bordered, foam bordered, non-adhesive, foam bordered, adhesive. Foams suitable for cavities. Cavity wound dressing is formed from 2 reagents which react together to make a pliable, slightly absorbent foam, which is poured into cavities to promote granulation (BNF A5.2.5).

**Table 10.3** Selection of wound dressings by wound type (BNF Appendix 8)

| Wound bed | Necrotic/ sloughy | Clinical signs of infection | Clean granulation | Epithelia- lization |
|---|---|---|---|---|
| Exudate level | | | | |
| Heavy | Alginate<br>Foam<br>Honey dressings<br>Hydrocolloid fibrous | Iodine dressings/ pastes<br>Honey dressings<br>Silver alginate<br>Silver foam<br>Silver hydrocolloid fibrous<br>Silver non-woven fabric | Alginate<br>Foam<br>Honey dressings<br>Hydrocolloid fibrous | N/A |
| Moderate | Activated charcoal<br>Alginate<br>Foam<br>Honey dressings<br>Hydrocolloid fibrous<br>Hydrogel + foam | Iodine dressings/ pastes<br>Honey dressings<br>Silver alginate<br>Silver activated charcoal<br>Silver foam<br>Silver hydrocolloid fibrous<br>Silver non-woven fabric | Alginate<br>Foam<br>Honey dressings<br>Hydrocolloid fibrous<br>Hydrogel + foam | N/A |
| Minimal | Honey dressings<br>Hydrocolloid<br>Hydrogel + foam/film | Honey dressings<br>Silver hydrocolloid | Foam<br>Honey dressings<br>Hydrocolloid-film<br>Low-adherent dressings | Thin hydrocolloid film<br>Low-adherent dressings |

For further information see BNF Appendix 5

### Related topics
📖 Wound assessment, p. 475; 📖 Management of chronic wounds, p. 480
📖 Wound debridement, p. 486.

### Further information
BNF Appendix 5 Wound management products. Available at: 🔊 www.medicinescomplete.com/mc/bnf/current/

Wounds International. Website for specialist information on wound care. Available at: 🔊 www.woundsinternational.com

# Leg ulcer assessment and management

### Principles of leg ulcer assessment and management

Prevalence of leg ulcers is between 1–2% of adult population ↑ with age. Healing rates range from 45–80% at 24wks for all ulcer types. Ulceration is characterized by alternating phases of ulceration, healing, and recurrence. Estimated that approx 25% of patients have open ulcers at any time. 75% of all leg ulcers are venous in origin, 25% are arterial, mixed aetiology, or neuropathic.

Many leg ulcer patients have never had the aetiology of their ulcer correctly diagnosed. Ulcer aetiology determines the management strategy.

### Specific assessment criteria

- Medical history (damage to arterial/venous system).
- History of previous ulceration, healing, and recurrence.
- Presence of foot pulses.
- Doppler ultrasound (ankle brachial pressure index (ABPI)).
- Wound related pain (persistent/temporary).
- Condition of surrounding skin.
- How the ulcer affects ability to sleep?
- How the ulcer affects patient's mood and social interaction?
- Level of social support available to patient with a leg ulcer.
- Does the patient understand causation of ulcer?

### Management principles

General management principles for patients with leg ulcers are:
- Identification and treatment of the underlying cause of the ulcer.
- Provision of optimum local conditions at wound site.
- Provision of graduated compression therapy.
- Prevention of avoidable complications and recurrence.
- Involvement of the patient in their care and achieving concordance with treatment and after care.

### Investigations

- Urinanalysis.
- Duplex scan.
- Bloods FBC, ESR.
- Wound swabs C & S.
- Ankle brachial pressure.
- Patch testing.

### Factors delaying healing

- Increasing age.
- Poor general mobility.
- Ulcer duration.
- Fixed ankle mobility.
- Ulcer size.
- Co-morbidities.

Correct treatment depends upon accurate differentiation between venous insufficiency and arterial disease. The clinical signs summarized in Clinical signs and symptoms of venous and arterial leg ulceration (📖 p. 499).

Older people with ulcers of venous origin are likely to have co-existing arterial disease. A differential diagnosis should be based on physical examination and Doppler assessment.

## Vascular assessment

Hand-held Doppler compares blood flow in the arm with blood flow in the lower limb to calculate the ABPI. Doppler ultrasound ↑ accuracy of ulcer assessment by excluding concomitant arterial disease and defining a safe level of compression bandaging. All patients should have their ABPI calculated prior to treatment (see Table 10.4). For arterial ulcers the ABPI reading provides an indication of severity of the arterial disease. ABPI readings should be re-assessed every 3mths to detect early vascular changes.

**Table 10.4** Significance of ABPI readings

| | |
|---|---|
| ABPI 1 or >1 | Normal arterial blood flow |
| ABPI <0.9 | Mild degree of arterial involvement |
| ABPI 0.8 | 80% arterial blood flow reaching the foot |
| | Standard compression contraindicated |
| ABPI <0.7 | Arterial insufficiency. Vascular referral required |
| ABPI <0.5 | Severe arterial disease. Urgent vascular referral |

Standard compression therapy should not be applied if ABPI <0.8 due to risk of necrosis. UK national guidelines recommend that all patients with ABPI <0.8 should receive specialist assessment.

*Note:* specialist advice important for those with arterial disease including diabetes and rheumatoid arthritis. The following should be included in leg ulcer assessment documentation (see 📖 Wound assessment, p. 475):
• Family history.
• Varicose veins, hypertension.
• DVT, phlebitis.
• Allergies/hypersensitivities.

## Ulcer history (see also Table 10.5)
• Duration of current ulcer.
• Ankle mobility.
• Onset of first ulcer.
• Ankle measurement.
• Number of episodes recurrence.
• Skin condition .
• Location, e.g. gaiter area, foot, toes.
• Eczema/dry skin.

- Type of ulcer, e.g. venous, arterial, neuropathic.
- Skin sensitivities/allergies. Signs of chronic venous insufficiency, e.g. ankle flare, lipodermatosclerosis.

Regular re-assessment is important.

*Referral criteria*
Patients should be referred to medical staff if:
- Younger, mobile individuals.
- Unresponsive ulcers within 3mths.
- Failure to heal within a year.
- ABPI below 0.6 (severe ischaemic disease).
- Individuals with contact dermatitis.
- Uncertain aetiology of ulceration.

## Clinical signs and symptoms of venous and arterial leg ulceration

**Table 10.5** Comparison of clinical signs and symptoms of venous and arterial leg ulceration (leg ulcer assessment)

|  | Venous ulceration | Arterial ulceration |
|---|---|---|
| Previous medical history | Previous leg fracture (DVT), skin staining, eczema, FH of leg ulcers, varicose veins. | History of (CVA), heart disease, PVD, hypertension, diabetes. |
| Site/position | Often near the ankle or between the ankle and knee (gaiter area). | Usually on the foot, between the toes, or close to the medial malleolus. |
| Appearance | Large, shallow wounds producing copious exudate. | Often small, deep wounds producing less exudate. |
| Surrounding skin condition | Characteristic pigmentation—lipodermatosclerosis, atrophy blanche. Contact dermatitis and eczema common. | Hairless, shiny skin. Skin colour ranges from white to dusky pink and purple. Dusky pink feet turn pale when raised above heart. |
| Pain/discomfort | Aching/heaviness of legs, localized ulcer pain. | Severe rest pain, constant ulcer pain, often worse at night. |

## Related topic
📖 Compression therapy for venous ulcers, p. 502.

## Further information
Wounds International. Best Practice Statement: Compression Hosiery. Available at: ℘ www.woundsinternational.com/pdf/content_28.pdf
Wounds UK (2009). Skills for Practice: Management of Chronic Oedema in the Community. Available at: ℘ www.woundsinternational.com/pdf/content_206.pd

# Venous leg ulcers

Venous ulcers are one of the common types of chronic wound. Patients frequently experience wound leakage, offensive odour, wound pain, and lack of sleep. This can ↑ dependence on carers, ↓ quality of life, and affect self-esteem (see 📖 Leg ulcer assessment and management, p. 496):

- *Venous leg ulcer:* a non-healing break in the skin of the lower leg caused by disease in the venous system.
- *Lipodermatosclerosis:* characteristic skin changes in lower extremities including fat necrosis, skin staining, fibrosis of skin, and subcutaneous tissues that become hard and 'woody'.
- *Atrophe blanche:* refers to the presence of white satellite scars in the ankle area commonly seen in venous stasis due to occlusion of dermal vessels causing tissue death.

## Assessment

Signs of venous hypertension are initially mild and become more pronounced (📖 Leg ulcer assessment and management, p. 496).

## Risk factors

- DVT.
- Increasing age.
- Vein trauma/surgery.
- Gender—female.
- Phlebitis.
- Sedentary lifestyle.
- Congenital valve defect.

## Clinical signs of venous hypertension

- Ankle oedema (dependent).
- Ankle flare (distended venous medial aspect of ankle).
- Varicose veins.
- Abnormal leg shape 'inverted champagne bottle'.
- Brown skin pigmentation.
- Lipodermatosclerosis.
- Atrophe blanche.
- Varicose eczema.

## Complications

- Recurrent infection.
- *Lymphodema* (📖 p. 505): refer to specialist services.
- *Malignant changes (rare):* refer for biopsy.
- Contact dermatitis refer for patch testing.

## Management

*Aim of venous leg ulcer management:* reversal of venous hypertension. Compression therapy is the cornerstone of treatment (📖 Compression therapy for venous ulcers, p. 502).

*Exudate*

Can produce high levels of exudate which ↓ with healing. Select dressings that will absorb excess exudate, but still maintain a moist wound environment to avoid dressing adhesion and trauma. Skin barriers can be an effective method of reducing damage and excoriation.

*Debridement*

(📖 Wound debridement, p. 486.) Infection or uncontrolled oedema are the commonest causes of slough accumulation on the ulcer surface and require removal. Uncomplicated venous ulcers generally do not require debridement. Surgical debridement seldom used as ulcers are shallow and risk of damage great.

*Pain*

Pain is common and often underestimated can contribute to sleep disturbance, anxiety, depression, and poor compliance with treatment. Important to assess and manage (📖 Pain assessment and management, p. 513).

*Skin care*

Varicose eczema and contact dermatitis are common. Patients are often sensitive to allergens, e.g. latex, preservatives, and perfumes. Corticosteroid creams may help. Contact dermatitis should be suspected when eczema does not respond to treatment. All topical products should be discontinued and patch tests performed. Development of irritant dermatitis and maceration often leads to new areas of ulceration.

*Prevention of recurrence*

Once healed follow-up care is essential as recurrence rates are high. Appropriate skin care, exercise, leg elevation, and avoidance of prolonged standing should be emphasized together with the permanent use of fitted compression stockings (BNF Appendix 8) to minimize recurrence.

*Useful dressing types (BNF Appendix 5)*

Refer also to local prescribing formularies for product choice and guidance.
- Alginate.
- Antimicrobial dressings.
- Foam.
- Hydrocolloid fibrous.
- Low adherent contact layers.
- Secondary absorbent pads.
- Clean ulcers with clean water or normal saline solution.
- Fluid absorption of dressings may be affected beneath compression bandages as lateral flow of fluid may be affected.
- Avoid bulky dressings that under compression can cause local pressure damage and tissue necrosis.
- Simple non-adherent dressings are recommended to minimize skin maceration.
- *To contain leakage distal to ulcer:* position dressings slightly off centre.
- Topical antimicrobials can used for short duration, if no improvement is seen by 2 wks, stop treatment and consider systemic antibiotics.
- Skin barriers may minimize skin excoriation/maceration.

## Related topics

📖 Wound assessment, p. 475; 📖 Management of chronic wounds, p. 480; 📖 Compression therapy for venous ulcers, p. 502; 📖 Wound dressings, p. 492.

## Further information

Scottish Intercollegiate Guidelines Network (2010). *Management of Chronic Venous leg ulcers guide-line.* 120. Available at: 🔗 www.sign.ac.uk/guidelines/fulltext/120/index.html

# Compression therapy for venous ulcers

The most effective treatment of venous leg ulcers is high compression therapy; can heal 50–80% of venous ulcers in a 12wk period. It is vital to involve the patient in all stages of care, especially decision-making around treatment decisions (📖 Leg ulcer assessment and management, p. 496; 📖 Venous leg ulcers, p. 499):

- Multi-layer systems are more effective than single-layered systems.
- High compression is more effective than low compression.

The aims of compression therapy are to:

- Reduce pressure in superficial venous system.
- Encourage venous return and tissue perfusion.
- Minimize oedema.
- Improve lymphatic drainage.

## Contraindications

- Arterial disease (ABPI >0.5).
- Co-existing vascular conditions.
- Patients with narrow ankles/calves.
- Patients with reduced sensation.
- Uncontrolled heart failure.

❶ Extreme caution should be exercised for patients with venous leg ulcer and diabetes (📖 p. 611) or rheumatoid arthritis (📖 p. 555).

Various methods of achieving graduated compression include:

- Compression bandages.
- Compression hosiery.
- Intermittent compression systems.

Choice depends on resources, size and shape of the patient's leg, patient mobility, and patient preference and local policy.

## Bandage types

(See 📖 BNF Appendix 5.8.)

*Highly extensible (elastic) bandage:* contain elastic materials and apply sustained compression over time by applying pressure inwards to the tissues at rest.

*Minimally extensible (inelastic) bandage:* contain inelastic materials providing a rigid structure—the pressure rises when the calf muscle expands against the rigid cuff during activity causing pressure to be forced into the tissues. Does not sustain pressure over long periods of time.

## Bandage application

❶ Should only be done by practitioners trained in compression therapy.

A venous ulcer with a reading of >0.8, standard compression should be applied which exerts a sub-bandage pressure of between 30–40mmHg at the ankle. The highest pressure should be exerted at the ankle, gradually falling to 50% at the knee. Reduced levels of compression may also be safely used in patients with mild arterial disease (ABPI 0.5–0.8). Table 10.6 outlines RCN/SIGN recommendations and a range of regimens that may be used.

**Table 10.6** Recommendations for use of compression in relation to arterial status

| ABPI (ankle to brachial pressure index) | Compression regimen | Comments |
|---|---|---|
| >0.8 | High compression | Bandage pressure approx. 40mmHg, e.g. Setopress®, Tensopress® Multi-layer, e.g.: Profore®. Caution in patients with concurrent conditions, e.g. diabetes and heart failure. |
| 0.5–0.8 | Reduced compression | Bandage pressure approx. 20–25mmHg, e.g. Litepress®, Elset® paste bandage + elastocrepe Rosidal K®, Comprilan®, Reduced multi-layer, e.g. Profore® Lite. Careful monitoring of vascular signs. |
| <0.5 | No compression | Patients should be referred for urgent vascular opinion. |

Three factors affect the amount of pressure exerted onto a limb.

### Factor 1. Bandage tension
The more the bandage is stretched on application the higher the sub bandage pressure. Generally elasticated bandages (highly extensible) are applied with 50% extension. The aim is to apply the bandage with constant extension.

### Factor 2. Limb circumference
For effective graduation, ankle circumference should measure approximately 50% of the calf circumference. A bandage applied with constant tension and 50% overlap will exert a higher pressure at the ankle than calf. Bony prominences are prone to high pressure. Apply orthopaedic wool to protect the skin and to increase the size of small ankles. To determine the bandage regimen, re-measure ankle circumference weekly and refer to manufacturer's guidance on bandage application according to ankle circumference.

*Factor 3. Bandage layers*
The more layers applied the higher the sub-bandage pressure gained. When applying a spiral application using 50% overlap 2 layers are being applied, conversely a figure of 8 application applies 4 layers.

## Practical application

* Measure ankle circumference.
* Cover ulcer with primary dressing.
* Avoid padding small areas, e.g. bony prominences.
* Apply bandage from base of toes to knee (refer to manufacturer's instructions).
* Avoid double turns of the bandage which doubles the pressure exerted in a single turn.
* Do not apply additional layers of bandage under knee in an attempt to use up bandage surplus.
* Ask patient to inform staff if bandage feels uncomfortable and remove if necessary.

*Prevention of recurrence after healing*
It is important that patients wear below-knee support hosiery. Compression hosiery maintains a compression force of between 30–40mmHg at the ankle and maintains venous return. Hosiery should be measured and fitted. Hosiery is tight and patients may initially have difficulty in getting it on, should be applied with care to prevent skin damage. A minimum of 1-year follow-up post healing to ↓ risk of recurrence.

## Related topics

📖 Wound assessment, p. 475; 📖 Management of chronic wounds, p. 480; 📖 Venous leg ulcers, p. 499.

## Further information

Scottish Intercollegiate Guidelines Network (2010). *Management of Chronic Venous leg ulcers guideline*. 120. Available at: 🔊 www.sign.ac.uk/guidelines/fulltext/120/index.html

# Lymphoedema

A long-term problem caused by obstruction of lymphatic drainage, causing oedema, affects one or more limbs and adjacent trunk. If not treated lymphoedema becomes resistant to treatment arising from chronic inflammation and subcutaneous fibrosis. Cellulitis causes a rapid ↑ in swelling. *Note:* swelling can usually be reduced, but can take weeks or months before discernible improvement and it may recur.

Secondary lymphoedema caused by:
• Tumour in axilla, groin, or intrapelvic area.
• Extensive axillary or groin surgery (including mastectomy involving axillary clearance).
• Post-operative infection/radiotherapy.
• Trauma.

*Note:* more likely to occur if surgery and radiotherapy on the same area.

## Aims of care
• Relieve discomfort by reducing swelling.
• Prevent build up of fluid.
• Prevent complications, e.g. cellulitis.

## Care and management
• Important to have good skin care and prevention of infection. Moisturize skin everyday with non-perfumed cream/oil, clean and treat small cuts, wear gloves for housework and gardening to reduce risk of cuts, insect repellant to avoid bites, sun protection.
• Treat fungal infections, e.g. athletes foot (📖 Fungal infections, p. 638).
• Avoid BP measurement, vaccination, and taking bloods on affected limb.
• Compression garments, e.g. sleeves, stockings, special bras need to be fitted. Use with extreme caution or not at all if skin fragile, limb is very swollen, or skin is pitted. Multi layer bandaging can provide support and immobility to affected limb.
• Support swollen arms when sitting with a pillow and slightly elevate when lying down (do not rest arm above shoulder height). Support affected legs when sitting and avoid standing for long periods.
• Gentle exercises following advice from lymphoedema specialist. Should always wear compression garment when doing exercise. Stop exercise if skin becomes red.
• Refer for manual lymphatic drainage (MLD) by trained specialist, patient can be taught by specialist to do simple lymphatic drainage (SLD). Gentle fingertip massage to promote drainage.
• Excess heat can exacerbate swelling. Advise to avoid saunas, direct heat, very hot showers and baths, etc.

## Related topic
📖 Breast cancer, p. 723.

## Key reference text

Lymphoedema Framework Best Practice for the Management of Lymphoedema International Consensus document (2006). The Management of Lymphoedema in Advanced Cancer and Oedema at the End of Life (2010). Available at: ℘ www.lympho.org

## Further information

British Lymphology Society. Available at: ℘ www.lymphoedema.org

Lymphodoema Support Network provides directory of services available for sufferers. Available at: ℘ www.lymphoedema.org/lsn

Lymphoedema Network (Europe). Available at: ℘ www.lymphoedema.org

# Chemotherapy in the home

Chemotherapy can be used for cure or palliation; aim to reduce the number of actively dividing cells in a tumour. Most cytotoxic drugs disrupt cell reproduction by damaging DNA or affecting mitosis. There is a narrow margin between therapeutic and lethal dose. Need to know:

- The name, action, and side effects of drugs the patient is receiving.
- Local policies and procedures for all aspects of cytotoxic drug administration including management of side effects and emergency situations including anaphylaxis and extravasation.
- Transport drugs in labelled, robust, tamper- and leak-proof container.
- Store drugs in the correct conditions and out of reach of children.
- Disposal methods for cytotoxic drugs and waste as set out in Hazardous Waste Regulations England and Wales (2011).
- Equipment available and access to spillage and extravasation kits.
- Links with 2° care and contact details for advice and support.
- Administration of drugs must comply with COSHH and HSE Protection legislation.
- Pregnant workers can choose not to be involved in activities involving exposure to cytotoxic drugs.

Cytotoxic drugs are teratogenic, mutagenic, and carcinogenic, and potentially hazardous to patients, staff, families, and the environment. Exposure occurs through ingestion, inhalation, and absorption through skin. Highest risk = reconstituting drugs, connecting and disconnecting IV tubing, and disposing of used equipment and patient excreta.

## Measures to reduce exposure to cytotoxic drugs

- Drugs should be supplied ready for administration.
- Gloves should be worn at all times when handling drugs and excreta and be changed regularly.
- Dispose of contaminated needles, syringes, should be intact. All drug containers, unused drugs and equipment such as gloves and aprons must be disposed on in leak proof container clearly marked *cytotoxic*. It is hazardous waste and must be disposed of separately from other types of waste. Consignment note needed so that disposal can be tracked[1]. Description should include waste codes for cytotoxic drugs, estimate of the weight of the waste in kg, chemical components of the waste and physical form of waste, i.e. liquid, solid mixed, and the hazard codes.
- Community pharmacists can receive hazardous waste from patients for disposal in the same way they receive other unwanted medication.
- Patient excreta may contain traces of drugs for up to 72hrs.
- *If there is a risk of splashing or generating an aerosol:* use eye and respiratory protection. Undertake a COSHH risk assessment for each handling activity to assess if a gown or plastic apron best protection.
- Avoid eating and drinking in areas where drugs are administered.
- Do not handle oral preparations never crush tablets or open capsules.

**Spillage** Kits should always be available. Use copious amounts of soap and water for skin contact. Eyes should be flooded with water or isotonic eye wash solution for 5min minimum and seek medical advice. Spillage of a large amount of cytotoxic drug incurring exposure should be reported to RIDDOR (Reporting Injuries, Diseases and Dangerous Occurrences Regulations 1995).

## Care and management

- Patients and their carers need education and information about safe handling, side effects of treatment, dose and duration of drug treatment, the importance of strict adherence to the drug regimen, who to contact, and what to do if they experience side effects.
- Absorption of oral drugs may be affected by food, gastrointestinal problems, e.g. nausea and vomiting or diarrhoea and concurrent medications.

**Venous access devices** For those having lengthy courses of treatment a central venous access device (CVAD) (e.g. Hickman line) is usual. Patients may be sent home with a small battery-operated pump connected to a central line for administration of chemotherapy.

- Prevention of infection is vital and strict asepsis.
- Monitor for signs of tissue infiltration/extravasation, i.e. infiltration of a drug into the subcutaneous tissues and subsequent tissue damage are major potential problems. Symptoms include erythema, discoloration, swelling, leakage, change in skin temperature, burning stinging and pain resistance to syringe or slowing of infusion rate, lack of blood return.
- Any prescribed pre-hydration fluids or anti-emetics should be given before chemotherapy is commenced.
- Before giving drug, withdraw blood and flush with NaCl 0.9% to ensure patency Note: sodium chloride not compatible with all drugs.
- Nurses looking after patients on chemotherapy should know drug properties, extravasation symptoms, and how to manage an emergency.

## Managing extravasation

Management of extravasation is controversial. Local protocols and procedures should be known before any drug administration. Administration of chemotherapy should always be done as part of the MDT, following training and with the support of the specialist oncology centre. General principles:

- Stop administration immediately.
- Leave cannula in place.
- Seek specialist medical help.
- Mark affected area with pen.

## Related topics

Palliative care in the home, p. 509; Syringe drivers, p. 521.

## Reference

[1]DH. (2013) Health Technical Memorandum 07-01 – Safe management of healthcare waste. Available at https://www.gov.uk/government/publications/guidance-on-the-safe-management-of-healthcare-waste

## Further information

NICE (2003). Infection control: prevention of health care associated infection in primary and secondary care (section on care of central venous catheters). Available at: www.nice.org.uk
Tadman M, Roberts D. (2007). *Oxford Handbook of Cancer Nursing*. Oxford: Oxford University Press.

# Palliative care in the home

The majority of people would like to die at home, but the minority achieve this. However, for most patients, 90% of the final year of life is spent at home or in a care home.

## Palliative care

Emphasizes the improvement of quality of life of patients with advanced illness and their families, through:
- The prevention and relief of distress.
- Early detection and assessment and treatment of symptoms and other problems, physical, psychosocial, and spiritual.

## General palliative care

Focus on patients with low to moderate palliative care needs, also those with complex needs supported by specialist palliative care.

## Specialist palliative care

Provided by practitioners for whom this is their main role often as part of MDT. Focus on patients with moderate to complex palliative care needs and their families by supporting GPs and primary care nurses to provide care and/or provide patient care themselves.

## End-of-life care

Usually the last year of life for patients with advance, progressive, incurable illness. *Aim:* to enable patients to live as well as possible until they die through the identification of patients and their families supportive and palliative care needs in the last phase of life and into bereavement.

## Terminal care

The management of patients from the time it is apparent the patient is in a progressive state of decline, i.e. last few days, weeks of life.

There is increasing emphasis in palliative care on using outcome measures to assess presentation and review management plan, e.g. symptom distress. Patients who are dying and their carers value:
- Person-centred care.
- Quality of life and effective symptom control.
- Choice, information, and control over care and decisions made.
- Being listened to and the time to discuss feelings and worries.
- Access to services.
- Continuity of care.

## National end-of-life care strategy

Details the End-of-Life Care Pathway applicable to all those approaching the end of life and into bereavement. *Dying Matters Coalition:* collaboration of key organizations involved in end-of-life care and organizes a dying awareness week each year.

### Gold Standard Framework (GSF)

Is a proactive model of care for end-of-life care that is provided by generalist staff in any registered setting, including general practice, care homes, and acute hospitals. GSF emphasizes a whole team approach (e.g. PHCT) for patients in the last year of life.

Three key processes:
- *Identify:* patients considered last year of life and stage, record on a register (e.g. surprise question).
- *Assess:* clinical and personal needs (e.g. Advance Care Planning).
- *Plan:* ahead and anticipate needs (e.g. pre-emptive prescribing).

Emphasizes the 7 Cs of:
- Communication record on palliative care register (e.g. if answer is 'no' to would you be surprised if this person died in the next 12mths: surprise question).
- Co-ordination of care.
- Control of symptoms.
- Continuity of care.
- Continued learning.
- Carer support.
- Care of the dying pathway.

### Advance Care Planning (ACP)

A process of discussion that intends to make clear a person's wishes. It anticipates a time when they might not have the capacity to make some decisions. ACP may cover any aspect of future health and social care.

### Preferred Priorities for Care (PfPC)

A tool that:
- Facilitates discussion(s) around end-of-life care wishes and preferences.
- Enable communication for care planning and decisions across care providers.
- Sharing the document (with consent) with key care providers can inform cross organizational care planning and clinical decision-making.
- Should a patient lose capacity information included within the PfPC can be used as part of an assessment of a person's best interests. (📖 Mental Capacity, p. 424) if the patient cannot make a decision about their care, it has to be taken into account.

### Advance Decision (advance directive to refuse treatment)

Enables the individual:
- To refuse a particular type of medical treatment or care if they become unable to make/communicate decisions for themselves.
- Can be verbal, but if an advance decision includes refusal of life sustaining treatment, it must be in writing, signed and witnessed, and include the statement 'even if life is at risk'.
- Will only come into effect if the individual loses capacity.
- Only applies if the treatment and any circumstances are those specifically identified in the advance decision.

- Is legally binding if valid and applicable to the circumstances.
- Can ask doctors not to give certain medical treatments.
- Cannot refuse basic nursing care or ask that nurses do not offer food and drink by mouth.
- Cannot refuse treatment that goes against a court order.

Completed forms are witnessed, and copies lodged with GP, friends, and family. Patients can change their minds. For people under 18, they do not have the same legal status. Young people's views must be considered in any decisions made about their own treatment.

### Do Not Attempt Cardiopulmonary Resuscitation

Completed by the clinician responsible for the individual (e.g. GP) often in discussion with the patient. If cardiac or respiratory arrest is an expected part of the dying process and CPR will not be successful, making and recording Do Not Attempt Cardiopulmonary Resuscitation (DNACPR) will help to ensure that the patient dies in a dignified manner and in their preferred place of care by, for example, avoiding emergency admission from a community setting to hospital.

(*Note:* see ☐ Prescribing, p. 130; ☐ Controlled drugs, p. 137.)

### Related topics

☐ Syringe drivers, p. 521; ☐ End-of-life issues, p. 530; ☐ Carers assessment and support, p. 412; ☐ Bereavement, grief, and coping with loss, p. 528; ☐ Controlled drugs, p. 137.

### Further information

Gold Standards Framework. Available at: ℘ http://www.goldstandardsframework.org.uk/

Macmillan Cancer Support Learning Zone with e-learning programmes and resources on cancer and palliative care. Available at: ℘ http://learnzone.macmillan.org.uk/

National Council for Palliative Care/National End of Life Care Programme Dying Matters coalition (23 January 2013) Advance decisions to refuse treatment A guide for health and social care professionals. Order hard copies by email to: information@eolc.nhs.uk

Palliative Care Guidelines NHS Scotland good practice in the management of adults with a life limiting illness. Available at: ℘ http://www.palliativecareguidelines.scot.nhs.uk/

Palliative Outcome Scale (POS) site. Available at: ℘ http://pos-pal.org/

Watson M, Lucas C, Hoy A, et al (2009). *Oxford Handbook of Palliative Care*, 2nd edn. Oxford: Oxford University Press.

WHO Palliative Care for Older People: Better Practices (2011). Available at: ℘ http://www.euro.who.int/en/what-we-do/health-topics/Life-stages/healthy-ageing/publications/pre-2009/better-palliative-care-for-older-people

# Services available for the dying patient and their carers

*PHCT provide generalist palliative care:* GP and DNs establish ongoing relationships with patients, assess need, provide direct care, liaise with specialists in palliative care, social care and 2° services.

Note: service provision is locally determined. Poor recognition of palliative care needs for patients with non-malignant advanced illness and their carers leads to less support than for people with cancers who have equivalent symptoms and problems.

## Services available

- *Out-of-hours* care where there is 24hr DN availability; greater likelihood of maintaining a patient at home.
- *Specialist palliative care services:* multi-disciplinary specialist palliative care team, e.g. consultant, social worker, clinical nurse specialist (e.g. Macmillan nurse), hospice home care team, symptom control team, pain control team, Marie Curie nurses.
- *Hospice services:* in-patient hospice care for symptom control, respite and end-of-life care; outpatient hospice day centre and clinics (e.g. Breathlessness Clinic) and outreach/hospice at home teams.
- Social care night sitters through social service or Marie Curie night sitter service. Some social services also fund or provide respite care, carers' support groups and financial advice.
- *Care homes and community hospitals:* provide respite and short stay support particularly for people who live alone. They also receive referrals from hospitals and hospices of people identified as in need of end-of-life care (EoLC). Often these care homes have GSF accreditation.
- Charities can help with respite care, extra nursing at home, financial support for people with advanced illness, and bereavement support.
- Online support and teaching e-ELCA contains 150 sessions on all aspects of EoLC for health and social care staff. ℘ www.e-lfh.org.uk/projects/e-elca Macmillan Cancer Support Learning Zone with e-learning programmes and resources on cancer and palliative care. ℘ http://learnzone.macmillan.org.uk/

## Related topics

📖 Palliative care in the home, p. 509; 📖 End-of-life issues, p. 530; 📖 Carers assessment and support, p. 412; 📖 Bereavement, grief, and coping with loss, p. 528.

## Further information

Advance Decisions to Refuse Treatment. Available at: ℘ http://www.adrt.nhs.uk/
Gold Standards Framework. Available at: ℘ http://www.goldstandardsframework.org.uk/
Palliative Adult Network Guidelines (2011). 3rd edn. Available at: ℘ http://book.pallcare.info or through local National Cancer Research Institute network.
Palliative Care Guidelines NHS Scotland. Available at: ℘ www.palliativecareguidelines.scot.nhs.uk/

# Pain assessment and management

Pain is an unpleasant sensory and/or emotional experiences linked to actual or potential tissue damage (e.g. muscle, nerve, bone). It is a subjective experience. It is always the patient who defines it and its severity.

Health professionals often underestimate patient's pain and overemphasize the risk of addiction or overmedication. Pain can go unrecognized especially in older people or those with cognitive impairment.

**Acute pain** The cause is often obvious although the amount of pain reported is often unrelated to injury.

## Chronic pain

For >3–6 million a significant source of suffering. >7% of adults in the UK and 70% of sufferers experience pain despite analgesia. Causes are multi-factoral. Living with pain can:
- Induce depression, sense of hopelessness and exacerbate anxiety.
- Disrupt sleep.
- Affect ability to perform everyday tasks and work.
- Damage relationships and challenge existential beliefs.

## Assessment

Open-ended questions to allow the patient to define the pain experience. Follow-up with questions to locate and monitor the pain, e.g.
- Where the pain is and if multiple pain sites, and how long experienced?
- Describe the pain, e.g. aching, stabbing, and pain intensity (e.g. numerical rating scale 0–10 with 'no pain' to 'worst pain', or hand with 1–5)?
- What triggers the pain and if these have changed over time?
- Is it worse at different times of day?
- What relieves the pain, e.g. analgesia, relaxation, distraction?
- Observational assessment essential patients with cognitive impairment, e.g. facial expressions grimacing; body movements rocking, guarding; vocalizations moaning; changes mental state increasing tearfulness.

## Pain assessment tools

Tools to initially assess pain and chart effectiveness of pain reduction strategies and interventions.
- *A body map:* to record location(s) and characteristics, useful multiple pain sites.
- *Visual analogue scales:* a line with 'no pain' and 'worst pain' at each extreme. Patient marks point online that reflects their pain severity.
- *Variations on the analogue scales include:* verbal rating scales, numerical rating scales or a hand is useful if patient has limited numeracy.
- Brief Pain Inventory measures location, intensity, triggers; McGill Pain Questionnaire useful if suspect nerve (neuropathic) pain (e.g. shooting pain). Useful individuals with cognitive impairment unable to verbalize. More complex tools can help identify complex patterns of pain and effectiveness of different treatments.
- If patient lacks capacity consider dementia specific scales, e.g. Abbey Pain Scale.

## Pain management

- Fear always increases the pain perception. Important that the patient is reassured supported and involved in decisions on pain control through education and discussion of possible options (see Table 10.7).
- Ensure when possible causes of pain are addressed, e.g. infection.
- Use WHO analgesia ladder: staged approach to pain control for progressive pain associated advanced illness (see Fig. 10.3).
- Morphine is gold standard opioid, 2nd-line opioid is oxycodone.
- To maintain freedom from pain in palliative care, pain relief should be given 'by the clock' not on demand, with breakthrough analgesia when managing moderate to severe pain.

### Management of pain in palliative care

Pain is multi-factorial and can arise from:

- Cancer-specific causes, e.g. bone metastases, nerve compression/ infiltration, muscle spasm, lymphoedema, raised intracranial pressure.
- Associated factors: e.g. constipation.
- Arising from treatment, e.g. surgery, radiotherapy.
- Co-morbidity, e.g. arthritis.

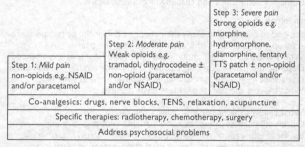

| Step 1: *Mild pain* non-opioids e.g. NSAID and/or paracetamol | Step 2: *Moderate pain* Weak opioids e.g. tramadol, dihydrocodeine ± non-opioid (paracetamol and/or NSAID) | Step 3: *Severe pain* Strong opioids e.g. morphine, hydromorphone, diamorphine, fentanyl TTS patch ± non-opioid (paracetamol and/or NSAID) |
|---|---|---|

| Co-analgesics: drugs, nerve blocks, TENS, relaxation, acupuncture |
|---|
| Specific therapies: radiotherapy, chemotherapy, surgery |
| Address psychosocial problems |

**Fig. 10.3** WHO Pain Relief ladder.

Reproduced with permission from Watson M. (2005). *Oxford Handbook of Palliative Care.* Oxford: Oxford University Press.

## Related topics

📖 Syringe drivers, p. 521; 📖 Symptom control in palliative care, p. 516.

## Further information

British Pain Society guidance on pain and management. Available at: ℅ www.britishpainsociety. org/pub-professional.htm

NICE (2012). *Opioids in palliative care: safe and effective prescribing of strong opioids for pain in palliative care of adults.* NICE Guideline 140. Available at: ℅ http://www.nice.org.uk/cg140

Oxford Pain Internet site. Available at: ℅ http://www.medicine.ox.ac.uk/bandolier/booth/painpag/

Payne S, Seymour J, Ingleton C. (2008). *Palliative Care Nursing: principles and evidence for practice*, 2nd edn. Maidenhead: Open University Press.

Watson MS, Lucas C, Hoy A, et al. (2009). *Oxford Handbook of Palliative Care*, 2nd edn. Oxford: Oxford University Press.

**Table 10.7** Management of specific types of pain

| Type of pain | Management |
|---|---|
| Bone pain | Try NSAIDs. |
| | Consider referral for palliative radiotherapy, strontium treatment (prostate cancer), or IV bisphosphonates (↓ pain in myeloma, breast and prostate cancer). |
| | Refer to orthopaedics if any lytic metastases at risk of fracture, for consideration of pinning. |
| Abdominal pain | Constipation is the most common cause. |
| | Colic—try loperamide 2–4mg qds or hyoscine hydrobromide 300mcg tds s/ling. Hyoscine can also be given via syringe driver. |
| | Liver capsule pain—use dexamethasone 4–8mg/day, titrating dose down to minimum that controls pain. |
| | Gastric distention—may be helped by an antacid ± an anti-foaming agent (e.g. Asilone®). Alternatively, a prokinetic may help, e.g. domperidone 10mg tds before meals. |
| | Upper GI tumour—coeliac plexus block may help. Refer to palliative care team. |
| | Consider drug causes—NSAIDs are a common iatrogenic cause. |
| | Acute/subacute obstruction |
| Neuropathic pain | Often burning/shooting. May not respond to simple analgesia. |
| | Titrate to the maximum tolerated dose of opioid. |
| | If inadequate, add a nerve pain killer e.g. amitriptyline 10–25mg nocte increasing as needed every 2wks to 75–150mg. Alternatives include carbamazepine, gabapentin, phenytoin, sodium valproate, and clonazepam. |
| | If pain is due to nerve compression caused by tumour, dexamethasone 8mg od may help. |
| | Other options: TENS; acupuncture; nerve block |
| Rectal pain | Topical drugs, e.g. rectal steroids. |
| | TCAs, e.g. amitriptyline 10–100mg nocte. |
| | Anal spasms—glyceryl trinitrate ointment 0.1–0.2% bd. |
| | Referral for local radiotherapy. |
| Muscle pain | Paracetamol and/or NSAIDs. |
| | Muscle relaxants, e.g. diazepam 5–10mg od, baclofen 5–10mg tds, dantrolene. |
| | Physiotherapy, aromatherapy, or relaxation. |
| | Heat pads. |
| Bladder spasm | Try oxybutinin 5mg tds or tolterodine 2mg bd. |
| | Amitriptyline 10–75mg nocte is often effective. |
| | If catheterized, try instilling 20mL of intravesical bupivacaine 0.25% for 15min tds. |
| Acute pain of short duration, e.g. dressing changes | Try short-acting opiate, e.g. meptazinol 200mg po given 20min. prior to procedure. |

Reproduced with permission from Simon, C., Everitt, H., and van Dorp, F. (2010). *Oxford Handbook of General Practice*, 3rd edn., Oxford University Press, Oxford.

# Symptom control in palliative care: nausea and vomiting

20–30% of patients with cancer will experience nausea and 70% in last week of life. Vomiting occurs in 20% of patients with cancer. 30% of patients receiving opioids will feel nauseated and/or retch and vomit in first week of treatment. Treatment decisions should be in consultation with patient, other members of the MDT and where available specialist palliative care services. Causes often multifactoral including:

- Metabolic, e.g. hypercalcaemia, renal failure (do blood biochemistry screen to check).
- Drugs, e.g. opioids. antibiotics, NSAIDs, iron, digoxin.
- Toxic, e.g. infection, chemotherapy, radiotherapy.
- Brain metastases.
- Dehydration.
- Dysphagia (*Note:* regurgitation can be mistaken for vomiting).
- Psychosomatic factors, e.g. anxiety, fear.
- Pain.
- Strong smells, e.g. from fungating wound.

When assessing impact of nausea and vomiting consider:

- Level of hydration.
- Functional impact on patient's and family/carer's everyday activities.
- Impact on patient's level of anxiety and depression.
- Whether patient's overall level of wellbeing means that they could benefit from chemotherapy to palliate symptoms, e.g. ovarian and colonic cancers can respond well.

## Care and management

- Identify presence nausea and/or vomiting, different management.
- Identify the cause (*Note:* if multifactoral = separate interventions).
- Correct reversible causes, e.g. constipation, dehydration.
- Refer to local formularies and protocols for care.
- Depending on symptoms use first line anti-emetic (Table 10.8). If fails to respond consider alternative medication and/or seek specialist opinion.
- Regular small amounts of fluid and food more likely to be tolerated.
- Support and reassurance to patient and family/carers.

❶ For prophylaxis of nausea and vomiting use oral medications. Always give anti-emetics regularly not prn. For established nausea and vomiting consider a parenteral route, e.g. syringe driver as persistent nausea may reduce gastric emptying and drug absorption.

## Non-drug measures to palliate nausea and vomiting

- Avoidance of food smells and strong odours.
- Diversion and relaxation techniques.
- Acupressure/acupuncture.

**Table 10.8** Anti-emetic therapy (refer to Palliative Adult Network Guidelines or NHS Clinical Knowledge Summaries and BNF for dosage advice, administration routes and possible interactions)

| Cause | First choice treatment | Second choice treatment |
|---|---|---|
| ↑ ICP, cerebral irritation/tumour/ metastases | Dexamethasone | Cyclizine<br>Metoclopramide |
| Abdominal and pelvic tumour | Cyclizine | Add dexamethasone |
| Gastric stasis | Metoclopramide or domperidone | Reduce gastric secretion PPI (e.g. omeprazole) |
| Chemically or metabolically induced and if beginning opioids | Metoclopramide or haloperidol (other drugs and metabolic causes haloperidol) | Dexamethasone or substitute with levomepromazine |
| Movement-related nausea and vomiting | Cyclizine | Hyoscine hydrobromide (consider transdermal patch) |
| Unknown cause | Haloperidol and/or cyclizine | Levomepremazine<br>Dexamethasone |

## Related topics

📖 Syringe drivers, p. 521; 📖 Palliative care in the home, p. 509.

## Further information

Essential information on drugs used in palliative care. Available at: ℘ http://www.palliativedrugs.com

NICE Palliative cancer care: nausea and vomiting. Available at: ℘ http://cks.nice.org.uk/palliative-cancer-care-nausea-vomiting

Palliative Adult Network Guidelines (2011) 3rd edn. Available at: ℘ http://book.pallcare.info or through local National Cancer Research Institute network

# Symptom control in palliative care: breathlessness

Breathlessness = breathing feels uncomfortable and/or difficult. The emotional experience of breathlessness is inextricable from the sensation and biomedical causes. Common in patients with primary lung cancer, but 19–64% of patients with other cancers particularly of breast, prostate, colon or rectum have symptoms, yet in 25% no evidence lung or pleural involvement. Reduces activity, social life, and self-esteem, few patients are continuously breathless, bouts triggered by exertion and emotion. Often characterized by:

- Rapid respiration.
- Nasal flaring and using accessory muscles to breathe.
- Feelings of panic and being unable to get enough breath.
- Fears of impending death.
- May be accompanied by cough, sputum, haemoptysis, fatigue, insomnia, pain, loss of appetite, anxiety, and depression.

## Breathlessness: possible physical causes

- *Primary or secondary cancer:* airway constriction/obstruction (always look for stridor), size and sit of tumour, inflammation, involvement of pleura, pericardium, vessel involvement (e.g. SVC obstruction), neural involvement, e.g. phrenic nerve palsy.
- *Indirect consequences of cancer :* PE, pneumonia, pneumothorax, ascites, fatigue/weakness, anaemia (<9.0g/dL), folic and B12 deficiency.
- *Respiratory muscle weakness* (severe) (e.g. MND), cachexia-anorexia, drug induced (corticosteroids, benzodiazepines), electrolyte imbalances/abnormalities.
- *Surgery:* e.g. pneumonectomy, lobectomy.
- Radiation-induced pneumonitis or fibrosis, pericarditis.
- Chemotherapy-induced pulmonary and cardiac toxicity, myelosuppression.
- *Co-morbidities:* heart failure, COPD.

## Care and management

Evidence for non-pharmacological nursing interventions for breathlessness suggest following help quality of life.

- Careful assessment of what relieves or exacerbates symptoms and if symptoms have rapid or gradual onset.
- Exploration of what breathlessness means to patients about their disease and their feelings about the future.
- Advice and support for patients and families on management strategies training in breathing control techniques, progressive muscle relaxation and distraction exercises.
- Goal setting alongside breathing and relaxation techniques.
- Early recognition of problems that need pharmacological/medical intervention.

## Treatments: non-pharmacological approaches

Relaxation strategies help 'undo' established reactions to breathlessness: and give patient a sense of control.

- To relax shoulders, upper back and neck, exhale slowly letting shoulders 'drop and flop' into a relaxed position.
- If accessory muscles used for breathing and to encourage slower breathing, rest hand on upper back and move slowly in downward.
- To promote improved respiratory muscle function alter positioning so that when sitting lean forward from the hips, with forearms resting above the knees.
- Controlled breathing techniques/breathing retraining, e.g. pursed lip breathing (PLB) and diaphragmatic breathing helps develop slower, relaxed, and more efficient breathing pattern.
- Activity pacing and planning.
- A fan (e.g. hand held).
- Rollator walking aid (improves positioning, pacing).
- Non-invasive ventilation (e.g. patients with MND).

## Pharmacological approaches and related treatments

(See BNF: prescribing in palliative care, ℬ www.bnf.org.uk.)

- *Opiates/opioids:* act by ↓ sensitivity of the respiratory centre to $CO_2$ altering the sensation of breathlessness and feelings of distress. Given immediate release (2.5mg morphine 4-hourly initially), some evidence modified release. Care in increasing dosage with elderly and renal impairment. No evidence for nebulized morphine.
- *Oxygen and air:* symptomatic relief of acute breathlessness and panic. Both air and oxygen reduce breathlessness in patients with cancer. Well-ventilated room and hand held fan helpful. Use nasal cannula to ↓ oral dryness and inhibition of conversation. (If $SaO_2$ within normal range reassure patient $O_2$ not required.)
- Benzodiazepines ease anxiety which may relate to breathlessness. No evidence relieves breathlessness. Opioids with benzodiapines provide a sedative effect for terminal breathlessness during the final hours or days of life. Anxiolytics may help relieve sleeplessness.
- High-dose steroids, corticosteroids for inflammatory aetiology, bronchodilators for airway obstruction, antibiotics, anticholinergics, nebulized saline, anticoagulants, and diuretics.

## Cancer directed therapies and interventions

- Hormones, chemotherapy, and radiotherapy → some symptomatic relief for patients with treatment sensitive primary and metastatic disease.
- Breathlessness from responsive anaemia, pleural effusions, airway obstruction, ascites, and superior vena cava obstruction can improve with targeted interventional treatments. Involve MDT in assessment.

## Further information

Bredin M, Corner J, Kristmasmy M, et al. (1999). Multicentre randomized controlled trial of nursing intervention for breathlessness in patients with lung cancer. Br Med J **318**: 901–4.

Bausewein C, Booth S, Gysels M, et al. (2008). Non-pharmacological interventions for breathlessness in advanced stages of malignant and non-malignant diseases. *Cochrane Database System Rev* Apr 16 **(2)**: CD005623.

# Symptom control in palliative care: fatigue

Fatigue is a common, distressing symptom on continuum from tiredness to exhaustion. Significant fatigue is present every day or nearly every day during same 2-wk period in the past month. Associated with pain, psychological factors (particularly depression), serious viral infection, age, anorexia, and cachexia, life events, genetic factors Characterized by:

- Longer duration than that of someone who is healthy and often all consuming and overwhelming.
- Sleep provides little recuperative effect.
- Unrelated to type of activity performed and unrelieved by rest.

## Treatment-related causes of cancer-related fatigue

- *Surgery:* linked to changes in muscle physiology, or may occur as part of a general stress response to surgery.
- *Radiotherapy:* commonly occurs from first day of treatment, intensifying over a course of therapy, plateauing between 2nd and 4th week.
- *Chemotherapy:* fatigue most frequent and distressing side effect.
- Hormone therapy and biological response modifiers.

Many instruments have been developed to assess cancer-related fatigue including symptom diaries, single-item, and multi-item measures.

## Pharmacological approaches to management of fatigue

(See BNF: prescribing in palliative care, ℘ www.bnf.org.uk.)

*Glucocorticoids* E.g. *dexamethasone:* may increase appetite and general wellbeing in 80% of patients. Trial for 7–10 days (dexamthasone 2–4mg od) if effective minimum maintenance dose, if no response stop (BNF 6.3).

*Progestational steroids* E.g. medroxyprogesterone acetate (MPA) or megestrol acetate (MA)—relieves anorexia and cachexia in patients whose fatigue related to cachexia (BNF 6.4).

*Erythropoietin therapy* Can increase energy levels in anaemic cancer patients receiving chemotherapy (BNF 9.1).

Antidepressants may be particularly useful in managing fatigue that is accompanied by depressive symptoms.

## Non-pharmacological approaches

- *Exercise:* evidence to suggest that moderate exercise promotes ↑ functional capacity and improved mood.
- *Diet:* advise to eat when hungry, frequent small amounts.
- *Pacing of activities:* prioritize and plan for activities.
- *Psychosocial interventions:* counselling, progressive muscle relaxation.

## Related topic

📖 Palliative care in the home, p. 509.

## Further information

Tadman M, Roberts D. (2007). *Oxford Handbook of Cancer Nursing.* Oxford: Oxford University Press.

# Syringe drivers

Palliative care, drugs are commonly administered by continuous subcutaneous infusion (CSCI) using portable battery-powered syringe drivers.
CSCI is an important alternative route of administration in certain circumstances. It delivers a measured volume of drugs at a predetermined rate,
used when:
- Terminally ill patient assessed as requiring continuous analgesic or
  continuous relief of other symptoms.
- To prevent the need for regular injections when medication cannot be
  swallowed or absorbed to provide effective symptom control.

Use of CSCI indicated if oral medication not tolerated, dysphagia, or intes-
tinal obstruction:
- Intractable vomiting.
- Severe dysphagia.
- Impaired consciousness.
- Patient too weak to swallow oral drugs.
- Decreased conscious level.
- Poor alimentary absorption (rare).
- Poor patient compliance.
- Patients preference.

Nurse should provide a full explanation to the patient and family carer
about what a syringe driver is, how it works, and why its use is indicated
and informed consent gained and recorded.

Advantages of using a syringe driver:
- Drug mixtures can be administered.
- Infusion timing is accurate.
- Allows mobility, independence, and enables patient to stay at home.

It is best to use one type of syringe driver with standardized procedures
across health organization to reduce risk of dose error. Always check
manufacturer's instructions before use, date of last service. Training is
essential before setting up and using a syringe driver. Always refer to
local policy and standard operating procedure.

*Note:* different syringe drivers deliver infusions in different ways. ALWAYS
check manufacturer's instructions.

McKinley T34 Medical Syringe Drivers are commonly used in community.
The McKinley T34 is calibrated in mL per hour and deliver the syringe
contents by continuous subcutaneous infusion over 24hr period only.

This is a clean procedure:
- Draw up medication and diluent.
- Invert syringe and observe for cloudiness, precipitation or change in
  colour. Discard if this happens and seek advice.
- Complete and attach an additive label to syringe, for monitoring
  purposes, with patient's details, date, time, drug, dose, and signature.
- Insert the battery and check the battery has at least 40% power.

- Before placing the syringe into the pump ensure the barrel clamp arm is down then press and hold the ON/ OFF key.
- The LCD display will read PRE-LOADING' and the actuator will start to move. Wait until it stops moving and the syringe sensor detection screen appears.
- Connect the extension line securely to the syringe. If it is a new infusion set, gently depress the syringe plunger to manually prime the line.
- Fit the syringe into the syringe driver pump.
- Select site for infusion, ensuring sites are regularly rotated and not compromised need to consider skin integrity and patient comfort; e.g. lateral aspects of upper arms, thighs or the abdomen.
- Check site is clean insert the needle safe infusion device into the skin according to the manufacturer's instructions or accepted best practice.
- Do not loop the line over the insertion site.
- Place a non-occlusive dressing over the site.
- Starting infusion—pump calculates and displays total syringe volume, duration of infusion (24 hours) and infusion rate (mL per hour). Press YES to confirm or ON/OFF to return to syringe options. Pump screen prompts, check line connected, press YES to start infusion. When running green LED displayed and screen indicated time remaining and rate.
- Locking—press and hold INFO key use 'progress' bar to lock.

Note: alarm system of some syringe drivers only operate if the plunger is obstructed so does not alert patient or nurse if flow is too rapid or if there are problems at the skin site.

## Medication

Diamorphine/morphine 1st line opioid for pain. Diamorphine can be administered SC in a smaller volume than morphine.

Oral morphine: SC diamorphine ratio 3:1 (See 🕮 BNF section on prescribing in palliative care and syringe drivers for detail on prescribing and dosages over time: 🕭 www.bnf.org.uk).

The following drugs may be mixed with diamorphine:
- Hyoscine hydrobromide.
- Levomepromazine.
- Haloperidol.
- Metoclopramide.
- Hyoscine butylbromide.
- Midazolam.
- Cyclizine (can precipitate with diamorphine in higher doses, and hyoscine butylbromide).
- Dexamethasone (advise separate driver can mix with diamorphine, but precipitates with cyclizine, midazolam, haloperidol, levomepromazine).

Contraindicated are chlorpromazine, prochlorperazine, and diazepam: these can cause skin reactions at the injection site; cyclizine and levomepromazine (methotrimeprazine) may also cause local irritation.

## General issues

(Training should be given according to local policies and protocols.)

- Accurate documentation of site, rate, flow, start time, and drugs used is imperative to avoid confusions and errors.
- Ensure patients and carers have explanations and supporting literature on problem-solving and guidelines for use.
- Care should be taken when mixing more than 2 drugs in a syringe. Ensure the diluent used is compatible with the drugs.
- The diluent of choice is water for injection except in the following where sodium chloride 0.9% for injection should be used—diclofenac, granisetron, ketamine, ketorolac, octreotide, and ondansetron.
- With combinations of 2 or 3 drugs in one syringe, a larger volume of diluent may be needed, e.g. 20mL or 30mL syringe.

## Problems

- *Infusion running too fast:* syringe correctly inserted, check rate and recalculate.
- *Infusion running too slow:* check syringe correctly inserted, start button, battery, syringe driver, cannula, and make sure injection site is not inflamed.
- *Site reaction:* firmness or swelling not always a problem. Change needle site if pain or obvious inflammation. A plastic/teflon needle may reduce local irritation if a nickel allergy.
- Check solution regularly for precipitation and discolouration and discard if it occurs. Check compatibility of drugs.
- *Light flashing:* this is normal. Flashing will stop when the battery needs changing. The syringe driver will continue to operate for 24hrs after the light has stopped flashing.
- *Alarm:* T34 alarms sound once infusion complete, press ON/OFF button to switch off. (MS26 alarm sounds when the battery is inserted). Silence by pressing Start/Test button. Check for empty syringe/kinked tube/blocked needle/tubing/jammed plunger.

## Related topics

&#x1F4D6; Chemotherapy in the home, p. 507; &#x1F4D6; Controlled drugs, p. 137.

## Further information

Dickman A. Schneider J. (2005). *The Syringe Driver: continuous subcutaneous infusions in palliative care*, 2nd edn. Oxford: Oxford University Press.

Watson M, Lucas C, Hoy A, *et al* (2011). Palliative Adult Network Guidelines, 3rd edn. Available at: &#x22FB; http://book.pallcare.info

# Symptom control in palliative care: depression and spiritual distress

Depression in palliative care is common (19%), but is often under-recognized. Time is precious for individuals with life-limiting illness; early detection and regular assessment are imperative.

## Core symptoms and signs

- *Persistent low mood:* slumped posture.
- Prolonged or chronic grief.
- *Loss of interest in everyday activities:* lack of movement.
- *Hopelessness, worthlessness, guilt:* flat affect.
- *Constant and unremitting suicidal thoughts, actions:* reduced emotional reactivity.

## Identifying patients 'at risk'

- Poorly controlled physical symptoms.
- Increasing disability/performance status.
- Advanced disease at diagnosis.
- Social isolation/absent social support.
- Younger patients at higher risk.
- Concurrent life stresses, e.g. recent bereavement.
- Personal or family history of depression.

## Barriers to detection

- Distinguishing normal sadness vs. depressive disorder (see Table 10.9).
- Overlap of somatic symptoms (e.g. appetite loss, fatigue, sleep disturbance, loss of libido) cause may be depression, physical disease, or treatment. Therefore somatic symptoms unhelpful in diagnosis.

Differential diagnosis with:

- Cognitive impairment associated with delirium (clouded consciousness, incoherent speech).
- Dementia (poor orientation, memory deficits).
- Adverse drug reaction/drug or alcohol misuse.
- Space-occupying lesion (e.g. cerebral metastases).
- Other psychiatric illness (e.g. anxiety disorders) or other physical illnesses, e.g. hypothyroidism, Parkinson's disease.
- Lack of specialist mental health services, particularly for individuals with differential diagnosis.

## Screening

See Box 10.3.

Aim to improve detection of cases of depression. No evidence that screening causes harm.

**Table 10.9** Characteristics of depression vs. appropriate sadness

| Depression | Sadness |
|---|---|
| Feels outcast and alone | Feels intimately connected to others |
| Feeling of permanence | Feeling that someday this will end |
| Regretful, rumination on past mistakes | Able to enjoy happy memories |
| Self-depreciation, self-loathing | Sense of self-worth |
| Constant and unremitting | Comes in waves |
| No hope/interest in the future | Looks forward to things |
| Enjoys few activities | Retains capacity for pleasure |
| Suicidal thoughts/behaviour | Will to live |

Reproduced from Rayner L, Price A, Hotopf M, et al. (2011). The development of evidence-based European guidelines on the management of depression in palliative care. *Eur J Cancer* **47(5)**: 702–12.

## Box 10.3 Screening for depression in palliative care patients

- Single-item: Are you depressed?
- Two-item: Have you been feeling down, depressed, or hopeless? Have you had little interest/pleasure in doing things?
- Hospital Anxiety and Depression Scale (HADS): 14 items, 7 anxiety, 7 depression, excludes somatic symptoms
- Brief Edinburgh Depression Scale (BEDS): 6 items, covering guilt, insomnia, fear, inability to cope, thoughts of self harm
- Note: single item and two items can be found within composite outcome scales, such as the Palliative Outcome Scale (POS) or the Edmonton Symptom Assessment Schedule (ESAS) (see resource Outcome Measurement in Palliative Care)

Reproduced from Rayner et al. (2011).[1]

Prevention emphasizes good palliative care with comprehensive assessment and optimal management of:
- Physical symptoms (e.g. pain, fatigue, constipation).
- Promoting psychological wellbeing (e.g. communication, coping strategies, spiritual issues).
- Social wellbeing (e.g. support in resolving conflicts, maintaining social roles and networks, i.e. attendance hospice day care).

## Management of depression in advanced illness

- Brief psychological therapy, e.g. CBT is increasingly used by nurses to improve outcomes in palliative care.
- *Anti-depressants:* selective serotonin uptake inhibitors (SSRIs) recommended 1st line treatment as well tolerated and effective. Commence low dose and slowly titrate up (e.g. citalopram or sertraline). SSRIs less sedative than tricyclic anti-depressant with few anti-muscarinic effects, low cardiotoxicity, and may have faster onset of action. Tricyclic anti-depressants (e.g. amitriptyline, BNF 4.3.1) all have anti-muscarine properties and maybe associated with symptoms of hypotension, dry mouth, and difficulty in micturition. Gradual dose increase to avoid unnecessary side effects.

## Spiritual care

Palliative care emphasizes care of the 'whole' person. Spiritual needs are understood broadly and include all the existential concerns of an individual and his/her family and close carers. Spirituality gives meaning and person to individuals' lives. It is how people make sense of their joys and difficulties in life. This may not include a belief in a particular God, but could include belief in a power greater than themselves. Spiritual care is important throughout the illness trajectory and into bereavement.

*Assessment and management*

- Identify spiritual needs by assessing and documenting individuals' spiritual needs (including faith). (See FICA assessment in Box 10.4.)
- Collate details of spiritual care services available (e.g. contact details for spiritual leaders of different denominations and traditional healers).
- Document in individuals' records services accessed and value.
- Encourage mutual training and education and organized visits with faith leaders and health care professionals.
- Refer to, and receive referrals from, faith leaders.

---

### Box 10.4 FICA

**F** Do you have a religious faith? Or a philosophy or a set of beliefs that help you?

**I** How important is your faith/beliefs to you?

**C** Are you part of a community that offers you support such as a: church, mosque, temple?

**A** How can we assist you? Are there things we need to be aware of—prayer times, diet? Can we contact anyone? What would best support you?

Spiritual Assessment developed by Dr Puchalski cited Watson, *et al.* (2011). Palliative Adult Network Guidelines (3rd ed.)[2] ◈ http://book.pallcare.info

# References

[1] Rayner L, Higginson IJ, Price A, *et al*. *The Management of Depression in Palliative Care: European Clinical Guidelines*. London: KCL, Department of Palliative Care, Policy and Rehabilitation/European Palliative Care Research Collaborative.

[2] Watson M, Lucas C, Hoy A, *et al*. (2011) Palliative Adult Network Guidelines, 3rd edn. Available at: ℜ http://book.pallcare.info

# Further information

Management of Depression in Palliative care: European Clinical Guidelines (2010). Summary guides for patients. Available at: ℜ http://www.epcrc.org/guidelines.php?p=depression

Marie Curie Spiritual and Religious Care Competencies for Specialist Palliative Care. Available at: ℜ www.mariecurie.org.uk/

NICE (2009). Depression in adults with Chronic Physical Health Problems: treatment and management. Available at: ℜ http://guidance.nice.org.uk/CG91

Rayner L, Price A, Evans A, *et al*. (2010). Antidepressants for depression in physically ill people. *Cochrane Database System Rev* Issue 3. Art. No.: CD007503.

Selman L, Harding R, Speck P, *et al*. (2011). Spiritual care recommendations for people from Black and minority ethnic (BME) groups receiving palliative care in the UK. London: Department of Palliative Care Policy and Practice, KCL. Available at: ℜ http://www.csi.kcl.ac.uk/files/Spiritualcarerecommendations-Fullreport.pdf

# Bereavement, grief, and coping with loss

Grief is a normal reaction to bereavement. Traditional models see it as a process where an individual moves to 'recovery'. Not a linear process, individuals likely to oscillate between loss and restoration, memories of the dead person and getting on with life. Normal manifestations of grief:

- *Physical:* hollowness in the stomach, tightness in throat and chest, SOB, sensitivity to noise, dry mouth, and muscle weakness.
- *Emotional:* initial response often shock and numbness. Also normal are feelings of anger, guilt, anxiety, disorganization, and helplessness. Sadness most common manifestation and may only really be experienced months later. Sense of relief and freedom, can → feelings of guilt.
- *Cognitive:* sense of unreality and disbelief, even denial often present in early bereavement. Short-term memory and concentration can be affected. Not uncommon to have sense of the presence of the deceased.
- *Behaviour :* appetite and sleep disturbed, individual may withdraw socially. May consider rapid changes in their life, e.g. new relationship, moving house, may be a way of avoiding pain of loss, but not advisable.

Health consequences of bereavement can include ↑ risk of mortality, mental health problems, alcohol abuse, depression, suicidal thoughts, ↓ immune response, disruption of family and working life, ↓ income.

Where there has been nursing involvement and relationship with the family/carers, appropriate for nurse to visit in the month after the death to see how the bereaved are, allow them to express how they are feeling, and remember the deceased. *Note:* care home staff can also experience bereavement.

## Bereaved children

Children understand what death is by 8yrs, and even by 2–3yrs will have some understanding. If possible prepare children for death with the opportunity to ask questions. Excluding children to protect them can increase the pain and feelings of being isolated. Specialist help may be appropriate.

## Complicated/abnormal grief reactions

Recognized patterns of abnormal grief (*Note:* impossible to generalize dependent on individual circumstances):

- *Inhibited grief:* absent or minimal expression.
- Delayed onset.
- Prolonged or chronic grief.

*Predisposing factors can include:* unexpected death, multiple/prior (unresolved) bereavements, ambivalent or dependent relationship with the deceased, poor social support, low self-esteem, history of mental illness.

*Warning signs of complicated grief*
- Presence pre-disposing factors.
- Long-term functional impairment.
- Exaggerated intense grief reactions.
- Significant self-neglect.
- Idealization of the deceased.

If abnormal grief is suspected monitor carefully, be a non-judgemental listener and keep in regular contact.
- Consider referral for bereavement counseling, e.g. CRUSE (available at ✍ www.crusebereavementcare.org.uk).
- Consider possibility of clinical depression refer to GP.

## Bereavement benefits and funeral payments

See 📖 Benefits for people with low income, p. 791; 📖 Benefits for illness, disability and carers p.795.

## Further information

Bereavement and widows' benefits Helpline Telephone: 📞 +44 (0)191 21 87608 Bereavement Service Helpline 08456088601

Child Bereavement Trust. Available at: ✍ www.childbereavement.org.uk/

Government Information on Death and Benefits. Available at: ✍ www.gov.uk/browse/benefits/bereavement

Support for bereaved partners CRUSE. Available at: ✍ www.crusebereavementcare.org.uk

Winstons Wish. Available at: ✍ www.winstonswish.org.uk/

# End-of-life issues

End-of-life issues include verifying death and the euthanasia debate, an individual's right to die.

## Verifying death and referral to coroner

Verifying death can be undertaken by nurses, death certification is issued by a medical practitioner who has been in attendance during the deceased's last illness (📖 Death confirmation and certification, p. 784). Verifying involves establishing absence of respiration, heartbeat, and pupil response. Referral of a death to coroner is in specific circumstances (examples Box 10.5). When no next of kin or families require financial assistance with burial payment refer to local authority Welfare Funeral Advisor. *Note:* in England and Wales death certification reforms will be implement 2014.

---

**Box 10.5 Examples of when a death should be referred to a coroner**

- Cause unknown.
- Doctor not attended in 14 days prior to death.
- Accidental injury, e.g. fall contributing to death.
- Industrial diseases, e.g. mesothelioma.
- Suicide.
- Suspicious or violent circumstances.
- All drug related deaths.
- Septicaemia.
- Poisoning.
- Creutzfeldt–Jakob disease.

Adapted from Watson et al. (2011). Palliative Adult Network Guidelines, 3rd edn. Available at: 🕮 http://book.pallcare.info

---

Advice to families on registering death: see 📖 Registration of births, marriages, and deaths, p. 786.

## Euthanasia/assisted suicide/assisted dying

- Euthanasia means the taking of direct action by a doctor to end a patient's life.
- Assisted suicide is when an individual is provided with the means and assistance (for example using drugs, equipment, and so forth).
- Assisted dying is often used to encompass either or both of the above refers to the act of intentional ending of life.

Focus of great debate, engendering on one hand strong feelings about the right to demand death and, on the other, strong feelings that life is so precious that we have a duty to preserve it at all costs. It is illegal in the UK, but the issue may be raised by patients and relatives. Always important to consider the views of patients and to act in the best interests of those who are not able to give consent.

Issues to consider when patient or relatives are asking for euthanasia:
• Whether all pain and symptom relief information has been shared and its implementation is effective.
• Whether there is reversible clinical depression.
• Patients, who are ill and unable to care for themselves, may feel a burden and under pressure to die quickly.
• The vulnerable deserve protection especially the frail old, disabled, and those with cognitive impairment.
• Patients' beliefs regarding euthanasia may be on the basis of inadequate information, since it is impossible to identify accurately when an individual patient will die naturally.
• Consider if previous experiences of seeing someone die has shaped the person's views and fears

Important to recognize where the primary intention is to prevent suffering it is not normally considered to be euthanasia, this includes the list in Box 10.6.

---

### Box 10.6 Euthanasia is not:
• Withholding or withdrawing futile, burdensome treatment. This includes nutrition and hydration if the patient is dying and is unable to swallow.
• Giving opioids, or any other medications, to control symptoms including pain, fear, and overwhelming distress.
• Sedating a patient in the terminal stages if all other practical methods of controlling symptoms have failed.
• Issuing a Do Not Resuscitate order.

Adapted from Watson M, Lucas C, Hoy A, *et al.* (2009). *Oxford Handbook of Palliative Care*, 2nd edn. Oxford: Oxford University Press.

---

### Related topics
📖 Consent, p. 77; 📖 Mental capacity, p. 424.

### Further information
BMA statement on assisted dying. Available at: 🔗 http://bma.org.uk/practical-support-at-work/ethics/bma-policy-assisted-dying

RCN (2011). When someone asks for your assistance to die. RCN guidance on responding to a request to hasten death. Available at: 🔗 http://www.rcn.org.uk/__data/assets/pdf_file/0004/410638/004167.pdf

# Injection techniques

Drugs are given via parenteral routes when they need to be absorbed quickly or when they would be altered by ingestion. Some drugs are released over a long period of time and need a parenteral route that will absorb the drug more steadily.

## Key principles
- Pre-plan before drawing up doses.
- Be familiar with medication and local policies/protocols.
- Do not prepare injectable medicines in advance of immediate use.
- Only administer an injectable medicine you have prepared yourself or which has been prepared in your presence.
- Ensure anaphylactic shock kit is easily accessible.
- Assess patient anxiety and if reassurance needed.
- Assess condition of proposed injection site, avoid sites that are oedematous, inflamed, and/or fibrosed.
- Where frequent injections are given, sites should be rotated to prevent damage, protect the administration route and maximize patient comfort (the use of rotation charts may be considered).
- Use aseptic non-touch technique.
- Skin cleansing only necessary if patient immune-compromised or skin visibly dirty. If necessary, clean site with an alcohol swab for 30s and allow to air dry for 30s.
- Use needles with engineered sharps injury protection where available.
- Ensure prompt disposal of sharps.
- Document procedure (drug name, dose given, site, batch, and expiry date).

### Implications of poor practice
- Haemorrhage in bleeding disorders (IM injections).
- Pain.
- Sciatic nerve injury (IM injections).
- Injection fibrosis.
- Infection.

## Intramuscular injections
### Sites and administration
- Deltoid, dorsogluteal, ventrogluteal, vastus lateralis, and rectus femoris.
- All site options for adults; ventrogluteal is advocated as first choice.
- Deltoid muscle only suitable for small volumes <1mL, other sites can tolerate higher volumes.
- Only dorsogluteal has close proximity to major nerve blood supply.
- Anterolateral thigh and deltoid sites recommended for vaccines in infants and children.

Recommend dose division between sites for volumes >3–4mL, Z track technique and stretching the skin of the injection site (bunching may be required in emaciated patients).

*Patient position*
- Only use dorsogluteal site when patient can lie in prone or lateral position.
- 'Toe in' position for prone administration or flexing the knee 20° in the side lying position.
- Land marking by palpating the ileum and trochanter is essential to reduce risk of sciatic nerve injury.
- Injection into the deltoid, rectus femoris, or lateralis can be administered while patient is seated and muscles relaxed.

*Administration*
- Needle length must be sufficient to penetrate the muscle layer, and reduce complications including abscess, pain, and bruising.
- Use at least 25mm (23G) blue needles or 38mm (21G) green needles for adults.
- For children, 16mm is recommended, although decisions depend on age and subcutaneous fat.

Hold syringe like a pen and insert at 90° in a dart-like motion up to the hub of the needle to ensure the full length is used.
- Aspirate with dorsogluteal procedures as needle insertion is close to the gluteal artery, but unnecessary with other sites.
- Inject at a rate of ~1mL per 10s.

## Subcutaneous injections
The SC route is used for slow, sustained absorption of medication.
- Use lateral aspects of upper arms and thighs, and abdomen.
- Absorption is most rapid from the abdomen, slower from arms and slowest from thighs and buttock area. Small volumes only (0.3–1mL).
- Introduction of shorter needles (e.g. 12mm and 16mm) allow injections to be given at 90° (45° for longer needles).
- Pinch skin to lift adipose tissue away from underlying muscle layer (avoid skin blanching). Leave the needle in place for at least 10s after the depressing contents. Teach patient to self-administer whenever possible.

Insulin injections are recommended in the abdomen for fast acting insulin, thighs for intermediate acting insulin or the evening dose of twice daily insulin regimens, and buttocks for intermediate or long acting insulin.
- For frequent injections, rotate sites and check for fat hypertrophy and scarring on a regular basis.
- For insulin injections rotate within each day daily.
- Cloudy insulin should be adequately mixed before injection.
- For insulin injections use a 31–29 gauge needle between 5–8mm.
- For other SC injections use a 25 gauge needle between 10–25mm.
- Use of alcohol swabs prior to frequent injections will harden the skin.
- Pinch skin to lift adipose tissue away from underlying muscle.
- Insert needle, bevel side up at a 90° angle.
- Do not aspirate.
- Leave needle in skin for 6–10s after depressing plunger.
- Hold skin fold until needle has been withdrawn.

## Intradermal injections

The ID route provides a local, rather than systemic effect and is used for diagnostic purposes such as allergy or tuberculin testing or for local anesthetics. BCG is always given by the ID route. Suitable sites are similar to those for SC injections, but also include ventral forearm and upper back. The preferred site for BCG is at the point of the insertion of the left deltoid muscle.

• Use a 25 gauge, 10mm needle.
• Stretch skin taut with thumb and forefinger of free hand.
• Insert needle bevel side up at a 10–15° angle for about 2mm.
• When testing for allergies, label area to monitor an allergic response.
• Never cover BCG vaccinations with a plaster or dressing.

## Administration of goserelin implant (Zoladex®)

Goserelin reduces the production of testosterone and oestrogen. It is also used in assisted reproduction. It is produced in ready-mixed sterile syringes and is administered every 28 days (3.6mg) or every 12wks (10.8mg).

• Consider application of topical anaesthetic agents.
• Position patient sitting or semi-recumbent.
• Administer SC in anterior abdominal wall below naval line.
• Cleanse proposed site with alcohol swab.
• Pinch skin to lift adipose tissue away from underlying muscle.
• Insert needle, bevel side up at a 30–45° angle, until hub of barrel touches the skin and depress plunger until it depresses no further.
• Remove the device and cover site with a sterile plaster.

## Further information

Forum for Injection Technique (2010). Diabetes care in the UK: the first UK injection technique recommendations. Available at: ℳ www.miltonkeynes.nhs.uk/.../Injection%20Technique%20 Recommendations.pdf

Malkin B. (2008). Are techniques used for intramuscular injection based on research evidence, available online. Available at: ℳ www.nursingtimes.net/nursing-practice/1952004.article

Public Health England. *Immunisation against infectious disease*. 'The Green Book', available online. Available at: ℳ https://www.gov.uk/governent/organisations/public-health-england/series/ immunisation-against-infectious-disease-the-green-book

Royal College of Paediatrics and Child Health (2002). Position statement on injection technique. Available at: ℳ www.rcn.org.uk/__data/assets/pdf_file/0010/78535/001753.pdf

UCLH (2010). *UCL Hospitals Injection Medicines Administration Guide*, 3rd edn. Oxford: Wiley Blackwell.

# Peripheral venepuncture

Venepuncture or phlebotomy is the introduction of a needle into a vein to obtain blood samples for haematological, biochemical, or bacteriological analysis. The antecubital fossa is the most commonly used site. In some circumstances the dorsal metacarpal veins in the hand are acceptable.

- ❶ Veins in the foot should not be used due to risk of DVT, and in diabetic patients, tissue necrosis.
- ❶ Complications of venepuncture include: pain, phlebitis, haematoma, arterial puncture, and nerve injury.
- ❶ Nurse should consider risks of needle stick injury and blood spillage.

The use of closed blood collection devices with engineered sharps injury protection is strongly advised. Make no more than two attempts to take blood; then ask more experienced colleague if necessary.

## Choosing a vein

- Palpate and visually inspect.
- Choose a vein which is visible, soft and bouncy, refills when depressed, is straight, has a large lumen, and is well supported.
- ❶ Do not use: dominant arm (where possible) infected areas, oedematous limbs, or limbs affected by CVA.
- ❶ Do not use limbs adjacent to mastectomy or ancillary node dissection or hard, cord-like, sclerosed, fibrosed, or thrombosed veins or same arm as an IV infusion or AV fistula sites (must be preserved for haemodialysis).

## Preparation

- *Gain consent:* has patient experienced an adverse outcome with venepuncture previously (such as fainting).
- *Any allergies to latex or plasters:* consider application of topical anaesthetic agents.
- Consider application of topical anaesthetic agents.
- Check patient has complied with any arrangements prior to sampling (e.g. when last ate or drank before fasting samples and time and dose of last medication before drug samples and hormone levels).
- Put on disposable apron and ensure patient is comfortable and arm supported. Wash hands and apply non-sterile gloves. Clean visibly dirty skin with soap and water and dry thoroughly.

## Procedure (antecubital fossa)

- Apply tourniquet to upper arm (7–10cm above proposed puncture site).
- Apply pressure to impede venous, but not arterial flow (check for pulse).
- Patient may assist venous filling by clenching/unclenching hand. Observe and palpate selected vein.
- Release tourniquet and check selected vein has decompressed (a thrombosed vein will remain hard and palpable).
- Cleanse proposed puncture site with an alcohol swab for 30s and allow to air dry for 30s.
- Select needle or winged infusion device (usually 21G).
- Assemble equipment according to manufacturer's instructions and reapply tourniquet.
- With arm in a downward position, apply traction to skin below puncture site. Align needle with vein and smoothly insert needle, bevel side up at a 20–40° angle. Secure device with tape if necessary and gently release skin traction.
- Attach collection tubes/bottles. If more than 1 sample is required, tubes/bottles should be filled in correct order to minimize cross contamination from additives.
- When blood withdrawal is nearly finished, release tourniquet.
- When sampling is complete, slip a cotton wool ball over puncture site and fully remove the needle.
- Once fully removed, apply digital pressure until bleeding stops and promptly dispose of needle and equipment in a sharps container.
- Cover site with a plaster or cotton wool ball/hypoallergenic tape and advise the patient to leave in place for ~1hr. Ask patient not to bend arm.
- Label collection tubes/bottles and check details against request form invert tubes/bottles to mix with additives (do not shake).
- Ensure safe and timely transport of specimens in biohazard container.
- Discuss arrangements for patients and carers to receive results.
- Document procedure.

## Further information

Dougherty L, Lister S. (eds) (2011). *The Royal Marsden Hospital Manual of Clinical Nursing Procedures*, 8th edn. Chichester: Wiley-Blackwell.

RCN (2010). Standards for infusion therapy. Available at: ℘ http://www.rcn.org.uk/__data/assets/pdf_file/0005/78593/002179.pdf

# Care of central venous catheters

Tunnelled devices inserted into the central venous system with the distal tip sitting within the superior or inferior vena cava or right atrium; enabling patients requiring long-term IV therapy (chemotherapy, total parental nutrition, blood products, fluids, medication, and blood sampling) to receive treatment without multiple venepunctures.

## Types of catheter

- Peripherally inserted central catheter (PICC)—inserted via the antecubital veins in arm and advanced until distal end sits in superior vena cava or proximal right atrium. Remains in position up to 6mths.
- Skin tunnelled long-term catheter (Hickman)—lies in subcutaneous tunnel before entering a central vein. Tip sits in the lower third of the superior vena cava or upper right atrium. Remains in position for over 2yrs.
- Totally implanted venous access device (portacath)—made up of a reservoir with a self-sealing septum which is attached to a silicone catheter. Remain in position for over 2yrs.

## Complications

- Thrombosis.
- Air embolism.
- Infection.
- Occlusion.
- Split line.
- Catheter dislodgement.

## General asepsis

- Aseptic technique essential for site care and accessing the system.
- Hands must be decontaminated by washing with antimicrobial liquid soap or alcohol hand rub.
- Clean gloves and a non-touch technique or sterile gloves.
- Disposable plastic apron should be worn.

## Site care

- Preferably, sterile, transparent, semi-permeable polyurethane dressing to cover catheter site. Transparent dressings should be changed every 7 days or sooner if indicated.
- If patient has profuse perspiration or if insertion site is bleeding or oozing, use sterile gauze dressing. Gauze dressings should be changed when damp, loosened, or soiled. Need for gauze to be reviewed daily and replaced by a transparent dressing as soon as possible.
- Individual sachets/packages of chlorhexidine gluconate solution should be used to clean site during dressing changes, and allowed to air dry.
- Observe for signs of infection—redness, swelling, discharge, and pain at exit site and pyrexia ▶ Liaise with 2° care if problems identified.
- Stabilize PICC and Hickman catheters with a stabilization device.

## General principles for catheter management

- Decontaminate injection port or catheter hub using either alcohol or chlorhexidine gluconate before and after accessing the system.
- External length of PICCs catheters should be measured to check device has not migrated before and after accessing the system.
- Preferably, a sterile 0.9% sodium chloride injection should be used to flush and lock catheter lumens. Flushing should be performed weekly unless occlusive problems indicate otherwise.
- Administer flush using push pause method. Usually a 10mL syringe should be used; smaller syringes may cause catheter to rupture. Clamp should be closed in the last second when flushing to prevent a backflow of blood into the line.
- Never force the flushing fluid into the catheter; if resistance is felt during flushing, or pain is reported, or swelling observed along the skin tunnel, or around the chest or in the neck area, stop flushing. Observe patient for breathlessness. ► Liaise with 2° care if problems identified.
- When recommended by the manufacturer, and prescribed by lead clinician, implanted ports or opened-ended catheter lumens should be flushed and locked with heparin sodium flush solutions.
- If needleless devices are used, the manufacturer's recommendations for changing the needleless components should be followed.
- When needleless devices are used, ensure all components of system are compatible and secured, to minimize leaks and breaks in system.
- When needleless devices are used, risk of contamination should be minimized by decontaminating access port with either alcohol or chlorhexidine gluconate before and after using it to access the system.
- Equipment should be luer lock.
- Showering preferable to bathing and swimming should be avoided.
- Patients should be educated in catheter care and signs of catheter related complications. ► Liaise with 2° care if problems identified.

## Furhter information

NICE (2012). Infection control: prevention of health care-associated infection in primary and community care. Available at: ℘ http://www.nice.org.uk/CG139

NPSA (2008). Risks with intravenous heparin flush solutions. Available at: ℘ www.nrls.npsa.nhs.uk/resources/?EntryId45=59892

RCN (2010). Standards for infusion therapy. Available at: ℘ www.rcn.org.uk/__data/assets/pdf_file/0005/78593/002179.pdf

# Recording a 12-lead electrocardiogram

An electrocardiogram (ECG) is the collection of electrical waveforms produced by the heart. Indications for recording a 12-lead ECG include chest pain, palpitations, and history of syncope. It is often undertaken by practice nurses on the request of the GP.

## Procedure

- To help produce a clear, stable trace without interference, make sure the room is warm and try to relax the patient.
- Position the patient in a semi-recumbent comfortable position—adjust the backrest on the couch as appropriate.
- Prepare the skin if necessary.
- Apply the limb electrodes and leads (*Note:* refer also to manufacturer's guidance as colours can vary):
  - *Red:* inner right wrist.
  - *Yellow:* inner left wrist.
  - *Black:* inner right leg, just above ankle.
  - *Green:* inner left leg, just above ankle.
- Apply the chest electrodes and leads (Fig. 10.4):
  - *V1:* 4th intercostal space, just to right of sternum.
  - *V2:* 4th intercostal space, just to left of sternum.
  - *V3:* midway between V2 and V4.
  - *V4:* 5th intercostal space, mid-clavicular line.
  - *V5:* on anterior axillary line, on same horizontal line as V4.
  - *V6:* mid-axillary line, on same horizontal line as V4 and V5.
- Ask patient to remain still and breathe normally.
- Print out ECG following manufacturer's recommendations.
- Correctly label ECG, e.g. patient's name, date of birth, date and time of recording, ECG serial number together with any relevant information, e.g. if patient was pain free or complaining of chest pain during recording.

## Accuracy, quality, and standardization

- *Accuracy:* ensure all the electrodes and leads are correctly applied.
- *Quality:* minimize interference, e.g. patient movement and electrical interference, as this can produce a 'fuzzy' trace.
- *Standardization:* e.g. standard calibration (1mV = 10mm), standard paper speed (25mm/s), and standard patient position.

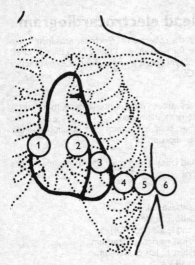

**Fig. 10.4** Positioning of chest electrodes and leads.

Reproduced with permission from Longmore M, Wilkinson I, Davidson E, *et al.* (2004). *Oxford Handbook of Clinical Medicine*, 6th edn. Oxford: Oxford University Press.

## Further information

Jevon P. (2009). *ECGs for Nurses*, 2nd edn. Chichester: Wiley-Blackwell.

# Tracheostomy and laryngectomy care

A tracheostomy is an artificial opening in the trachea into which a tube is inserted. The larynx (voice box) remains intact and the connection between the lungs and the mouth maintained. May be:

- Temporary (performed to secure the airway in head and neck injuries or in event of acute stridor due to obstruction).
- Long term (due to progressive neurological conditions or carcinoma of the naso-oropharynx or larynx).

Laryngectomy may be performed, dependent on the stage of disease. This entails removal of the larynx, where the trachea is sutured to the skin to create a permanent opening, which disconnects the lungs from the mouth. Laryngectomy stomas don't usually have a tube inserted.

## Patients at risk of death or harm if inappropriate care provided!

- Laryngectomy patients are neck breathers—in emergencies, standard oral airway manoeuvres will not work as there is no connection between the mouth, nose or pharynx, and lungs.
- Tracheostomy patients who have not had their larynx removed still have an upper airway available.

## Potential complications include:

- Problems with altered body image.
- Communication problems.
- Risk of infection.
- Scarring.
- Dysphagia.
- Occlusion.
- Haemorrhage.
- Pneumonia.
- Displaced tracheostomy tube.
- Tracheal damage.

## Discharge home and assessment

Patients, parents, and carers taught care, management, and action in emergency in hospital.

Important for primary care nurses to liaise with hospital staff pre-discharge.

Tracheostomy care needs a multi-disciplinary approach, particularly from dieticians, physiotherapists, and speech and language therapists. Local policy and guidance should be consulted prior to visiting the patient and providing tracheostomy care.

Assessment should consider:
- Rationale for tracheostomy.
- Presence or absence of larynx.
- Requirement for supplementary oxygen.
- Type and size of tube.
- Type and characteristics of secretions.
- Cough effort.
- Ability to swallow.
- Frequency of suctioning and cleaning of inner cannula.
- Condition of stoma site and requirement for dressing.
- Availability of spare and emergency equipment.
- Type of humidification device.
- Routine observations.
- Oral health assessment.
- Tube and any humidification device care.
- Patients communication methods.
- Advice in emergency.

Patients require electric and foot suction pump (for emergencies), and inform power supplier patient requires continuous supply for medical equipment.

### Types of tracheostomy tubes

Dependent on individual patient requirements. Whenever possible, patients will have double cannulated tube (to reduce risk of occlusion). A cuffed tube may be used to provide protection from aspiration in those with swallowing difficulties. Cuff inflation should be checked twice daily using a cuff pressure manometer. Fenestrated tubes may be used to encourage weaning or for voicing. Fenestrated tubes are supplied with two inner cannulae; one is fenestrated and one is not.

### Humidification

Artificial humidification essential to prevent drying of secretions.
- Heat and moisture exchanger (HME) (e.g. Thermovent, Swedish nose) and stoma filters (e.g. Buchanan Bib) commonly used for patients self-ventilating on air in community.
- HMEs need checking regularly to ensure not occluded by secretions and changed daily.

### Suctioning

Some patients may be able to project mucus by forced expirations, but most will require suctioning. Procedure should only be performed when patient is unable to clear own airway effectively. Routine tracheostomy suctioning should be limited to the lumen of the tube.

*Note:* some patients may require deep bronchial suctioning, but this should only be performed following medical instruction.
- Standard infection control precautions should be applied, including use of PPE (including goggles).
- If fenestrated tube *in situ*, a plain inner tube should be inserted prior to suctioning.

- Diameter of catheter should be no more than half the internal diameter of tracheal tube.
- Maximize removal of secretions with minimal tissue damage and hypoxia.
  - Use lowest effective pressure (below 120mmHg, and no more than 200mmHg as a maximum and only if necessary in adults).
  - No longer than 10s at a time.
  - Multi-eyed catheters cause least trauma.
  - Do not apply suction to catheter when inserting tube.
  - Observe for signs of respiratory distress.

## Stoma care and securing the tracheostomy tube

Frequency dependent on individual patient requirements.

Standard infection control precautions, including use of PPE (including goggles).

- Two people according to local policy; one person holds the tube in place whilst the other removes tapes/tube holder and dressing.
- Clean stoma with normal saline; apply barrier film to surrounding skin.
- ❶ Cotton wool should *never* be used to cleanse stoma.
- Use of dressings not always necessary; if indicated, use a manufactured tracheostomy dressing.
- Tube must be secured at all times to prevent airway obstruction.
- Velcro tube holder or cotton ties (2 pieces ~50–80cm in length).
- You should be able to place 1–2 fingers between the tapes/tube holder when the neck is in the neutral position.
- Observe patient for at least 15min for signs of respiratory distress (respiratory rate, colour, and chest movements).

## Cleaning the inner tube

- Inspect condition x3 per day; more frequently if in respiratory distress.
- Replace with spare inner cannula whilst cleaning taking place.
- Clean with warm water and air dry.
- Do not use brushes to clean plastic tubes.

## Further information

Great Ormond Street Hospital. Living with a tracheostomy. Available at: ℘ www.gosh.nhs.uk/medical-conditions/procedures-and-treatments/living-with-a-tracheostomy

National Tracheostomy Safety Project. Available at: ℘ www.tracheostomy.org.uk

NHS Quality Improvement Scotland (2007). Best practice statement, caring for the patient with a tracheostomy. Available at: ℘ www.health careimprovementscotland.org/previous_resources/best_practice_statement/tracheostomy_care.aspx

Resuscitation Council (UK) (2012). The emergency management of tracheostomies and laryngectomies. Available at: ℘ www.resus.org.uk/

# Ear care

Nurses carrying out ear care should ensure they have received formal skills training. Require:

- Understanding of anatomy and physiology of the ear.
- The ability to carry out an ear examination using an otoscope.
- The recognition of a normal tympanic membrane.
- Documentation and referral process if abnormalities identified.
- Assessment of wax/debris in ear canal and removal management.
- Referral process for patients with ear and/or hearing problems.

## Routine ear examinations

Ear examination to identify normal or abnormal anatomy should be carried out in the following cases:

- Annual checks on patients >65yrs who wear hearing aids.
- Annual checks on patients who have required wax removal (irrigation, manual removal, microsuction) in the past.
- Patients presenting with ear-related symptoms—hearing loss, discharge, pain, vertigo, tinnitus, itching, blocked feeling/fullness in ear.
- Problems with hearing aid (i.e. whistling) or patients over the age of 60yrs with an audiology appointment.

Examination aims to identify any abnormalities, e.g. infections and wax/debris build up. Nurses undertaking ear examinations should be clear when and where to refer for medical or other assessment.

- Take a comprehensive history.
- Examine external ear(s) checking for previous surgery/abnormalities.
- Examine ear(s) using an otoscope:
- Speculum size should be appropriate for ear canal.
  - Use a single-use only speculum where available.
  - Hold the otoscope in a pencil grip and turn light to full beam.
  - Examine good ear first.
  - Pull pinna upwards and backwards to straighten ear canal.
  - Assess whether wax is present and its colour and consistency.
  - Assess condition of ear canal.
- Examine whether the tympanic membrane is visible and its colour, transparency, and condition.

Patients over the age of 60yrs can usually be referred directly to the audiology department providing they do not suffer any other ear-related problems and there is no wax in their ears (☐ Deafness, p. 649).

## Cerumen/wax

- Cerumen/ear wax is a mixture of lipids, produced by the sebaceous glands to protect the epithelial lining of the external auditory meatus (ear canal). It only needs to be removed if it is causing a hearing deficit and/or discomfort, or restricts the view of the tympanic membrane preventing examination.
- Assess for colour, consistency, odour, and location. Wax that is dull and dark in colour tends to be harder.

- Use clinical judgement to consider options for wax removal assessing both the wax and patient suitability. The first line treatment option is softening agents with natural migration.
- Only consider irrigation when conservative methods have failed.
- Patients for whom irrigation is contraindicated may require referral to ENT. Risks associated with ear irrigation include perforation to tympanic membrane and otitis externa.

## Irrigation should not be carried out when

- A past history of tympanic membrane perforation.
- A recent history of otalgia (earache) or present middle ear infection.
- Had previous untoward experiences following this procedure.
- Had previous ear surgery (e.g. mastoidectomy or cleft palate).
- Grommets in place or history of recurrent grommet insertions.
- Hearing in only one ear.
- Recurring otitis externa.

## Irrigation procedure

- Soften wax prior to removal; for example, olive oil 1 drop twice daily to the ear(s) for 5–7 days prior to treatment.
- Always use an electronic ear irrigator.
- Metal syringes should not be used as their design, combined with the inability to control water pressure, increases the risk of ear damage.
- Put on disposable apron and ensure patient is comfortable.
- Check temperature of water to approximately 37°c (variation may cause dizziness).
- Set water pressure to minimum and ensure single-use only jet tip applicator firmly in place.
- Gently pull pinna upwards and backwards. Place tip of applicator into ear canal entrance.
- Warn patient you are about to start and to immediately report symptoms of pain, dizziness, or nausea.
- Ask patient to hold receiver under affected ear. Switch on machine and direct stream of water onto posterior wall of ear canal.
- Periodically inspect ear canal with otoscope.
- ❶ STOP irrigation if patient feels water at the back of throat, could indicate perforation.
- A maximum of 1 reservoir of water per procedure per ear.
- After removal of wax, or when maximum volume of water is used, dry excess water from the external auditory meatus.
- Examine with otoscope and assess need for further treatment.
- Document procedure and condition of ear canal and tympanic membrane following treatment.
- Patients requiring ear irrigation should always receive education and advice, which may reduce contributory factors and therefore the need for ear irrigation in the future.

## Further information

NICE (2012). Clinical Knowledge Summaries (NHS Evidence) guidance on ear wax. Available at: 🕮 http://cks.nice.uk/earwax

# Enteral tube feeding

Enteral tube feeding (ETF) is the delivery of nutritionally complete feed (containing protein or amino acids, carbohydrate ± fibre, fat, water, minerals, and vitamins) directly into the gut via a tube. Many types of feeding tubes can be used and choice will depend on expected period of feeding, clinical condition, and anatomy. The routes most often used are:
• Nasogastric (NG) tubes.
• Percutaneous endoscopic gastrostomy (PEG) tubes.

The 1° reason for initiating ETF is dysphagia, which may result from CVA, MS, or MND. Other reasons for tube feeding include:
• Increased nutritional requirements (e.g. cystic fibrosis).
• Psychological problems (e.g. anorexia nervosa).
• During specific treatment (e.g. for short enteral access during surgery for head and neck cancer).

Most commonly, ETF is initiated in hospital and the patient subsequently discharged into the community.

## Nasogastric tubes

A narrow-bore tube passed into the stomach via the nose. Usually short-term use only. Not generally suitable for patients with vomiting, gastro-oesophageal reflux, poor gastric emptying, ileus, or intestinal obstruction. Tubes should be placed by appropriately training staff only. Position should be verified on initial placement, before each use, and after any episode of coughing, retching, or vomiting.
• Potentially dangerous in patients with an unsafe swallow.
• Complications include aspiration due to misplacement on insertion or movement out of position at a later stage:
  • ❶Tube position should be monitored by aspiration of gastric contents and use of pH graded indicator paper. A pH <5.5 is consistent with gastric placement. If aspirate cannot be obtained or the pH is >5.5 feeding should not commence. Length of tube at point of exist from nostril should also be measured before each use.
  • *Nasal fixation tapes*: check daily and observe patient for signs of respiratory discomfort or regurgitation.
  • Location and securing of tube can be irritating.
  • Tube blockage and unplanned removal are other complications.
• ❶ Use of blue litmus paper to check acidity of aspirate is *not* sensitive enough to distinguish between levels of acidity.
• ❶ Introducing a small quantity of air into the stomach and checking for a bubbling sound over the epigastrium is unreliable.

## PEG tubes

Placed by endoscopic technique under local anaesthetic with antibiotic prophylaxis, passed through the abdominal wall directly into the stomach, held in place with a retention device. Often performed as an outpatient.

Usually for medium to long-term feeding. Patients and carers can manage feeds using PEG, must be their choice, should only happen with direct access to nursing and dietician support and regular review.

Compared to NG tubes, less oesophageal reflux (Aspiration pneumonia, 📖 Pneumonia, p. 701).

- First change of dressing the morning after PEG placement.
- Until granulation of the stoma canal, sterile dressing to be changed daily (~7 days).
- Dressings should be removed and external fixation plate opened and tube removed from grove.
- Inspect wound area, clean and dry completely.
- In order to avoid adhesions (buried bumper syndrome) tube should be pushed approximately 2–3cm ventrally and carefully pulled back up to resistance of the internal fixation flange. Then a Y-compress is applied under the tube and external fixation plate is secured with free movement of at least 5mm and a sterile dressing applied.
- After initial wound healing, wound cleansing and dressing every 2–3 days.
- Washing with soap and water or showering is possible after initial wound healing (1–2wks after insertion of PEG).
- Remove dressings before washing, residual soap rinsed away and tube dried well before a new dressing is applied.
- To prevent material fatigue, the C-clamp should be repositioned daily or preferably left open if not needed. Tube tip should be cleaned daily using water and a small brush.

❶ Most common complication is wound infection. Other complications include occlusion of the tube, tube porosity, and fracture with subsequent leakage, development of cellulitis, eczema, hyper-granulation tissue, and buried bumper syndrome.

Once a stable stoma has formed at least 4wks after insertion of the PEG system, a changeover to use of a button system can be done for cosmetic reasons, at the request of the patient

### Types of enteral feeds

Feeds are provided on prescription. Most enteral feeds ready to use liquid microbial-free preparations that contain energy, protein, vitamins, minerals, trace elements, and fluid ± fibre.

❶ Only specially prepared feeds and water should be administered through the feeding tube.

*Mode of delivering enteral tube feeding*

Bolus feeding is as effective as continuous (16–24hr) feeding. Mode of delivery determine by patient circumstances, bolus feeding a safe alternative, while issues of gastric emptying, metabolic stability, and control of glucose levels favours continuous feed administration. During feeding, and 45min after feeding, patient head and shoulders should be elevated to reduce the risk of aspiration.

*Infection control*

Whenever possible pre-packaged, ready-to-use feeds should be used in preference to feeds requiring decanting, reconstitution, or dilution.

Educate patients and carers on preparation and storage of feeds, administration of feeds, and care of insertion site and enteral feeding tube.

• Minimal handling, an aseptic, no-touch technique to connect administration system to enteral feeding tube.
• Ready-to-use feeds may be given for a whole administration session, up to a maximum of 24hrs.
• Reconstituted feeds administered over a maximum 4hr period.
• Administration sets and feed containers single use only.
• To prevent blockage, the enteral feeding tube should be flushed with fresh tap water before and after feeding or administering medication.
• Enteral feeding tubes for patients who are immunosuppressed should be flushed with either cooled freshly boiled water or sterile water from a freshly opened container.

## Drug administration

The use of enteral feeding tubes as a route of drug administration is ↑common. Using a feeding tube to administer a drug should be a last resort, and whenever possible an alternative route should be used. Medication administration common cause of feeding tube blockage; flush with 30mL of water before first medication and after last medication and at least 10mL of water between different medications.

Liaison between the prescriber and the pharmacist is essential.

• Medication should be regularly reviewed.
• 50mL enteral syringe should be used (a smaller syringe may produce too much pressure and split the tube).
• Liquids/soluble tablets are preferred formulation for administration.
• Crushing tablets or opening capsules should be a last resort.
• *Medicines that should not be crushed include:* enteric coated, modified/slow release, cytotoxics, and hormones.
• ❶ Interaction between enteral feeds and drugs maybe clinically significant, e.g. phenytoin, ciprofloxacin, theophylline, tetracyclines, digoxin, and rifampicin.

## Nutritional review

Review nutritional status regularly to enable re-instigation of oral nutrition as appropriate. Use Malnutrition Screening Tool (MUST) recommended

## Further information

BAPEN (2004). Administering drugs via enteral feeding tubes: a practical guide. Available at: ℘ www.bapen.org.uk/pdfs/d_and_e/de_pract_guide.pdf

Löser C, Aschl G, Hébuterne X, et al (2005). ESPEN guidelines on artificial enteral nutrition – percutaneous endoscopic gastrostomy (PEG). Available at: ℘ www.espen.org/espenguidelines. html

NICE (2006). Nutrition support in adults: Oral nutrition support, enteral tube feeding and parenteral nutrition. Available at: ℘ www.nice.org.uk/nicemedia/live/10978/29979/29979.pdf

NPSA (2005). Reducing harm caused by the misplacement of nasogastric feeding tubes. Available at: ℘ www.nrls.npsa.nhs.uk/EasySiteWeb/getresource.axd?AssetID=129696

# Care of people with long-term conditions

# Continuity of care

Continuity of care is characterized by an on-going relationship with a nurse/clinician and coordinated care as the patient moves between health and social care providers. Patients with a LTC and their carers should have:
- Care that is focused on their individual needs and sustained over time.
- Confidence that their nurse and MDT know them.
- Trust in their judgement and advice.
- Care that is coordinated.

Where there is good continuity of care there are better health outcomes, e.g. ↓ duplication of services and unnecessary interventions, ↑ self-management and concordance with treatments, patient satisfaction and cost control. There are three components to continuity:
- *Relationship continuity:* a working relationship between nurse/clinician that allows shared decision-making and flexibility of response to reflect patient and carer's needs.
- *Management continuity:* co-ordination and communication (often by named clinician 🕮 Care/case management models, p. 112), between services and caregivers, and across organizations that enables patient to navigate health and social care systems.
- *Informational continuity:* supports management continuity and ensures assessments, treatment reviews, and records (including patient-held records) are accessible and shared.

## Threats to continuity of care
- Increased specialization in primary care.
- Patients with multiple health and social care needs whose care is not coordinated by one of the services/professionals involved in their care.
- Time limited services designed to provide extra support, e.g. intermediate care (🕮 Services to promote hospital discharge and prevent unplanned admission, p. 18) need an ongoing link to primary and community care services to prevent breaks in service provision.
- Incompatible IT and record systems.

Note: integrated systems of care, and improved working relationships between different health professionals do not automatically mean that continuity of care is achieved. There is a need to audit service delivery from the patient perspective.

## References

Cowie L, Morgan M, White P, Gulliford M. (2009). Experience of continuity of care of patients with multiple long-term conditions in England. *J Hlth Serv Res Policy* **14**: 82–7.

Rand Europe, Ernst & Young LLP (2012). *National Evaluation of the Department of Health's Integrated Care Pilots*. London: Department of Health. Available at: ℘ www.gov.uk/government/uploads/system/uploads/attachment_data/file/215103/dh_133127.pdf

# Osteoarthritis

Osteoarthritis (OA) is the biggest cause of joint-related pain and mobility problems in adults. ♀ > ♂ with onset in middle age (average 50yrs). The main reason for patients seeking help is pain. A very variable condition involving the whole joint → pain, stiffness, and joint instability.

- Knee OA more common than hip OA. Together affect 10–20% population >65yrs.
- OA of the hands develops gradually with swellings on the back of joints—Herbeden's nodules.
- OA of the neck: spondylosis may not present with pain or symptoms.

## Causes

- *Age:* OA is uncommon before 45yrs.
- *Obesity:* especially with knee.
- *Joint injury:* e.g. sports related or earlier operation.
- Occupational.
- *Hard repetitive activity may injure joints:* e.g. sport and physical labour.
- Hereditary.

## Problems associated with OA

There is a wide variation of experience.

- Painful and stiff joints with pain ↑ on exercise.
- Joint may give way because of weak muscles.
- Symptoms vary with some having periods of remission.
- Advanced OA pain is severe and constant.
- Compromised mobility and difficulty completing ADL.
- Depression.

## Support and advice to ↓ pain and progression

- *Assess impact of OA on everyday life:* function, occupation, mood, relationships, and leisure.
- *Advise patient about disease and health promotion:* healthy diet (📖 Nutrition and healthy eating, p. 304), smoking cessation (📖 Smoking cessation, p. 315).
- Reduce stress on joints by maintaining ideal weight.
- *Exercise to strengthen muscles to stabilize and protect joints:* consider referral to physiotherapist for advice and teaching of exercises.
- *Pace activities:* do physically demanding work intermittently.
- *Wear flat heels* and footwear with thick soft soles to act as shock absorbers.
- *Walking sticks:* use on opposite side to OA joint. Can ↓ weight and stress on hip and knee.
- *Home modifications:* to avoid trips and falls, and ↓ need to bend and strain (📖 Assistive technology and equipment for home nursing, p. 778). Consider OT referral.
- *Psychological support:* OA does *not* always worsen, symptoms may reach a peak a few years after first onset, and plateau or lessen.
- *Activities to optimize joint movement and maintain general health:* regular aerobic exercise, e.g. walking and cycling (for OA knee, but latter may worsen patella femoral OA) and swimming (for OA back and hip).

**Treatment**

- Expert patient, peer support groups (📖 Expert patient, p. 303).
- *Non-pharmacological interventions:* weight loss (📖 Weight management: obesity, p. 307), exercise (📖 Exercise, p. 313), and activity as described earlier, footwear adaptation, walking stick, transcutaneous electrical nerve stimulation (TENS), local heat and cold treatment.
- *Analgesia:* paracetamol first choice 1g qds and/or topical NSAIDs for use on knee/hands. OA only. Topical NSAIDs have fewer side effects than oral (NB also refer to local formulary advice for prescribing).
- *Glucosamine and chondroitin from health shops and chemists:* evidence mixed so not recommended by NICE.
- *Opioids, oral NSAIDs or COX2 inhibitors:* as second line agents in addition to or instead of paracetamol. Use lowest effective dose for shortest possible time. Proton pump inhibitor, e.g. omeprazole, should be prescribed with NSAIDs.
- *Low-dose antidepressants:* e.g. amitriptyline, are a useful adjunct, especially if sleep disturbed by pain.
- *Surgery:* hip and knee replacement for severe pain or immobility.

**Related topics**

📖 Expert patient, p. 303; 📖 Rheumatoid arthritis, p. 555; 📖 Healthy ageing, p. 325.

**Further information**

Arthritis Care. Available at: 🖰 www.arthritiscare.org.uk
Arthritis Research Campaign. ☎ 0870 850 5000. Available at: 🖰 www.arc.org.uk
Disabled Living Foundation. Available at: 🖰 www.dlf.org.uk
NICE (2008). *Osteoarthritis; the care and management of osteoarthritis in adults (CG59)*. Available at: 🖰 www.nice.org.uk/CG59

# Rheumatoid arthritis

Rheumatoid arthritis (RA) is an immunological chronic disease of connective tissue with no cure, believed to be triggered by environmental factors in patients that have a genetic predisposition. It is characterized by inflammation of peripheral joints and tendons. Affects ~1% of the UK population, can occur at any age, but most commonly at 40–50yrs; 3× as many ♀ are affected as ♂. It is a variable disease characterized by exacerbations and remissions. For some it is a rapid progressive disease.

## Onset and symptoms of RA

Important treatment for RA is started as soon as possible as this affects the progression of the disease and damage caused by the inflammation process. Any patient with symptoms that might be RA should see GP for onward referral to rheumatology service.

- Often starts slowly; discomfort and intermittent swelling of joints.
- Symmetrical small joint involvement; pain, stiffness, swelling, and functional loss (especially in the hands).
- Pain in the morning, often people do not seek help until they experience difficulty in movement.
- Irreversible damage occurs early if untreated. In addition to joint-related pain people may experience fatigue, stiffness, and anaemia.
- Eyes may become dry and irritable (use artificial tears BNF 1.8.1).
- Rheumatoid nodules may appear on elbows, hands, and feet.

## Care and support to ↓ pain and progression

It is difficult to tell a patient how their RA will progress and for many it will be characterized by exacerbation and periods of remission. RA sufferers may experience depression and fatigue is a common symptom.

- Encourage exercise to maintain function and muscle strength, *but* if joints feel warm, become painful or swollen, rest.
- Devise exercise programme that patient can do, e.g. gentle exercises, gym, swimming is often the best exercise.
- Choose footwear that cushions foot and acts as shock absorber.
- Mixed evidence about diet and RA, encourage healthy low-fat diet.
- Expert patient, peer support groups (🕮 Expert patient, p. 303).
- Medication likely to involve analgesics, including paracetamol, NSAIDs), disease modifying anti-rheumatics (see Arthritis Research Campaign[1] for more detail, and corticosteroids.
- Advise patient about possible side effects of medication (see Table 11.1 for monitoring and side effects).
- People with RA may have ↑ risk of stroke and CVD.
- May need referral for surgical review, e.g. to relieve trapped nerve and tendons or full joint replacement.
- Refer to physiotherapist for exercises, and possible joint support and strapping. Consider OT referral for home modifications.

**Table 11.1** Specific disease-modifying drugs—side effects and monitoring

| Drug | Routine monitoring | Side effects to monitor |
|------|--------------------|--------------------------|
| ⚠ Before starting baseline urea and electrolytes (U&Es), creatinine, estimated glomerular filtration rate (eGFR), LFTs, FBC, and urinalysis checked | | |
| *Methotrexate* (7.5–25mg weekly) Common practice to give folate 5mg the day after methotrexate (i.e. weekly) as well | FBC, U&E, and LFT weekly until dose and monitoring are stable. Then monthly for at least 1yr. Frequency of monitoring may be ↓ by specialist if disease/dose stable after 1yr CXR within 1yr of start of treatment. Check baseline lung function if lung disease | Ask to report symptoms/ signs of infection, especially sore throat If severe respiratory symptoms <6mths after starting, refer to A&E If mean corpuscular volume (MCV) > 105fL check B12/folate |
| ❶ Advise patients *not* to self-medicate with aspirin or ibuprofen. Avoid alcohol | | |
| *Sulfasalazine* (1g bd/ tds) maintenance | FBC and LFT monthly for first 3mths. Then every 3mths Urgent FBC if intercurrent illness during initiation If stable after a year, frequency of monitoring may be ↓ by specialist. | Rash (1%) Nausea/diarrhoea often transient Bone marrow suppression in 1–2% in the first months. If MCV >105 fL check B12/ folate |
| *Intramuscular gold* (Myocrisin ℳ) 50mg monthly | FBC, and urinalysis at the time of each injection CXR within 1yr of start of treatment | Ask patients to report: Symptoms/signs of infection especially sore throat Bleeding/bruising Breathlessness/cough Mouth ulcers/metallic taste or rashes |
| *D penicillamine* (500–750mg/day) maintenance | FBC, urinalysis 2-weekly for 3mths and 1wk after any ↑ dose. Then monthly | Altered taste (can be ignored) Rash |
| *Azathioprine* (1.5–2.5mg/kg/day) maintenance | FBC and LFT weekly for 6wks, then every 2wks until dose/monitoring stable for 6wks. Then monthly | GI side effects, rash, bone marrow suppression Avoid live vaccines |
| ❶ If allopurinol is co-prescribed, ↓dose to 25% of the original. | | |

| Drug | Routine monitoring | Side effects to monitor |
|------|--------------------|-----------------------|
| Ciclosporin (1.25mg/kg bd) maintenance | FBC and LFT monthly until dose/monitoring stable for 3mths, then every 3mths<br><br>U&E, creatinine/eGFR every 2wks. until dose stable for 3mths, then monthly<br><br>Lipids 6-monthly | Rash, gum soreness, hirsutism, renal failure ↑ creatinine (if ↑ by >30% from baseline, withold and discuss with rheumatologist), ↑ BP<br><br>Monitor BP |
| Hydroxychloroquine (200–400mg/day) maintenance | Baseline eye check and annual check of visual symptoms and visual acuity | Rash, GI effects, ocular side effects (rare) |
| Leflunomide (10–20mg/ day) maintenance | FBC and LFT monthly for 6mths then, if stable every 2mths | Rash, GI, ↑ BP, ↑ ALT<br><br>Check weight and BP at each review |

Reproduced from Simon, C, Everitt H, van Dorp F (2010). *Oxford Handbook of General Practice* 3rd edn. Oxford: Oxford University Press. With permission of Oxford University Press.

LFT, liver function test; ALT, alanine transaminase.

- Disabled 'blue' parking badge if mobility affected (☐ Benefits and Support, Table 14.7 p. 798).
- Financial support (☐ Benefits for illness, disability and carers, p. 795).

## Reference

[1]Arthritis Research Campaign. Available at: ℘ http://www.arthritisresearchuk.org/arthritis-information/drugs/dmards.aspx

## Further information

Arthritis Care. Available at: ℘ www.arthritiscare.org.uk
Disabled Living Foundation. Available at: ℘: www.dlf.org.uk
NICE (2009). *Rheumatoid Arthritis (CG79)*. Available at: ℘ www.nice.org.uk

# Osteoporosis

A progressive, systemic, skeletal disease, characterized by low bone mass and micro-architectural deterioration of bone tissues, →↑ in bone fragility and susceptibility to fracture, significant cause of mortality, pain, and disability particularly in older people and can result in:

- Vertebral deformity.
- Loss of height.
- Limitations in daily activities.

The lifetime risk of osteoporotic fracture in women is 40% and in men 13%. It is often diagnosed after the first fracture. Main morbidity and costs link to hip fracture. The aim is to ↓ osteoporotic fractures.

## Bone mineral density

Osteoporosis = bone mineral density (BMD) >2.5 SD below the young adult mean (T score −2.5). BMD measurement by dual energy X-ray absorptiometry (DEXA) scan can quantify risk of fracture. A T score −2.5 or less indicates treatment with a bisphosphonate should be started.

## Risk factors

- Age (about 50% of those >75yrs).
- ♀ Post-menopause oestrogen deficiency and ↑ risk if:
  - Premature menopause (<45yrs).
  - Prolonged 2° amenorrhoea.
- 1° or 2° hypogonadism in ♂.
- ♂ alcohol misuse.
- *Glucocorticoid use:* patients taking any doses of oral steroids should take calcium/vitamin D supplements.
- Maternal history of hip fracture, <75yrs.
- Low body mass index (<19kg/m$^2$).
- *Other disorders associated with osteoporosis:* anorexia nervosa, malabsorption syndromes, 1° hyperparathyroidism, post-transplantation, chronic renal failure, chronic liver disease, hyperthyroidism, Cushing's syndrome.
- Prolonged immobilization
- *Previous fragility fracture:* especially hip, spine, wrist.
- Loss of height, thoracic kyphosis.

If there are risk factors for osteoporosis refer to GP for DEXA scan.

## Prevention of osteoporotic fractures

Each primary care organization should have:
- Lead clinician for falls prevention/osteoporosis programme/monitor organization's performance.
- Establish local osteoporosis interest group to facilitate multidisciplinary implementation.
- Access to adequate levels of diagnostic and specialist services including falls clinics.
- Promotion of care pathways and auditing to standards of care.

Since 2012 included in Quality and Outcomes Framework (📖 Quality and outcomes framework, p. 66).

## Preventive interventions

- Maintain body weight.
- *Nutrition* (📖 Nutrition and healthy eating, p. 304):
  - Calcium reference nutrient intake 1000mg/day for adult, 1200mg >50yrs, 1300mg/day for 9–18yrs, 500–8000mg for children, 210–270mg/day for infants. Found in dairy products and green leafy vegetables, flour products, some fish.
  - Vitamin D helps absorb calcium. Found in dairy products and fish oils, but major source sunlight on skin. Requirement is 15–20min/day during summer months, but avoid burning.
  - ❶ Elderly people in care homes are at higher risk of VitD deficiency.
- *Exercise and physical activity*: recommendation 30min/day for 5 or more days/wk. Weight-bearing, high impact exercise most beneficial, e.g. running, jumping, climbing stairs or exercise referral for frailer and older people (📖 Falls prevention, p. 327).
- *Stopping smoking*: →↑ toxic effect on bone; ↓ fracture rate by 25% (📖 Smoking cessation, p. 315).
- *Moderate alcohol intake*: 3–4U/day for men, 2–3U/day for women. Alcohol is damaging to bone turnover (📖 Alcohol, p. 319).
- HRT postpones post-menopausal bone loss and ↓ fractures. *But* concerns around risk of breast cancer → not first choice for prevention (📖 Menopause, p. 323).
- Hip protector pads, although often poorly tolerated.
- *Bisphosphonates*: e.g. alendronate 10mg od or 70mg once weekly

## Further information

National Osteoporosis Society: online resources for primary care. Helpline ☎ 0845 4500230. Available at: ℘ www.nos.org.uk

NICE (2012). *Osteoporosis: assessing the risk of fragility fracture (CG146)*. Available at: ℘ www.nice.org.uk/CG146

# Low back pain

Common complaint; 80% of the adult population will experience low back pain at some time in their lives. 50% of these will have recurring symptoms.
- *Acute low back pain:* new episode of <6wks duration.
- *Chronic low back pain:* pain lasts >3mths, if >1yr poor outlook.

Some back pain involves irritation of the nerve roots (radicular pain). *Sciatica* occurs when pain radiates down buttocks and leg caused by irritation of sciatic nerve.

## Causes
- Postural.
- Pregnancy.
- Prolapsed disc.
- Trauma.
- 📖 Osteoporosis, p. 558.
- Degenerative joint disease, osteoarthritis (including ankylosing spondylitis).

NB Refer to GP if <20yrs, >55yrs, pain is non-mechanical, worse when supine or at night, involves thoracic pain; previous history of cancer, taking steroids, HIV, also being generally unwell, observable structural deformity, accompanied with weight loss, neurological symptoms and impairment, or muscle weakness in leg and foot.

## Care and support for acute back pain
- *Discount possibility of fracture or other treatable causes:* e.g. following trauma.
- *Regular and effective pain relief:* paracetamol, NSAIDs.
- Hot and cold compresses to affected area (will not benefit everyone).
- *Encourage to be as active as possible:* do not lie flat on back for prolonged periods unless advised by doctor.
- *Evidence mixed on manipulation:* osteopath/chiropractor may help.
- If no improvement in 6wks should see physiotherapist for exercises.

## Care and support for patients with chronic back pain
Patient should see GP and possible orthopaedic/rheumatology referral to discount need for surgery and/or possible referral to pain clinic if available locally.
- Overall aim to improve self-management (📖 Expert patient, p. 303), and reduce and manage pain.
- Encourage patient to practise back exercises and maintain activity.
- Chronic pain can lead to loss of sleep, depression, and reduced QoL psychosocial support, analgesia should be used when exacerbations and amitriptyline at night can give relief.
- For chronic pain use painkillers, e.g. paracetamol regularly and add NSAID for acute exacerbations.
- TENS can be helpful.

### Health promotion and prevention
- Improve posture, and overall physical fitness and activity levels.
- Exercise (□ Exercise, p. 313) and interventions that improve back strength: cycling and swimming (avoiding breast stroke), yoga, Alexander technique.
- Advice from physiotherapist on back exercises and correct lifting techniques.
- Review household and work furniture: use chairs that support lumbar spine, firm mattresses, etc. Workplace assessment by OH department. May determine need for specialist furniture/equipment.
- Reduce weight if BMI >25 (□ Weight management: obesity, p. 307).

### Related topics
□ Pain assessment and management, p. 513; □ People with depression, p. 438; □ Talking therapies, p. 429; □ Expert patient, p. 303; □ Osteoarthritis, p. 553.

### Further information
Backcare. ☎ 0845 1302704. Available at: ✆ www.backcare.org.uk
NICE (2009). Low back pain early management of persistent non-specific low back pain (CG 88). Available at: ✆ http://publications.nice.org.uk/low-back-pain-cg88

# Measuring lung function

The early identification and management of chronic obstructive pulmonary disease (📖 Chronic obstructive pulmonary disease, p. 574). COPD requires the use of spirometry. The management of asthma (📖 Asthma in adults, p. 566) requires the use of peak flow meters. Practice nurses, with appropriate training, are often the most frequent users of this equipment in practices.

## Peak flow

Measures how hard and how quickly a patient can exhale. Peak flow is used to monitor the progress of disease and effects of treatment for patients with asthma. *Note:* it is not a good measure of airflow limitation as it tends to over-estimate lung function. Peak flow meters are available on NHS prescription. Patients with asthma, and all patients with severe asthma, should have an agreed written action plan and their own peak flow meter, with regular checks of inhaler technique and compliance. They should know when and how to increase their medication and when to seek medical assistance. Asthma action plans can ↓ hospitalization and deaths from asthma

### Measuring peak expiratory flow rate (PEFR)
- Ask the patient to stand up (if possible) and hold peak flow meter horizontally. Check indicator is at zero and track clear.
- Ask patient to take a deep breath and blow out forcefully into peak flow meter ensuring lips are sealed firmly around mouthpiece.
- Read PEFR off meter. The best of three attempts is recorded.
- Consider using a low range meter if predicted or best PEFR is <250L/min.
- Normal values: see Table 11.3.

## Spirometry

Measures the volume of air the patient is able to expel from the lungs after a maximal inspiration.
- *Forced expiratory volume in 1s ($FEV_1$):* volume of air patient is able to exhale in first second of forced expiration.
- *Forced vital capacity (FVC):* total volume of air patient can forcibly exhale in single breath.
- *$FEV_1$/FVC:* ratio of $FEV_1$ to FVC expressed as a %.

*Measuring FEV₁ and FVC*

- Note patient's sex, age, and (measured) height so that measurements can be compared with predicted normal values.
- Sit the patient comfortably.
- Ask patient to breathe in as deeply as possible and hold breath long enough to seal lips around mouthpiece.
- Ensure patient does *not* purse lips and ideally ask them to pinch their nose.
- Patient should then breathe out forcibly as hard and as fast as possible until there is nothing left to expel. In patients with severe COPD—this can take up to 15s.
- Repeat procedure and repeat again → three readings of which best two should be within 100mL or 5% of each other.

Readings are interpreted against normal values—see Table 11.2 for interpretation, and Table 11.3 and Table 11.4 for normal valves. If results are borderline normal then repeat in a few months.

**Table 11.2** Interpretation of spirometry results

|  | Restrictive lung disease, e.g. fibrosing alveolitis | Obstructive lung disease, e.g. COPD |
|---|---|---|
| $FEV_1$ (% of predicted normal) | ↓ (<80%) | ↓ (<80%) |
| FVC (% of predicted normal) | ↓ (<80%) | Normal or ↓ |
| $FEV_1/FVC$ | Normal (>70%) | ↓ (<70%) |

Reproduced from Simon C, Everitt H, van Dorp F. (2010). *Oxford Handbook of General Practice*, 3rd edn. Oxford: OUP. With permission of Oxford University Press.

## Essential reading

British Thoracic Society (2005). *Spirometry in Practice: A Practical Guide to Using Spirometry in primary care*. London: BTS. Available at: ℜ www.brit-thoracic.org.uk

## Further information

Association for Respiratory Technology and Physiology (UK) ARTP/BTS Further details and list of approved training centres from ☎ 0121 697 8339. Available at: ℜ www.artp.org.uk
British Thoracic Society Guidelines. Available at: ℜ www.brit-thoracic.org.uk
NICE (2010) *Management of Chronic Obstructive Pulmonary Disease: Management of Adults in Primary and Secondary Care (CG101)*. London: NICE. Available at: ℜ http://publications.nice.org.uk/chronic-obstructive-pulmonary-disease-cg101/guidance

# Normal spirometry and peak flow values

**Table 11.3** Predicted PEFR measurements in L/min (EU scale)

| Height (ft) | 3' | 3'4" | 3'8" | 4' | 4'4" | 4'8" | 5' | 5'4" | 5'8" | 6' |
|---|---|---|---|---|---|---|---|---|---|---|
| m | 0.9 | 1 | 1.1 | 1.2 | 1.3 | 1.4 | 1.5 | 1.6 | 1.7 | 1.8 |
| PEFR (L/min) | 88 | 105 | 136 | 172 | 220 | 265 | 313 | 371 | 427 | 487 |

### Women

| Ht (ft) | 4'10" | 4'11" | 5' | 5'1" | 5'2" | 5'3" | 5'4" | 5'5" | 5'6" | 5'7" | 5'8" | 5'9" | 5'10" |
|---|---|---|---|---|---|---|---|---|---|---|---|---|---|
| m | 1.47 | 1.5 | 1.52 | 1.55 | 1.57 | 1.6 | 1.62 | 1.65 | 1.67 | 1.7 | 1.72 | 1.75 | 1.77 |
| **Age** | | | | | | | | | | | | | |
| 15y | 379 | 382 | 385 | 389 | 391 | 394 | 397 | 400 | 402 | 405 | 407 | 411 | 413 |
| 20y | 402 | 406 | 409 | 413 | 416 | 419 | 422 | 425 | 428 | 431 | 434 | 437 | 439 |
| 25y | 415 | 419 | 422 | 426 | 429 | 433 | 435 | 439 | 441 | 445 | 447 | 451 | 453 |
| 30y | 419 | 424 | 427 | 431 | 433 | 437 | 440 | 444 | 446 | 450 | 452 | 456 | 458 |
| 35y | 418 | 423 | 425 | 430 | 432 | 436 | 439 | 443 | 445 | 449 | 451 | 454 | 457 |
| 40y | 413 | 417 | 420 | 424 | 427 | 431 | 433 | 437 | 439 | 443 | 445 | 449 | 451 |
| 45y | 405 | 409 | 412 | 416 | 418 | 422 | 425 | 428 | 431 | 434 | 436 | 440 | 442 |
| 50y | 394 | 399 | 401 | 405 | 407 | 411 | 414 | 417 | 419 | 423 | 425 | 428 | 430 |
| 55y | 383 | 387 | 389 | 393 | 395 | 399 | 401 | 404 | 407 | 410 | 412 | 415 | 417 |
| 60y | 370 | 373 | 376 | 379 | 382 | 385 | 387 | 391 | 393 | 396 | 398 | 401 | 403 |
| 65y | 356 | 360 | 362 | 366 | 368 | 371 | 373 | 376 | 378 | 381 | 383 | 386 | 388 |
| 70y | 343 | 346 | 348 | 351 | 353 | 356 | 358 | 361 | 363 | 366 | 368 | 371 | 372 |

### Men

| Ht (ft) | 5'2" | 5'3" | 5'4" | 5'5" | 5'6" | 5'7" | 5'8" | 5'9" | 5'10" | 5'11" | 6' | 6'1" | 6'2" |
|---|---|---|---|---|---|---|---|---|---|---|---|---|---|
| m | 1.57 | 1.6 | 1.62 | 1.65 | 1.67 | 1.7 | 1.72 | 1.75 | 1.77 | 1.8 | 1.82 | 1.85 | 1.87 |
| **Age** | | | | | | | | | | | | | |
| 15y | 479 | 485 | 489 | 494 | 498 | 503 | 506 | 511 | 515 | 520 | 523 | 528 | 531 |
| 20y | 534 | 540 | 545 | 551 | 555 | 561 | 565 | 571 | 575 | 580 | 584 | 589 | 593 |
| 25y | 568 | 575 | 580 | 587 | 591 | 598 | 602 | 608 | 612 | 618 | 622 | 628 | 632 |
| 30y | 587 | 594 | 599 | 606 | 611 | 617 | 622 | 628 | 633 | 639 | 643 | 649 | 653 |
| 35y | 594 | 601 | 606 | 613 | 618 | 625 | 629 | 636 | 640 | 646 | 650 | 657 | 661 |
| 40y | 592 | 599 | 604 | 611 | 615 | 622 | 627 | 633 | 637 | 644 | 648 | 654 | 658 |
| 45y | 582 | 590 | 594 | 601 | 606 | 612 | 617 | 623 | 627 | 634 | 638 | 644 | 647 |
| 50y | 568 | 575 | 580 | 586 | 591 | 597 | 601 | 608 | 612 | 618 | 622 | 627 | 631 |
| 55y | 550 | 557 | 561 | 568 | 572 | 578 | 582 | 588 | 592 | 598 | 602 | 607 | 611 |
| 60y | 529 | 536 | 540 | 546 | 550 | 556 | 560 | 566 | 570 | 575 | 579 | 584 | 588 |
| 65y | 507 | 513 | 517 | 523 | 527 | 533 | 536 | 542 | 545 | 551 | 554 | 559 | 562 |
| 70y | 484 | 490 | 493 | 499 | 503 | 508 | 511 | 517 | 520 | 525 | 528 | 533 | 536 |

❶ For normal values in age groups/heights not represented on these charts or for conversion from the old Wright scale peak flow meters see ℛ www.peakflow.com

Adapted from Gregg I, Nunn AJ. (1989). *BMJ* 298, with permission of the BMJ Publishing Group.

**Table 11.4** Predicted FEV$_1$ and FVC measurements (in L)

❶ These values apply for Caucasians. ↓ values by 7% for Asians and 13% for people of African Caribbean origin.

**Women**

| Height | ft | 4'11" | 5'1" | 5'3" | 5'5" | 5'7" | 5'9" | 5'11" |
|--------|-----|-------|------|------|------|------|------|-------|
|        | m | 1.5 | 1.55 | 1.6 | 1.65 | 1.7 | 1.75 | 1.8 |
| **Age** | | | | | | | | |
| 38–41y | FEV$_1$ | 2.3 | 2.5 | 2.7 | 2.89 | 3.09 | 3.29 | 3.49 |
|        | FVC | 2.69 | 2.91 | 3.13 | 3.35 | 3.58 | 3.80 | 4.02 |
| 42–45y | FEV$_1$ | 2.2 | 2.4 | 2.6 | 2.79 | 2.99 | 3.19 | 3.39 |
|        | FVC | 2.59 | 2.81 | 3.03 | 3.25 | 3.47 | 3.69 | 3.91 |
| 46–49y | FEV$_1$ | 2.1 | 2.3 | 2.5 | 2.69 | 2.89 | 3.09 | 3.29 |
|        | FVC | 2.48 | 2.7 | 2.92 | 3.15 | 3.37 | 3.59 | 3.81 |
| 50–53y | FEV$_1$ | 2 | 2.2 | 2.4 | 2.59 | 2.79 | 2.99 | 3.19 |
|        | FVC | 2.38 | 2.6 | 2.82 | 3.04 | 3.26 | 3.48 | 3.71 |
| 54–57y | FEV$_1$ | 1.9 | 2.1 | 2.3 | 2.49 | 2.69 | 2.89 | 3.09 |
|        | FVC | 2.27 | 2.49 | 2.72 | 2.94 | 3.16 | 3.38 | 3.6 |
| 58–61y | FEV$_1$ | 1.8 | 2 | 2.2 | 2.39 | 2.59 | 2.79 | 2.99 |
|        | FVC | 2.17 | 2.39 | 2.61 | 2.83 | 3.06 | 3.28 | 3.5 |
| 62–65y | FEV$_1$ | 1.7 | 1.9 | 2.1 | 2.29 | 2.49 | 2.69 | 2.89 |
|        | FVC | 2.07 | 2.29 | 2.51 | 2.73 | 2.95 | 3.17 | 3.39 |
| 66–69y | FEV$_1$ | 1.6 | 1.8 | 2 | 2.19 | 2.39 | 2.59 | 2.79 |
|        | FVC | 1.96 | 2.18 | 2.4 | 2.63 | 2.85 | 3.07 | 3.29 |

Reproduced from Simon, C, et al, *Oxford Handbook of General Practice*, 3rd ed. (2010), with permission of Oxford University Press

For women ≥70yrs use the formulae:
- FEV$_1$ = (0.0395 × height (m) × 100) − (0.025 × age (yrs)) − 2.6.
- FVC = (0.0443 × height (m) × 100) − (0.026 × age (yrs)) − 2.89.

**Men**

| Height | ft | 5'3" | 5'5" | 5'7" | 5'9" | 5'11" | 6'1" | 6'3" |
|--------|-----|------|------|------|------|-------|------|------|
|        | m | 1.6 | 1.65 | 1.7 | 1.75 | 1.8 | 1.85 | 1.9 |
| **Age** | | | | | | | | |
| 38–41y | FEV$_1$ | 3.2 | 3.42 | 3.63 | 3.85 | 4.06 | 4.28 | 4.49 |
|        | FVC | 3.81 | 4.1 | 4.39 | 4.67 | 4.96 | 5.25 | 5.54 |
| 42–45y | FEV$_1$ | 3.09 | 3.3 | 3.52 | 3.73 | 3.95 | 4.16 | 4.38 |
|        | FVC | 3.71 | 3.99 | 4.28 | 4.57 | 4.86 | 5.15 | 5.43 |
| 46–49y | FEV$_1$ | 2.97 | 3.18 | 3.4 | 3.61 | 3.83 | 4.04 | 4.26 |
|        | FVC | 3.6 | 3.89 | 4.18 | 4.47 | 4.75 | 5.04 | 5.33 |
| 50–53y | FEV$_1$ | 2.85 | 3.07 | 3.28 | 3.5 | 3.71 | 3.93 | 4.14 |
|        | FVC | 3.5 | 3.79 | 4.07 | 4.36 | 4.65 | 4.94 | 5.23 |
| 54–57y | FEV$_1$ | 2.74 | 2.95 | 3.17 | 3.38 | 3.6 | 3.81 | 4.03 |
|        | FVC | 3.39 | 3.68 | 3.97 | 4.26 | 4.55 | 4.83 | 5.12 |
| 58–61y | FEV$_1$ | 2.62 | 2.84 | 3.05 | 3.27 | 3.48 | 3.7 | 3.91 |
|        | FVC | 3.29 | 3.58 | 3.87 | 4.15 | 4.44 | 4.73 | 5.02 |
| 62–65y | FEV$_1$ | 2.51 | 2.72 | 2.94 | 3.15 | 3.37 | 3.58 | 3.8 |
|        | FVC | 3.19 | 3.47 | 3.76 | 4.05 | 4.34 | 4.63 | 4.91 |
| 66–69y | FEV$_1$ | 2.39 | 2.6 | 2.82 | 3.03 | 3.25 | 3.46 | 3.68 |
|        | FVC | 3.08 | 3.37 | 3.66 | 3.95 | 4.23 | 4.52 | 4.81 |

For men ≥70yrs use the formulae:
- FEV$_1$ = (0.043 × height (m) × 100) − (0.029 × age (yrs)) − 2.49.
- FVC = (0.0576 × height (m) × 100) − (0.026 × age (yrs)) − 4.34.

# Asthma in adults

Asthma is a lung disease, with intermittent narrowing of the bronchi, causing shortness of breath, wheezing, and cough. 7% of the population has medically diagnosed asthma, although significantly more have a wheeze or suffer from wheeze with breathlessness. Characterized by:
- *Airflow limitation:* usually reversible spontaneously or with treatment.
- Airway hyper-responsiveness to a wide range of stimuli.
- Inflammation of the bronchi.

During the asthma attack muscles in the bronchi contract, the lining swells, becomes inflamed, and produces excess mucus. The inflammatory process, if left unchecked causes irreversible damage to airways. Asthma is a major cause of hospitalization.

Symptoms consistent with asthma >1 of the following:
- Wheeze.
- Breathlessness.
- Cough.
- Tightness of chest.

Symptoms are variable, intermittent, worse at night, and provoked by triggers, which can include:
- Exercise.
- Household allergens, including house mites, fur, and feathered pets.
- Emotion.
- FH of atopy.
- Unexplained low $FEV_1$ or PEFR.
- Weather (fog, cold air, thunderstorms).
- Air pollutants (smoke and dust).

Diagnosis is made on clinical history and recognition of a characteristic pattern of symptoms/signs. Refer for specialist opinion when diagnosis unclear or atypical features.

## Aims and principles of management
- To control symptoms and impact on everyday life.
- To restore normal or best possible long-term airway function.
- To reduce risk of severe attack.
- Reduce need for reliever medication.
- To minimize absence from work.
- To involve patient in active management.
- To use lower effective doses of medications, minimizing side effects.

## Primary care asthma services
When asthma care is delivered by GPs and nurses trained in asthma management there is evidence it improves diagnosis, prescribing, patient education, monitoring, and continuity of care. General practices should:
- Keep a register of asthma patients to ensure adequate follow-up.
- Recall asthma patients at least annually for review.
- Offer services that are flexible and reflect patient preference, e.g. telephone follow-up over clinic attendance.
- Follow-up any who fail to attend for review.

Practice nurses, with training, often run the register and review programme. Audit materials are available with the national guidelines[1]. High quality performance is recognized in QOF ( Quality and outcomes framework, p. 66).

Patients who have had near fatal asthma attacks or brittle asthma i.e. they are well-controlled but then experience sudden unexpected severe attacks should always be reviewed by specialists.

## Review and monitoring
- Check and record symptoms and control since last seen, e.g.: RCP 3[2] questions are useful for monitoring patients:
  - Have you had any difficulty sleeping because of your asthma symptoms (including cough)?
  - Have you had your usual asthma symptoms during the day (cough, wheeze, chest tightness, or breathlessness)?
  - Has your asthma interfered with your usual activities (e.g. housework, sport etc.)?
- Review PEFR ( Normal spirometry and peak flow values, p. 564).
- Review medication use, problems, inhaler technique.
- Check smoking status and advise to cease.
- Check influenza vaccination up-to-date.
- Identify and address any other health or psycho-social problems that may be impacting on asthma management.
- Address any problems, education needs, and queries.
- Agree management plan and next review date.

## Patient self-management
See also  Expert patient, p. 303 Patients should have:
- Education and information (including written) about asthma tailored to them including:
  - Nature of the disease and treatment.
  - Identification of areas where patient most wants improvement.
  - Development of self-monitoring/self-assessment skills and when to consult GP.
  - Recognition and management of acute exacerbations.
  - Appropriate allergen or trigger avoidance.
- Written action plan, negotiated in the light of their asthma goals, including recognizing symptoms of asthma worsening, peak flow levels and actions to take.
- Patient-held record of asthma reviews.
- PEFR monitoring, often home monitoring helpful in managing symptoms ( Measuring lung function, p. 562).

Asthma UK produces a range of material to support this self-management.

*Secondary non-pharmalogical prophylaxis*
- In committed families wishing to try house dust mite avoidance, suggest barrier bed covering, removal of carpets, removal of soft toys from beds, high temperature washing of bed linen, dehumidification.
- Smoking cessation (📖 Smoking cessation, p. 315) by patient and household members reduces symptoms and severity.
- Weight reduction in obese patients to improve asthma control (📖 Weight management: obesity, p. 307).

*Pharmacological treatment*
See 📖 Drug treatment of asthma, p. 569.

## References

[1]British Thoracic Society/SIGN Asthma Guideline: 2012 🔗 http://www.brit-thoracic.org.uk/guidelines/asthma-guidelines.aspx

[2]Thomas M, Gruffydd-Jones K, Stonham C, et al. (2009). Assessing asthma control in routine clinical practice: use of the Royal College of Physicians '3 Questions'. *Primary Care Resp J* **18**: 83–8.

## Further information

Asthma UK. Advice line: ☎ 0800 121 62 55, Monday–Friday, 09.00–17.00 hours Triple A test: online test that helps patient review their asthma control. Available at: 🔗 www.asthma.org.uk/

# Drug treatment of asthma

Asthma management aims to control symptoms (including nocturnal symptoms and exercise-induced asthma), prevent exacerbations and achieve the best possible lung function, with minimal side effects of treatment A stepwise approach is used to abolish symptoms and to optimize peak flow. See Fig. 11.1.

- The aim is to achieve early control and maintain control by stepping up treatment as necessary and down when control is good. Start at the step most appropriate to severity of symptoms.
- Exacerbations should be treated early. A rescue dose of prednisolone 30–40mg od for 1–2wks may be required at any step and any time.

## Inhalers

The effective inhaler is one that the patient is able to use. Inadequate technique may be mistaken for drug failure. Use a metered dose inhaler whenever possible.

- Patients should be advised to inhale slowly and hold breath for 10s after inhaling.
- Patients should be told explicitly of dose, frequency, and maximum number of inhalations in 24hrs in action plan.
- Advise to seek medical help if prescribed dose failing to relieve symptoms or relieving for <3hrs.
- Check technique at each review.
- A spacer or breath-activated devices may improve delivery for patients that find activation difficult. Follow manufacturer's instructions for care.
- Asthma UK online animations of correct inhaler technique for different devices[1].

## Short-acting bronchodilators (beta-2 agonists)

Usually taken through a small, hand-held inhaler. Beta-2 agonists relax muscles to allow bronchodilation. Work quickly with fewer side effects than alternatives. Use prn unless evidence of benefit with regular doses.
❶ Using more than one canister a month or more than 10–12 puffs/day is a marker of poorly-controlled asthma

## Inhaled corticosteroids

Suppress inflammation in lungs and are recommended for prophylactic treatment of asthma. Five corticosteroids are available as inhaled formulations for the treatment of asthma: beclometasone dipropionate, budesonide, fluticasone propionate, mometasone furoate, and ciclesonide. Effective for achieving overall treatment goals, can be beneficial even for patients with mild asthma. Consider if patient has:

- Exacerbations of asthma in the last 2yrs.
- Using inhaled beta-2 agonists >3× a week.
- Symptomatic three or more times a week, or one or more nights a week.

### Add-on therapy

*Long-acting beta-2 agonists (LABA)* Inhaled preparations (e.g. salmeterol) improve lung function and symptoms. Do not use without inhaled steroids, only continued if demonstrable benefit.

*Theophylline* Improves lung function/symptoms, side effects common.

*Leukotriene receptor antagonists* E.g. montelukast, improve symptoms and lung function and reduce exacerbations.

*Sodium cromoglycate and nedocromil sodium* Some evidence of benefit in adults.

### Related topics

📖 Asthma in adults, p. 566; 📖 Asthma in children, p. 242; 📖 Expert patient, p. 303.

### Essential reading

British Thoracic Society & Scottish Intercollegiate Guidelines Network (2008 revised 2012). British Guideline on Asthma Management. Available at: 🖰 www.brit-thoracic.org.uk/.

NICE (2012). Inhaled corticosteroids for the treatment of chronic asthma in adults and in children aged 12 years and over (TA138). Available at: 🖰 http://publications.nice.org.uk/inhaled-corticosteroids-for-the-treatment-of-chronic-asthma-in-adults-and-in-children-aged-12-years-ta138/evidence-and-interpretation

### Reference

[1] Asthma UK. Advice line: ☏ 0800 121 62 55, Monday–Friday, 09.00–17.00 hours. Available at: 🖰 www.asthma.org.uk/

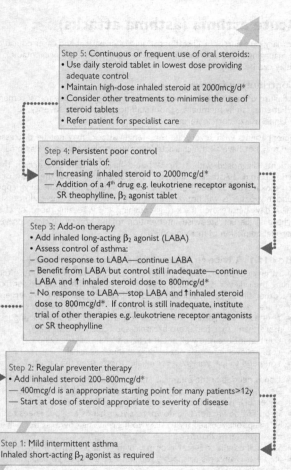

Step 5: Continuous or frequent use of oral steroids:
• Use daily steroid tablet in lowest dose providing adequate control
• Maintain high-dose inhaled steroid at 2000mcg/d*
• Consider other treatments to minimise the use of steroid tablets
• Refer patient for specialist care

Step 4: Persistent poor control
Consider trials of:
— Increasing inhaled steroid to 2000mcg/d*
— Addition of a 4th drug e.g. leukotriene receptor agonist, SR theophylline, $\beta_2$ agonist tablet

Step 3: Add-on therapy
• Add inhaled long-acting $\beta_2$ agonist (LABA)
• Assess control of asthma:
– Good response to LABA—continue LABA
– Benefit from LABA but control still inadequate—continue LABA and ↑ inhaled steroid dose to 800mcg/d*
– No response to LABA—stop LABA and ↑ inhaled steroid dose to 800mcg/d*. If control is still inadequate, institute trial of other therapies e.g. leukotriene receptor antagonists or SR theophylline

Step 2: Regular preventer therapy
• Add inhaled steroid 200–800mcg/d*
— 400mcg/d is an appropriate starting point for many patients>12y
— Start at dose of steroid appropriate to severity of disease

Step 1: Mild intermittent asthma
Inhaled short-acting $\beta_2$ agonist as required

\* Beclometasone dipropionate or equivalent.

**Fig. 11.1** Summary of stepwise management in adults.

Reproduced from British Guidelines on the Management of Asthma. Available at: ℘ www.brit-thoracic.org.uk. With kind permission of the British Thoracic Society.

# Acute asthma (asthma attacks)

Primary care nurses in all settings should offer patient and carer education in managing acute asthma. Many deaths from asthma are preventable and delay can be fatal).

## Contributory factors

- Failure of practitioners to assess severity using objective measurement.
- Patients, family members, school staff not recognizing severity.
- Underuse of corticosteroids.

*Note:* patients with severe life-threatening attacks may not be distressed and may not have all the characteristic abnormalities of severe asthma.

Patients diagnosed with asthma should have written guidance in their action plan (📖 Asthma in adults, p. 566) on what to do in the event of an acute exacerbation (see Box 11.1). Asthma attacks do not usually happen suddenly, patients will notice asthma getting worse over several hours or a few days before the attack (e.g. coughing and wheezing more, or chest tightness). Earlier stepwise intervention in the community can prevent hospital admission of many people.

---

### Box 11.1 Advice to patients (and parents)

If asthma symptoms slowly get worse don't ignore them! Quite often, using the reliever is all that is needed to get the asthma under control. At other times, the symptoms become more severe and more urgent. You are having an asthma attack if any of the following happen:

- Your asthma is getting worse (e.g. you are coughing or wheezing more than usual, feel more breathless, or chest feels tighter).
- You cannot breathe well and it is hard to talk, eat, or sleep.
- Your reliever inhaler is not helping as much as usual.
- You need to use your reliever inhaler more often than usual.

Action is needed in the following steps:

- *Step 1:* take one to two puffs of your reliever inhaler immediately, preferably using a spacer.
- *Step 2:* sit down, don't lie down, rest your hands on your knees to help support yourself try to slow your breathing down, as this will make you less exhausted.
- *Step 3:* if condition is stable or improving wait 5–10min.
- *Step 4:* if symptoms disappear, you should be able to go back to whatever you were doing.
- *Step 5:* if you *do not* start to feel better, continue to take two puffs (one at a time) of your reliever inhaler every 2min. Take up to 10 puffs.
- *Step 6:* if the reliever has no effect, call ambulance.
- *Step 7:* continue to take reliever inhaler every few minutes until help arrives, preferably using a spacer.

Carers, parents, relatives, and school staff need to be made aware that signs such as being unable to complete a sentence in one breath, too breathless to feed or speak, continual coughing in children indicate severe attack and the ambulance should be called.

Attending doctor (or nurse with appropriate training), in the home or surgery, increases treatment in line with the step-up model, but arranges hospital admission if symptoms fail to respond or immediately if signs of any one of the following occur: life-threatening asthma; silent chest; cyanosis; feeble respiratory effort; bradycardia; <33% predicted peak flow; hypotension; confusion; exhaustion; bradycardia; dysrhythmia.

## Risk factors for fatal or near fatal asthma attacks

- Previous admission especially if within year.
- Requires 3 or more classes of asthma medication.
- Heavy use of beta-2 agonists.
- Repeated attendance as A&E for asthma care.
- *Brittle asthma:*
  - *Type 1*—wide PEF variability (>40% diurnal variation for >50% of time over >150 days).
  - *Type 2*—sudden attacks despite asthma apparently being well controlled.
- Asthma, poorly treated and monitored, did not have written action plans, failed to return for review, often with associated psychosocial problems, e.g. psychosis, depression, alcohol, or drug abuse,
- Learning difficulties, employment problems, income problems, social isolation, childhood abuse, severe domestic, marital or legal stress.

British guidelines, British Guideline on Asthma Management[1], support a well-structured asthma management programme in primary care.

## Related topics

📖 Measuring lung function, p. 562; 📖 Asthma in adults, p. 566; 📖 Asthma in children, p. 242.

## Essential reading

[1]British Thoracic Society and Scottish Inter-Collegiate Guidelines Network (2011). *British Guideline on Asthma Management*. and *Managing asthma in adults : A booklet for patients and their families and carers*. London: BTS/SIGN. Available at: ℬ www.brit-thoracic.org.uk; 2005 electronic update www.sign.ac.uk.

## Further information

Asthma UK. Advice line: ☎ 0800 121 62 55, Monday–Friday, 09.00–17.00 hours, Available at: ℬ www.asthma.org.uk/

# Chronic obstructive pulmonary disease

Chronic obstructive pulmonary disease (COPD) is a term used to describe a number of conditions, including chronic bronchitis and emphysema. An estimated 3 million people have COPD in the UK. Most are not diagnosed until they are in their 50s. Predominantly caused by smoking and characterized by airflow obstruction that is not fully reversible. Usually progressive in the long term with exacerbations that occur, when there is a rapid and sustained worsening of the patient's symptoms beyond normal day-to-day variations. No single diagnostic test for COPD. Diagnosis relies on a combination of history, physical examination, and confirmation of airflow obstruction using spirometry.

## Airflow obstruction

- Defined as reduced $FEV_1$ and reduced $FEV_1/FEC$ ratio (📖 Measuring lung function, p. 562) measured by spirometry.
- Caused by inflammation of large and small airways, increased mucus production, damage to alveoli.

Advanced lung destruction causes respiratory failure, i.e. disorder of such extent not meeting metabolic requirements. Other consequences include cor pulmonale, right-sided heart failure, and oedema.

Breathlessness can be very frightening. COPD patients can be very anxious and restrict activities, this sets up a vicious cycle leading to further restrictions. Often also leads to depression.

## Indications for a COPD diagnosis to be considered

- >35yrs.
- SOB on exertion (see dyspnoea scale in Table 11.5).
- Smoker or ex-smoker.
- Chronic cough, producing sputum.
- Increased chest problems in winter.
- Wheeze.

*Note*: uncommon in COPD: chest pain and haemoptysis. May also require other investigations, e.g. chest X-ray, and referral.

## Severity of airflow limitations

- *Mild*: cough, but little or no breathlessness. No abnormal signs or use of services, $FEV_1$ 50–80% predicted.
- *Moderate*: breathlessness, wheeze on exertion, cough with or without sputum, known to GP, $FEV_1$ 30–49% predicted.
- *Severe*: SOB on exertion, marked wheeze and cough, known to services with frequent problems/hospitalizations, $FEV_1$ <30% predicted.

## Key principles in management

- *On diagnosis*:
  - Coded on GP patient records to be added to practice COPD register (📖 Quality and outcomes framework, p. 66).
  - Baseline spirometry reading, dyspnoea scale, and BMI recorded.

**Table 11.5** MRC dyspnoea scale

| Grade | Degree of breathlessness related to activities |
|---|---|
| 1 | Not troubled by breathlessness except on strenuous exercise |
| 2 | Short of breath when hurrying or walking up a slight hill |
| 3 | Walks slower than contemporaries on level ground because of breathlessness, or has to stop for breath when walking at own pace |
| 4 | Stops for breath after walking about 100m or after a few minutes on level ground |
| 5 | Too breathless to leave the house, or breathless when dressing or undressing |

Reproduced with permission from NICE (2007). Medical Research Council dyspnoea scale. Available at: ℞ www.nice.org.uk/usingguidance/commissioningguides/pulmonaryrehabilitationserviceforpatientswithcopd/mrc_dyspnoea_scale.jsp

- *Key principles in management:*
  - Help patient stop smoking if still a smoker (◻ Smoking cessation, p. 315).
  - Effective inhaled therapy (including inhaler technique).
  - Annual flu and pneumococcal vaccination.
  - Weight reduction if BMI >25, nutritional supplements if <18.5.
  - Exercise: lack of exercise decreases $FEV_1$ pulmonary rehabilitation of proven benefit.
  - Advice on action to take in an exacerbation.
  - Provide sources of advice and support in living with breathlessness, e.g. British Lung Foundation, leaflets on travel, sex, and breathlessness, etc.
  - Document efficacy of drug treatment on quality of life and lung function.
- Follow-up review at least annually in mild/moderate, 6-monthly for severe COPD.

## Related topics
◻ Measurement of lung function, p. 562; ◻ Management in stable COPD, p. 576; ◻ Management of exacerbation COPD, p. 579.

## Essential reading
NICE (2010). *Chronic obstructive pulmonary disease. Management of chronic obstructive pulmonary disease in adults in primary and secondary care* (CG101). Available at: ℞ www.nice.org.uk/cg101.

## Further information
British Lung Foundation. Advice line: ☏ 03000 030 555. Email: helpline@blf.org.uk. Available at: ℞ www.blf.org.uk

# Management in stable chronic obstructive pulmonary disease

The lung damage cannot be repaired, but the symptoms and their impact can be managed. Key elements are smoking cessation, effective inhalation therapy, pulmonary rehabilitation, optimum BMI (low BMI indicator of poor prognosis), and immunization.

Review people with mild or moderate COPD at least once a year and those with very severe COPD at least twice a year (see Table 11.6). People with stable severe COPD do not normally need regular hospital review, but there should be locally agreed mechanisms to allow rapid hospital assessment when necessary

**Smoking cessation** A key issue to prevent further lung damage. Offer help to quit at every consultation if patient is still a smoker (📖 Smoking cessation, p. 315).

**Effective inhaled therapy** Stepwise increase according to COPD severity and frequency of exacerbations (see Fig. 11.2).

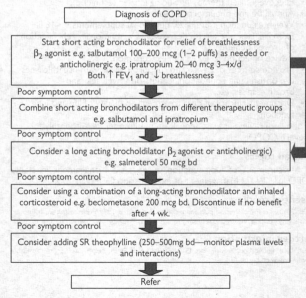

Fig. 11.2 Drug management of COPD. Reproduced from Simon C, Everitt H, van Dorp F. (2010). *Oxford Handbook of General Practice*, 3rd edn. Oxford: OUP.
With permission of Oxford University Press.

## Other medication

- Prescribe according to other problems, e.g. diuretics in cor pulmonale.
- Long-term oxygen therapy (LTOT; 📖 Oxygen therapy in the community, p. 581) in chronically hypoxic COPD.

***Immunization*** Offered pneumococcal vaccination and an annual influenza vaccination. A QOF indicator (📖 Quality and outcomes framework, p. 66).

***Weight management*** BMI >25 or <18.5 may require referral to dietician. ↑ BMI places additional strain on cardiovascular system and mobility. ↓ BMI requires nutritional supplements (📖 Weight management: malnutrition, p. 309).

### Pulmonary rehabilitation

Shown to reduce dyspnoea, improve QoL, and reduce disability and use of health services irrespective of age, of impairment or smoking status. Usually, a 6-wk programme led by specialist and therapy services. Includes aerobic exercise, always of lower extremities (brisk walking, cycling) and may include upper extremities. Often includes educational programme and opportunity for tailored advice on smoking cessation, nutrition, minimizing impact on activities of daily living, physical relationships, etc.

***Education*** Comprehensive disease education for patient and family to understand nature, symptoms, management, and management of exacerbations.

### Advice on exacerbations

See 📖 Management of chronic obstructive pulmonary disease exacerbation, p. 579.

### Regular review and follow-up

(See Table 11.6.)
GP practice COPD registers aid this, also QOF indicator (📖 Quality and outcomes framework, p. 66).

**Table 11.6** Guidance on review and follow-up consultations

| Mild/moderate COPD | Severe COPD |
|---|---|
| *Measurements:* | *Measurements:* |
| FEV₁ and FVC (📖 Measuring lung function, p. 562) | FEV₁ and FVC |
| BMI (📖 Nutrition and healthy eating, p. 304) | BMI (📖 Nutrition and healthy eating, p. 304) |
| MRC dyspnoea score (📖 Chronic obstructive pulmonary, p. 574) | MRC dyspnoea score (📖 Chronic obstructive pulmonary disease, p. 574) |
| | O₂ saturation of arterial blood |
| *Assessment of:* | *Assessment of:* |
| • Smoking status and desire to quit | • Smoking status and desire to quit |
| • Adequacy of symptom control: | • Adequacy of symptom control: |
|   • Breathlessness |   • Breathlessness |
|   • Exercise tolerance |   • Exercise tolerance |
|   • Estimated exacerbation frequency |   • Estimated exacerbation frequency |
|   • Presence of complications |   • Presence of cor pulmonale |
|   • Effects of each drug treatment |   • Need for LTOT |
|   • Inhaler technique |   • Patient's nutritional state |
|   • Need for referral to specialist and therapy services |   • Presence of depression |
|   • Need for pulmonary rehabilitation |   • Effects of each drug treatment |
| |   • Inhaler technique |
| |   • Need for social services and OT input |
| |   • Need for referral to specialist and therapy services |
| |   • Need for pulmonary rehabilitation |

Adapted with permission from NICE Guidance (2011). *Quick Reference Guide Chronic Obstructive Pulmonary Disease*, Clinical guideline 101, p.15.

## Essential reading

NICE (2010). *Chronic Obstructive Pulmonary Disease. Management in adults in primary and secondary care* (CG101). Available at: 🔗 www.nice.org.uk/cg101.

## Further information

British Lung Foundation. ☎ Advice line: 03000 030 555. Email: helpline@blf.org.uk. Available at: 🔗 www.lunguk.org

# Management of chronic obstructive pulmonary disease exacerbation

An exacerbation is acute in onset, and/or a sustained worsening of symptoms from stable state of one or more of the following:

- ↑ dyspnoea, use of accessory muscles at rest, pursed lip breathing.
- ↑ and/or infected sputum.
- ↑ fluid retention.
- ↑ wheeze/cough/sore throats.
- ↓ exercise tolerance and or activities of daily living.
- ↑ fatigue.
- Tight chest.
- Acute confusion.

Respiratory infections and pollutants can cause exacerbations, 30% have no identifiable cause.

## Self-management of exacerbations

All patients with COPD diagnosis should be advised on actions to take on identifying an exacerbation. Patients should respond quickly. At review/follow-up they will have been prescribed antibiotics and oral corticosteroids and advised:

- To start oral corticosteroids if dyspnoea interferes with usual activities.
- To start antibiotics if sputum purulent.
- How to adjust bronchodilator therapy to control symptoms.
- Which health professional/service to contact if symptoms do not improve in a specified timescale.

## Initial management of exacerbations

- Increased frequency of bronchodilator use (may use nebulizer, oxygen therapy). Note: *check inhaler technique.*
- Oral antibiotics if purulent sputum.
- Short course of prednisolone for 7–14 days for all patients with significant increase in breathlessness unless contraindicated.
- Decide whether to manage at home or refer to hospital, based on severity, co-morbidity, ability to cope at home availability of other services, e.g. rapid response team for 24-hr care at home for short periods. Local care pathways inform decision making (see Table 11.7).
- If treated at home, may require pulse oximetry to establish blood $O_2$ saturation levels if severe dyspnoea. Establish on optimum therapy, review and referral to other services/therapies as appropriate.

## Related topics

📖 Measurement of lung function, p. 562; 📖 COPD, p. 574; 📖 Management in stable COPD, p. 576.

## Essential reading

NICE (2010). *Chronic Obstructive Pulmonary Disease. Management in adults in primary and secondary care* (CG101). Available at: 🖝 www.nice.org.uk/cg101.

**Table 11.7** Factors to consider when managing a COPD patient with acute exacerbation

| Factor | Favours treatment at home | Favours treatment in hospital |
|---|---|---|
| Able to cope at home | Yes | No |
| Breathlessness | Mild | Severe |
| General condition | Good | Poor/deteriorating |
| Level of activity | Good | Poor/confined to bed |
| Cyanosis | No | Yes |
| Worsening peripheral oedema | No | Yes |
| Level of consciousness | Normal | Impaired |
| Already receiving LTOT | No | Yes |
| Social circumstances | Good | Living alone/not coping |
| Acute confusion | No | Yes |
| Rapid rate of onset | No | Yes |
| Significant co-morbidity (particularly cardiac disease and insulin-dependent diabetes) | No | Yes |
| $SaO_2$ <90% | No | Yes |
| Changes on the chest radiograph | No | Present |
| Arterial pH level | <7.35 | ≥7.35 |
| Arterial $PaO_2$ | <7kPa | ≥7kPa |

Reproduced with kind permission from NICE (2004). *Quick Reference Guide Chronic Obstructive Pulmonary Disease*. Clinical Guideline 101, p. 17. London: NICE.

## Further information

British Lung Foundation. ☎ Advice line: 03000 030 555. Email: helpline@blf.org.uk. Available at: 🖰 www.lunguk.org

# Oxygen therapy in the community

$O_2$ is a prescription-only therapy. It is combustible/explosive near naked flames and cigarettes. Inform patients and carers of risks and strongly advise not to smoke near oxygen supply. $O_2$ is used therapeutically in 3 ways:
- LTOT.
- Ambulatory.
- Short burst.

Appropriate $O_2$ use can prolong and enhance life. Inappropriate use at best is expensive and, at worst, is life-threatening.

## Long-term oxygen therapy

Only prescribed after assessment by a respiratory physician (e.g. in chronically hypoxic COPD (📖 Chronic obstructive pulmonary disease, p. 574) LTOT can:
- Improve life expectancy.
- Reduce hospitalization.
- Improve QoL.

NICE guidance (2011) specifies people potentially requiring LTOT:
- Patients with very severe airflow obstruction ($FEV_1$ < 30% predicted).
- Patients with cyanosis.
- Patients with polycythaemia.
- Patients with peripheral oedema.
- Patients with a raised jugular venous pressure.
- Patients with oxygen saturations ≤ 92% breathing air.

Assessment should also be considered in patients with severe airflow obstruction ($FEV_1$ 30–49% predicted). LTOT must be:
- Used for ≥15h/day.
- Given at prescribed flow rate only.

## Ambulatory oxygen uses

- LTOT patients able and willing to leave their homes. Can improve exercise tolerance for some patients.
- Patients with exercise-induced $O_2$ desaturation.
- Specialist assessment necessary to determine need and flow rate.

## Oxygen services

Companies in England provide home $O_2$ services for the NHS, each covering certain geographical areas. All hold contracts with the NHS. Arrangements can be made to have $O_2$ supplied to holiday destinations in England or Wales. The British Lung Foundation website has advice on travelling with a lung condition.

*Scotland and Northern Ireland* Home oxygen supplied on FP10s by pharmacy contractors.

## Further information

British Lung Foundation (2012). *What should I expect from a home oxygen service?* Helpline: ☎ 03000 030 555. Email: helpline@blf.org.uk. Available at: 🖰 www.lunguk.org

IMPRESS (Improving and Integrating Respiratory Services) 2011 Rationalising oxygen use to improve patient safety and to reduce waste The IMPRESS step-by-step guide. Available at: 🖰 www.impressresp.com

NHS Choices. Home oxygen treatment. Available at: 🖰 http://www.nhs.uk/Conditions/home-oxygen/Pages/Introduction.aspx

# Nebulizers

A nebulizer converts a drug solution into a continuous fine aerosol mist, inhaled by tidal breathing over 5–10min directly into the lung. Drug solution is prescription-only medicines (POM), and patients advised not to use more frequently than prescribed or change dosage. Many patients can get the same effect by taking four to six puffs from an aerosol inhaler with a spacer.

## Indications for use

- Acute exacerbations of acute asthma and COPD.
- Long-term bronchodilator treatment in asthma and COPD to those shown to benefit from higher medication doses (usually after 2-wk trial).
- When patient unable to use other inhalation devices.
- Delivery of antibiotics for cystic fibrosis, bronchiectasis.
- To deliver pentamidine for prophylaxis and treatment of *Pneumocystis* pneumonia.
- *Palliative care:* palliation of breathlessness or cough (⬛ Palliative care in the home, p. 509).

If prescribed for home use, patients and family should have:
- Instruction in use, cleaning, and maintenance.
- Regular follow-up by respiratory specialists and their contact details.
- ❶ Advise not to treat acute exacerbations at home without also seeking professional help.
- Details of how to service equipment.

## Equipment

There are four parts—face mask/mouthpiece, nebulizer chamber for the drug solution, tubing to connect to the compressor or oxygen to drive the nebulizer chamber.

- *Jet nebulizers:* most commonly used as more efficient in drug delivery. Requires an electric compressor.
- *Main source:* through loan from hospital respiratory services. In England and Wales nebulizers and compressors not available on NHS drug tariff. In Scotland some nebulizers available on GP10A. Equipment may be available at local equipment stores depending on local protocols and services.
- *Mouthpiece:* preferred delivery method as face masks (mostly used with children) inefficient.

## Care and maintenance

- Chamber and mouth piece washed in hot soapy water after every use, rinsed well, dried with kitchen towel, and left disassembled to air dry. Change every 3mths for disposable kits or annually if durable.
- Tubing changed on a regular basis as becomes damp during use and difficult to dry.
- Compressor left on for a few minutes, following disconnection of nebulizer to blow-out any water droplets.
- Compressor should be serviced yearly, and filters changed according to manufacturer's instructions.

## Further information

British Thoracic Society. Available at: ℅ www.brit-thoracic.org.uk
British Lung Foundation (2012). *Nebulisers fact sheet.* Available at: ℅ www.blf.org.uk/Page/Nebulisers

# Coronary heart disease

CHD is one of the main diseases of the heart and circulatory system, and the most common cause of premature death in the UK. 1:5 men and 1:8 women die from CHD. In the UK, there are an estimated 2.7 million people living with the condition and 2 million people affected by angina (the most common symptom CHD). From 50yrs, the chances of developing CHD are similar for men and women. Mortality is falling, but morbidity is rising. Atherosclerosis can be caused by lifestyle habits and other disease conditions.

## Risk factors
- Socio-economic.
- Age: risk increases with age.
- FH of CHD, diabetes, hyperlipidaemia, or hypertension.
- Low birth weight.
- Ethnicity: e.g. Indian subcontinent increased risk.
- Gender: ♂ are more likely to develop CHD at an earlier age than ♀.
- Smoking.
- Hypertension.
- Hyperlipidaemia.
- Diabetes (📖 Diabetes, p. 611).
- Diet.
- Obesity (📖 Weight management overweight, p. 307).

## Primary prevention
Attempts to reduce a person's/population's overall risk of developing CHD. Local policies are essential on:
- Smoking cessation (📖 Smoking cessation, p. 315).
- Promoting healthy eating (📖 Nutrition and healthy eating, p. 304).
- Taking regular exercise (📖 Exercise, p. 313).
- Controlling weight and/or reducing obesity.
- Controlling high BP (📖 Hypertension, p. 589).
- Controlling raised cholesterol (📖 Hyperlipidaemia (high/raised cholesterol), p. 593).
- Controlling blood sugar in diabetes (📖 Type 2 diabetes, p. 621).
- Managing stress (📖 Managing stress, p. 317).
- Alcohol (📖 Alcohol, p. 319), within recommended limits.
- Identifying those at most risk of CHD by calculating risk score.

## Secondary prevention

Almost half of people that die from a MI are already known to have CHD. Targeting people with CHD for risk factor modification is effective in reducing risk of recurrent CHD.

Management and treatment can be jointly managed between nurse and doctor, and should focus on:
- Identification of those at risk, registration, and ongoing follow-up.
- Providing information on how to modify lifestyle/risk factors.
- Best practice according to evidence-based care guidelines.
- Stopping smoking ([📖] Smoking cessation, p. 315).
- Medicine management (refer to local protocols).
- Management of hypertension 50yrs or more (>150/90mmHg) with antihypertensive drugs. See QOF ([📖] Quality and outcomes framework, p. 66) guidelines.
- Anti-platelet therapy can reduce cardiovascular morbidity and mortality. Aspirin (75–300mg/od for maintenance treatment reduce gastric intolerance with dispersible/ enteric coated preparations, PPIs or H$_2$ inhibitors), warfarin or aspirin if >60yrs and with atrial fibrillation. *Note:* caution if on anticoagulant therapy, risk of GI bleed. Avoid concomitant use of aspirin and warfarin except on specialist advice
- Statins and dietary advice.
- After myocardial infarction: in addition to offering a statin and antiplatelet treatment also offered:
  - An angiotensin-converting enzyme inhibitor.
  - A *beta-blocker*—not recommended for people MI more than 1yr ago, have preserved left ventricular function, but have not yet been taking 2° prevention.
- Blood sugar control if diabetic.
- Not all people need referral to a cardiologist, depends on previous history and symptoms.

## Related topics

[📖] Diabetes, p. 611; [📖] Models and approaches to health promotion, p. 298; [📖] Exercise, p. 313; [📖] Cardiac rehabilitation in the community, p. 595; [📖] Quality and outcomes framework, p. 66.

## Further information

British Heart Foundation. Available at: ℘ www.bhf.org.uk
NICE CKS (2008). CVD risk assessment and management. Available at: ℘ http://cks.nice.org.uk/cvd-risk-assessment-and-management#!topicsummary

# Angina

Angina pectoris is the classic symptom of chest pain and is due to transient myocardial ischaemia. CHD is the most common cause. Less commonly, angina is caused by valve disease (e.g. aortic stenosis), hypertrophic obstructive cardiomyopathy, or hypertensive heart disease. Typically caused by exertion or emotion, and relieved by rest. Almost 2 million people in the UK suffer from angina and the incidence is higher in ♂ than in ♀, and ↑ with age.

## Symptoms of stable angina

⚠ *Always considers possibility of MI.* Some or a combination of:
- Heaviness in central chest.
- Squeezing, crushing, or gripping pain.
- Radiating pain to neck, jaw, back, or arms (usually the left).
- Breathless on exertion.
- Musculoskeletal pain.
- Nausea, sweating, palpitations, and/or breathlessness during attacks.
- Referred pain from thoracic spine.
- Anxiety.
- Pain in other sites, e.g. pleural pain, acute cholecystitis.

## Assessment

- What precipitates attack, e.g. exertion, cold weather, large meals, stress.
- Past medical history and family history.
- Lifestyle, i.e. smoking, alcohol intake, drug history.
- Dietary assessment and the possibility of gastro-oesophageal reflux.

## Clinical examination

- BP.
- *Pulse:* rate and rhythm.
- Presence of heart murmurs, arrhythmias, and heart failure (joint examination with GP).
- Evidence of anaemia, hyperlipidaemia, and vascular disease (joint examination with GP).
- BMI.

## Investigations

❶ Health care professionals should follow local protocols for diagnostic testing and referral.
- 12-lead ECG (📖 Recording a 12-lead ECG, p. 589) and exercise ECG to define risk.
- Coronary angiography.
- FBC, fasting lipid profile, and fasting blood sugar.

## Management and treatment
- Advise on lifestyle factors, especially smoking cessation, diet, alcohol consumption.
- Education about angina and heart attacks (see Box 11.2).
- Cardiac rehabilitation may be helpful for patients with severe angina and after surgery.
- All patients with angina should be referred for an exercise tolerance test. (Advise patients to take usual medication prior to test.)
- Patients who drive should inform DVLA.
- If job involves heavy work, may need to review, some groups need to notify occupational health departments, e.g. pilots, seamen.

Medication includes (*Note:* refer to local protocols for medicines management):
- Anti-platelet therapy.
- Nitrates: glyceryl trinitrate (GTN) or nitrate spray (see Box 11.2) prn for symptom relief (sub-lingual GTN alternative to GTN spray, but deteriorates after 8wks).
- Beta-blockers unless contraindicated.
- Calcium channel-blockers if beta-blockers contraindicated.
- Potassium channel openers (BNF 2.6.3).
- Statins (not suitable for people with liver disease, pregnant, or breastfeeding).

❶ If angina worsens, occurs on minimal exertion, or at rest, or nocturnally, is more frequent and with persistent pain that lasts longer than 15min patient at ↑ risk of MI and needs urgent hospital admission.

## Nurse run clinics
Refer to local protocols for nurse-run clinics.
- Maintain register for call and recall of patients (📖 Quality and outcomes framework, p. 66).
- Review medication use and compliance, and blood results.
- Management of co-existing disease, e.g. hypertension and diabetes.
- Stop smoking advice and support.
- BP control.
- Lipid management.
- Exercise and dietary advice.
- Education about symptoms of heart attack and seeking help.

## Related topics
📖 Hypertension, p. 589; 📖 Cardiac rehabilitation in the community, p. 593; 📖 Adult basic life support, p. 742.

## Further information
NICE CKS (2012). Angina. Available at: ℘ http://cks.nice.org.uk/angina#!topicsummary
British Heart Foundation. Available at: ℘ www.bhf.org.uk/
NHS Choices. Angina. Available at: ℘ www.nhs.uk/Conditions/Angina/Pages/Introduction.aspx

**Box 11.2 Advice for patients on using GTN or nitrate spray when having an angina attack**

Sometimes you may experience pain or discomfort and often this will be angina that you can manage at home with your GTN. If you have symptoms consistent with angina:

- Stop what you are doing, sit down and rest.
- Take your GTN spray and tablets, according to your doctor or nurse's instructions. Pain should ease within a few minutes—if it doesn't, take a second dose.
- *If the pain does not ease within a few minutes after your second dose, call 999 immediately.*
- If you're not allergic to aspirin, chew one adult tablet (300mg). If no aspirin, or unsure if you're allergic to aspirin, rest until ambulance arrives.
- Even if your symptoms don't match these, but you suspect you're having a heart attack, call 999 immediately.

Adapted from British Heart Foundation. Available at: ℜ www.bhf.org.uk/heart-health/conditions/angina.aspx

# Hypertension

Hypertension (in people without diabetes) is defined as sustained systolic BP of >140mmHg, and/or sustained diastolic BP of >90mmHg on at least three separate occasions. Often symptomless, 40% of adults in England and Wales have raised BP. Major risk for CHD and CVA. *Hypertension = major risk factor for cardiovascular disease, stroke, and renal failure.* Aim to detect and treat hypertension before damage occurs. Hypertension:

- ↑ with age.
- ↑ in people of Afro-Caribbean origin.
- ↑ people of South Asian origin who are commonly insulin-resistant and have a high prevalence of type 2 diabetes.

## NICE definitions of hypertension

- *Stage 1 hypertension:* clinic BP is 140/90mmHg or higher, and subsequent ambulatory blood pressure monitoring (ABPM) daytime average or home blood pressure monitoring (HBPM) average BP is 135/85mmHg or higher.
- *Stage 2 hypertension:* clinic BP is 160/100mmHg or higher, and subsequent ABPM daytime average or HBPM average BP is 150/95mmHg or higher.
- *Severe hypertension:* clinic systolic BP is 180mmHg or higher, or clinic diastolic BP is 110mmHg or higher.

## Assessment

Hypertension produces no symptoms, is often picked up at routine screening (see also 📖 New patient health check, p. 342), occasionally patient may complain of headache or visual disturbance.

- Regularly maintain and calibrate sphygmomanometer. Use a cuff of correct width (check manufacturer's instructions). Most adults 12 × 26cm bladder. Large adults with arm circumference >33cm use 12 × 40cm bladder. Thin adults and children <26cm use 10 × 18 bladder (if using automated BP monitoring device ensure it is validated).
- Before measuring BP palpate radial or brachial pulse, if pulse irregularity then measure BP manually.

### Postural hypotension

In people with symptoms of postural hypotension (falls or postural dizziness):

- Measure BP with the person either supine or seated. Measure BP again with person standing for at least 1min prior to measurement.
- If the systolic BP falls by 20mmHg or more when person is standing, consider to GP for possible referral to specialist care.

- When measuring BP, provide a relaxed, temperate setting, with the person quiet and seated (reduce the white coat effect).
- Seat the patient with arm at the level of the heart.

- Measure BP to nearest 2mmHg. Measure diastolic pressure when sounds completely disappear.
- Measure BP in both arms. If the difference in readings is more than 20mmHg, repeat measurements. If difference in readings between arms > 20mmHg on the second measurement, measure subsequent BP in arm with higher reading.
- If BP measured in clinic is 140/90mmHg or higher: take a second measurement during consultation. If second measurement is substantially different from first, take third measurement. Record lower of the last two measurements.
- If the clinic BP is 140/90mmHg or higher, offer ambulatory BP monitoring to confirm diagnosis of hypertension.
- Consider starting antihypertensive drug treatment/referral to GP immediately, for people with severe hypertension.
- Establish significant and family history.
- Examine fundi (*note:* only nurses with advanced clinical assessment skills, e.g. nurse practitioners).
- Refer to specialist care same day if BP 180/110mmHg or more, with signs of papilloedema and/or retinal haemorrhage.
- Consider referral in people with signs and symptoms suggesting a 2° cause of hypertension.
- Calculate CVD risk (see Joint British Risk Prediction Chart[1]).

### Investigations
Performed according to practice/local protocols.
- Resting ECG.
- Chest X-ray (CXR).
- Urinalysis for proteinuria and haematuria.
- Urea and creatinine.
- Fasting lipid profile and fasting glucose.
- FBC and LFT.

### General practice nurse run clinic, or as part of routine appointments and checks
Aim (refer to local protocols):
- To monitor and treat people with hypertension.
- To ↓ the risk of related cardiovascular morbidity and mortality.
- To identify risk factors and offer personalized advice and management.

*Achieved by*
- Maintaining register for call and recall of patients with hypertension (📖 Quality and outcomes framework, p. 66).
- Lifestyle advice on diet and exercise with supporting literature and links to local initiatives, e.g. support groups, walking groups.
- Review alcohol consumption.
- Discourage excessive consumption of coffee and other caffeine-rich products encourage low or substitute sodium salt intake.
- Smoking cessation advice.
- Do not offer calcium, magnesium, or potassium supplements as a method of reducing BP.

- Relaxation therapies can ↓ BP (see 📖 Cardiac rehabilitation in the community, p. 593).
- Control BP to less than 140/90mmHg. Once BP controlled regular monitoring at 3–6-monthly and yearly recalculation of CVD risk, BP check, and blood tests and medication review.

*Anti-hypertensive treatment*
See also NICE 2011 guidelines[2]. Medication ↓ risk of CVD and death.
- Same treatment for people with isolated systolic hypertension (systolic BP 160 mmHg or higher) as people with both raised systolic and diastolic BP.
- Patients at ↑ cardiovascular risk or existing CVD or target organ damage with persistent BP of >140/90mmHg.
- If possible, offer drugs taken only od.
- >80yrs same antihypertensive drug treatment as people aged 55–80yrs, take account of comorbidities.
- An ACE inhibitor should not be combined with an angiotensin II receptor blocker (ARB).

*Initiating anti-hypertensive treatment (see Fig. 11.3)*
*Step 1 treatment*
- ACE inhibitor and calcium channel blocker (CCB) (*note*: side effects can cause flushing, dizziness and constipation) for:
  - Patients <80yrs with stage one hypertension, and one or more symptoms of target organ damage, established CVD, renal damage, diabetes, cardiovascular risk equivalent to 20%.
  - Patients of any age with stage 2 hypertension.
- <55yrs an ACE inhibitor or a low cost ARB. If ACE inhibitor is not tolerated offer low cost ARB.
- >55yrs and black people (African or Caribbean family origin) of any age—CCB. If CCB not suitable, e.g. because of oedema, intolerance, evidence of heart failure, offer thiazide-like diuretic.
- If a diuretic is being started or changed offer a thiazide-type diuretic in preference to a conventional thiazide diuretic. (Does not apply if patient with stable BP who is on conventional thiazide diuretic.)
- Beta-blockers should only be considered for younger people if ACE inhibitors and ARBs are contraindicated or not tolerated

*Step 2 treatment* (That is, BP not controlled by step one treatment):
- Offer CCB in combination with either ACE inhibitor or ARB.
- If CCB unsuitable, e.g. because of oedema, intolerance, evidence of heart failure, offer thiazide-type diuretic.
- For black people (African or Caribbean family origin) offer ARB in preference to ACE inhibitor in combination with a CCB.
- If beta-blocker (side effects include poor sleep, tiredness, and impotence) used in stage one, add CCB, rather than thiazide-type diuretic to ↓ risk of diabetes.
- *Before* considering step 3 treatment, review medication and patient concordance.

*Step three treatment*
- ACE inhibitor or ARB with a CCB and a thiazide-like diuretic.
- BP that remains 140/90mmHg or higher after step 3 treatment consider as resistant hypertension, refer to NICE guidelines for step 4 treatment and refer for specialist advice.

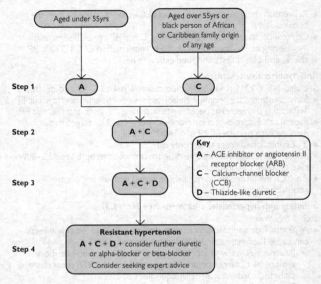

**Fig. 11.3** Summary of hypertension guidelines.

Reproduced from NICE (2011). *Clinical management of primary hypertension in adults* (CG 127). With permission from NICE.

## Related topics

📖 Coronary heart disease, p. 584; 📖 Expert patient, p. 303; 📖 Exercise, p. 313; 📖 Smoking cessation, p. 315.

## References

[1] Joint British Risk Prediction Chart. Available at: 🖱 www.eguidelines.co.uk/eguidelinesmain/guidelines/summaries/cardiovascular/jb_chd.php

[2] NICE (2011). *Clinical management of primary hypertension in adults* (CG 127). Available at: 🖱 http://www.nice.org.uk/nicemedia/live/13561/56008/56008.pdf

## Further information

Blood Pressure UK. Available at: 🖱 www.bloodpressureuk.org

British Heart Foundation. Available at: 🖱 www.bhf.org.uk

British Hypertension Society. Available at: 🖱 www.bhsoc.org

# Hyperlipidaemia (high/raised cholesterol)

## Cholesterol

A fatty substance produced mainly by the liver. It has a vital role in cell membrane function. ↓ cholesterol is beneficial in 1° and 2° prevention of CVD. A target cholesterol level of less than 5 is recommended. In the UK, two out of three adults have a total cholesterol level of 5 or above.

- *Low-density lipoprotein cholesterol (LDL):* high levels associated with ↑ risk of CVD.
- *High-density lipoprotein cholesterol (HDL):* high levels protect against MI and low levels associated with ↑ risk of CVD.
- *Triglycerides (TGs):* independent risk factor for CVD. If >10mmol/L refer to specialist.
- *Ratio of total cholesterol HDL:* used to predict risk, high risk if 6 or more.

## Assessment

- Blood cholesterol concentration not constant, 1:4 ↑ cholesterols normal on repeat testing. Check two or more samples at different times.
- *For screening and routine follow-up:* take non-fasting samples testing total blood cholesterol and total cholesterol: HDL ratio.
- *Suspected familial hypercholesterolemia* (take fasting samples testing total cholesterol, LDL cholesterol, HDL cholesterol and TGs): total cholesterol >6.5mmol may need specialist referral.
- Screen 40–75yrs and or family history of CVD.
- *Other risk factors:* e.g. CHD, DM, renal disease, hypertension.
- *Calculate 10-year CVD risk:* see Joint British Society cardiac risk assessment charts. (Available at: ℘ www.bhsoc.org).
- *Smoking status:* 🕮 Smoking cessation, p. 315.
- *Review diet and calculate BMI:* 🕮 Adult body mass index chart, p. 306.

## Aims

- ↓ LDL and raising HDL.
- ↓ LDL cholesterol to <3.0mmol/L or by 30%, whichever is lower.

## Non drug-based interventions and health promotion advice

- ↓ overall dietary fat intake (foods enriched with plant sterol/stanol esters inhibit the cholesterol absorption from the GI tract and can ↓ serum cholesterol in those on an average diet by 10%).
- ↓ saturated fat intake, use low fat mono/polyunsaturated spreads and oils, 2–3 portions of fish (one oily), lean meat, and low salt food:
  - Total fat intake 30% or less of total energy intake.
  - Saturated fats 10% or less of total energy intake.
  - Dietary cholesterol < 300mg/day.
  - Replace saturated with monounsaturated and polyunsaturated fats.
- *Eat at least* (🕮 Nutrition and healthy eating, p. 304):
  - 5 portions of fruit and vegetables per day.
  - 2 portions of fish per week, including a portion of oily fish.

- *Lifestyle advice* (as with 📖 Cardiac rehabilitation in the community, p. 593), stop smoking, alcohol (📖 Alcohol, p. 319) within normal limits, exercise (📖 Exercise, p. 313) promotion.
- Reinforce all advice with written material and patient information leaflets (PILs).

### Medication-based intervention

*Statins* Reduce overall death rate by 12%, first stroke by 17%, major coronary events by 23%. Statins most effective if taken in the evening (*contraindications*: pregnancy, breastfeeding, and active liver disease).

*Primary prevention of CVD* Appropriate for adults who have a 20% or greater 10-yr risk of developing CVD. Estimate risk using an appropriate risk calculator (see NICE[1]), or clinical assessment when appropriate risk calculator not available or appropriate (e.g. older people, people with DM, people in high-risk ethnic groups). For those with familial hypercholesterolaemia: *Treatment* Simvastatin 40mg. If potential drug interactions, or simvastatin 40mg is contraindicated, a lower dose or alternative preparation, such as pravastatin appropriate:

*Secondary prevention* Recommended for adults with clinical evidence of CVD and people with diabetes mellitus.
- *Simvastatin 40 mg:* if there are potential drug interactions, or contraindications, a lower dose or pravastatin.
- *Aim:* reduce total cholesterol below 4mmol/L or LDL cholesterol below 2mmol/L. Consider ↑ to simvastatin 80mg or drug of similar efficacy if total cholesterol <4mmol/L or LDL cholesterol <2mmol/L not attained (NICE guidelines for further prescribing advice[2]).
- People with acute coronary syndrome should be treated with a higher intensity statin. Take into account the patient's preference, comorbidities, multiple drug therapy, and the benefits and risks of treatment.
- To assess progress in groups with CVD an 'audit' level of total cholesterol of 5mmol/L should be used. Although evidence suggests that less than half will achieve total cholesterol less than 4mmol/L or LDL cholesterol less than 2mmol/L.

### Follow-up and review of patients
- Ask how patient is managing on medication.
- Measure liver function within 3 months and at 12 months, but not again unless clinically indicated.

❶ Advise people to seek medical advice if they develop muscle pain, tenderness or weakness, refer for GP review.

### Related topics
📖 Coronary heart disease, p. 584; 📖 Hypertension, p. 589; 📖 Cardiac rehabilitation in the community, p. 595.

### References

[1]NHS Choices High Cholesterol. Available at: ℘ www.nhs.uk/conditions/Cholesterol/Pages/Introduction.aspx

[2]NICE (2010). *Lipid modification Cardiovascular risk assessment and the modification of blood lipids for the primary and secondary prevention of cardiovascular disease* (CG67). Available at: ℘ http://publications.nice.org.uk/lipid-modification-cg67/guidance

# Cardiac rehabilitation in the community

Cardiac rehabilitation appropriate for anyone who has had MI, coronary angioplasty, or heart surgery. Can also help some people who have angina (📖 Angina, p. 586) or heart failure. In the UK, ~838,000 ♂ and 394,000 ♀ have had MI at some point. A multidisciplinary approach that can benefit patients regardless of age and condition that aims to:
• Promote recovery from MI.
• Reduce CHD related symptoms (e.g. 📖 Angina, p. 586) or need for cardiac surgery.
• Reduce risk of death in people with heart disease and provide long-term preventative care, can ↓ morbidity by 25%.

Many of the problems people with heart disease suffer are not physical, but are due to anxiety and misunderstanding about their condition, ∴ it is important that patients receive adequate, consistent, and accurate advice.

After an acute MI, future management plans and advice on 2° prevention should be part of every discharge summary. Patients should have an agreed care plan. Cardiac rehabilitation programmes run out of hospitals provide a mix of exercise promotion sessions, patient education, and psychosocial interventions that lasts between 6 and 12wks. Uptake is variable and ♀ less likely to receive cardiac rehabilitation than ♂. Up to 38% of patients in England, Wales, and Northern Ireland who need cardiac rehabilitation do not have access.

❶ A proactive approach to patient participation and monitoring is needed. Treatment and care should take into account patients' individual needs and preferences. After an MI, decisions about a patient's care and treatment should always be in partnership with their health care professional. If the individual agrees, families and carers should have the opportunity to be involved. In some areas primary care nurses run programmes.

## Assessment
• Individual risk factors (see 📖 Coronary heart disease, p. 584).
• Physical needs, e.g. self-caring.
• Exercise tolerance testing.
• *Psychological needs:* patients are often anxious, weepy, and depressed following an MI. Should be reassured that this is a normal response.
• *Social needs:* e.g. family support systems.

## Care and management in liaison with GP and other health professionals
• *Exercise:* patients should be advised to undertake regular physical activity sufficient to increase exercise capacity. Advise to be physically active for 20–30min/day to point of slight breathlessness. Patients not achieving this should be advised to increase activity in gradual, stepwise way, aiming to increase exercise capacity. They should start at level

that is comfortable, and increase duration and intensity of activity as they gain fitness. (📖 Exercise, p. 313).

- *Smoking cessation* (📖 Smoking cessation, p. 315): all patients who smoke should be advised to quit and be offered assistance from a smoking cessation service.
- *Diet*: Mediterranean-style diet (↑ bread, fruit, vegetables and fish; ↓ meat; replace butter and cheese with vegetable and plant oil products).
- *Cardiac rehabilitation*: should be equally accessible and relevant to all. Particular attention should be paid to groups with known low uptake—BME groups, older people, people from lower socio-economic groups, ♀, and people from rural areas and people with multi-morbidities (including mental health problems).
- *All patients who have had an acute MI should be offered treatment with a combination of the following drugs:* ACE inhibitor, aspirin, beta-blocker, statin. See NICE guidelines[1] for prescribing guidance.
- Patient education and support on medication management and concordance, supported with PILs and review progress.
- Returning to work after an uncomplicated MI: 4–6wks for sedentary workers; light manual workers 6–8wks; heavy manual workers 3mths.
- No driving for 1mth after MI and inform car insurer; only inform DVLA if HGV and PSV licence holder.
- *Flying*: most airlines will not carry passengers <2wks post-MI and then only if able to climb flight of stairs without difficulty
- *Sexual activity*: resume after 6wks, may experience loss of libido (specific guidance in BHF).
- *Psychological aspects*: many patients experience depression and anxiety—may benefit from advice on relaxation and talking therapies.
- *Educational support*: including information on basic working of heart accompanied by PILs and written information.
- Needs of family and carers.
- Patient support and/or self-help groups/use of self-help manuals.

## Related topics

📖 Coronary heart disease, p. 584; 📖 Angina, p. 586; 📖 Hypertension, p. 589; 📖 Talking therapies, p. 429.

## Reference

[1]NICE (2007) *Secondary prevention in primary and secondary care for patients following a myocardial infarction* (CG48). Available at: ℘ http://guidance.nice.org.uk/CG48

## Further information

British Heart Foundation Heart Health. Available at: ℘ www.bhf.org.uk/heart-health/recovery/sex-and-heart-conditions.aspx

British Heart Foundation. ☏ Helpline 0300 330 3311 for information on local cardiac rehabilitation programmes.

Cardiac rehabilitation useful resource for health professionals. Available at: ℘ www.cardiacrehabilitation.org.uk

# Chronic heart failure, tachycardia, and related problems

## Chronic heart failure

The cardiac output is insufficient to meet demands of the body. Most of the evidence on treatment is for heart failure due to left ventricular systolic dysfunction (LVSD). The most common cause of heart failure in the UK is coronary artery disease, and many patients have had MI. For both patients and their carers heart failure can be a financial burden and have adverse effects on their quality of life.

~900,000 people in the UK have heart failure and almost as many have damaged hearts, but no symptoms. Incidence and prevalence of heart failure increases with age, average age at first diagnosis 76yrs.

All patients with suspected heart failure should be included in practice register and have specialist assessment (📖 Quality and outcomes framework, p. 66).

## Heart failure

Poor prognosis—30–40% of patients diagnosed with heart failure die within a year. Thereafter, the mortality rate is <10%/yr heart failure accounts for a total of 1 million in-patient bed days, and 5% of all emergency medical admissions to hospital.

### Causes

- *High output:* heart working at normal or ↑ rate, but needs of body exceed what heart can supply, e.g. hyperthyroidism, anaemia, Paget's disease, AV malformation.
- *Low output:*↓ heart function; can be due to mitral regurgitation, fluid overload. Pump failure 2° to cardiac muscle disease ischaemic heart disease (IHD) (46%), cardiomyopathy, hypertension, valve disease, atrial fibrillation and other tachycardias.

### Risk factors

- Smoking (📖 Smoking cessation, p. 315)
- Alcohol (📖 Alcohol, p. 319) acts as cardiac toxin.
- Diabetes (📖 Diabetes, p. 611).
- Obesity (📖 Weight management : overweight, obesity, p. 307).
- High cholesterol (📖 Hyperlipidaemia (high/raised cholesterol), p. 593).
- Pregnancy (📖 Pregnancy, p. 378).

### Types of heart failure

- *LVSD:* failure of left ventricle results in respiratory symptoms.
- *Heart failure with preserved ejection fraction (HFPEF):* usually due to the left ventricle become stiff, causing difficulty in filling with blood.
- Heart failure due to valve disease.

*Symptoms*

Patients complain of:
- Breathlessness at rest and/or on exertion.
- Fatigue.
- Paroxysmal nocturnal dyspnoea and orthopnoea.
- Ankle oedema.
- Abdominal discomfort from liver distention and nausea.

*Care and management*
- Reassure patient and family that treatment for heart failure can help make heart stronger, improve symptoms, reduce risk of flare-up, to live longer and fuller lives.
- Discuss symptoms and the underlying reasons and support with written information. Encourage self-management and consider possible referral to expert patient programme.
- Patient may benefit from case management approach and involvement of specialist nurse/community matron involvement.
- Lifestyle advice on smoking, alcohol, exercise, and healthy eating, including ↓ salt intake.
- Immunization against influenza and pneumonia.
- Benefits and mobility aids, and possible social care support.
- Patients with chronic heart failure often experience anxiety and depression. Ensure they and their family has access to emotional support.
- Ensure other related conditions are well managed: hypertension (📖 Hypertension, p. 589), diabetes (📖 Type 2 diabetes, p. 621), coronary heart disease (📖 Coronary heart disease, p. 584), and high cholesterol Hyperlipidaemia (high/raised cholesterol), p. 593.
- Medication for symptom control and to improve prognosis: ACE inhibitor unless contraindicated with a diuretic. Once stabilized, a beta-blocker prescribed although if symptoms persist patient may be prescribed digoxin or spironalactone (see NICE guidance for chronic heart failure[1]).
- As part of the MDT review patients at least every 6mths or more often as required. Include physical assessment, medication review, and functional ability.
- Palliative care (📖 Palliative care, p. 509) for people with end-stage heart failure.

## Tachycardia/palpitations

Sensation of rapid irregular or forceful heart beats, heart rate >100/min. May or may not be a significant symptom. ❶ Potentially serious if:
- Pre-existing cardiovascular disease.
- FH of syncope.
- Arrhythmias, sudden death, and/or falls.

Other causes include underlying disease, caffeine, alcohol, smoking, and fatigue. Patient may complain of:

- Chest pain, breathlessness, funny turns, sweating, or hyperventilation.
- May last seconds, minutes, or longer.
- May affect driving or work.

Requires medical assessment and investigation, including blood tests, ECG and related cardiac tests, e.g. 24-hr ECG exercise tolerance test. May require specialist assessment and treatment according to cause. Recommend stopping smoking, ↓ alcohol, and caffeine.

## Atrial fibrillation (AF)

Common disturbance of cardiac rhythm may be episodic or chronic. The most common sustained cardiac arrhythmia. ❶ If left untreated is a significant risk factor for stroke and other morbidities. 1:6 cases no apparent cause 'lone AF', other causes include hypertension, complication of CHD, hyperthyroidism, PE, cardiomyopathy. Routine investigations for AF include ECG (📖 Recording a 12-lead electrocardiogram, p. 539).

Patients can be asymptomatic, but may complain of chest pain, palpitations, dyspnoea, and fatigue. Requires medical assessment as previously described and may be admitted or referred to specialist according to severity or complications. Treatment may include digoxin, beta-blockers, anticoagulation therapy. Review lifestyle and advice on healthy eating and exercise.

## Reference

[1]NICE (2010). *Chronic heart failure: management of chronic heart failure in adults in primary and secondary care* (CG108). Available at: ℘ www.nice.org.uk/CG108

## Further information

British Heart Foundation. Available at: ℘ www.bhf.org.uk/heart-health/conditions/heart-failure. aspx

NICE (2006). *Atrial fibrillation: The management of atrial fibrillation* (CG36). Available at: ℘ www. nice.org.uk/CG36

NHS Choices. Heart Failure. Available at: ℘ www.nhs.uk/conditions/Heart-failure/Pages/Introduction. aspx

NHS Choices. Atrial Fibrillation. Available at: ℘ www.nhs.uk/Conditions/Atrial-fibrillation/Pages/ Introduction.aspx

# Patients on anticoagulant therapy

Anticoagulants ↓ the formation of new blood clots and the extension of existing clots. Most commonly used with patients with AF, following heart surgery, or at risk of PE and/or DVT. Warfarin antagonizes the effects of vitamin K; and takes 48–72hrs to work. Patients on oral anticoagulants often managed by nurses working to an agreed protocol.

## Management and patient information

See Tables 11.8 and 11.9 for dose regimens and recall periods during maintenance therapy.

- Check FBC (before and during therapy).
- Check international normalized ratio of prothrombin time (INR; daily and/or alternate days until therapeutic range achieved, then 4–8-weekly) on a morning sample.
- Check interactions with other prescription drugs. Many drugs prescription, over-the-counter, or herbal can interact with warfarin.
- Check urine and stools (if practical) for occult blood regularly.
- Check BP measurement.

## Lifestyle advice

- Take warfarin at same time each day.
- Should always carry their yellow anticoagulant treatment booklet or anticoagulant alert card (issued in hospital) with them. Medi-alert band with anticoagulant name advisable.
- Inform doctor, dentist, or pharmacist about anticoagulant treatment.
- Avoid aspirin or NSAIDs.
- Eat normal diet and avoid sudden changes before blood being taken. Make patient aware of:
  - Avoiding cranberry, grapefruit juice as has ↑ anticoagulant effect.
  - Foods high in vitamin K affect anticoagulant effect, e.g. leafy vegetables, broccoli, and liver and ↓ INR readings.
- Limit alcohol intake as this ↑ INR readings. Maximum of one or two drinks a day, and never binge drink.
- Avoid activities that could cause abrasion, bruising, or cuts (e.g. contact sports, gardening, sewing), or at least use protection.
- Take extra care when brushing teeth or shaving, and consider using a soft toothbrush and an electric razor.
- Avoid insect bites; consider use of an insect repellent, as appropriate.
- Avoid vigorous nose blowing.
- Report bleeding gums, bruises, nosebleeds, joint swelling, sudden severe back pain increased menstrual loss, abdominal pain, and if pregnant.
- Never stop medication without reference to doctor.
- Call 999 if:
  - Prolonged bleeding.
  - Vomiting with blood.
- Advise about signs and symptoms of PE.

## Self-testing and self-management

The availability of training and support for self-testing or self-management varies across the UK.

- *Self-testing:* where person tests their own INR, but contacts a health care professional for dose adjustment.
- *Self-management:* is where person tests their own INR and also adjusts dose of warfarin themselves (based on individualized algorithm).

### Suitability for self-testing

People who require long-term anticoagulation can be considered for warfarin self-testing or self-management. May suit people that are frequently away from home, in employment or in education, or find it difficult to travel to clinics. Previous stability of INR is not essential, people with an unstable INR may benefit from the possibility of increased frequency of testing NB Self-testing devices cost from £400 to £800 and are not reimbursable on the NHS. Important that:

- Person is both physically and cognitively able to perform self-monitoring test or designated carer is able to do so.
- Supportive educational programme is in place to train person and/or carers.
- Person's ability to self-test or self-manage can be regularly reviewed.
- There is access to appropriately-trained health care professionals for ongoing advice and support (including if they plan to travel abroad).

## Related topics

📖 Coronary heart disease, p. 584; 📖 Cardiac rehabilitation in the community, p. 595.

## Further information

British Heart Foundation. Available at: ℘ www.bhf.org
NICE CKS (2009) Anticoagulation-oral. Available at: ℘ http://cks.nice.org.uk/anticoagulation-oral#!topicsummary

**Table 11.8** Dose regimen for starting warfarin in the community

| INR on day 5 | Dose on days 5–7 | INR on day 8 | Dose from day 8 | Instructions |
|---|---|---|---|---|
| ≤1.7 | 5mg | ≤1.7 | 6mg | Give warfarin 5mg od for 4 days then check INR. |
| | | 1.8–2.4 | 5mg | |
| | | 2.5–3 | 4mg | Adjust dose as in table. Recheck INR on day 8 and adjust dose as in table. |
| | | >3 | 3mg for 4 days | |
| 1.8–2.2 | 4mg | ≤1.7 | 5mg | |
| | | 1.8–2.4 | 4mg | |
| | | 2.5–3 | 3.5mg | Thereafter, check INR weekly (unless 4-day interval stated) and adjust dose accordingly until dose is stable in the target range. |
| | | 3.1–3.5 | 3mg for 4 days | |
| | | >3.5 | 2.5mg for 4 days | |
| 2.3–2.7 | 3mg | ≤1.7 | 4mg | |
| | | 1.8–2.4 | 3.5mg | |
| | | 2.5–3 | 3mg | ❶ High INR |
| | | 3.1–3.5 | 2.5mg for 4 days | INR ≥8 (lower if other risk factors for bleeding)—admit to hospital even if not bleeding. |
| | | >3.5 | 2mg for 4 days | |
| 2.8–3.2 | 2mg | ≤1.7 | 3mg | |
| | | 1.8–2.4 | 2.5mg | |
| | | 2.5–3 | 2mg | |
| | | 3.1–3.5 | 1.5mg for 4 days | INR >3.7 and <8—omit warfarin 1–2 days and recheck INR. Restart when INR <5 and retitrate dose. |
| | | >3.5 | 1mg for 4 days | |
| 3.3–3.7 | 1mg | ≤1.7 | 2mg | |
| | | 1.8–2.4 | 1.5mg | |
| | | 2.5–3 | 1mg | |
| | | 3.1–3.5 | 0.5mg for 4 days | |
| | | >3.5 | omit for 4 days | |
| ~3.7 | 0mg | <2 | 1.5mg for 4 days | |
| | | 2–2.9 | 1mg for 4 days | |
| | | 3–3.5 | 0.5mg for 4d | |

Reproduced from Oates A, Jackson PR, Austin CA, et al. (1998) A new regime for starting warfarin therapy in outpatients, *Br J Clin Pharmacol* **46**: 157–61. With permission of Wiley-Blackwell.

**Table 11.9** Warfarin therapy. Recall periods during maintenance therapy

| INR | Recall interval and action |
| --- | --- |
| 1 high INR<br>❶ If INR>8—admit | Recall 7–14 days. Stop treatment for 1–3 days (max. 1wk in prosthetic valve patients) and restart at a lower dose |
| 1 low INR | ↑ dose and recall in 7–14 days |
| 1 therapeutic INR | Recall 4wks. |
| 2 therapeutic INRs | Recall 6wks (max. interval if prosthetic heart valve) |
| 3 therapeutic INRs | Recall 8wks* |
| 4 therapeutic INRs | Recall 10wks* |
| 5 therapeutic INRs | Recall 12wks* |

❶ Warfarin is a dangerous drug. In every case weigh up the pros and cons of prescribing.

* Except prosthetic heart valves where maximum recall interval is 6wks.

Reproduced from Simon C, Everitt H, van Dorp F. (2010). *Oxford Handbook of General Practice*, 3rd edn. With permission of Oxford University Press.

# Anaemia

A common problem when the blood fails to produce sufficient red blood cells and haemoglobin (♂ Hb <13g/dL, ♀ Hb 11 <12g/dL or <11g/dL if pregnant). Mainly affects ♀ of child-bearing age, teenagers, and young children. Also 1/6 ♀ >85. Younger people often asymptomatic and always consider as a possibility in older people. Anaemia occurs when:

- Decreased red blood cell production.
- *Increased loss or rate of destruction:* bleeding or haemolysis.
- *Decreased tissue requirement for oxygen:* hypothyroidism.

The presence of anaemia may indicate a more serious underlying problem.

## Causes

- Iron deficiency anaemia (most common form of anaemia).
- *Vitamin deficiency:* e.g. B12 or folic acid.
- Blood loss through haemmorhage, menstrual loss, or internal bleeding.
- *Excessive use:* e.g. pregnancy, lactation, cancer.
- Defective bone marrow (aplastic anaemia).
- *Infection:* e.g. malaria.

Patients may complain of tiredness, palpitations, SOB, dizziness, recurrent infections. They may appear pale (*note:* non-specific sign may be racial, familial, or cosmetic), complain of night cramps. Severe anaemia can cause angina, headaches. Long-term anaemia that arises from iron or B12 deficiency can cause burning sensation in the tongue, oral dryness, and mouth ulcers. Diagnosis of which kind of anaemia is achieved through a blood test (MCV see 📖 Biochemical and haematological values, p. 780).

## Iron deficiency anaemia

Most common form of anaemia. Lack of iron prevents bone marrow producing sufficient Hb for red blood cells. May be resolved by diet: good sources of iron include fruit, wholemeal bread, beans, and lean meat. However, other problems may be present, e.g. malabsorption-related problems (e.g. coeliac disease) may mean iron is not absorbed.

- *Persistent bleeding:* arising from problems, such as gastritis, peptic ulcer, IBD, haemorrhoids, and prolonged use of medication, e.g. NSAIDs.
- GI malignancy.
- *Non-GI blood loss:* menstruation (20–30%), blood donation (5%), haematuria, epistaxis.

### Care and management

Oral iron supplements, e.g. ferrous sulphate 200mg bd. *Note:* medication can cause constipation and black stools. Hb should improve incrementally by 1g/dL/wk, review 2–3wks after starting treatment, takes ~3mths to replenish iron stores. Repeat blood test required. If there is failure to improve, refer to GP for medical review and possible referral. If iron is not being absorbed, parenteral route or transfusion may be considered or further investigations required.

## Vitamin B12 deficiency

B12 found in liver, kidney, fish, meats, and dairy products. Absorption occurs by active and passive mechanisms, latter is dependent on presence of intrinsic factor, a protein produced by gastric cells. May be first noticed with mouth ulcers or neuropathy. Vitamin B12 deficiency produces anaemia identical to folate deficiency and potential damage to peripheral and central nervous system.

*Care and management* When the cause is inadequate intake, advise on healthy diet (vegans may be particularly at risk). If cause is malabsorption, e.g. following gastric surgery or pernicious anaemia, it is treated with vitamin B12 injections IM. Initially, 1mg on alternate days for 1–2wks until blood count is normal, and then, maintenance dose of 1mg/2–3mths.

## Pernicious anaemia

Autoimmune disease caused by lack of intrinsic factor due to gastric atrophy, usually develops in people >50yrs. Presence of intrinsic factor antibodies confirm diagnosis. Patient may or may not present with symptoms related to anaemia. Care and management as for vitamin B12 deficiency above. *Note:* people with pernicious anaemia have ↑ risk of stomach cancer and should be advised to seek medical advice if they experience dyspepsia and/or stomach pain.

## Folate deficiency

Folates are vitamins essential to the development of the central nervous system. Insufficient folate at conception and early pregnancy (Ⅲ Pregnancy, p. 378) leads to neural tube defects (Ⅲ Neural tube defects, p. 289) in newborns. In adults deficiency causes megaloblastic anaemia, and there is some evidence there are links with arterial disease and dementia. Folate is found in liver, yeast, nuts, spinach and other green vegetables. Causes often arises from inadequate diet, including alcohol misuse, also anticonvulsants.

*Care and management* Folate supplements with folic acid 5mg od for 4mths. Treat cause. If malabsorption problems or as a prophylactic in renal disease may need a higher dose; refer to GP.

To prevent neural tube defects ♀ who are planning a pregnancy or are pregnant should take folate supplements up to 12wks gestation 400 micrograms od (consult with GP if on anticonvulsants or previous medical history). Also see Ⅲ Pre-conceptual care and advice, p. 376.

## Related topics

Ⅲ Nutrition and healthy eating, p. 304; Ⅲ Alcohol, p. 319.

## Further information

NHS Choices Causes of iron deficiency anaemia. Available at: ℘ www.nhs.uk/Conditions/Anaemia-iron-deficiency-/Pages/Causes.aspx

Goddard AF, James MW, McIntyre AS, et al.; British Society of Gastroenterology. Guidelines for the management of iron deficiency anaemia. *Gut* **60**: 1309–16. doi:10.1136/gut.2010.228874. Available at: ℘ www.bsg.org.uk/clinical-guidelines/small-bowel-nutrition/guidelines-for-the-management-of-iron-deficiency-anaemia.html

# Leukaemias and lymphomas

Little is known about causes of leukaemia, but exposure to radiation, people with certain genetic disorders, including Down's syndrome, have a higher risk of developing leukaemia. Infection may be involved, *but* no specific infections have been found to cause leukaemia. Treatments at specialist centres and MDT teams and will involving systemic chemotherapy, and adjuncts such as radiotherapy, bone marrow transplant, etc., according to type, stage and clinical decision-making. See 📖 Chemotherapy in the home, p. 507 for advice to patients. Prognosis for acute leukaemias is 80% survival at 5yrs for children and for adults 20–60% depending on age and type of leukaemia. Long-term consequences/side effects of treatment can include:
- Heart and lung problems (cardiomyopathy and lung fibrosis).
- Growth delay in children, hypothyroidism, and integrity.
- Impaired kidney function.
- Psychological problems for patients and family members.
- Secondary malignancies may appear after several years.

## Acute lymphoblastic leukaemia (ALL)

Cancer that affects the lymphocyte producing cells in the bone marrow. In ALL there is an accumulation of immature lymphocyte precursor cells (blast cells) in the bone marrow. ALL is responsible for 85% of childhood leukaemia. In adults it is most common between 15–25 and >75yrs.

## Acute myeloid leukaemia (AML)

Most common leukaemia of adulthood incidence ↑ with age, median age at diagnosis 60yrs. Patients may complain of:
- *Fatigue and breathlessness because of anaemia:* 📖 Anaemia, p. 604.
- *Bruising and bleeding from mucous membranes:* gums and gut because of low platelet counts (signs of spontaneous bleeding children need same day referral to paediatric haematology services).
- Persistent infections and fever caused by ↓ white cell counts, high metabolic rate, and ↑ numbers of abnormal cells.

## Chronic lymphocytic leukaemia (CLL)

Occurs in older people. After diagnosis patients that are well managed in the community with low levels of lymphocytosis, are often managed in primary care with regular FBC and clinical review q6m. Refer if experiencing:
- Weight loss, night sweats, fever.
- Lymphadenopathy and/or hepatosplenomegaly.
- Rising lymphocyte count.
- Anaemia or thrombocytopenia.

Note: for many patients with CLL, the diagnosis is benign and prognosis can be >10yrs.

## Lymphoma: cancers of the lymphatic system

Lymphoma is the fifth most common cancer in the UK. Classified according to type of cell involvement, often start in lymph nodes or spleen but can spread to any organ in the body.

*Hodgkin's lymphoma* Most common in young people 20–30yrs. Risk factors include immunodeficiency, also exposure to Epstein–Barr virus that causes glandular fever may slightly increase risk of developing Hodgkin's. The majority achieve a cure.

*Non-Hodgkin's lymphoma (NHL)* Associated with ageing, more common in people aged >55yrs. NHLs can be divided into either B-cell lymphomas (the majority) or T-cell lymphomas. Histology and age are key factors in prognosis. Patients may initially present with:
- Peripheral lymphadenopathy in neck axilla, groin.
- Weight loss.
- Night sweats.
- Loss of appetite and fatigue.
- Pain in the lymph nodes after drinking alcohol (rare).
- Pruritus.
- Abdominal swelling and/or pain.

All patients suspected of having lymphoma need urgent referral to haematology. Once diagnosed, staging of the disease describes size and degree of spread:
- *Stage 1:* 1 group of lymph nodes affected.
- *Stage 2:* 2 or more lymph node groups affected on the same side of diaphragm.
- *Stage 3:* lymph nodes above and below diaphragm affected.
- *Stage 4:* lymphoma has spread to organs, e.g. liver, bones, or lungs.

The treatment is according to individual situation. Some people with low-grade non-Hodgkin lymphoma will not require immediate treatment straightaway.

## Related topic

📖 Early signs of cancer, p. 333.

## Further information

Leukaemia Research. Available at: 🖰 www.lrf.org.uk
Lymphoma Association: Helpline 0808 808 5555 (Mondays to Thursdays 09.00–18.00 hours, Fridays 09.00–17.00 hours. Available at: 🖰 www.lymphoma.org.uk
Macmillan Cancer Support. Available at: 🖰 www.macmillan.org.uk/Home.aspx
CLIC Sargent for Children with Cancer. Available at: 🖰 www.clicsargent.org.uk/

# Varicose veins, thrombophlebitis, and deep vein thrombosis

## Varicose veins

Veins (usually in the calf, leg, and/or groin) become visibly swollen, distorted, twisted, or lengthened. Occur because of incompetent valves that allow the blood to flow backwards from the deep to the superficial venous system, causing back pressure and further dilatation. 1:5 people will have varicose veins and ♀ > ♂.

*Risk factors*
- Age (unusual in <20yrs).
- Parity.
- Occupations that require a lot of standing.
- Obesity in ♀.
- Family history.
- 2° causes include pregnancy, DVT, pelvic tumour.

Patients may complain of:
- Cosmetic appearance of legs, but otherwise be asymptomatic.
- Aching legs, feeling heavy and uncomfortable, especially in warm weather.
- In severe cases, skin can become itchy and thin and may develop into varicose eczema and venous ulcers.
- Complications associated with varicose veins include; haemmorhage, oedema, skin pigmentation, white scars, and thrombophlebitis.

*Care and management*
- *Prevention:* advice on regular exercise, walking helps circulation, healthy diet, ↓ weight. Avoid standing for long periods and sitting cross legged. If possible raise legs higher than chest when sitting.
- Support stockings to ↓ swelling.
- Bleeding varicose veins controlled by raising foot about level of heart and applying compression, on recovery, advise on compression hosiery and consider referral to GP for possible surgical review.
- *Treatment in 2° care:* sclerotherapy involves closing off veins by chemical injection, surgery. Vein stripping for recurrent or more severe varicose veins.

## COC pill

♀ with varicose veins are *not* at ↑ risk of DVT, but are at ↑ risk of thrombophlebitis. History of thrombophlebitis a contraindication to the COC pill, stop if using (📖 Contraception general, p. 359).

## Thrombophlebitis

Superficial vein thrombosis or phlebitis involves inflammation and thrombus formation in the superficial veins (often saphenous vein and its linked veins) patients complain of severe pain, erythema, pigmentation, and hardening of the vein. Cause often linked to presence of varicose veins, occurs because of:

- Damage to the blood vessel because of trauma or infection.
- Stasis of blood flow.
- Hypercoagulability of blood.
- Infected thrombophlebitis can be a complication of IV cannulation, IV drug use, or skin infection. People with diabetes or those taking immunosuppressant drugs are more susceptible. Requires urgent hospital referral.

*Care and management for uncomplicated superficial thrombophlebitis*
- Treat pain with analgesia, e.g. NSAIDs or paracetamol.
- Compression stockings.
- Local heat may provide some relief, e.g. warm towel to affected limb.
- Encourage use of affected limb and continue activities, leg elevation will aid venous flow and ↓ swelling. Bed rest is not advisable → ↑ risk of DVT.

Continue treatment till pain and erythema have settled (2–6wks). Anticoagulants not used. If suspect this DVT requires same day/urgent assessment in ED/ Medical Assessment Unit (MAU).

## Deep vein thrombosis

Formation of a thrombus in a deep vein that partially or completely obstructs blood flow. Usually occurs in in the deep veins of the calf (distal DVT) or in veins above the knee (proximal DVT), rarely occur elsewhere. Affects 1:2000 people, 1:500 >80yrs. Can be asymptomatic. Patients complain of:
- Unilateral leg pain.
- Swelling and/or tenderness with or without pitting oedema.
- Warmth and distended superficial veins.
- *With severe obstruction:* colour change to red or purple.

*Multiple risk factors*
- Age >40yrs.
- Smoking.
- Obesity.
- Immobility.
- Pregnancy.
- Surgery.
- Trauma.
- Recent long distance travel (e.g. long-haul flights).
- COC pill.
- HRT.
- Malignancy.
- Heart failure.
- Inflammatory bowel disease.

- Chronic illness.
- Clotting disorders.

Difficult to establish DVT from clinical observation: <50% patients suspected of having DVT have this confirmed by diagnostic imaging. All suspected cases are referred for same-day/urgent assessment in local ED/MAU. PE is a serious life-threatening complication of a DVT and without treatment 20% of proximal DVTs develop PE.

*Care and management of patients with confirmed DVT*
- Following initial anticoagulation on heparin, oral anticoagulation to ↓ risk of recurrence for 3–6mths post-DVT.
- Graduated elastic compression stockings should be worn >2yrs.
- Patients with history of DVT risk recurrence in high-risk situations e.g. surgery, pregnancy, immobility, and should receive prophylactic treatment with anticoagulants in such situations.

**Further information**

NHS Choices. Varicose veins. Available at: ℘ www.nhs.uk/Conditions/Varicose-veins/Pages/Whatarevaricoseveins.aspx

NICE (2012). *Venous thromboembolic diseases: the management of venous thromboembolic diseases and the role of thrombophilia testing* (CG144). Available at: ℘ http://guidance.nice.org.uk/CG144

# Diabetes: overview

In England there are >3 million people with diabetes. An ageing population and increasing obesity mean that the number of adults with diabetes is projected to increase. By 2020 an estimated 3.8 million adults, 8.5% of the adult population, will have diabetes and by 2030 this is estimated to rise to 4.6 million or 9.5% of the adult population. ~half of this increase is due to the changing age and ethnic group structure of the population and half due to ↑ levels of obesity.

It is characterized by raised blood sugars and abnormalities of carbohydrate and lipid metabolism due to lack of, or ineffective, endogenous insulin. Inadequate treatment can lead to devastating complications. Diabetes is classified according to aetiological differences *not* descriptions based upon age at onset or type of treatment.

The majority of patients with type 1 diabetes have autoimmune destruction of the pancreatic beta cells; they will develop diabetic ketoacidosis (DKA) if not given insulin. Some patients with type 2 diabetes can develop DKA under certain circumstances (severe infection or other illness) and many require treatment with insulin.

Type 1 diabetes and type 2 diabetes are the most common types, the latter estimated as accounting globally for approximately 90% of diabetes cases.

Patients have a very high risk of cardiovascular disease and all risk factors should be treated aggressively.

### Signs and symptoms
- Sudden onset.
- Weight loss.
- Thirst.
- Blurred vision.
- Polyuria.
- Urinary ketones may be present.

For all children and adults with suspected ketoacidosis or who are unwell are referred for same day specialist assessment. Diagnosis of diabetes can be made on the basis of fasting blood glucose only.
- *Normal:* fasting plasma glucose (FPG) <6.1mmol/L. (see 📖 Biochemical and haematological values, p. 780).
- *Impaired fasting glucose (IFG):* FPG between 6.1 and 6.9mmol/L.
- *Diabetes mellitus:* FPG ≥7.0mmol/L or OGTT ≥11.1mmol/L.

## Type 1 diabetes: autoimmune disorder
- 20% of people with DM. Person has *no* insulin supply and needs insulin injections to survive.
- Diagnosis < 35yrs *and* continual insulin treatment within 6/12mths of diagnosis *OR* diagnosis >35yrs (Note: in high-risk racial groups use cut-off of 30yrs) *and* continual insulin treatment from diagnosis.

*Management*

See 📖 Principles of diabetic care and control, p. 615. Initial management by specialist services then in primary care. Overall aim is to develop flexible regimen for self-management:

- Will need insulin injections for survival.
- Referral to dietician helpful for learning carbohydrate estimation.
- Advise on healthy living, specifically smoking cessation and exercise.
- All drivers must notify DVLA and their insurance company when starting insulin.
- Enter patient details on practice register (📖 Quality and outcomes framework, p. 66).
- Discuss general aspects of diabetes and history of illness.
- Establish patient's level of knowledge of illness and educational needs.
- Measure BP, height, and weight, and calculate BMI.
- Test urine for protein and ketones; arrange mid-stream specimen of urine (MSU) if proteinuria.
- Take blood for glucose, HbA1c, U&Es, LFTs, lipid profile.
- Examine feet for diabetic complications and consider podiatry referral.
- Consider initial psychological, educational, and lifestyle issues.
- Ensure retinal screening organized.
- Provide PIL and link to Diabetes UK.
- Arrange regular and early reviews.

*Note:* impaired glucose tolerance and impaired fasting glucose = risk factors CVD.

## Type 2 diabetes

Patient produces insufficient insulin becomes insulin resistant. ❶ Can be asymptomatic. There is generally a more gradual onset and many people remain undiagnosed. Diagnosis < 35yrs *and* not on continual insulin treatment within 6/12mths of diagnosis *or* diagnosis >35yrs (in high-risk racial groups use a cut-off of 30yrs) *and* not on continual insulin treatment from diagnosis.

Silent killing disease—life expectancy reduced by 20–40% in the 40–70-yr age range. Those at risk:

- Older age group >65yrs.
- FH strong.
- *Obesity:* 80% overweight; BMI—>25kg/m² (for Asians, >23kg/m²).
- Ethnicity important (South Asian, Afro Caribbean, and Hispanics).
- Past medical history (PMH) of gestational diabetes, or if they had big babies >4kg.

*Signs and symptoms*

- Weight loss.
- Thirst.
- Polyuria.
- Irritability and/or lethargy.
- Genital itching/thrush.
- Blurred vision.
- Recurrent UTIs.
- Tingling in the feet.
- No urinary ketones present.

## Care and management

(See also ▢ Principles of diabetic care and control, p. 615; ▢ Type 2 diabetes, p. 621.) As already described and aim to ↓ glycaemic load of meals, fat and calorie intake, and risk of CHD. Initially, diet control, but insulin often needed in later stages of disease. Always tailor glycaemic targets to individual. Check specific manufacturer's guidance when using therapies in people with diabetes and CKD. Always consider the risk of hypoglycaemia when using specific medicines in older people.

## Diabetes in pregnancy

See ▢ Common problems in pregnancy, p. 385.

## Secondary causes of diabetes

- *Drugs:* steroids and thiazides.
- *Pancreatic disease:* pancreatitis, surgery, cancer, cystic fibrosis, haemochromatosis.
- *Endocrine disease:* Cushing's disease, thyrotoxicosis, agromegaly.

## Acute complications

DKA, in type 1, due to lack of insulin the body, or hyperosmolar non-ketotic coma (HONK) in type 2 due in part to dehydration. If blood glucose levels are high (>12mmol/L) always assess patient for signs of dehydration, check urinary ketones, drowsiness, infection, etc.

> Mortality rates are significant, especially in young or older people. If ketoacidosis suspected, urgent referral for same day specialist assessment or admission to hospital.

*Hypoglycaemia/hypoglycaemia unawareness*

*Emergency management*

See ▢ Insulin therapies, p. 618. Education about preventing and treating hypoglycaemia is required. Consider safety aspects with regards to operating machinery or driving, etc. Changing medication to run blood glucose levels at upper end of normal range for 6–8wks can help regain warning signals in hypoglycaemic unawareness.

*Protracted vomiting/dehydration/drowsiness* Refer to A&E.

*Diabetic foot* If cellulitis, abscess, or wet gangrene, refer for same day assessment.

## Chronic complications

- *Microvascular or small vessel disease:* retinopathy can cause blindness, neuropathy can lead to amputation, and nephropathy to renal failure.
- *Macrovascular or large vessel disease:* causing MI, strokes, erectile dysfunction, or peripheral vascular disease again leading to amputation.

## Health promotion and advice for those at risk of DM

Prevention is possible in high-risk groups.

- *Daily physical activity:* ↓ insulin resistance—regularity is important.
- *Healthy eating:* 5–10% weight loss can improve metabolic profiles for those at risk (📖 Nutrition and healthy eating, p. 304).
- Goal is to maintain as near normal weight/BMI as possible, or at least no weight gain.

### Related topics

📖 Principles of diabetic care and control, p. 615; 📖 Insulin therapies, p. 618; 📖 Hypertension, p. 589; 📖 Coronary heart disease, p. 584.

### Further information

Diabetes UK. ☎ 0845 120 2960, Monday–Friday, 09.00–17.00 hours. Email: careline@diabetes.org. uk. Available at: 🖱 www.diabetes.org.uk

NICE (2009). *Management of Type 2 Diabetes* (CG 87). Available at: 🖱 http://publications.nice.org. uk/type-2-diabetes-cg87

SIGN (2010). *Management of diabetes*. Available at: 🖱 www.sign.ac.uk/guidelines/published/index. html#Diabetes

# Principles of diabetic care and control

Good diabetic care and control can be managed in the community.

## Overall aims of diabetic care

- Alleviation of symptoms.
- Minimization of complications.
- Enhanced quality of life.
- Reduction of early mortality.
- Open access for patients to advice and support and specialist services, e.g. podiatrist, dietician, clinical nurse specialist.
- Support and education with supporting materials of patient and their family/carer.

Care planning should be inclusive process that reflects ongoing partnership between health care professionals and person with diabetes. The process of agreeing a care plan helps to achieve active involvement in deciding, agreeing, and 'owning' how their diabetes will be managed Two national patient education programmes aim to give people the skills and confidence to manage their condition:

- *Dose adjustment for normal eating (DAFNE):* educational programme helps people with type 1 diabetes adjust their insulin injections to fit lifestyles. Available at: ℘ www.dafne.uk.com
- *The Diabetes Education & Self-Management for Ongoing & Newly Diagnosed (DESMOND):* a structured education programme for those with type 2 diabetes. Available at: ℘ www.desmond-project.org.uk

*Each diabetic patient requires at least a 6-mth review and this includes a thorough formal annual medical review (more frequent if complications, e.g. cardiovascular disease, neuropathy, eye disease, etc.).*

- Asking about patient problems, new symptoms since last visit.
- Weight and BMI measurements and diet.
- BP.
- Smoking status.
- Blood test (HbA1c aim for 6.5% or 48mmol/mol).
- Urinary albumin test.
- Serum creatinine test.
- Cholesterol levels.
- Eye check (retinopathy screening).
- Feet check.
- Review medication and side effects.
- Skin care and rotation of injection sites.
- Activity.
- Self-management skills.
- Other illnesses/problems.
- *Immunizations:* influenza /pneumococcal vaccination.
- In ♀ if contraception required or thinking of starting a family.

### Review of possible complications from diabetes

Complications often occur when a person's control, BP, and lipids are high. There are ~73 lower limb amputations a week in England because of complications of diabetes, 80% are potentially preventable.

- *CVD:* ↑ risk of MI and stroke symptoms (2–5×), monitor BP closely; any reduction in BP = reduced risk of cardiovascular complications.
- *Eyes:* blurred vision, and cataracts are more common and diabetes a risk factor for glaucoma. Retinopathy most common cause of blindness in people of working age. Sight threatening in 5–10% of diabetics. Referral to ophthalmologist/optometrist for retinal screening, visual acuity. Annual check to detect retinopathy before visual loss occurs. Emergency if unexplained drop in visual acuity or loss of vision, retinal detachment, haemmorhage.
- *Renal complications:* UTIs may exacerbate renal failure. 25% diabetics have renal damage. Ensure annual renal function check. Will need specialist referral if proteinuria or micro-albuminuria or raised serum creatinine (>150µmol/L) (📖 Biochemical and haematological values, p. 780).
- *Neuropathy:* ask about symptoms such as erectile dysfunction, tingling or pain. Can cause depression. Consider referral to GP.
- *Feet:* 5% develop an ulcer in any year arising from peripheral neuropathy and peripheral vascular disease. Recommend daily foot checks for colour change, skin breaks, swelling, numbness. Important to have well-fitting shoes, good foot hygiene, and nail care. Should be referred to emergency foot care services if problems. Check pedal pulses and nerves and general condition. High risk if absent pulses, deformity, skin changes, previous ulcer. Consider regular podiatry if poor vision, immobility or poor social conditions/foot hygiene. 'Putting feet first', by Diabetes UK a best-practice guide to diabetes foot care.
- *Skin changes:* there is a predisposition to skin changes and skin-based infections, e.g. boils, pruritus, as well as neuropathic and or ischaemic ulcers.

### Monitoring blood glucose

Good blood glucose (glycaemic) control is achievable and reduces risk of micro vascular complications (see Table 11.10). All people on insulin should test their blood glucose levels and people on certain tablets, such as sulfonylureas, to identify any periods of low blood glucose levels.

- Explain range of monitoring devices available to patient.
- Assess skills and meters if used annually or if problems arise.
- Agree targets for pre-meal glucose levels.

Evaluate the reliability of results against HbA1c results helps achieve control through:

- Informing food choices and portion quantities.
- Assisting medication dosing decisions.
- Identifying periods of high or low blood glucose levels.

*Urine monitoring* Adequate for those who cannot cope with more complex methods.

**Table 11.10** Indices of control

| Measure | Target |
|---|---|
| Fasting blood glucose (mmol/L) | 4–7 (postprandial <9) mmol/L—adults<br>4–8 (postprandial <10) mmol/L—children |
| Urine | –ve (postprandial sugars <0.5%) |
| HbA1c (normal 4.0–6.0% or 20–42mmol/mol)—measure every 2–6mths depending on control | 6.5% or 48 mmol/mol (but set realistic targets for each individual) |
| Serum cholesterol (mmol/L)—2° prevention, type 2 DM or type 1 DM with risk factors for CVD, metabolic syndrome or microalbuminuria | ↓ total cholesterol by 25% or to <4mmol/L, whichever is the lower value or ↓ LDL cholesterol by 30% or to <2.0mmol/L, whichever is the lower value |
| BMI | 25–30kg/m² |
| BP—without macrovascular disease | <135/85mmHg |
| BP—with macrovascular disease | <130/80mmHg |

Reproduced from Simon C, Everitt H, van Dorp F. (2010). *Oxford Handbook of General Practice*, 3rd edn. With permission of Oxford University Press.

*HbA1c (glycosylated haemoglobin)* Represents a measure of control over previous 6–8wks. Use HBA1c measure at least 2× a year and in conjunction with person's own self-monitoring blood glucose results (see Table 11.10).

## Documentation: maintain a structured record that the patient holds

• Document jointly agreed main points arising from review.
• Agreed targets to next consultations.
• Services involved/new referrals.
• Changes in treatment/therapy.

## Related topics

📖 Diabetes: overview, p. 611; 📖 Type 2 diabetes, p. 621; 📖 Insulin therapies, p. 618; 📖 Hypertension, p. 589; 📖 Coronary heart disease, p. 584; 📖 Hyperlipidaemia, p. 593; 📖 Wound assessment, p. 475.

## Further information

Diabetes. Available at: ℛ http://www.diabetes.co.uk
Diabetes UK. ☎ Helpline: 0845 120 2960. Available at: ℛ www.diabetes.org.uk
NHS Choices. Standards for diabetes care. Available at: ℛ http://www.nhs.uk/NHSEngland/NSF
NICE (2011). *Diabetes in adults : Quality Standards(Q26)*. Available at: ℛ http://guidance.nice.org.uk/QS6

# Insulin therapies

Insulin is first line treatment for type 1 diabetes. Also used when diet and oral therapy failed for type 2 diabetes. Usually started by specialist clinic with ongoing care involving of primary care team. Joint guidelines between local 1° and 2° care sectors will apply. Insulin requirements may be increased by infection, stress, exercise, accidental or surgical trauma, puberty, and during second and third trimesters of pregnancy.

Drivers must notify the DVLA and insurance company on starting insulin.

## Information, education, and advice

Therapy with insulin should be part of a treatment package that supports:
- Structured education.
- Access to telephone support.
- Regular self-monitoring, adjusting doses.
- Understanding diet.
- Managing hypoglycaemia.
- Managing acute changes in plasma glucose control values.
- Injection technique including site selection.
- Care and managing sick days.

See 🕮 Principles of diabetic care and control, p. 615 plus:
- Injection techniques and rotating sites.
- Storing and using insulin, maintaining supplies.
- Disposal of sharps (🕮 Managing health-care waste, p. 105).
- Plus avoiding, recognizing, and managing hypoglycaemia.
- *DAFNE:* skills-based education programme for people with type 1 diabetes (available at: ᗐ www.dafne.uk.com).
- Ask patients to keep a record of blood sugar values, time and date taken, and to measure blood sugar before meals at least od and at different times of the day (>if using multiple injection regimens/after dose changes or during illness).
- Record episodes of hypoglycaemia.
- Target blood glucose 4–8mmol/L pre meals with hypoglycaemic episodes kept to a minimum (4mmol/L if <18yrs).

## Insulin regimens

There are three groups of insulin—animal, human, and analogues. Most use human insulin and insulin analogues, a small number of people still use animal insulin.

The dose of insulin is adjusted on an individual basis, by gradually ↑ dose, but avoiding hypoglycaemia.

### Common insulin regimens
- Intermediate- and or short-acting insulin od (type 2 only).
- Short-acting insulin mixed with intermediate-acting insulin before breakfast and before evening meal.

- Short-acting insulin mixed with intermediate-acting insulin before breakfast, short- or rapid-acting insulin before evening meal and intermediate-acting insulin before bed.
- Short- or rapid-acting insulin tds before meals and intermediate-acting insulin before bed.
- Combinations of oral therapy, and od or bd long- or intermediate-acting insulin.

Rapid-acting insulin should be used as an alternative to meal time soluble insulin where nocturnal or late between meals hypoglycaemia is a problem or to eliminate the need for snacks between meals.

## Administration

Two main delivery devices used include preloaded, disposable insulin pens and cartridge, re-usable pens. Most available on prescription. Conventional syringe and needle infrequently used for self-administration. Continuous SC insulin infusion pumps used in some patients where multiple dose therapy has failed. Increased absorption can occur if limb involved in increased exercise post injection.

See Diabetes UK online video on how to inject insulin safely. Available at: ℘ www.diabetes.org.uk/Guide-to-diabetes/Treatments/Insulin/Video—how-to-inject-insulin-safely
- Deep SC injection into abdomen, thigh, buttock, and upper arm.
- Minimize fat hypertrophy (affects insulin absorption) by rotating sites.

## Storing insulin

- Keep spare insulin in fridge.
- Raise cold insulin to room temperature before administering.
- Insulin pen in use can be kept at normal room temperature for 1mth.

## Advice on illness/sick days

- Never stop or omit insulin.
- Drink extra fluids.
- Maintain dietary intake even if not eating (e.g. soup, milk, ice cream, fruit juice, sugar, honey, fruit juice).
- Measure and record blood sugar values qds. Follow medical/specialist advice on increasing insulin units if blood sugar values >10mmol/L.
- Check urine if blood sugar >than 13mmol/L. Seek urgent medical advice if unable to take glucose, persistently vomiting, dehydrated, or ketotic.

## Poor control

*Possible causes* Inter-current illness, changes in diet, alcohol intake, and level of exercise, non-adherence to insulin regimen, problems with injection sites, psychosocial factors. Ask patient to record blood sugar before meals and before bed to inform decision possibly to change dose, Requires medical/specialist advice.

## Hypoglycaemia

Advise patients to:
- Check their blood sugar and regularly if they are on a long journey (more than 2h).
- Carry glucose and sandwiches on long journey.
- *If hypoglycaemia occurs:* stop activities, take action and only resume activities when fully recovered.

Hypoglycaemia may present with range of symptoms including coma, fits, odd/violent behaviour, tachycardia, increased BP. May or may not have been warning signs of sweating, hunger, tremor. *Note:* children may be atypical and complain of headache or have behavioural changes. Blood sugar <2.5mmol/L (on blood testing strip).

### Management

- Treat with fast-acting carbohydrate (e.g. 2–3 glucose tablets; 90–180mL fizzy drink squash; or 50–100mL Lucozade®) Glucogel. Follow with longer-acting, starchy carbohydrate (e.g. a sandwich or biscuits), if it is a while before next meal or if meal due add some extra carbohydrate (e.g. bread, potatoes or pasta).
- If unable to take oral carbohydrate give IM glucagon 1mg adults (children <25kg/0.5mg) Follow with fast-acting carbohydrate when conscious. Seek medical advice.
- Repeat glucose testing in < 15min then monitor hourly over next 4h and every 4h for the next 24h.
- Review reasons for hypoglcaemia.

### Further information

Diabetes UK. Available at: ℬ www.diabetes.org.uk/home.htm

NICE (2004). *Type 1 Diabetes: diagnosis and management* (CG15). Available at: ℬ http://www.nice.org.uk/cg15

NICE (2008). *Type 2 diabetes* (CG66). Available at: ℬ ww.nice.org.uk/cg66

SIGN (2010). *Management of Diabetes 116* www.sign.ac.uk/pdf/sign116.pdf

# Type 2 diabetes

Prevalence of type 2 diabetes is ↑ across all groups, particularly among black and minority ethnic groups. Risk factors include obesity, physical inactivity, family history of diabetes, older age groups. People of African, African-Caribbean, South Asian, and Middle Eastern descent have a higher than average risk as do less affluent people. Preventive strategies are at a societal level and population level as well as at the individual in promoting health lifestyles to increase activity, reduce weight problems and ↑ awareness of risks.

## Management

Aim is to maintain target HbA1c for each individual, reduce likelihood of acute and chronic complications, prevent hypoglycaemia, prevent premature deaths from diabetes-related conditions and improve quality of life.

- Tight control of type 2 DM ↓ macrovascular and microvascular complications.
- *When setting a target HbA1c:* involve person in decisions about HbA1c target level, maybe> 6.5% set for people with type 2 diabetes in general. Encourage person to maintain individual target unless side effects or their efforts impair their quality of life.
- For a person with a higher HbA1c any reduction in HbA1c towards agreed target is advantageous to future health.
- Optimal results are obtained if HbA1c is maintained at 6.5–7.5%. Blood monitoring at 2–6mthly intervals until stable then 6-monthly.
- Treatment of hyperglycaemia is always combined with modification of other risk factors for vascular complications, e.g. monitoring for and controlling hypertension 📖 p. 589; 📖 Hyperlipidaemia (high/raised cholesterol), p. 593 📖 Smoking cessation, p. 315; 📖 Nutrition and healthy eating, p. 304.
- Plan of care always negotiated and agreed with patient (and family).
- Education is an important aspect as is knowledge of self-help groups, expert patient programmes.
- Regular recall and review helps to improve quality of care and subsequent outcomes for people with diabetes.

### Management by diet, weight control, and ↑ exercise

Management by diet tried for at least 3mths before medication is considered.

#### Healthy eating

Diet is the cornerstone of diabetic treatment. All diabetic patients should see a dietician. Supplement with opportunistic healthy eating advice. Provide in a form that is sensitive to the person's needs, culture and beliefs, and readiness to change. Integrate with diabetes management plan, including increasing physical activity. Recommend high-fibre, low-glycaemic index sources of carbohydrate, low-fat dairy products and oily fish.

Discourage use of foods marketed specifically for people with diabetes.

Individualize recommendations for carbohydrate and alcohol intake, and meal patterns. Aim to reduce risk of hypoglycaemia, particularly if using insulin:

Initial body weight loss target = 5–10% in an overweight person.

Lesser amounts are still beneficial. Diet information available from Diabetes UK.

*Weight management* Anti-obesity drugs only prescribed for patients with type 2 DM if they have BMI ≥27kg/m$^2$ and they have previously made serious attempts to lose weight by diet and exercise.

*Physical activity* ↑ physical activity is also beneficial (↓ weight, ↓ lipids, and ↑ insulin sensitivity), although not always possible. See 🕮 Exercise, p. 313.

## Management with oral hypoglycaemic agents (Fig. 11.4)

Biguanides or sulphonlylureas prescribed as first line treatment only effective if some insulin production. If control poor may be added to with other oral hypoglycaemics. Insulin considered if control not achieved or planning pregnancy.

- *Sulphonylureas:* e.g. gliclazide 40–80mg od.
  - *Acts by augmenting insulin secretion*—all are equally effective. If one sulphonylurea does not work another is not likely to either.
  - *Sulphonylureas should be taken before meals*—warn patients about possible hypoglycaemia if meals are omitted.
  - Started at the minimum dose and ↑ until either blood sugar is control-led or the maximum dose is reached. ≥1mth between adjustments.
  - Main side effect is weight gain, advise as above.
- *Biguanides:* metformin 500mg od–qds.
  - 1st line oral treatment for obese patients (BMI >25).
  - Contraindicated for older patients, those with serious heart disease, liver or renal failure (even mild) or high alcohol intake as ↑ risk of lactic acidosis.
  - Hypoglycaemia is not a problem.
  - Started with the minimum dose and ↑ monthly until control is achieved or maximum dose reached.
- *Glitazones:* used for
  - Patients who are obese and cannot tolerate metformin.
  - Combination therapy with metformin and/or sulphonylurea.
  - For patients with poor control on metformin and/or sulphonylurea.

### Starting insulin therapy

If other measures do not keep HbA1c to <7.5% (or other agreed target), discuss benefits and risks of insulin treatment, begin with human insulin taken at bedtime or bd according to need. If the person needs help with injecting insulin consider a once-daily long-acting insulin.

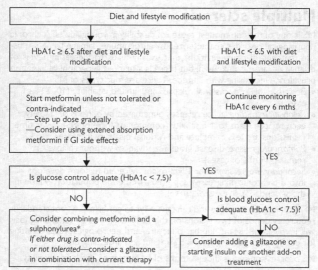

**Fig. 11.4** Using oral hypoglycaemic agents in type 2 DM. Reproduced from Simon, C, Everitt H, van Dorp F. (2010). *Oxford Handbook of General Practice*, 3rd edn. With permission of Oxford University Press.

*A rapid-acting insulin secretagogue is an alternative for those with poor control and erratic lifestyle

## Regular recall and review

This should include:
- Opportunity for emotional and psychological support.
- Regular HbA1c blood monitoring.
- Regular surveillance for and management of cardiovascular risk factors.
- Early detection of long-term complications.
- Advice and information.

## Further information

Diabetes UK. ☎ 0845 120 2960. Available at: 🖰 www.diabetes.org.uk
NICE (2008). *Type 2 diabetes* (CG66). Available at: 🖰 ww.nice.org.uk/cg66

# Multiple sclerosis

MS is one of the commonest causes of disability in young adults. A chronic neurological disorder characterized by autoimmune damage to neural tissue (patches of demyelination) that usually leads to increasing levels of disability. Cause is unknown, but there is a marked geographical variation prevalence increasing with latitude. There are four types of MS:

- *Benign:* involves occasional relapses and limited disability (10–20% of cases).
- *Relapsing/remitting:* acute relapses punctuated by periods of stability, each relapse leads to ↑ disability (commonest form of MS). Over time remissions are less complete and residual disability increases.
- *Primary progressive:* disease gradually advances without relapse or remission (10% of cases).
- *Secondary progressive:* after 15yrs relapsing/remitting form develops into the chronic progressive type (60% of the MS population will be in the secondary progressive phase).

MS is difficult to diagnose and can take >1yr to confirm. Current standards require evidence of two lesions on the CNS separated by time. Diagnosis will involve: MRI scans, lumbar puncture, and neurological tests. Waiting for confirmation of diagnosis is a stressful and unsettling time.

MS progression is classified in terms of its increasing levels of disability.

NICE guidelines for diagnosis and management of MS[1] for MS identifies four phases:

- Diagnostic phase.
- Minimal impairment phase.
- Moderate disability phase (e.g. patient walks with stick).
- Severe disability phase.

The speed of progression is unpredictable, can be a rapid or slowly developing disease. Poorer outcomes are associated with ♂ that are older at onset of disease that have frequent relapses with poor recovery, and cerebellar involvement.

## Common problems

Many patients often experience escalating physical disability depending on where the neurological damage occurs. Partners and family and carers are often adversely affected by the problems patients with MS have, and may need support. Most common issues encountered are:

- Continence problems (see 🕮 Urinary incontinence in women, p. 448) and 🕮 Urinary incontinence in men p. 453 arising from bladder and bowel dysfunction.
- *Fatigue:* one of the commonest and most debilitating problems.
- Cognitive impairment: memory loss and concentration problems.
- Balance and vertigo problems.
- Depression (🕮 Depression, p. 435) anxiety, and mood swings.
- Pain.
- Tremor and spasm.

- Visual disturbance.
- Mobility problems (□ Mobility for disabled people, p. 798).
- Sexual dysfunction (fertility is not affected) (□ Sexual problems, p. 718).

Symptoms can be exacerbated by heat or exercise.

## Care and management

All care will be with the MDT and in collaboration with specialist neurology services. The range of complications that can arise as a result of MS means much of care involves their identification and management. Patients require long-term coordinated care and emotional support and accurate information and advice about their health, prognosis, entitlement to disability benefits, and access to housing, transport, education, and leisure. Some areas have access to MS CNSs for ongoing patient support. MS charities provide guidance and standards for health and social care.

- Supplementing diet with linoleic acid 17–23g/day (polyunsaturated fats) may help slow progression of disability. Sources include sunflower, cornflower, and safflower oils.
- Influenza vaccination should be offered to all patients.

As there is no cure for MS, modifying therapies are used with the aim of slowing down the effects of the disease. The evidence for these is mixed. Therapies include:

- Beta-interferon and glatiramer acetate (2° care-led treatment).
- Cannabis for pain and spasticity (only through participation in trials).
- Neural therapy (injection of local anaesthetic into key points).
- Reflexology and massage (□ Complementary therapies, p. 782).
- Psychotherapy, e.g. for depression (□ Talking therapies, p. 429).
- Physiotherapy, speech therapy, and occupational therapy.

## Related topics

□ Sources of information on benefits and support, p. 789; □ Carers assessment and support, p. 412.

## Reference

[1]NICE (2003). *Diagnosis and management of MS in primary and secondary care (CG8)*. Available at: ℘ www.nice.org.uk/cg8

## Further information

Multiple Sclerosis Trust. Available at: ℘ www.mstrust.org.uk
Multiple Sclerosis Society. ☎ Helpline: 0808 800 8000. Available at: ℘ www.mssociety.org.uk

# Motor neurone disease

MND is a rapidly progressive neurodegenerative disease. Onset usually between 40–70yrs. Causes largely unknown: possible genetic and environmental, familial in 5%.

## Three main forms of MND
- *Amyotrophic lateral sclerosis (ALS):* most common (50%).
- *Progressive muscular atrophy (PMA):* least common (25%).
- *Progressive bulbar palsy (PBP):* 25% of cases.

Life expectancy varies depending on the form: ALS: 2–5yrs, PMA: 5yrs+, PBP: 6mths–3yrs.

## Presentation
Symptoms vary according to form, but include:
- Muscle weakness and wasting.
- Weight loss.
- Weak grip.
- Stumbling.
- Fasiculation (small involuntary contractions) of skeletal muscles.
- Emotional lability.
- Dysarthria and dysphagia with nasal speech, poor swallow, and regurgitation if upper motor neurones involved.

> Consciousness and intellect are unaffected.

## Aims of care
- Symptomatic relief, maintain for QoL, speed of response essential.
- Ensure early referral to MDT and MND Nurse Specialist. MDT should have ensured home physiotherapy/OT assessment for adaptations/mobility aids (Ⓠ Assistive technology, p. 776).
- Full community care assessment process (Ⓠ Integrated or single assessment processes, p. 114).
- Awareness of state benefits for disability and attendance (Ⓠ Benefits for illness, disability and carers, p. 795).
- Carers assessment and support (Ⓠ Carers assessment and support, p. 412) needs addressed.
- *Pharmacological:* riluzole (BNF 4.9) is only disease-modifying therapy that may prolong life.

### Dysphagia
- Control head position with pillows +/- collar.
- Modify diet and thicken fluids.
- Ensure SLT (Speech and Language Therapist)/dietician assessment.
- Initiate discussions of gastrostomy (Ⓠ Enteral tube feeding, p. 546) early before patient too unwell to tolerate procedure.

*Dyspnoea*
- Due to poor respiratory function/anxiety.
- Symptom control, e.g. $O_2$ therapy at night (📖 Oxygen therapy, p. 581), opioids may relieve coughing and choking.
- Psychotherapy and relaxation techniques (📖 Talking therapies, p. 429).
- Physiotherapy exercises may aid breathing.
- Position upright.
- Discuss options for ventilation including non-invasive ventilation (NIPPV), consider advantages of prolonging life against prolonging discomfort.

*Pain*
Due to joint immobility, spasm and cramps, pressure areas, constipation.
- Ensure physiotherapy referral, pressure area relief equipment and mattress, drugs, e.g. baclofen/quinine for spasm and cramps.
- *Dysarthria:* early referral to SLT and dietician, provide communication aids.
- *Emotional lability (different from depression):* treated with amitriptyline.

*Key issues to consider*
- Maintaining emotional, physical, and financial support throughout course of disease for patient, family, and carers.
- Ensure there is regular symptom review involving PHCT.
- Ensure there are opportunities for discussion about end of life, and support patient and carer, e.g. palliative/respite care/withdrawal of treatment and ventilation.
- Discuss and a document patient wishes/advance directives/preferred place of care.

MND Association can help with information, advice, equipment loan, and financial support.

**Related topics**

📖 People with depression, p. 435; 📖 Carers assessment and support, p. 412; 📖 Talking therapies, p. 429; 📖 Counselling skills, p. 123; 📖 Palliative care in the home, p. 509; 📖 End-of-life issues, p. 530.

**Further information**

Motor Neurone Disease Association. Available at: ℜ www.mndassociation.org
NICE (2001). Motor neurone disease-riluzole (TA20). Available at: ℜ www.nice.org.uk/TA20
NHS Choice. Motor Neurone Diseases. Available at: ℜ http://www.nhs.uk/Conditions/Motor-neurone-disease/Pages/Symptoms.aspx

# Parkinson's disease

Parkinson's disease (PD) is a chronic, incurable progressive, degenerative, neurological disorder. Causes are largely unknown, although environment and genetic susceptibility are possible factors. Symptoms appear from the age of 50yrs, but in young-onset PD can appear <40yrs.

*Note:* Parkinsonism is seen in other conditions—multi-system atrophy, progressive supranuclear palsy, Lewy body dementia, encephalitis, side effects of drugs, e.g. haloperidol, chlorpromazine.

## Pathology

- Degeneration of dopaminergic neurones in substantia nigra, part of the basal ganglia (regions in the brain that control voluntary movement).
- 80–90% depletion of dopamine in substantia nigra.
- Presence of Lewy bodies.

## Risk factors

- Old age.
- Identical twin with early onset PD.
- Family history.
- Exposure to herbicides, pesticides, heavy metals, proximity to industry, rural residence, repeated head trauma.

## Presentation

Slow insidious onset:

- *Bradykinesia:* can include resting tremor (pill rolling) rigidity, disorders of posture—neck and trunk flexion, balance problems.
- *Gait disturbance:* festination, freezing, shuffling.
- *Rigidity:* limbs resist passive extension throughout movement.
- Loss of facial expression.
- Monotonous and hypophonic speech.
- Dribbling, dysphagia.
- Micrographia (small handwriting).

## Aims of care

Symptomatic relief, maintain QoL, ↓ progression and ↓ side effects of medication. The mainstay of treatment is pharmacological. Drugs include levodopa, dopamine agonists, COMT inhibitors, MAO-inhibitors, and anticholinergics. After 3–5yrs use, effectiveness of levodopa is reduced and should usually not be started until symptoms disrupting QoL.

> *Note:* rarely achieves complete control of symptoms.

- ↑ functional disability → early referral to specialist MDT and nursing support.
- Reduce or delay long-term complications of drug therapy (e.g. on/off effect by delaying start of L-dopa).
- Help come to terms with diagnosis.
- *Reduce distress:* symptoms worse when stressed.

- Legal obligation for patient to inform DVLA and insurers of diagnosis.
- Complementary therapies (📖 Complementary therapies, p. 782) may help relaxation.

## Management in later stages

- *Manage drug effects and motor complications*: risk of falls.
- *Identify and address behavioural/psychological issues*: depression, sleep disorders, psychosis. Consider referral to mental health team.
- *Monitor BP*: risk of orthostatic hypotension → review PD drugs and advise to avoid sitting out in sun, getting up quickly, or sitting in one position for long periods. Sit down immediately if feeling dizzy. Encourage leg exercises that maintain ankle flexion and dorsiflexion.
- Monitor other complications: constipation (📖 Constipation in adults, p. 457), urinary incontinence (in women 📖 p. 448; and in men 📖 p. 453)/retention, impotence, poor nutrition.
- MDT should have ensured:
  - Home OT/physiotherapist assessment for home adaptations and mobility aids (📖 Assistive technology, p. 776).
  - Full community care assessment (📖 Integrated or single assessment processes, p. 114).
  - Awareness of state benefits for disability (📖 Benefits for illness, disability and carers, p. 795) and attendance.
  - Carers assessment and support (📖 Carers assessment and support, p. 412) needs addressed.

## Related topics

📖 People with depression, p. 435; 📖 People with dementia, p. 438; 📖 Falls prevention, p. 327.

## Further information

NICE (2006). *Parkinson's Disease: national clinical guidelines for diagnosis and management in primary and secondary care.* (CG35). Available at: ℜ www.nice.org.uk/cg35

Parkinson's Disease Society. Available at: ℜ www.parkinsons.org.uk

NHS Choices. Parkinson's disease. Available at: ℜ www.nhs.uk/Conditions/Parkinsons-disease/Pages/Introduction.aspx

# Frailty

Frailty can be defined as 'a precarious balance between the assets maintaining health and the deficits threatening it'[1]. With age physical, cognitive, emotional, and social factors become increasingly interdependent influencing health and wellbeing. A state of increased vulnerability ↑ the risk of falls, delirium, and disability. Associated with advanced age, *but* being old does not = frailty. It may overlap with disability and co-morbidity may appear suddenly, an older individual who has been coping can have multiple needs following a single incident, e.g. illness. Up to 50% of >85yrs are frail. Frailty is predictive of ill health, move to care home, and death.

## Indicators consistent with frailty in older people

- Extreme fatigue, unexplained weight loss, and frequent infections.
- Muscle weakness (sarcopenia).
- *Falls:* balance and gait impairment present. Spontaneous falls occur in more severe frailty when vision, balance, and strength affect ability to walk (⚏ Falls prevention, p. 327).
- Fear of further falls = develop severely impaired mobility.
- *Delirium:* rapid onset of fluctuating confusion /impaired awareness. ~30% of older people admitted to hospital develop delirium.
- Fluctuating disability people have independent days, and days on which (professional) care is often needed.

## Frailty measures

Measures designed to identify frail older people include the assessment of mobility, hand grip strength, and pulmonary function. The Edmonton Frail Scale[2] is a multidimensional assessment instrument; includes the timed-up-and go test, and a test for cognitive impairment. It takes <5min, is valid, reliable. Frailty tools may improve:

- Identification of individuals requiring complex care.
- The way in which health and social care practitioners' coordinate their goals and care plans.
- Evaluation of care according to person-centred outcomes, rather than disease or care outcomes.
- Monitoring of the effects of interventions and to chart significant changes in individual's wellbeing and vulnerability.

Interventions that may help reduce the impact of frailty include:

- *Strength and balance training:* can successfully increase muscle strength and functional abilities.
- *Nutritional interventions:* to address the impaired nutrition and weight loss of frailty.
- Strengthening of social networks and support (⚏ Social support, p. 24).

## References

[1]Clegg A, Young J, Iliffe S, et al. (2013). Frailty in elderly people. *Lancet* **381**: 752–62.
[2]Rolfson DB, Majumdar SR, Tsuyuki RT, et al. (2006). Validity and reliability of the Edmonton Frail Scale. *Age & Ageing* **35**: 526–9.

# Chapter 12

# Common adult health problems

# Bacterial skin infections

Skin infections can range from minor to life-threatening conditions.

## Impetigo

- A superficial cutaneous infection caused by *Staphylococcus aureus* and/or beta-hemolytic *Streptococcus*.
- Vesicles that rupture easily, producing golden yellow exudates, forms a crust when dry.
- *Commonly involved sites:* face, neck, but can be more extensive.
- Impetigo can occur as a 2° infection on excoriated skin conditions, e.g. eczema, scabies.
- Contagious.
- Children in poor living conditions, overcrowding, or with poor hygiene are at greater risk of developing impetigo.

### Treatment and advice

- Localized infection treated with fusidic acid (3 or 4 x day for 7 days (BNF 13.10.1)).
- Before initial application advise patient to remove crusty areas by soaking in soapy water if not painful.
- For extensive areas, or sever infection oral antibiotics, e.g. (flucloxacillin QDS x 7 days or erythromycin if allergic to penicillin).
- Saline soaks to cleanse area and remove crusts.
- Encourage basic hygiene practice to limit the contact and spread of infection, e.g. not sharing towels, face cloths.
- Exclusion from group child care/school until lesions crust over (☐ Infectious diseases in childhood, p. 283).
- Advise to return if no significant improvement in 7 days. Bacterial culture for diagnosis if not clearing.

## Infection of the hair follicles

There are three types:

### Follicullitis

- A superficial active pustular inflammation of hair follicles caused by *Staphylococcus aureus*.
- *Triggered by:* shaving, waxing, tar ointments, oil-based ointments.

### Furuncle (boil)

- A deep infection of the hair follicle caused by *Staphylococcus aureus*.
- Characterized by inflammation, nodule with peeling of the overlying skin. The area will be tender.
- The nodule will erupt and discharge the contents.
- Common areas affected are areas affected by sweat and/or friction (nose, face, axilla, buttocks).
- Patients who are immunosuppressed or have diabetes are more prone to boils.

## Carbuncle

- Deep infection of a group of hair follicles by *Staphylococcus aureus*.
- Common site—nape of neck.
- Characterized by a dome-shaped area of erythema developing into a deep, painful abscess.
- May rupture spontaneously.

### Treatment

- Exclude diabetes.
- Warm cloths applied 4x day to help pain and help drainage.
- Pain killers e.g. paracetamol for pain.
- Systemic antibiotics for all carbuncles, if ↑ temperature, presence of secondary infection, if on face, if in severe pain or discomfort, as per local guide lines, (flucloxacillin usually first line treatment or erythromycin; BNF 5.1).
- In recurrences longer courses of 4–6wks of antibiotics may be required and bacterial culture from lesion and carrier sites.
- Large carbuncle or in sensitive area may require incision (often in ED rather than GP surgery).
- OTC antiseptic washes and emollients may help to avoid recurrences.
- Referred to specialists if not responding to primary care treatment and management.

## Cellulitis

- Infection of the subcutaneous tissues with *Streptococcus pyogenes*.
- Most commonly the lower legs are affected, becoming erythematous, oedematous, and painful. Blisters may be noted.
- The patient will become systemically unwell and pyrexial.
- The organism enters the tissue through a fissure caused by eczema, tinea pedis, leg ulceration, although entry port not found.
- It is often a recurrent problem.

### Treatment

Acute phase requires medical assessment and may need IV antibiotics and/or admission to hospital if systematically unwell. Otherwise treated in primary care.

- Antibiotics (flucloxacillin, penicillin V; BNF 5.1 table 1) orally or in severe infection benzylpenicillin and flucloxacillin IV.
- May require prophylactic antibiotics if recurrent.
- Advise analgesia prn, fluids, if site on leg—elevate.
- Monitored to assess treatment effectiveness.
- Emollient therapy (BNF 13.2.1) helps prevent fissures in dry skin.

## Further information

NHS Choices. Boils and carbuncles. Available at: ℘ www.nhs.uk/Conditions/Boils/Pages/Introduction.aspx

NICE CKS Impetigo (2009), Boils (2011), Cellulitis –acute (2012). Available at: ℘ http://cks.nice.org.uk/

# Skin cancer

Primary cutaneous cancer is most commonly of the keratinocytes or melanocytes. Caused by genetic factors, exposure to sunlight, sometimes exposure to carcinogens (see 📖 Skin cancer prevention, p. 331). Incidence rates are increasing rapidly.

## Types of skin cancer

There are 2 main types of skin cancer:
- Malignant melanoma (majority).
- *Non-melanoma skin cancer:* basal cell carcinoma, squamous cell carcinoma.

## ABCDEFGs of melanoma

A useful guide for determining which moles are potential melanomas and teaching patients warning signs:
- *Asymmetry:* an unusual shape or a non-symmetrical shaped mole should be evaluated further.
- *Border:* a benign mole will usually have a smooth, clearly demarcated border. If an ill-defined or irregular border is noted, evaluate further.
- *Colour:* pigment variation indicative of malignancy and should be evaluated.
- *Diameter:* most melanomas are >6mm.
- *Elevated/Evolutionary changes:* in colour, size, symmetry, surface characteristics, and symptoms.
- *Firm.*
- *Growing:* for >1mth.

These changes usually take place over a relatively short time from weeks to months. Other signs can include mole or growth that crusts, bleeds, or is itchy, or sore that won't heal.

## Malignant melanoma

Malignant melanoma is a malignancy of the melanocytes. It is the most serious form of skin cancer.
Good prognosis depends on early detection and treatment. 4 types:
- *Superficial spreading malignant melanoma:* an enlarging brown/black macular/popular lesion may be irregular with colour variation.
- *Nodular melanoma:* a pigmented papule that enlarges and ulcerates.
- *Acral melanoma:* brown/black macules on the non-hair bearing skin of the palms, soles, and nail beds.
- *Lentigo maligna melanoma:* an irregularly shaped, flat, pigmented lesion on sun damaged skin. Most frequently occurs on the face or other sun exposed sites.

### Treatment

- All suspected cases of melanoma referred to 2° care.
- Surgical removal of suspected lesion to establish the histological diagnosis. May require further surgery to ensure adequate margins around the excised lesion. Laser therapy and immunotherapy also used.
- Patient assessed for the presence of metastatic disease.
- The patient is followed up by 2° care for at least 5yrs.

## Non-melanoma skin cancer

### Basal cell carcinoma

- Most common type of skin cancer. Also known as rodent ulcer, locally invasive, low grade tumours of the basaloid cells that rarely metastasize. Usually occur on sun exposed skin of older patients, but can affect younger patients.
- There are different types of basal cell carcinoma:
  - *Nodular basal cell carcinoma (BCC):* slow growing with a characteristic translucent or pearly surface. Dilated vessels may be visible. The area may ulcerate.
  - *Cystic BCC:* similar to nodular, but there will be more dilated vessels.
  - *Superficial spreading BCC:* thin lesions that gradually increase in surface area. They may be reddened, slightly raised, with some scaling.
  - *Morphoeic BCC:* white/yellow morphoeic plaques resembling an enlarging scar. Ulceration and crusting are usual.

### Squamous cell carcinoma

- An invasive tumour of the keratinocytes that can metastasize.
- There are different types of squamous cell carcinoma (SCC):
  - *Actinic keratosis:* these are pre-malignant lesions, if left untreated a small percentage will develop into SCC. Appear in sun exposed sites as tiny, palpable lesions.
  - *Bowen's disease (SCC in situ):* may appear on non-sun exposed sites. Appears as a persistent, erythematous, indurated, plaque.
  - *Nodular SCC:* hard nodule which increases in size rapidly.
  - *Ulcerated SCC:* nodular area on the edge of an ulcer or an ulcer on a scar.

### Treatment

All suspected BCC and SCC are referred to dermatology. Treatment is dependent on the site, type, and size of lesion, but may include: cryosurgery, curettage and electrosurgery, fluorouracil topically applied, excision, radiotherapy, surgery, photodynamic therapy.

Patients need to be offered clear information about the diagnosis, prognosis, and any changes required to their lifestyle.

### Further information

Cancer Research: skin cancer. Available at: ℘ www.cancerresearchuk.org

NICE (2010). *Skin tumours including melanoma (CGSTIM).* Available at: ℘ www.nice.org.uk/CSGSTIM

NICE. CKS Melanoma and pigmented lesions (2011). Available at: ℘ http://cks.nice.org.uk/

# Eczema/dermatitis

Dermatitis is an acute and/or chronic pruritic inflammation of the skin. Only about 20% seek medical help for these conditions. See 🕮 Eczema in childhood, p. 266.

## Clinical features

### Atopic eczema

Usually presents between 3–12mths of age (🕮 Eczema in childhood, p. 266). There is an inherited predisposition to eczema, and hay fever. It may start on the face and scalp. In older children and adults eczema is often localized to the flexures. Eczema can continue through into adulthood.

### Seborrhoeic dermatitis

Associated with an overgrowth of pityrosporum ovule yeasts in adults. The distribution is characterized by pink, orange/brown, scaly patches on the scalp, eyebrows, eyelashes, nasolabial folds, external ear, centre of chest, and centre of back.

### Discoid (nummular) eczema

Characterized by well-demarcated, round, scaly plaques. There may be numerous vesicles present that produce exudate and crusting.

### Contact dermatitis

Eczema can be associated with exposure of the skin to certain irritants or allergens.

### Pompholyx

Eczema on the hands and feet may present as crops of vesicles with severe itching. There may be peeling and cracking of the skin.

### Gravitational (venous, varicose, stasis) eczema

Occurs on the lower legs of patients with venous hypertension.

## Management

### Emollients (BNF 13.2)

Patients with eczema usually have dry skin and therefore should be prescribed an emollient package:

- *Bath additive (e.g. Balneum®, Hydromol®, Oilatum®):* 10–20mL of the oil should be added to the bath.
- *Soap substitute (e.g. aqueous cream, emulsifying ointment):* soap has a drying effect on the skin and should not be used.
- *Moisturizer (e.g. 50:50 white soft paraffin: liquid paraffin, Oilatum® cream, Epaderm®):* the moisturizing emollient should be applied after the bath and then frequently throughout the day.

### Topical steroids (BNF 13.4)

There are different strengths of topical steroids (mild, moderate, potent, and very potent). The weakest steroid that is effective should be the steroid of choice. Usually a mild steroid is sufficient to treat eczema on the face. Many patients are aware of the potential side effects of over use of topical steroids and therefore allow time for advice and questions. It is only applied to the affected areas and not mixed with emollient.

### Topical immunomodulators

Imunomodulators are recommended if the eczema has not responded to topical steroids or is severe. They are prescribed by dermatology specialists. The treatment acts by blocking the molecular mechanisms of inflammation (BNF 13.5.3). The patient may experience burning or stinging of the skin for about 20min when the treatment is applied.

### Antihistamines

Antihistamines, e.g. chlorphenamine are useful for short-term use in acute phases of the eczema for their sedative effect. They are used an hour before bed time, daytime use should be avoided.

### Infection

- *Bacterial:* Staphylococcus aureus, characterized by pustules, yellow crusting, or weeping. Sometimes presents as a flare up not responding to usual medication. Treated with systemic flucloxacillin (BNF 5.1.1) or erythromycin (BNF 5.1.5).
- *Viral:* herpes simplex, characterized by painful, small umbilicated vesicles. Requires medical assessment as widespread inflection (ezcema herpeticum) may be life threatening. The patient will be unwell and will require systemic aciclovir (BNF 5.3.2) as inpatient.

## General advice

- Avoid the use of soaps and detergents on the skin.
- Extremes of temperature, cold winds, or hot environment with a low humidity may exacerbate eczema.
- Cotton clothing should be worn next to the skin.
- Nails should be kept short to reduce damaging the skin if scratching.
- Eczema in a family can cause an increase of stress for other family members.
- Dietary manipulation is indicated if there is a history of specific food allergy. It should be undertaken with medical and dietician advice.

## Further information

National Eczema Society. Available at: ℗ www.eczema.org
NICE. CKS Dermatitis-contact (2013). Available at: ℗ www.cks.library.nhs.uk
Scottish Intercollegiate Guidelines Network (SIGN) (2011). *Management of atopic eczema in primary care (National clinical guideline 125)*. Available at: ℗ www.sign.ac.uk

# Fungal infections

Fungal infection in humans is largely attributable to 2 groups:

- Dermatophytes—multicellular filaments or hyphae.
- Yeasts—unicellular forms replicating by budding.

Infection can occur from direct contact with infected animals, humans, or soil, or contact with a contaminated object for example shared towels.

## Dermatophyte (tinea) infection

Tineas are superficial infections in keratinized tissue (hair, nails, stratum corneum). 3 types—trichophyton, microsporum, epidermophyton. Diagnosis usually clinical, but can be confirmed by skin scrapings, or nail clippings (depending on site) sent for mycology. General advice should be given on good hygiene.

### Tinea corporis (ringworm)

- Single or multiple pink scaly plaques on trunk or limbs, which gradually increase in size. As expands the centre clears to look like a ring.
- Localized area treated with an imidazole cream (BNF 13.10.2) applied bd for 2–4wks or terbinafine cream for 7–10 days. Continued 7 days after visibly clears.
- Extensive areas need systemic treatment with itraconazole, griseofulvin, or terbinafine (BNF 5.2) for 2–4wks started after confirmation of diagnosis from mycology.

### Tinea pedis (athlete's foot)

- There are 5 patterns of tinea on the feet:
  - Itchy, scaling, and maceration between toes, usually 4th and 5th.
  - Plaques of tinea similar to tinea corporis on dorsum of the foot.
  - White itchy scaling on the soles of 1 or both feet.
  - Scaling on the sides of the foot.
  - Vesicles on the instep usually on 1 foot.
- Treated with an imidazole cream bd for 2–4wks or terbinafine for 7 days. Continue for 7 days after clears (BNF 13.10.2).
- Oral treatment if widespread, severe, or treatment failed.

### Tinea cruris (ringworm in the groin)

- Common in young men, may be associated with tinea pedis.
- Itchy, pink scaly patches with central clearing on insides of thigh, scrotum rarely affected.
- Treated with imidazole cream bd for 2–3wks or until clear.

### Tinea manium

- Uncommon.
- Affects hand with powdery scaling.
- Treatment topical imidazole creams for 2–3wks.

## Tinea unguium

- Nail(s) becomes thickened, discolored white or yellow.
- Treated if patient requests, or is causing other recurrent infections.
- After diagnosis confirmed by mycology, oral, pulsed itraconazole (200mg bd for 7 days repeated after 21 days for fingernails and 2 more for toes) (BNF 5.2).

## Tinea capitis (scalp ringworm)

- Most common in children. Rare in adults. Causes discrete bald areas with short broken off hairs. The underlying skin is scaly and red.
- Treated systemically. Griseofulvin 15–20mg/kg body weight/day od with food for 6wks (BNF 5.2).
- Sometimes also a kerion, a red boggy swelling discharging pus. Treated by softening crusts with olive oil. Swab for MC&S. Treat with flucloxacillin if *Staphylococcus aureus* is present as well as the griseofulvin.

# Yeast infections

## Candida (thrush) skin infections

- Common.
- Caused by the opportunistic pathogen *Candida albicans*.
- Advise on good hygiene, allow air to circulate, etc.
- *Common when:* broad-spectrum antibiotics used or poor nappy hygiene, but other reasons should be investigated, e.g. if immunosuppressed, patient with diabetes. Usually flexures are affected and pattern is symmetrical. Treated with a topical imidazole cream (BNF 13.10).

## Cheilitis topical

- Infections causing inflamed and cracked grooves at corner of mouth.
- Common when wearing poorly fitted dentures. Advise the patient to clean the dentures after each meal, sterilize at night, and see dentist.
- Clotrimazole cream (BNF 13.10.2) bd.

## Oral candidiasis

Seen as white plaques; requires oral forms of anti-fungal (BNF 12.3.2).

## Genital candidiasis

♀ see (📖 Vaginal and vulval problems, p. 737). ♂: redness, sore glans penis, ± ulceration of foreskin. Not usually transmissable. Treated with 1% clotrimazole (OTC/BNF 13.10).

## Intertrigo

- In skin folds due to heat and humidity. Common if overweight.
- The area will be painful, red with red satellite lesions.
- Clotrimazole and 1% hydrocortisone cream clears infection reduces symptoms, but recurrence is common.

## Paronychia

- Infection of nail fold and loss of cuticle. Creates chronic infection.
- *To induce growth of new cuticle:* advise to keep hands dry by wearing cotton gloves inside rubber gloves when washing up, etc. and apply petroleum jelly to affected nail several times a day to protect the area.

## Pityrosporum skin infections

### Pityriasis versicolor

A scaly rash that occurs most commonly in young adults due to pityrosporum orbiculare. Characterized by pigmentary skin changes, either hypo- or hyperpigmented and occasionally red patches.

- If localized use clotrimazole cream bd (BNF 13.10.2) for 2wks. Referred to dermatologist if extensive.
- Reassure patient as pigmentary changes may take 3mths to go.

## Further information

British Association of Dermatologists. Available at: ℡ www.bad.org.uk for professional guidelines and patient information leaflets

NICE. CKS Candida infections. Available at: ℡ http://cks.nice.org.uk/

# Psoriasis

Psoriasis is a chronic, relapsing, inflammatory, hyperproliferative skin disease. Whilst rarely fatal, it affects psychological, socio-economic, and physical wellbeing. It affects 2–3% of the population. It appears at any age, most commonly between 20–30yrs. Affects ♀ = ♂. Genetically predetermined, but also caused by infection, stress, drugs, e.g. lithium, anti-malarials, beta-blocking agents, systemic glucocorticoids, environment, e.g. usually worsens in the winter, however a small percentage worsen in the summer.

## Clinical features

- *Chronic plaque psoriasis:* well demarcated, raised pink plaques, dry silver/white scales. Commonly on elbows, knees, and lower back.
- *Scalp psoriasis:* may be dry and scaly or in more severe cases will be inflamed, with thickened, scaly, well demarcated plaques.
- *Guttate psoriasis:* multiple red papules and small psoriatic lesions. Usually on the trunk in a 'raindrop' distribution commonly following a streptococcal infection.
- *Flexural psoriasis:* well demarcated, red, smooth plaques affecting the submammary, axillary, and anogenital areas.
- Pustular psoriasis.
  - Localized—multiple small, sterile pustules, with erythema and hyperkeratosis on the palms and soles. As they dry, brown patches develop.
  - Generalized—multiple tiny pustules on generalized erythrodermic skin. The skin is unstable and requires emergency dermatology care.
- Erythrodermic psoriasis—involves entire skin surface. Patient febrile, ↑ white cell count, ankle oedema, and problems controlling their temperature. Requires emergency dermatology care.
- Psoriatic arthropathy—less than 10% of patients with psoriasis will also have psoriatic arthropathy. The most common form seen is characterized by distal interphalangeal involvement.
- The distribution of psoriasis is largely symmetrical.
- Can be itchy although it is often considered not to be. Scratching removes overlying scale, elicits pinpoint bleeding—'Auspitz sign'.
- Often occurs at sites of trauma—'Koebner phenomenon'.

## Management

Consider the following:
- The severity and effect on QoL.
- Previous therapies, other drug therapies, time available for treatments.
- The physical ability of the patient to apply topical treatments.
  Treatments for psoriasis fall into 3 groups.

### Topical treatments

Used for mild to moderate psoriasis, or with other therapies.
- *Emollients* (BNF 13.2.1): regular use reduces scaling, itching, and ↑ penetration of other topical medications.

- *Vitamin D3 analogues* (BNF 13.5.2): effective in plaque psoriasis. Colorless and odorless. Significant ↓ condition after 4wks.
- *Coal tar* (BNF 13.5.2): ↓ in use as concerns about oncogenic potential. Have a strong smell so are not acceptable to all patients. Used in shampoos, bath emollient, lotions, and scalp treatments.
- *Retinoid* (BNF 13.5.2): tazarotene gel is used for mild-to-moderate psoriasis.
- *Dithranol* (BNF 13.5.2): short contact cream preparations available for home use. Only applied to the plaques as local irritation to non-affected skin. Leaves an unwanted staining on the skin.
- *Keratolytics* (BNF 13.5.2): ↓ scale, ↑ penetration of other drugs.
- *Corticosteroids* (BNF 13.4): may be used in combination with other products listed earlier. Important to explain side effects to prevent misuse of the product.

*Phototherapy*

Natural sunlight may be beneficial. Phototherapy (artificial sunlight) indicated for moderate-to-severe psoriasis, administered in dermatology clinic. Commercial sun beds should not be used as an alternative.

- *UVB:* a 10wk course of 2–3 times per week. Well tolerated, but risk of sun burn type reaction and potential to increase skin cancer risk.
- *Psoralen and UVA (PUVA):* combination of a photosensitizing drug, methoxypsoralen, and UVA. More effective than UVB. Localized PUVA may be administered for palmer–plantar psoriasis. Patients must wear eye protection for 24hrs after taking drug to minimize the risk of cataracts.

*Systemic treatments*

Considered when 10–15% body coverage, patient not responded to other treatments, or causing severe negative impact on quality of life. Treatments are under the supervision of the dermatology consultant although care may be shared with 1° care. Types (BNF 13.5.3) include:

- *Methotrexate:* a cytotoxic agent, licensed for severe, uncontrolled psoriasis. Administered orally once weekly. Regular monitoring of FBC, electrolytes, renal function, and LFTs throughout treatment. Patients have hand-held monitoring records.
- *Acitretin:* a retinoid. Useful in treating palmer–plantar psoriasis. LFTs, FBC, and fasting lipids will be monitored throughout treatment.
- *Ciclosporin:* a potent immunosuppressant with effects on the T cells. It is used for widespread unresponsive psoriasis. During therapy patients will have BP, renal function, GFR, fasting lipids monitored.
- *Biologics:* designed to block specific molecular steps in the pathogenesis of psoriasis. Considered only if patient is unresponsive or intolerant to all other treatments or else has life threatening psoriasis.

**Further information**

NICE. CKS Psoriasis (2012). Available at: ℜ http://cks.nice.org.uk
Psoriasis Association. Available at: ℜ www.psoriasis-association.org.uk

# Viral skin infections

## Warts (verrucae)

Warts appear as firm, rough, pink- or brown-coloured papules with black pinpoint dots on the surface.

- Benign, cutaneous tumours caused through the infection of the epidermal cells with HPV.
- Characterized by hyperkeratosis and thickening of the epidermis.
- Common in children.

### Treatment and advice

- The majority will resolve with no treatment within 2yrs.
- Topical wart treatments containing salicylic acid, glutaraldehyde, or formaldehyde may be bought OTC or prescribed. The topical treatments need to be used for 3mths (BNF 13.7) or until it resolves.
- Liquid nitrogen cryotherapy is sometimes used as 2nd line therapy, it has the same effectiveness as the topical treatments. It can be painful.
- Patients can use a swimming sock to cover any warts on their feet to reduce the risk of spreading the virus.

## Molluscum contagiosum

- Discrete, umbilicated pearly white or pink papules caused by the pox virus.
- Common in children and young adults.
- Most commonly seen on the face and neck, but can occur on any part of the skin.

### Treatment and advice

- The lesions will resolve spontaneously within 6–24mths.
- Picking and squeezing the lesions may cause the lesions to spread.

## Herpes simplex

- Primary infection with type 1 occurs either in the epidermis or buccal mucosa usually within the first 5yrs of life.
- The virus remains dormant in dorsal root ganglion until reactivated.
- A recurrence commences with a prodromal sensation of itching, burning, or tingling. A few hours later there will be small grouped vesicles these will burst, crust, and heal in 7–10 days.
- Triggers for reactivation—fever, sunlight, menstruation, stress.
- *Eczema herpeticum:* eczema becomes secondarily infected with the herpes simplex virus. The patient will be unwell and will require systemic aciclovir.

### Treatment and advice

- Usually no treatment is required.
- Topical aciclovir (OTC/BNF 5.3.2) applied 2-hrly (at start of episode) for 2 days will reduce the episode, but will not prevent future attacks.

## Genital herpes

(See 📖 Sexually transmitted infections, p. 715.)

### Herpes varicella zoster (chickenpox)

- Infectious droplet infection from the upper respiratory tract.
- There is a prodromal illness that is often mild; first signs of infection are lesions.
- Characterized by pink macules which develop into papules, tense vesicles, pustules, and then crusts.
- The condition is very itchy, chlorphenamine syrup and calamine lotion (OTC) may reduce the irritation.
- Pock-like scarring can occur.
- It usually affects children under the age of 10yrs (📖 Infectious diseases in childhood, p. 283), but adults can also be affected.
- Treatment is not usually required unless immunocompromised or pregnant and non-immune. These groups should urgently see GP. Pregnant ♀ commenced on oral aciclovir if >20wks and within 24hrs of first developing rash. Hospital assessment if other symptoms or if smokes, has lung disease, or late in pregnancy. Immunocompromised often require hospital admission for IV aciclovir.

### Herpes zoster (shingles)

- Reactivation of the varicella zoster virus, allowing replication and migration along nerve endings—prodromal phase of pain and tenderness.
- All ages, but more common in >50yrs and in immunocompromised patients.
- The acute phase is characterized by erythema and vesicles followed by weeping and crusting.
- Healing occurs within 3–4wks, however, the pain may continue for months or years, more common in older people.
- It is unilateral and confined to 1 or 2 adjacent dermatones with a cut off at or near midriff.

*Treatment and advice*

- Skin hygiene advice and non-adherent dressings on rash.
- Antiviral drugs (BNF 5.3.2) used only for groups at risk of complications, e.g. >50yrs, immunocompromised, who present within 72hrs of onset of rash.
- Calamine lotion and regular analgesia if required.
- Post-herpetic neuralgia pain can be severe and debilitating. Nerve painkillers required, e.g. amitriptyline (BNF 4.7.3) may require the advice of pain specialists.
- If the skin around the eye is affected patients are referred to an ophthalmologist.

### Related topic

📖 Infectious diseases in childhood, p. 283.

### Further information

NICE. CKS Herpes simplex-ocular (2012). Available at: ℘ http://cks.nice.org.uk
NICE. CKS Warts and verrucae (2009). Available at: ℘ http://cks.nice.org.uk

# Pigmentation and hair problems

## Albinism

- Rare genetic condition in which melanocytes produce reduced or no pigment in skin, hair, and eyes.
- 1 in 20,000.
- Affects all races.
- Two main types:
  - Ocular-albinism, affects just eyes.
  - Oculo-cutaneous albinism, effects skin, eyes, and hair. Most common type (with sub varieties).

Associated with vision problems such as photophobia, nystagmus, strabisimus, requires specialist follow-up and support. Often people prefer dim lighting and/or wearing sunglasses. It requires high level skin protection in sun as vulnerable to sun burn (🕮 Skin cancer prevention, p. 331) and skin cancers. Can have a psychological impact and isolating effect.

## Vitiligo

Vitiligo appears as white patches due to loss of melanocytes in skin. It affects 1 in 100 people and men and women equally. 50% start before 20yrs. It is thought to be autoimmune response; 30% have FH. The areas most commonly affected—face, neck, hands, arms, elbows, and knees. A small percentage of people repigment.

### Management

No cure. May be referred to specialist for steroid therapy or PUVA to arrest spread or restore original skin colour. High risk of sunburn, so advise the use of high-factor sunscreens (can be prescribed BNF 13.8.1). May also benefit from skin camouflage (BNF 13.8.2) and psychological support.

## Alopecia or hair loss

Male pattern baldness is common. Alopecia means hair loss. May be due to side effects of other therapies, e.g. cytotoxic therapy or other conditions, e.g. ringworm.

### Alopecia areata

- Thought to be an auto-immune response of the hair.
- Sometimes FH.
- Affects men and women equally. 3 types named according to severity:
  - Alopecia areata, mild patchy hair loss on the scalp.
  - Alopecia totalis, loss of all scalp hair.
  - Alopecia universalis, loss of scalp and all body hair.

### Management

No cure. If <50% hair loss then 80% chance of re-growth. Severe cases referred to dermatology. Options include steroid creams, steroid injections, and topical contact immunotherapy. Some wigs may be available on the NHS. Counselling and emotional support may be required.

## Hirsutism or excess hairiness

Additional hair in male pattern on face, torso, and limbs, affects 1 in 100 women. Mostly idiopathic although may be associated with therapies, e.g. steroids, or syndromes, e.g. polycystic ovary syndrome. Patients are referred to a specialist as required, topical treatments available on consultant prescription only. Advice to those with idiopathic hirsutism includes home therapies of cosmetic bleaching, removal by creams, shaving, waxing, electrolysis. Laser therapy is available in some areas for those with severe problems.

### Hypertrichosis

- Excess hairiness in non-male pattern.
- Often caused by drug therapies, e.g. ciclosporin.
- If idiopathic advised as for hirsuitism.

## Further information

Albinism Fellowship. Available at: ◌ www.albinism.org.uk

Alopecia Online UK. Available at: ◌ www.alopeciaonline.org.uk

British Association of Dermatologists guidelines for the treatment of alopecia areata. Available at: ◌ www.bad.org.uk/health care/guidelines/

British Association of Dermatologists. Information Leaflet on Hirsutism. Available at: ◌ www. bad.org.uk

Changing Faces (includes skin camouflage). Available at: ◌ www.changingfaces.org.uk/Home

Vitiligo Society. Available at: ◌ www.vitiligosociety.org.uk/

# Allergies

An allergic reaction is an exaggerated response by the immune system to an allergen. Common allergens are house dust mite excreta, grass and tree pollen, moulds, pet hair, wasp and bee stings, industrial and household chemicals, medicines, e.g. penicillin, and foods such as milk and eggs. Less common allergens include latex, nuts, and fruit. The first exposure to the allergen causes the immune system to produce immunoglobulin E (IgE) antibodies which attach to mast cells. In subsequent exposures the allergens attach to the IgE antibodies and the cell releases histamines, causing widened blood vessels, leakage of fluid into tissues, and muscle spasms. Particular conditions associated with allergic problems include asthma (📖 p. 566), eczema (📖 p. 266), conjunctivitis (📖 Common problems affecting eyes, p. 697).

## Signs and symptoms

Common allergic symptoms include itching, watering eyes, sneezing, swelling, urticaria, and wheezing. See 📖 Anaphylaxis, p. 751.

## Assessment and management

### Investigations

Depends on the type and severity of symptoms and associated conditions, e.g. asthma. Referred to specialist allergy clinic if diagnosis in doubt, investigation and management of anaphylaxis, food allergies, occupational allergies.

### Management strategy

- Allergen avoidance, e.g. exclude pets, documentation of medication allergies especially penicillin, avoid pollen (keep windows shut, avoid grassy areas in pollen release season, wear wraparound sunglasses, wash hair/shower after being out, cover bed during day), check food labels for food allergens.
- Medication for symptoms or condition as required.
- Education and information on allergen avoidance and management.
- In severe allergic reactions, provision and education in the use of pre-loaded syringes of adrenalin for self administration or administration by family, carers, school staff. Also advice on wearing medic alert bracelets.

## Allergic rhinitis (including hayfever)

It is characterized by an irritation and inflammation of nose and eyes. Common disorder, often seasonal or perennial triggered by allergens affecting 16% of the UK population. Incidence ↑. Hayfever— is an allergic rhinitis caused by pollen. Sufferers may experience:

- Blocked stuffy nose, like having a permanent cold.
- Allergic conjunctivitis/itchy watery red eyes.
- Hayfever sufferers may have wheeze.
- Headaches and ear ache.
- Sleep disturbed and snoring.
- Poor concentration.
- ↓ sense and smell.

*Care and management*
- ↓ exposure to possible allergens (hayfever common causes grass pollen, June–August, and silver birch pollen, April).
- Steam and inhalations may provide temporary relief.
- *Medication:* low-dose steroid nasal sprays and nose drops, but need to be used on a daily basis. Decongestants also helpful, but short-term use only (BNF 12.2.1, 12.2.2). Check patient understands how to apply correctly or application will not be effective.
- *Hayfever:* treated with systematic antihistamine (BNF 3.4.1), and/or topical nasal spray (BNF 12.2.1), and/or eye drops (BNF 11.4.2). Most preparations available OTC. Severe symptoms may require a short course of oral steroids. Treatment should begin 2–3wks before pollen season: see BBC pollen index. Available at: ℘ www.bbc.co.uk/weather/pollen. Self-help advice includes wraparound sunglasses, avoid drying clothes outside.
- Consider referral to allergy clinic for testing and specialist review.

## Bee/wasp sting allergy
About 3 in 100 people who are stung have some kind of allergic reaction; minorities of these have severe reactions. Local or mild generalized reactions are treated with antihistamine. Severe reactions are usually followed up in allergy clinics. These individuals may be given pre-loaded syringes of adrenaline (epinephrine) (BNF 3.4.3) and taught how and when to use them (including all family, carers, others, e.g. school staff). May also be considered for a desensitization (to the allergen, i.e. insect venom) programme at the specialist clinic.

## Food allergies and intolerances
Present in about 5–7% of children, but less in adult population. A limited number of foods cause real allergic reactions—nuts (especially peanuts) wheat, eggs, fish, shellfish, and cows' milk. Some such as nut allergies provoke an acute, severe reaction and will be managed as severe reactions to stings as previously described.

There are a wide range of other types of food intolerances many caused by enzyme deficiencies (e.g. 📖 Coeliac disease, p. 666) or reactions to additives that do not involve an allergic response, but cause symptoms such as rashes, abdominal pain, vomiting, diarrhoea, palpitations. Referred to specialist allergy clinic for identification and advice on management. Advice for prevention of food allergy or intolerances developing includes breastfeeding, delaying introduction of solid food as per guidelines (see 📖 Bottle feeding, p. 178), avoid foods with preservatives and additives.

## Further information
Allergy UK: ☎ 01322 619 898. Available at: ℘ www.allergyuk.org
NICE Choices. Hayfever. Available at: ℘ www.nhs.uk/Conditions/Hay-fever/Pages/Introduction. aspx
NICE. CKS Allergic rhinicitis (2012). Available at: ℘ http://cks.nice.org.uk

# Deafness

Nearly 9 million in the UK are deaf or hard of hearing, being deaf can lead to depression and isolation. Categorized as:

- Mild deafness is when a person has difficulty following speech in noisy situations.
- Moderate deafness is when a person has difficulty following speech without a hearing aid.
- Severe deafness is when they use lip-reading to supplement use of hearing aid.
- Profound deafness means that there is so little ability to hear sounds, that BSL will be first language or may prefer lip reading for communication.

There are multiple possible causes:

- *Age:* >50% of people >60yrs have a hearing loss and 71% of >70yrs will have some hearing loss.
- *Noise:* prolonged and repeated exposure to loud noise at work/leisure. *Note:* young adults particularly vulnerable through personal stereos/ and loud dance music.
- *Conduction problems:* ear wax, trauma, perforated ear drum, and inflammation/infection.
- *Genetic:* 1 in every 1000 babies born moderately/profoundly deaf, 50% are thought to be due to genetic causes.

## Presentation in adults  (see 📖 Hearing screening, p. 155)

Slow onset with increasing difficulties in understanding people, e.g. when there is background noise. Questions to ask as part of assessment:

- Do people seem to be mumbling?
- Are you often saying pardon?
- Do you always hear the phone/door bell?
- Are conversations sometimes difficult to follow?
- Do other family members complain that the TV is on too loud?

## Management

Check that problem not caused by ear wax (📖 Ear care, p. 544), or presence of infection. If there is no obvious cause referral to GP for audiology or specialist ENT assessment to find cause for deafness, quantify hearing loss, and assess for possible hearing aid. Principles in working with people with hearing loss:

- Always face the deaf person in a well-lit room when talking to them.
- Write down important information.
- Mark nursing and medical notes with sign/sticker to alert other staff to hearing problems.
- Hearing aids are a significant step for many people and can take time to adjust to. Encourage to wear for short periods (10min) of time to build confidence.
- *Loop systems:* often available in public places for people with hearing aids helps to cut out background noise.

- Advise on telecommunications products that use both speech and text, which help with media like films and TV.
- Alerting devices are available to help improve deaf person's awareness of things happening around them, e.g. flashing light doorbell alert. May be purchased through RNID or supplied as part of Community Care support (📖 Assistive technology, p. 776).
- Hearing dogs (🖱 www.hearing-dogs.org.uk) trained to alert owners to significant sounds, have full access to public places under Disability Discrimination Act.

## Tinnitis

Ringing or buzzing heard in ear or head, occasional tinnitus common in 15% of population, for minority (2%) severe and can interfere with life and ability to sleep. Cause is often unknown. It can be very distressing and depressing. Possible management:
- Mask with background music/radio.
- White noise aid available from ENT depts.
- *Surgical sectioning of cochlear nerve:* last resort and causes permanent deafness.

Deaf people are eligible for benefits if the disability interferes with ability to work (📖 Benefits for illness, disability and carers, p. 795).

## Related topic

📖 Deafness in children, p. 263.

## Further information

British Deaf Association. Available at: 🖱 www.bda.org.uk/
Hearing dogs for the deaf. Available at: 🖱 www.hearingdogs.org.uk
Royal Association for Deaf People. Available at: 🖱 www.royaldeaf.org.uk/

# Mouth and throat problems

## Mouth ulcers

Common problem can make it difficult to eat, drink, and talk. Caused by:

* Traumas, e.g. tooth brushing, minor burns from hot drinks—last for approx. a week unless trauma recurs/persists, e.g. a rough tooth.
* *Apthous ulcers:* painful white ulcers commonly believed to be associated with stress (but no evidence to support this) and poor health. May first appear at puberty, take longer to heal and likely to recur until there is an improvement in health.
* Ulcers caused by herpes infection, or inflammatory bowel disease usually linked to other symptoms.
* Iron or vitamin B12 deficiency (📖 Anaemia, p. 604).

All red or white patches in the mouth and ulcers persisting for >3wks need medical assessment to exclude malignancy.

### Care and management

* Advise on good dental hygiene and regular dental check-ups.
* Healthy diet avoiding food and drink that may exacerbate symptoms, e.g. highly spiced foods.
* ↓ *pain:* paracetamol, iced water rinses, OTC anaesthetic gels, wafers.
* Adcortyl in Orabase® or Corlan® pellets (BNF 12.3) can be effective in treatment.

## Gingivitis

Inflammation of the gums often occurs with a buildup of plaque, mild cases patients may only have reddened gums can also be caused by:

* Trauma to gum.
* Pregnancy.
* DM.
* Smoking.
* Stress.
* Side effects of medication, e.g. phenytoin.
* Diet.

Gingivitis can lead to receding gums, halitosis, infection, abscesses, or loss of teeth. Occasionally patient may have acute ulcerative gingivitis (Vincent's angina) this will need antibiotic treatment.

### Care and management

As for mouth ulcers, see dentist to clean teeth and address any dental problems, also:

* Antiseptic toothpaste and mouth washes.
* Smoking cessation (📖 p. 315).

## Sore throat (including laryngitis and tonsillitis)

70% sore throats have viral cause and 90% resolve in a week. Antibiotics are unnecessary for most patients. Patients complain of pain on swallowing, fever. Adolescents with persistent sore throat need review for possible glandular fever (📖 Viral infections, p. 672). *Note:* anyone with stridor, breathing difficulty, or dehydration needs medical assessment.

*Care and management*
• Pain relief, e.g. ibuprofen.
• ↑ fluid intake and try aspirin (not in <16yrs) or salt gargles.
• Laryngitis as above, recommend resting voice and steam inhalations.
• Antibiotics only *if* evidence of systemic illness 2° to the sore throat, unilateral peri-tonsillitis, a history of rheumatic fever or patient is at ↑ risk of acute infection, e.g. immunodeficiency or child with DM.
• Patient with tonsillitis may be considered for tonsillectomy if patient has >4–6 episodes of sore throat/tonsillitis per year, effects interfere with normal functioning and schooling.
• Persistent sore throats may be a symptom of throat cancer and require medical assessment.

## Sinusitis

This is an acute or chronic inflammation of sinuses >90% of patients with maxillary sinusitis will clear in <1wk without antibiotics. Frontal sinusitus is associated with brain abscess and cavernous sinus thrombosis, and should ∴ be treated with amoxicillin or erthromycin. It is more common in adults and those with nasal abnormalities, cystic fibrosis (📖 p. 262), allergic rhinitis, and smokers. Acute sinusitis may follow upper respiratory tract infection, although 10% may come from dental problems. Characterized by:
• Acute headache and facial pain often worse bending or coughing.
• Fever.
• Blocked nose and/or purulent discharge.
• Loss of smell and taste.

*Care and management*
• Advise:
  • Stopping smoking and avoiding smoky environments.
  • Pain control, e.g. paracetamol.
  • Decongestant nose drops or sprays.
  • Steam inhalations.
• ENT referral considered for chronic sufferers for surgery to drain sinuses.

## Related topics
📖 Allergies, p. 647.

## Further information
NHS Choices. Mouth Ulcers. Available at: 🔗 www.nhs.uk/Conditions/Mouth-ulcer/Pages/Introduction.aspx
NICE. CKS Aphthous ulcer (2012), sinusitis – acute and chronic (2009), sore throat – acute (2012). Available at: 🔗 http://cks.nice.org.uk

# Adrenal disorders

The adrenal gland produces adrenaline and noradrenaline. The steroids have 3 main functions—virilization, conversion of tissue proteins to glucose, and salt and water retention. Adrenocortical disorders include:

## Cushing's syndrome

This is caused by high levels of adrenocortical hormones. In the majority of cases this is the result of the administration of prednisolone or other corticosteroids. Other rare causes include a pituitary adenoma. Cushing's syndrome has high morbidity and mortality. Signs and symptoms include redistribution of body fat to create a moon face and truncal obesity, hypertension, hirsuitism, acne, bruising and striae, osteoporosis, glycosuria and hyperglycaemia.

### Management

Steroids are reduced or stopped. If the cause is not due to prescribed steroids then patient is referred to an endocrinologist.

## Addison's disease

This is the result of adrenal cortical insufficiency. Most cases due to surgery, cessation of therapeutic steroids, autoimmune disorders. TB is a major cause outside of the UK. Early symptoms are—languor, debility, weight loss, pigmentation of the skin and mucous membranes. It can present as a crisis in a coma.

### Management and treatment

Patient referred to endocrinology. Treatment usually involves replacing deficient steroids. Treated patients have a normal lifespan. Advise patients to tell any health professional treating them about their condition and to wear a warning bracelet in case of emergency. Patients can apply for a medical exemption to NHS prescriptions (☐ Prescribing, p. 130).

## Further information

Addison's Disease Self-help Group. Available at: ℰ www.adshg.org.uk
NHS Choices. Cushing's Syndrome. Available at: ℰ www.nhs.uk/Conditions/Cushings-syndrome/Pages/Introduction.aspx

# Pituitary disorders

The pituitary gland secretes many hormones (adrenocortitrophic hormone (ACTH), anti-diuretic hormone (ADH), growth hormone, melanocyte-stimulating hormones (MSH), follicle-stimulating hormone (FSH), luteinizing hormone (LH), thyroid-stimulating hormone (TSH), oxytocin, and prolactin) and affects the function of most other glands in the endocrine system. Pituitary disorders are relatively rare in the UK.

## Hypopituitarism

↓ production of all pituitary hormones. It is caused by tumour, surgery, trauma, and necrosis from postpartum haemorrhage. Signs and symptoms include—hypogonadism, hypothyroidism, debility, weight loss.

### Management

Patients are referred to neurology or endocrinology. Treatment is lifelong hormone-replacement therapy supervised by a specialist.

## Pituitary tumours

These are relatively rare, can affect any part of the pituitary and be either malignant or non-malignant. Many pituitary adenomas are tiny and accidental findings on CT scans. These are usually left and watched.

### Sign and symptoms

Associated with the pressure effects on surrounding structures, e.g. chronic headache and visual disturbances. Also:

- Hypopituitarism.
- Hyperprolactaemia with associated galactorrhoea.
- ↓ libido.
- Menstrual disturbances.
- ↓ fertility.
- Impotence.

### Management

Patients are referred to neurology. Treatment options include surgery and radiotherapy. Prolactinomas will be treated medically.

## Acromegaly

Hyper-secretion of the growth hormone. This is a rare condition (40–60 per million) that has an insidious course over many years. Signs and symptoms include:

- Intercranial pressure effects, e.g. headaches.
- Changes in appearance:
  - Coarse, oily skin.
  - Change in facial appearance with coarsening of features.
  - ↑ foot size.
  - ↑ teeth spacing.
- Other effects:
  - Deepening of voice.
  - Sweating.
  - Paraesthesiae.
  - Proximal muscle weakness.
  - Progressive heart failure.
  - Goitre.

*Management*

Patients are referred to endocrinologist. Treatment options include surgery and medication, e.g. bromocriptine or radiotherapy.

## Diabetes insipidus

Impaired water reabsorption by the kidney caused either by ↓ ADH secretion or by trauma, tumour, or inherited. Signs and symptoms include: polydipsia, polyuria, dilute urine, dehydration. It is managed according to the cause.

## Further information

Pituitary Foundation: ☎ 0845 450 0375. Available at: ✆ www.pituitary.org.uk

# Thyroid

The thyroid concentrates iodine in order to produce the hormones thyroxine ($T_4$) and triiodothyronine ($T_3$). Thyroxine controls many body functions, including heart rate, temperature, and metabolism. It also plays a role in the metabolism of calcium in the body. Thryoid disorders present in 4% of the population.

Enlargement or lumps in the pre-tracheal neck region require medical assessment. Solitary thyroid nodules can be benign (~90%) or malignant (~10%). Goitres are enlarged thyroid glands that can be:

- *Physiological (associated with teenagers, pregnancy):* do not require treatment.
- *Nodular:* does not require treatment unless thyrotoxic, compressing other structures, or cosmetically unacceptable.
- *Toxic or inflammatory:* require treatment and referral to an endocrinologist.

## Hyperthyroidism

This affects 2% ♀ and 0.2% ♂. Peak age: 20–49yrs. Graves' disease is the most common cause of hyperthyroidism. It is an autoimmune disease associated with smoking and stressful life events in which antibodies to the TSH receptor are produced. Other causes include:

- Thyroiditis.
- Amiodarone.
- Kelp ingestion.
- *Toxic nodular goitre:* older women with past history of goitre.

### Signs and symptoms

- Weight loss.
- Tremor.
- Palpitations.
- Hyperactivity.
- Eye changes, exophthalmos.
- AF.
- Emotionally labile.
- Infertility.

In older people symptoms may be less obvious and include confusion, dementia, apathy, and depression.

### Management

Referred to an endocrinologist (and ophthalmologist if eye problems). Treatment options include beta-blockers to control symptoms, thionamides, e.g. carbimazole (warn patient to immediately stop taking the drug and seek medical help if they develop a sore throat or other infection) and radioactive iodine (may take 4mths for effects to become apparent). Women of childbearing age should avoid pregnancy during and 4mths after radioactive iodine treatment. Surgery is an option for patients with large goitres or who decline radioactive iodine. Long-term monitoring of thyroid function is necessary.

# Hypothyroidism (myxoedema)

A deficiency of thyroid hormones which results in a lowered rate of all metabolic processes. Common: 10% ♀ >60yrs. ♀:♂~ratio 8:1.

## Causes

Chronic autoimmune thyroiditis, that occurs after treatment with radioactive iodine, thyroidectomy. Onset tends to be insidious and may go undiagnosed for years.

Patients with hypercholesterolaemia, infertility, depression, dementia, obesity, and other autoimmune diseases, Turner's syndrome or congenital hypothyroidism are screened using thyroid function tests (TFTs).

## Signs and symptoms

Non-specific symptoms may include:
- Depression.
- Fatigue.
- Lethargy or general malaise.
- Weight gain.
- Constipation.
- Hoarse voice or dry skin/hair.
- Mental dulling.

## Management

If the TSH concentration is greater than 10mU/L (confirmed on repeated testing) commenced on treatment with levothyroxine. Specialist advice sought if very elderly prior to prescribing. <50yrs initial dose of 50–100mcg of thyroxine is prescribed (to be taken before breakfast) and TFTs re-checked after 6wks. Once TSH is within the normal range then TFT is monitored annually. If >50yrs or pre-existing heart disease, has 25mcg of thyroxine and dose ↑ every 4wks, according to TFTs. Patients taking thyroxine replacement are entitled to apply for medical exemption from NHS prescription charges (☐ Prescribing, p. 130).

## Related topic

☐ Hyper- and hypocalcaemia, p. 658.

## Further information

British Thyroid Foundation. Available at: ✂ www.btf-thyroid.org
NICE. CKS Hypothyroidism (2011). Available at: ✂ http://cks.nice.org.uk

# Hyper- and hypocalcaemia

See 📖 Thyroid, p. 656; 📖 Common musculoskeletal problems, p. 688.

Most of the calcium in the body is in bone and needed for constant renewal. Calcium is important in normal neuromuscular activity and blood coagulation. Check calcium levels on an *uncuffed* blood sample to avoid falsely high readings (📖 Peripheral venipuncture, p. 535). Assessment of serum calcium concentration includes consideration of serum albumin levels (📖 Biochemical and haematological values, p. 780).

## Hypocalcaemia

↓ level of serum calcium. Causes include: hypoparathyroidism (may be 2° to thyroid or parathyroid surgery), insensitivity to parathyroid hormone, osteomalacia, over-hydration, and pancreatitis. Signs and symptoms include tetany, neuromuscular excitability, carpo-pedal spasm (wrist flexion and fingers drawn together).

### Management

Calcium supplements prescribed and referred to specialist for investigation of cause.

## Hypercalcaemia

↑ level of serum calcium (>2.6mmol/L). It affects ~1:1000. Causes include: 1° hyperparathyroidism, malignancy (10% tumours), chronic renal failure. More rarely: familial benign hypercalcaemia, milk alkali syndrome (high use of antacids for indigestion), thyrotoxicosis, vitamin D treatment. Signs and symptoms are often very non-specific, but can include:

- Lethargy.
- Weakness.
- Weight loss.
- Low mood.
- Mild aches and pains.
- Nausea.

### Management

This is according to the cause.

## Further information

NICE. CKS Hypercalcaemia (2010). Available at: ℰ http://cks.nice.org.uk

# Anal conditions

**Anal cancer** Squamous cell cancer. It is more common in ♀. Risk ↑ by HPV, anal intercourse, smoking, lowered immunity, e.g. HIV. Patient may present with bleeding, pain, small lumps or ulcers around anus pruritus or change in bowel habit. Symptoms require medical assessment and referral to specialist treatment as appropriate. Treated by surgery, radiotherapy and/or chemotherapy as determined by size and stage.

## Anal fissure

Is when the anal mucosa is torn or ulcerated, occurs at any age, can be acute or chronic, i.e. >6wks. Most are caused by constipation, but also child birth and IBD. Patient may complain of pain on defaecation, anal spasm, fresh rectal bleeding (noticed on toilet paper).

*Care and management*
Usually heal within a few weeks without medical treatment, but preventing constipation (📖 Constipation in adults, p. 460). Advise to: have high fibre diet, and good fluid intake → soften stools, ↓ pain by use of topical treatments such as OTC haemorrhoid preparations, encourage good personal hygiene. Warm baths may provide relief. If no relief advise to consult GP, may require specialist surgical opinion.

## Anal itch

Pruritis ani often occurs if anus is moist or soiled, e.g. fissures, incontinence, poor hygiene. *Note:* there is the possibility of thread worm, haemorrhoids, dermatological problems (📖 Eczema/dermatitis, p. 636).

*Care and management*
Advise on personal hygiene particularly after bowel movement, OTC anaesthetic cream, and avoiding spicy food may help.

   *Note:* any signs of trauma around anus in child should consider possibility of child abuse (📖 Identifying the child in need of protection, p. 232).

## Haemorrhoids (piles)

Approx. 50% of people in UK will develop a haemorrhoid at some stage in their life. They occur when the veins in anus distend and swell. Patients complain of discomfort, fresh red bleeding, feeling of incomplete emptying, mucous, pruritis ani. Risk factors: constipation, straining, obesity, pregnancy, portal hypertension. Classified according to severity:

- *1st degree:* small swelling inside the anal canal, not visible external to anus or palpable, most common, but may enlarge to become 2nd degree.
- *2nd degree:* prolapse from anus (often on defaecation), but spontaneously reduce.
- *3rd degree:* prolapse from anus, can be felt as small soft lumps, possible to reduce and push back with a finger.
- *4th degree:* permanently prolapsed.

**Possible complication of 3rd and 4th degree**  Thrombosis and strangulation.

*Care and management*
- As with anal fissures (see 📖 p. 659).
- Encourage patients not to wait to open their bowels.
- Often clear up on their own or with OTC ointments.
- Advise consult GP if problem persists, or pain or bleeding.

**Peri-anal abscess** Affects people of any age and is an infection in a peri-anal gland, patients may complain of gradual onset of pain becoming more severe, defaecation and sitting very painful. This requires medical assessment for urgent referral for surgery to drain abscess (see 📖 Post-operative wound care, p. 478). *Note:* peri-anal abscesses can be difficult to diagnose.

**Peri-anal haematoma** Due to ruptured peri-anal vein, presents with sudden onset of severe pain and visible 'dark blue berry' under skin next to the anus. Treated with analgesia, settles spontaneously over a week.

## Pilonidal sinus

An obstruction of hair follicles between the buttocks (natal cleft) → foreign body reaction that includes pain, swelling abscess, and or fistula formation often with foul smelling discharge. Most commonly occurs ivn teenagers and young adults and more common in ♂. Risk factors include:
- Sedentary occupation (especially if involves long hours driving).
- Obesity.
- Persistent irritation or trauma in affected area.
- FH.

*Care and management*
Surgery to excise and drain sinus tract. Post-operatively encourage personal hygiene. These post-operative wounds (📖 p. 478) can take weeks to heal. Alginate dressing then a foam dressing *in situ* to prevent premature closure of wound edges although contraindicated if signs of infection (📖 Wound assessment, p. 496). Progressively reduce foam dressing as wound heals and contracts. These can recur.

## Rectal prolapse

Relatively common and people may live with it for years before seeking help. Occurs either in the very young or those >60yrs. In adults there are 2 types:
- *Mucosal:* bowel musculature stays in position, but redundant mucosa prolapses out of the anus. Occurs in adults with 3rd degree haemorrhoids.
- *Complete:* descent of the upper rectum into the anal canal. Often caused by weak pelvic floor muscles following child birth.

Referred for specialist assessment for surgery or where this is not possible a supporting ring may be used.

**Skin tags** Seldom cause any problems. Cause unknown.

## Further information

Macmillan Cancer Support. Anal Cancer. Available at: ℅ www.macmillan.org.uk/
NICE. CKS: Haemorrhoids (2012). Available at: ℅ http://cks.nice.org.uk/
World Wide Wounds. Pilonidal sinus disease. Available at: ℅ www.worldwounds.com

# Dyspepsia, gastro-oesophageal reflux disease, and peptic ulceration

## Dyspepsia

Very common, characterized by recurrent epigastric pain, heartburn, or acid regurgitation, can include bloating, nausea, and vomiting. Cause often unknown, but can be due to gastric oesophageal reflux disease (see 📖 p. 661), gastric and peptic ulceration, or rarely cancer. Can also be exacerbated by:

- Medication (e.g. $Ca^{2+}$ agonists, nitrates, theophyllines, bisphosphonates, SSRIs, corticosteroids, and NSAIDs).
- Previous gastric surgery or history of ulceration.

*Note:* people presenting with 'indigestion' may in fact have cardiac pain.

Requires urgent medical assessment if any of the following with dyspepsia:
- Bleeding and/or iron deficiency anaemia.
- Dysphagia.
- Recurrent vomiting and/or weight loss.

*Helicobacter pylori bacteria* (major cause of gastric ulceration) present in approx. 50% of UK middle aged population so does not always trigger disease. In patients with non-specific symptoms consider referral to GP for tests (e.g. urea breath test, faecal antigen test) and eradication therapy of antibiotics and anti-secretory medication according to set regimen.

### Care and management

- Review with patient possible triggers to avoid, e.g. medication, particular foods or actions such as bending, posture, etc.
- Lifestyle advice, e.g. weight loss, smoking cessation, alcohol.
- *Self-care:* antacids and alginates for symptomatic treatment (BNF 1.1).
- Eating smaller meals, not eating before bed and propping up bed head can help control symptoms.
- If *H. pylori* has been excluded then patient may be prescribed low-dose proton pump inhibitor (e.g. omeprazole BNF 1.3) for a month following by the use of self-care alternatives, e.g. antacids/alginates using antacids as the need arises. Also referred to 2° care patients with unresolved/ongoing symptoms.

## Gastro-oesophageal reflux disease

Heartburn common symptom of gastro-oesophageal reflux disease (GORD) can also experience reflux of acid in the mouth, nausea and vomiting, nocturnal cough. Symptoms caused by regurgitation of gastric contents irritating oesophagus. It affects approx. 5% population. GORD can cause oesophagitis, oesophageal strictures, oesophageal haemorrhage, and anaemia.

*Risk factors* Include: diet rich in fatty foods, alcohol, smoking, hiatus hernia, Barrett's oesophagus (intestinal metaplasia), obesity pregnancy.

*Care and management*
As for dyspepsia.

## Gastritis

Inflammation of the stomach mucosa when there is no ulcer present although may lead to subsequent ulceration if *H. pylori* is the cause. Vitamin B12 deficiency can cause symptoms and certain medication, e.g. NSAIDs.

*Care and management* As for dyspepsia.

## Hiatus hernia

Hiatus hernia is common and present in 30% of >50yrs. 50% of these have GORD. It occurs when proximal stomach herniates/protrudes through a tear or weakness in the diaphragm into the thorax. Major risk factor is obesity.
- Sliding hiatus hernia (80% of sufferers).
- Rolling hiatus hernia where a bulge of the stomach herniates into the chest alongside the oesophagus.

*Care and management* As for dyspepsia and GORD.

## Peptic ulceration

Peptic ulceration includes gastric (GU) and duodenal ulceration (DU).
- *GU:* usually affects middle-aged and older ♂, may be asymptomatic or complain of epigastric pain made worse with food, but helped with antacids and/or lying flat.
- *DU:* affects young/middle aged ♂, can affect any adult, maybe asymptomatic or relapse and remit. Epigastric pain is typically relieved by food and worse at night.

*Complications* Includes bleeding, perforation requiring emergency admission, pyloric stenosis—scarring from chronic DU. Results in unrelieved and copious vomiting of food which requires medical assessment and referral for surgery.

*Risk factors* Include *H. pylori* (main cause in both types of ulcer >90% in DU), NSAID use, smoking.

*Care and management*
- Investigation and treatment as for dyspepsia.
- If possible stop NSAIDs, lower dose or safer option, e.g. paracetamol.
- Medication may include PPI, or H2 receptor agonist (BNF 1.3).
- Lifestyle advice as described earlier, eat little and often, avoid eating 3hrs before bed.
- Referred to 2° care if symptoms persist/unrelieved.

## Further information

CORE. Charity for research and awareness into gut and liver disease. Available at: ℘ www.core-charity.org.uk/

NICE (2004). *Managing adults with dyspepsia in primary care (CG17)*. Available at: ℘ http://guidance.nice.org.uk/CG17

# Irritable bowel syndrome

Irritable bowel syndrome (IBS) is an extremely common GI problem. 5–19% of ♀ and up to 12% of ♂ although majority will not seek professional help. Stress/food intolerance/infection are often thought to precipitate symptoms that can occur at any age though most commonly first presents between 30–50yrs. Characterized by abdominal pain and change in bowel habit although can include the following: cramps, constipation or diarrhoea, feeling bloated, flatus, mucus, urgency to open bowels, nausea/vomiting.

It is a socially isolating condition, often misunderstood or not taken seriously and leads to poorer QoL compared to those without symptoms.

❶ Patient should see GP for confirmation of diagnosis of IBS and to discount other possible causes, e.g. colonic cancer, inflammatory bowel disease (Crohn's disease (CrD)), infection, endometriosis.

## Care and management
- *Reassurance:* IBS is not a life-threatening condition, support patient and provide information about condition.
- Reduce incidence and impact of symptoms on patient's life.
- Review with patient possible triggers (e.g. particular foods, social situations), plan how to avoid these. For some exclusion diets are successful, e.g. exclude dairy products, citrus, caffeine, alcohol, gluten, eggs.

### General advice
- Some patients find small and frequent meals help reduce symptoms.
- Healthy diet that is rich in fibre. Probiotics often recommended, but evidence weak, consider referral to dietician.
- Smoking cessation (📖 p. 315).
- Exercise (📖 p. 313).
- Self-management and expert patients (📖 p. 303).

### For specific symptoms
- *Constipation if diet insufficient:* consider bulk forming laxatives.
- *Abdominal pain:* peppermint oil and antispasmodics, e.g. mebeverine (BNF 1.2).
- *Diarrhoea:* loperamide (BNF 1.4). Sometimes possible to anticipate events and situations that precipitate symptoms and take anti-diarrhoeals prophylactically.
- *Psychological support:* talking therapies/counselling (📖 Talking therapies, p. 429).

Patients will need specialist referral if symptoms are severe, change and/or do not respond to treatments.

## Further information
Irritable bowel syndrome network. Available at: ℳ www.theibsnetwork.org/
NICE. CKS Irritable Bowel Syndrome (2013). Available at: ℳ http://cks.nice.org.uk/

# Inflammatory bowel disease

Ulcerative colitis (UC) and CrD are chronic, relapsing inflammatory non-infectious conditions of the gut. Approx. 1:1000 in UK develop UC and 1:1500 people develop CrD. Cause is unknown although environmental and genetic factors, infections, and possibly foods are thought to adversely affect susceptible individuals. Symptoms described in Table 12.1. All patients with suspected UC or CrD referred to specialist gastro-enterology for assessment.

> ❶ Emergency referral to hospital by GP if any of the following: severe abdominal pain, severe diarrhoea >8/days and bleeding, dramatic weight loss, fever, and signs of systemic disease.

## Care and management

Both conditions are lifelong and characterized by flare-ups and periods of remission. Patients can become socially isolated and depressed. Most patients have ongoing hospital follow-up and the MDT always provides care across 1° and 2° care settings.

- *UC:* most patients will have symptoms controlled by medication to reduce the impact of inflammation and prolong periods of remission. Mainstay of treatment are 5-ASA derivatives, aminosalicylates, e.g. mesalazine and corticosteroids, e.g. prednisolone (BNF 1.5). CrD patients receive similar medication regimen plus antibiotics and monocloncal antibodies (e.g. infliximab). *Note:* NSAIDs can exacerbate symptoms.
- *Surgery:* for CrD to remove damaged part of the colon and/or as for UC when symptoms cannot be managed medically → ilestomy/ileo-anal pouch (🕮 Stoma care, p. 466).
- Advise patients on:
  - Side effects of steroid treatment and consider increased risk of osteoporosis (🕮 p. 558).
  - *Diet:* healthy diet important to maintain fluid intake during bouts of diarrhoea, frequent eating can exacerbate discomfort during acute phases of disease. Patients may need dietary supplements. Enteral nutrition sometimes prescribed for children and adolescents failing to grow.
  - Smoking cessation (🕮 p. 315).
  - Patients who have had ileal resection will have B12 levels checked and possible supplementation.
  - Contraception (🕮 p. 359) for women with active IBS, e.g. COC, not advised due to malabsorption, but effective contraception must be used if taking monoclonal therapies and for 6mths after.
  - Fertility may be suboptimal in ♀ with active IBD and pregnancy has to be planned when IBD controlled, and after 6mths when monoclonal or methotrexate therapies ceased.
  - Self-management and expert patients (🕮 p. 303).
  - *Psychological support:* talking therapies (🕮 p. 429).

**Table 12.1** UC and CrD symptoms vary according to extent and severity of inflammation

| Ulcerative colitis | Crohn's disease |
|---|---|
| • At any time 50% will be asymptomatic. | • Diarrhoea often with blood and mucous, mouth ulcers. |
| • *Mild:* 30% have mild symptoms, usually limited to rectum (proctitis) with diarrhoea and or rectal bleeding may be mistaken for haemorrhoids. | • Abdominal pain, weight loss. |
| | • Fever and general tiredness. |
| • *Moderate:* symptoms more severe with frequent stools with blood (4–6 liquid stools a day), pain relieved with defaecation. General tiredness, fatigue, weight loss. Other symptoms may occur: skin rashes, uveitis, arthritis, inflammation of the liver. | • Peri-anal sores and/or abscess with discharge (may be first indication of CrD). |
| | • Can also have related symptoms that included uveitis, pain, arthritis, skin rashes liver inflammation. |
| • *Severe:* profuse diarrhoea, bleeding, high fever, abdominal tenderness and distention, tenesmus (constant desire to defaecate). ↓ appetite and weight, fatigue. | • *Complications include:* strictures caused by scar tissue = impedes the passage of food → pain and vomiting. |
| • Severe episodes uncommon, but can cause serious illness, danger of perforation or haemorrhage (requiring surgical intervention). | • Perforation of the gut wall (potentially life threatening). |
| • Patients with UC have an increased risk of developing cancer. | • Creation of fistulas (often peri-anal between colon and other organs = leakage). People with CrD have a small ↑ risk of cancer. |

## Further information

Crohn's and Colitis UK. Available at: ℜ www.crohnsandcolitis.org.uk/
NICE. CKS Crohn's disease (2012). Clinical Knowledge Summaries (Prodigy) guidelines. Available at: ℜ http://cks.nice.org.uk/#azTab

# Coeliac disease

A common autoimmune GI disease. UK prevalence approx. 1:300 (many undiagnosed). Lifelong inflammatory disease of the upper small intestine triggered by eating gluten: protein found in wheat, rye, and barley (occasionally oats). It occurs at any age, causing villous atrophy → malabsorption problems. Peak occurrence in childhood and then further peak in mid-adulthood.

## Risk factors

- Environmental.
- FH (risk increases 1:10 if family member has coeliac disease).

Patients are often either asymptomatic or have non-specific symptoms. The following summarizes how coeliac disease can present (can be mistaken for IBS or wheat intolerance):

- *Infants and children:* in babies being weaned may fail to thrive, suffer from diarrhoea and vomiting and be generally pale and irritable with swollen abdomen. Older children may present with loss of appetite, anaemia and vitamin deficiencies, may have steatorrhoea. *Note:* lack of growth may be most significant symptom.
- *Adults:* majority complain of tiredness and fatigue, weight loss, and bowel symptoms, e.g. constipation, diarrhoea, flatus. May have mouth ulcers, sore tongue and mouth. Some patients develop dermatitis herpetiformis (itchy skin condition) and/or osteoporosis related bone pain.

### Associated health issues and complications

- Due to mal-absorption of calcium ↑ risk of osteoporosis.
- Link between coeliac disease and type 1 diabetes and hypothyroidism.
- Small ↑ risk of GI malignancy, reduced after gluten-free diet for 3–5yrs.

*Lactose intolerance:* common in undiagnosed people once inflammation of the intestine subsides then intolerance usually goes.

> All people with suspected symptoms of coeliac disease will need referral for specialist assessment and confirmation of diagnosis.

## Care and management

Gluten-free diet will give complete remission from symptoms within weeks. Patient will need to remain on a gluten-free diet for life.

- Reassure that there is a wide choice of alternative gluten-free foods and refer to dietician for specialist support and advice.
- Patient may initially need vitamin supplements.
- ♀ planning a family should take folic acid until 12wks gestation.
- Skin symptoms can take up to a year to settle.

## Further information

Coeliac UK: Helpline ☎ 0845 305 2060. Available at: ✍ www.coeliac.co.uk
NICE (2009). *Recognition and assessment of coeliac disease (CG86).* Available at: ✍ www.nice.org.uk/CG86

# Colorectal cancer

Colorectal cancer is the fourth most common cancer in the UK. Highest rates in Scotland. Lifetime risk 1:25. Incidence increases with age and 99% occurs in people >40yrs. Risk factors include: ↑ age, FH, IBD (📖 Inflammatory bowel disease, p. 664). Diets high in fibre ↓ risk.

## Screening

See 📖 Bowel cancer screening, p. 334.

## Symptoms

Patients should have a medical assessment if:

- Change in bowel habit.
- Rectal bleeding.
- Complain of abdominal or rectal mass.
- General effects such as weight loss, anaemia, malaise especially if a FH of bowel cancer.

Suspicious lower GI tract symptoms urgently referred to specialist.

## Care and management

Treatment is usually surgical, also radiotherapy and/or chemotherapy (📖 Chemotherapy in the home, p. 507). Care provided by MDT.

- *Patient education, support, and advice:* patients with tumour confined to bowel wall have >90% chance of survival.
- May have stoma (📖 p. 466) post-operatively.
- May benefit from review of diet and referral to dietician.
- Advise on smoking cessation (📖 p. 315) and diet.
- Link to support organizations.
- Consider referral to community palliative care services for patients with advanced disease.
- Genetic advice for family members and possible referral for screening, e.g. colonoscopy.

## Further information

Beating Bowel Cancer. Available at: ℛ www.beatingbowelcancer.org/
British Association of Cancer United Patients. Available at: ℛ www.bacup.org.uk
Cancer Research UK (2012). Bowel Cancer Key Facts. Available at: ℛ www.cancerresearchuk.org/h
Macmillan Cancer Support. Bowel Cancer. Available at: ℛ www.macmillan.org.uk/
NICE (2011). Colorectal cancer: the diagnosis and management of colorectal cancer (CG131).
Available at: ℛ http://guidance.nice.org.uk/CG131

# Appendicitis, diverticulitis, hernias, and intestinal obstruction

## Appendicitis

Appendicitis is an infection in the appendix. It is the most common surgical emergency in the UK. Affecting mainly people aged 10–30yrs. Always requires emergency admission (although 50% suspected appendicitis admissions turn out to be something else, e.g. UTI, food poisoning, ectopic pregnancy, diverticulitis or false alarm). Complications can include peritonitis from perforation, abscess and ♀ infertility.

Commonly patient will complain of:
- Abdominal colicky pain becoming progressively worse and more constant and localizing in right iliac fossa, worse on walking and movement (may walk stooped).
- Tenderness and guarding when palpated.
- Dysuria, may be blood or leucocytes in urine.
- Nausea and vomiting.
- Anorexia.
- Fever and generally flushed and unwell.
- May have nausea and vomiting.

It requires medical assessment and emergency referral. *Note:* in ♀ child-bearing age an ectopic pregnancy is a possibility and pregnancy test are undertaken to exclude this.

## Diverticulosis

A common condition that occurs when the colon wall is weaker in some areas than others and small 'pouches' (i.e. diverticula) are forced outwards through the outer layer of the colonic wall. Common in >30% of people >60yrs, the majority have no or only mild symptoms. Diagnosis confirmed through endoscopy or barium enema. Predisposing factors include low roughage diet, history of constipation, and increasing age. Encourage patients to:
- ↑ fibre and fluid intake (may benefit from bulk forming agents, e.g. bran, ispaghula, and methylcellulose).
- ↑ activity will ↓ constipation.
- Anti-spasmodic medication and peppermint oil can ↓ colicky pain.

## Diverticulitis

This occurs when there is infection and inflammation precipitated by faeces trapped in the diverticula and bacterial infection. A complication of diverticulitis is peritonitis. Patients complain of:
- Altered bowel habit.
- Abdominal colicky pain.
- Nausea and flatulence (may be improved with defaecation).

Patients require medical assessment. Acute diverticulitis treated with antibiotics (e.g. co-amoxiclav), painkillers, anti-spasmodics, laxatives, and diet. In severe cases or patients at higher risk (e.g. older person, someone who is immunosuppressed) may be admitted to hospital. Diverticulitis recurs in up to a third of cases. Advise on diet and prevention as for diverticulosis.

# Hernias

Hernias occurs when there is an abnormal protrusion of peritoneal contents through a weakness in the abdominal wall. Common problem: inguinal hernia most common, occurs in ♂>♀, and at any age. It may be precipitated by a chronic cough, constipation, urinary obstruction, heavy lifting previous abdominal surgery. Patient complain of:

- Lump in the groin which in ♂ can track down into the scrotum.
- Discomfort when straining or standing for long periods.

Hernias require medical assessment. Usually requires surgery, high success rate with little recurrence advised because hernia may enlarge and ↑ discomfort, risk of strangulation → emergency surgery. Small hernias may not require surgery. Trusses are used for patients who are a poor surgical risk or are awaiting surgery. Lifestyle advice: to maintain ideal weight, healthy diet, and learn correct lifting and handling procedures.

*Hiatus hernia*: see 📖 Dyspepsia gastroesophageal reflux disease, and peptic ulceration, p. 661.

## Incisional hernia (post- abdominal surgery)

Bulging at the side of operation site occurs when there is a breakdown of the muscle closure at an abdominal wall. It is a late complication in up to 10% of surgical cases. It may have been preceded by wound infection or haematoma. It does not always need surgical intervention. If causing pain, discomfort or risk of obstruction or strangulation then referred to 2° care for surgical review/treatment.

*Umbilical hernia*: most common in infants, in adults may present as a bulge next to the umbilicus. It requires medical assessment and may be referred for surgical assessment, as strangulation or obstruction risk is high.

## Intestinal obstruction

Arises from mechanical obstruction or failure of peristalsis, It requires urgent medical assessment and referral for surgical intervention. Types:

- *Obstruction external to bowel:* e.g. adhesions, volvulus, external malignancy, strangulated hernia.
- *Obstruction internal to the bowel:* e.g. cancer of the bowel, infarction, inflammatory bowel disease, diverticulitis.
- *Obstruction in the lumen:* constipation/impaction, large polyps, intussusception, swallowed foreign body, gallstone ileus.
- *Ileus functional obstruction:* e.g. post op, DM, uraemia, anticholinergic drugs.

Patients complain of anorexia, nausea and vomiting, abdominal pain and distention, though no guarding or rebound, uncomfortable, and restless.

## Further information

Bladder and Bowel Foundation. Diverticulitis. Available at: ℜ www.bladderandbowelfoundation. org/default.asp

NHS Choices. Hernia. Available at: ℜ www.nhs.uk/conditions/hernia/Pages/Introduction.aspx

# Problems of the liver, gallbladder, and pancreas

See 📖 Viral hepatitis, p. 676.

## Cirrhosis

Characterized by fibrosis/scarring of the liver due to progressive cumulative damage. It is more common in people >40yrs and in ♂, 3000 deaths a year. Uncertain prognosis: 50% living for >5yrs. Causes can include:

- Excessive alcohol intake (misconception this is the only cause).
- Chronic hepatitis B or C infection.
- Autoimmune chronic active hepatitis.
- Active hepatitis.
- Primary biliary cirrhosis and other chronic diseases of the bile duct, e.g. sclerosing cholangitis, biliary atresia in children.
- Congenital disease.
- Prolonged exposure to drugs or toxins.
- Vascular disease.

Patients with cirrhosis can be asymptomatic, but they may experience:

- Anorexia.
- Lethargy, fatigue, and general feeling of being unwell.
- Nausea and vomiting.

In the later stages of the disease:

- Jaundice.
- Itching.
- Ascites and oedema.
- Haematemesis.
- Confusion arising from encephalopathy.
- Weight loss.
- Hepatomegaly.

Patient requires specialist gastroenterological care. Complications include hypertension, liver cancer, liver and renal failure. Ongoing care:

- Avoid alcohol and advice on diet and nutrition.
- Pruritis (itching) may be relieved by colestyramine (BNF 1.9.2).
- Ensure flu and pneumoccal immunization.

To reduce the risk of developing cirrhosis patients should be advised to:

- Drink alcohol (📖 p. 319) within normal limits.
- Safe sex to avoid risk of hepatitis B (see 📖 Sexual health, p. 711).
- Consider immunization against hepatitis A and B (📖 Viral hepatitis, p. 676).

## Portal hypertension

It is a consequence of chronic liver disease/cirrhosis. Other rarer causes are parasitic disease (common in Middle East), pancreatic disease, and clotting disorders. BP ↑ in portal vein which carries blood from bowel and spleen to liver → collateral circulation. It causes oesophageal varices, which can ooze blood causing anaemia, maleana, or haemorrhage and/or haematemesis. Early treatment of varices can be very effective, but bleeding is a medical emergency.

## Gallstones

Made of cholesterol and bile pigments, 9% of those >60yrs have gallstones and prevalence ↑ with age. ♀>♂, associated with obesity, affluence, also pregnancy. Can be asymptomatic or complain of vague intermittent discomfort. Patient with obstructed, inflamed, infected bile duct may experience:

- *Biliary colic:* severe upper abdominal pain causing jaundice, nausea and vomiting. Requires medical assessment for analgesia and possible emergency admission.
- *Acute cholycystitis:* pain and tenderness in epigastrium. Requires medical assessment for antibiotics, analgesia, and possible referral to 2° care.

### Care and management

- Low-fat diet and maintain ideal weight.
- Patients referred to secondary care may be offered lithotripsy, endoscopic retrograde cholangiopancreatography, cholycystectomy.
- Post surgery patients may still experience symptoms that may settle over time.

## Pancreatitis An inflammation of the pancreas.

### Acute pancreatitis

Sudden onset of acute epigastric pain often with nausea and vomiting can be self-limiting. Range of possible causes: most commonly alcohol, gallstones, and medication. Patient admitted as medical emergency. To avoid further attacks:

- Advise to avoid triggers, e.g. alcohol.
- Advise low-fat diet.
- Ensure avoidable causes are addressed, e.g. gallstones.

### Chronic pancreatitis

Causes gradual destruction and fibrosis with loss of pancreatic function, mal-absorption, and DM (📖 p. 611). Alcohol (📖 p. 319) is the commonest cause also cystic fibrosis (📖 p. 262). It is characterized by chronic ill health, fatigue, and weight loss, pain radiating to the back sometimes relieved by sitting forwards, steatorrhoea, jaundice, pain and vomiting, DM.

### Care and management

- *Diet:* low fat, high protein, high calories with fat soluble vitamins.
- Pancreatic enzyme supplementation.
- No alcohol.
- Pain control.
- Referred to 2° care for possible surgery.
- Management of diabetes (📖 Principles of diabetic care and control, p. 615).

## Further information

British Liver Trust. Available at: ℘ www.britishlivertrust.org.uk
NICEs CKS Pancreatitis-acute (2012). Available at: ℘ http://cks.nice.org.uk/
Pancreatitis Supporter's Network. Available at: ℘ www.pacnreatitis.org.ukInfectious diseases

# Viral infections

Viruses are the smallest known type of infectious agent and consist of genetic material surrounded by 1 or 2 protective protein shells. Viruses enter through mucous membranes, latch on or enter cells and then multiply. Spread can be airborne (coughing, sneezing), passed on by touch, or though body fluids, e.g. blood, saliva, semen. The body's own immune system then has to deal with the virus. Vaccinations have been developed for many common viral infections, e.g. childhood infections, which sensitize the immune system to rapidly produce antibodies to destroy those viruses. Viral infections are the usual causes of colds, rashes, diarrhoea, influenza, sore throats, cold sores, etc. Most are mild, short lasting, but can cause the person to feel very unwell. They do not respond to antibiotics. More serious if the person is immune-compromised or vulnerable in some other way. *Note:* immunocompromised people and pregnant ♀ should seek medical advice if exposed to conditions such as chickenpox or parvovirus infection.

## Self-help advice for viral infections
- Keep comfortable, warm, and rested.
- Avoid unnecessary contact with others to ↓ spread (*Note:* self-certification for first 7 days from work).
- Drink plenty of liquids.
- Take paracetamol or similar for aches, pains, and fevers.
- Seek medical advice if illness appears to be getting worse after a few days, or complications, e.g. ear infection, sinusitis, exacerbation of asthma, COPD.

## Common viral infections
- *Common cold:* as above in self-help advice.
- *Childhood infections:* e.g. mumps, measles, rubella (🕮 Infections in children, p. 282).
- *Skin infections:* (🕮 Viral skin infections, p. 643).
- *Seasonal influenza* (flu): (see 🕮 Targeted immunizations for adults, p. 347).

3 main types: C causes a mild form, like a cold and immunity for life, A and B alter to produce new strains. Symptoms: fever, headache, muscle ache, weakness, and mucus in respiratory tract. Patients are at risk of severe symptoms if COPD, DM, CHD, immunosuppressed, older people, immobile—pre-winter vaccination available. It is treated by rest, fluids, and paracetamol. Antiviral used with high-risk groups (>65yrs, pregnant, LTC, immunocompromised) when flu incidence high to shorten duration of symptoms and ↓ risk of complications. HPA monitors incidence of influenza and alerts practitioners when antivirals can be used. Complications treated as required. 2° chest infection common.

*Herpes virus:*
- *Herpes zoster:* chickenpox (see 📖 Viral skin infections, p. 642).
- *Herpes zoster:* shingles (see 📖 Viral skin infections, p. 642).
- *Herpes simplex HSV 2:* genital (📖 Sexually transmitted infections, p. 715).
- *Herpes simplex HSV1:* commonly causes cold sores, herpetic stomatitis, and keratitis. Prodromal period (<6hrs) of tingling or itching, small vesicles appear, persist for a few days, then dry forming yellowish crust. Healing occurs 8–12 days after onset. Remains dormant in nerve ganglia, recurrent eruptions can occur triggered by sunlight, illness, stress, or unknown. Cold sores can be treated in prodromal phase by OTC topical aciclovir. Eye involvement requires medical assessment and referral to specialist Can cause severe infections, e.g. in patients with eczema or immunosuppression requiring systemic treatment as inpatient.
- Glandular fever (infectious mononucleosis). It is caused by Epstein–Barr virus. It is most common in teenagers and young adults. Characterized by high temperature, sore throat, malaise, fatigue, and swollen lymph glands. Diagnosis through symptoms and blood test (FBC and Paul Bunnell and/or glandular fever antibodies). Treated with rest, fluids, and paracetamol. It may last some months.

## Further information

Herpes Virus Association. Available at: 🖰 www.herpes.org.uk
HPA A–Z Seasonal Influenza. Available at: 🖰 www.hpa.org.uk
NHS Choices. Flu. Available at: 🖰 www.nhs.uk/conditions/flu/pages/introduction.aspx
NHS Choices. Glandular Fever. Available at: 🖰 www.nhs.uk/conditions/glandular-fever/Pages/Introduction.aspx
NICE CKS (2010). Glandular Fever. Available at: 🖰 cks.nice.org.uk/glandular-fever#azTab

# Methicillin-resistant *Staphylococcus aureus*

## *Staphylococcus aureus*

- A Gram-positive bacterium which is carried as a skin commensal by about 30% of the population, usually in moist sites such as nose (anterior nares), axillae, and perineum. It causes infections such as boils and styes and is the commonest cause of wound infections.
- Most strains are resistant to penicillin and some strains are resistant to several classes of antibiotics, including meticillin, these are known as MRSA.
- Over use of antibiotics has played a significant part in ↑ resistance to antibiotics (HPA provides annual updated guidance on best practice in antibiotic prescribing, see 📖 Prescribing, p. 130).

## MRSA

82% of those with MRSA infection are ≥60yrs and are <1% of patients living at home, but about 22% of care home residents.

- *Colonization:* carrying MRSA, but no symptoms.
- *Infection:* MRSA causing harm, e.g. boils.
- Most MRSA in those who have had direct contact with hospitals, care homes, or other health care facilities.
- Some strains of MRSA have a particular ability to spread and cause epidemics; referred to as EMRSA.
- Very occasionally there is no history of health care contact; these strains are referred to as community-associated MRSA (CA-MRSA).
- MRSA is not a notifiable disease, but MRSA bacteraemias must be reported as part of a national surveillance programme.
- Prevention of transmission from those MRSA+ is very important.
- Patients who are colonized with MRSA can come home from hospital or go to a care home if their general condition allows. PHCT and care home staff should be informed of patient's status.

### MRSA treatment

- Only on advice of local microbiologist or member of local infection-control team.
- Most asymptomatic requiring no treatment.

### MRSA de-colonization

May be required for those screened positive prior to hospital admission. Regimen detailed in HPA guidance. Nasal: 2% mupirocin in paraffin base tds for 5 days, skin 4% chlorhexidine gluconate body-wash/shampoo 3 tds for 5 days (alternatives: 7.5% povidone iodine or 2% triclosan od × 5 days).

## MRSA in care homes

In the UK 22% of older residents in care homes are colonized with MRSA, but clinical infections in such settings are uncommon. For those who have open lesions, invasive devices, or catheters, a single room, with a wash hand basin is preferable although sharing with another resident who has MRSA would be acceptable. The local Infection Control team can help to evaluate the risk to other residents and provide advice on infection control measures. Staff who require treatment for MRSA carriage should follow local policies and be referred to their GP.

## Infection control measures

The spread of MRSA can be prevented by:
- Hand washing, hand washing, and more hand washing (with liquid soap), especially after giving patient care, and after removing protective clothing (gloves and aprons).
- Judicious use of antibiotics (according to local policy).
- Aseptic handling of catheters or any invasive device/procedure.
- Cleaning equipment after use (hot, soapy water is best).
- Covering patients' wounds, pressure sores, and skin lesions on staff or patients with an impermeable dressing.
- Controlled handling of contaminated dressings and linen.
- Washing laundry at 65°C.

## Related topics

📖 Personal protective equipment, p. 98; 📖 Wound assessment, p. 475; 📖 HIV, p. 686; 📖 Tuberculosis, p. 680.

## Further information

Health Protection Agency (HPA) (2012). Management of infection guidance for primary care. Available at: ℘ www.hpa.org.uk/Topics/InfectiousDiseases/InfectionsAZ/PrimaryCareGuidance/

Health Protection Agency (2012). Methicillin Resistant *Staphylococcus aureus* (MRSA) Screening and Suppression. Quick Reference Guide for Primary Care. Available at: ℘ www.hpa.org.uk/Topics/InfectiousDiseases/InfectionsAZ/PrimaryCareGuidance/#MRSA

NHS Choices. MRSA Infection. Available at: ℘ http://www.nhs.uk/Conditions/MRSA/Pages/Introduction.aspx

NICE CKS (2009). MRSA in primary care. Available at: ℘ cks.nice.org.uk/mrsa-in-primary-care#!topicsummary

# Viral hepatitis

Hepatitis is inflammation of the liver. Viral infection is responsible for around half of all cases of acute hepatitis and is a notifiable disease (📖 Infectious disease notification, p. 103). Incidence is about 100,000 cases annually in the UK.

## Hepatitis A (HAV)

- *Spread*: faecal-oral route. Patients are infectious 2wks before feeling ill.
- *Incubation*: 2–7wks (average 4wks).
- *Risk factors*: travel to high-risk areas, living or working in an institution, poor hand hygiene, poor access to toilet and hand washing facilities, IV drug use, and high-risk sexual practices.
- *Signs and symptoms*: may be asymptomatic (especially young children); fever; ↓ appetite; nausea ± vomiting; pale stools ± diarrhoea; fatigue; jaundice; dark urine; abdominal pain.
- *Investigations*: LFTs, hepatitis serology.
- *Management*: supportive. Advised to avoid alcohol until LFTs are normal. Most recover in <2mths. There is no carrier state and hepatitis A does not cause chronic liver disease. After infection immunity is lifelong.

### Prevention

Vaccination is indicated for travellers (📖 Travel health care, p. 350) to high-risk areas, people with chronic liver disease or working in high-risk situations. Hepatitis A vaccine (and combined with typhoid) is a single dose with booster 6–12mths later.

## Hepatitis B (HBV)

Common. It is endemic in much of Asia and the Far East.

- *Spread*: blood and bodily fluids.
- *Incubation*: 6–23wks (average 17wks).
- *Risk factors*: travel to high-risk areas; babies of infected mothers; sexual partners of infected patients or patients with high-risk sexual practices; IV drug users; health care workers.
- *Signs and symptoms*: may be asymptomatic or present with fever, malaise, fatigue, arthralgia, urticaria, pale stools, dark urine, and/or jaundice.
- *Investigations*: LFTs, hepatitis serology.
  - HBsAg is present from 1–6mths post-exposure. If present >6mths after the acute episode defines carrier status.
  - HBsAg suggests high infectivity. Present from 6wks–3mths after acute illness.
  - Anti-HBs antibodies appear >10mths after infection. Imply immunity.
- *Management*: advised to avoid alcohol. Referred for specialist advice. Treatment is supportive for acute illness. Chronic hepatitis is treated with antiviral medication to slow the spread and damage to the liver.
- *Prognosis*: ~85% recover fully, 10% develop carrier status, 5–10% develop chronic hepatitis—may lead to cirrhosis and/or liver carcinoma.

*Prevention*
- Advise patients re: 'safe sex' practices.
- High-risk groups (including health workers, travellers to high risk areas 📖 Travel health, p. 350) immunized. MSM offered immunization at first visit to sexual health services (see 📖 Targeted immunization in adults, p. 347).
- Passive immunization with human immunoglobulin is used to protect non-immune high-risk contacts of infected patients.

## Hepatitis C (HCV)

Most common type—a major cause of liver damage. Most patients are unaware they have it. Treatment can clear virus in >50%.

- *Spread*: contact with infected blood; mother → baby. *Not* easily spread through sexual contact. In 10% no source of infection is identified.
- *Incubation*: 2–25wks (average 8wks).
- *Patients at high risk of infection and should be offered HCV test*: unexplained jaundice, ever an IV drug user, blood transfusion pre-1992 or blood products pre-1986, had dental or medical treatments in countries with poor infection control, child of HCV mother, regular sex with HCV+ person, accidental exposure to blood, has had tattoos, piercings, acupuncture, etc. where infection control poor.
- *Signs and symptoms*: as for HBV often asymptomatic.
- *Screening*: anti-HCV antibody detectable 3–4mths post-infection. Positive antibody results are followed by HCA RNA blood test. Positive antibody test advised not to donate blood or carry organ donor cord. Positive HCA RNA referred to specialist.
- *Treatment*: referred to specialist. Treated with interferon and ribavirin. Successful in clearing virus in about 40% of people. Advised to avoid alcohol and how to avoid infecting others.

## Hepatitis E (HEV)

- *Spread*: faeco-oral route.
- *Incubation*: 2–9wks (average 40 days).
- *Risk factors*: travel to developing countries (especially pregnant women).
- *Symptoms and management*: similar clinical presentation to HAV infection. Diagnosis is made after serological confirmation. Treatment is supportive. There is no chronic state. No vaccine exists. Mortality in pregnancy can be as high as 20%.

## Further information

Health Protection Agency (HPA). Topics A–Z: Hepatitis A, B, C, E. Available at: ℘ www.hpa.org.uk
Hepatitis C Trust. Available at: ℘ http://www.hepctrust.org.uk/
NHS Choices. Hepatitis. Available at: ℘ www.nhs.uk/conditions/Hepatitis/Pages/Introduction.aspx

# Pandemic influenza

Pandemic influenza is different from seasonal influenza. Caused by a novel influenza virus type A spreading rapidly to people, who are unlikely to have any immunity, covers large geographical areas and a significant proportion of the population in each country. It is likely to have more severe effects than seasonal flu. E.g. 'Hong Kong flu' of 1968–9 estimated to have caused a million deaths across the globe. Transmission is by droplet. It can occur at any time of the year. No vaccine is available until the virus has been identified (and may take 4–6mths to develop) likewise current anti-virals may or may not be effective.

## Pandemic threat

Recent pandemic viruses thought to originate in birds through the spread of the highly pathogenic avian flu (A/H5N1) to humans involved in close contact with poultry. Intercontinental virus spread is rapid, e.g. severe acute respiratory syndrome (SARS) in 2003 affected 8000 people in 30 countries across 6 continents in 4mths, and 900 people died. Another pandemic is likely although when can't be predicted, may come in several waves. Estimated that 14.5 million people will be affected in the UK. UK is part of international network of flu surveillance to monitor evolution of flu virus and detect anything unusual. DH England coordinates the pandemic alert status for the UK.

## Preparation and action in a pandemic

UK has flu pandemic contingency plans. A key principle is *social distancing* in order to slow down spread and give more time for vaccines and anti-virals to be developed. May include:
- Voluntary home isolation of cases.
- Voluntary quarantine of contacts of known cases.
- Restrictions of mass gatherings.
- Travel restrictions.
- School closure.

Each health organization, LA and general practice has local contingency plans. These plans are activated on identification of the new virus in the UK. Each GP practice is advised to have a named flu coordinator in order to plan for:
- Clinical management of patients with influenza.
- Management of patient demand, including those without influenza.
- Priority vaccination programme as directed by chief medical officer (CMO).
- Minimizing risk of infection spread.

In the event of a pandemic many primary care nurses are likely to be directed to work specifically on the implementation of local plans.

## Key primary care principles

- Those with or likely to have flu should be kept physically apart from those without flu, where possible, e.g. telephone triage, separate waiting area in surgeries.
- Avoid working practices and procedures which risk enhancing transmission of flu.
- Plan for reducing patient movements and contacts, e.g. telephone triage, prescriptions collected from pharmacy not surgery.
- Sensible barrier precautions to be used in close contact with a flu-infected patient:
  - Fluid-repellent surgical face mask (changed when moist or moving to non-infected patient), aprons to reduce transmission of droplets to clothes, gloves if sufficient supply, but not strictly necessary.
  - Coughing and sneezing patients should also use mask in consultations.
- Strict adherence to infection control practices in patient contact, e.g. regular and effective hand washing, equipment, premises.

## Key advice to patients and public

- To reduce transmission:
  - Cover nose and mouth when coughing or sneezing, using a tissue when possible, dispose of dirty tissues promptly and carefully.
  - Avoid non-essential travel and large crowds whenever possible.
  - Maintain good basic hygiene, e.g. wash hands frequently with soap and water.
  - Clean hard surfaces (e.g. door handles) frequently using a normal cleaning product.
  - Make sure children follow this advice.
- *On symptoms of influenza:* stay at home, do not go to GP or hospital, rest, take plenty of fluids, and paracetamol.
  - In uncomplicated illness usually resolves in 7 days with rest, fluids, and paracetamol, but cough, malaise, and lassitude can persist for weeks.
  - Pre-existing medical conditions may worsen and require further medical treatment.

## Further information

Department of Health (2012). Health and social care response to flu pandemics. Available at: ℜ www.gov.uk/government/publications/health-and-social-care-response-to-flu-pandemics

Department of Health (2011). The UK Influenza Preparedness Strategy 2011. Available at: ℜ www.gov.uk/government/publications/responding-to-a-uk-flu-pandemic

Royal College of General Practice (2008). *Helping Practices Plan for a Pandemic.* Available at: ℜ www.rcgp.org.uk

UK Health Protection Agency. Pandemic Influenza includes contingency planning, infection control in a pandemic, pandemic influenza clinical management guidelines. Available at: ℜ www.hpa.org.uk/Topics/InfectiousDiseases/InfectionsAZ/PandemicInfluenza/

World Health Organization. Available at: ℜ www.who.int

# Tuberculosis

TB is a serious, but treatable infectious disease caused by inhaling *Mycobacterium tuberculosis*. It is transmitted in the air by tiny droplets of mucus and saliva produced when an infectious person coughs, sneezes, or talks. About 11,000 cases a year in Britain, ½ in London, where rates have doubled in the past decade. Anybody can catch tuberculosis, but more likely amongst:

- Socially excluded groups in large cities.
- People from areas of the world with a high prevalence of TB.
- Homeless/hostel dwellers.
- People with a history of imprisonment and/or overcrowding.
- Problem drug/alcohol users.
- People that are HIV+/immunocompromised.

## Key issues

- Need to prevent the emergence of multi-drug resistant (MDR) TB, which is more difficult and more costly to treat.
- TB is still highly stigmatized and patients can feel isolated and find it difficult to communicate their problems.

## Prevention

BCG immunization is now recommended to:

- All infants living in areas where the incidence of TB is equal to or >40/10,000 (📖 Childhood immunization, p. 156).
- Infants whose parents or grandparents were born in a country with a TB incidence of 40/100,000 or higher.
- Previously unvaccinated new immigrants from high prevalence countries for TB.
- Those at risk due to:
  - Their occupation, e.g. health care workers, veterinary staff.
  - Contacts of known cases.
  - Intend to live or work in high TB prevalence countries.

Children at school are screened for these risk factors. Those who have them who are at risk are offered tuberculin skin tested and vaccinated as appropriate (📖 Childhood immunization, p. 156).

Apart from infants <3mths, tuberculin skin test is by intradermal injection of Mantoux (BNF 14.4) for hypersensitivity to TB prior to BCG. Those with +ve results are not given BCG injection, but are investigated for TB.

## Common symptoms

- Persistent cough, night sweats, fever, loss of appetite, weight loss, and fatigue.
- TB of the lymph glands will cause enlargement of the glands.
- TB affecting other parts of the body (most commonly the kidneys, bones, or joints) causes other symptoms. Children may not have such specific symptoms, but may be generally unwell.

Patients presenting in general practice will have the following investigations:
- CXR.
- Sputum samples—keep in the fridge and send for culture (tick AFB, acid-fast bacilli on the form). Culture confirms diagnosis and drug sensitivities.
- Bloods to include FBC, renal, liver, ESR, CRP, + urates.
- Tuberculin skin test +ve (may be –ve in immunocompromised).

## Management
- Referred to the local TB service, often based at a Chest OPD.
- TB is a notifiable disease (☐ Infectious disease notifications, p. 103) and this initiates contact tracing by TB specialist nurses.
- Medication prescribed by the TB service to monitor compliance:
  - Most people are completely cured by a course of 3–4 antibiotics for the 1st 2mths. Then 2 antibiotics for a further 4mths.
  - Antibiotics used are rifampicin, isoniazid, pyrazinamide, and ethambutol.
  - All have potentially serious side effects (including jaundice) and require blood monitoring.
  - Following 2wks Rx or 3 negative sputums most cases are non-infectious.

## Concordance and compliance
- Concordance and compliance for the whole length of Rx is very important to prevent further transmission and drug resistance.
- Non-compliance is best managed by directly observed therapy (DOT) in which drugs are taken in the presence of a health professional, e.g. primary care nurse—usually on a 3x weekly regimen.

*Contact tracing:* depends on screening by sputum microscopy. 'Close' usually household contacts are screened first. If transmission is found 'casual' contacts—friends, colleagues, school year groups may be screened.

## Related topic
☐ Targeted immunization in adults, p. 347.

## Further information
British Lung foundation. Available at: ℘ www.blf.org.uk/
Health Protection Agency. Topics A–Z: Tuberculosis. Available at: ℘ www.hpa.org.uk/infections/topics_az/tb/
NHS Choices. Tuberculosis. Available at: ℘ www.nhs.uk/Conditions/Tuberculosis/Pages/Introduction.aspx
NICE (2011). *Tuberculosis: (CG117).* Available at: ℘ http://guidance.nice.org.uk/CG117

# Foodborne disease

(*Note:* see 📖 Home food safety and hygiene, p. 311.)

Foodborne disease is an important issue: >80,000 reported foodborne gastrointestinal problems each year in England and Wales. Incidents are under reported. Food poisoning is defined as: '*Any disease of an infectious or toxic nature caused by or thought to be caused by the consumption of food or water*' (Food Safety Act 1990).

## Factors which most commonly contribute to outbreaks

- Preparation of food > half a day in advance of needs.
- Storage at ambient temperature.
- Inadequate cooling.
- Inadequate reheating.
- Use of contaminated processed food.
- Undercooking.
- Contaminated canned food.
- Inadequate thawing.
- Cross-contamination from raw to cooked food.
- Infected food handlers and poor hygiene. People do not play a significant role in outbreaks except in *Staph. aureus* food poisoning; they tend to be victims, not sources.

*Note:* meat and poultry account for 75% of outbreaks.

## Notification

All cases of suspected food poisoning are statutorily notifiable to the environmental health dept. of the LA. Providing information about food eaten, signs, symptoms, and incubation period (see Table 12.2) may suggest the micro-organism involved (📖 Infectious disease notifications, p. 103).

## Personal care

- Give symptomatic care and treat signs such as dehydration.
- Do not advise anti-diarrhoeal drugs (e.g. kaolin, codeine phosphate, loperamide) as contraindicated in children and rarely needed in adults. *Note:* can aggravate nausea and vomiting and occasionally ileus.
- Antibiotics are rarely indicated, may prolong the carrier state.

## Infection control measures

- Hand washing before and after contact with patient and vomit/urine/faeces is essential (applies to family members).
- Handling contaminated material wear PPE, e.g. gloves, aprons.
- Discard excreta directly into the drainage system.
- Anyone with gastroenteritis should not attend work or school until free from diarrhoea and vomiting, and, if necessary, clearance tests have been completed.
- Obtain faeces for microscopy and culture if the patient has been abroad, is severely ill, comes from an institution or works as a food handler or has symptoms for >1wk.

## Further information

Food Standards Agency (2008). *Management of outbreaks of foodborne illness in England and Wales* www.food.gov.uk/business-industry/guidancenotes/hygguid/outbreakmanagement#.UaCLw0BvOZc

NHS Choices. Food poisoning. Available at: ℘ www.nhs.uk/Conditions/Food-poisoning/Pages/Introduction.aspx

Health Protection Agency (HPA). Infections topics A–Z. Available at: ℘ www.hpa.org.uk

**Table 12.2** Causes and characteristic clinical features of food poisoning

| Organism | Common source | Incubation period | Signs and symptoms | | | | | Duration |
|---|---|---|---|---|---|---|---|---|
| | | | Vomiting | Diarrhoea | Abdominal pain | Prostration | Pyrexia | Other | |
| *Bacillus cereus* (toxin in food) | Inadequately heated rice | 1–16hrs | Profuse | Slight | Often present | Moderately severe | Absent | | 12–24hrs |
| *Campylobacter jejuni* (infection) | Undercooked poultry and meat; unpasteurized milk | 3–5 days | Slight | Often profuse | Often severe | Often severe | Often present | Blood-stained faeces often | Days or weeks |
| *Clostridium botulin* (toxin in food) | Contaminated canned food | 12–96hrs usually 18–36hrs | Slight | Absent | Absent | Severe | Absent | Nausea, vertigo, aphonia, respiratory paralysis and death can occur | Death in 24hrs to 8d, or slow convalescence over 6–8mths |
| *Clostridium perfringens* (toxin in intestine) | Spores on contaminated meat | 8–22hrs | Absent | Moderate | Colicky pains often present | Slight | Absent | | 24–48hrs |
| *E. coli* (infection and toxin) | Undercooked beef and beef products, milk and vegetables | 12–72hrs | Slight | Moderate | Slight | Slight | Absent | *E. coli* 0157 bloody diarrh o ea | 1–7 days |

| | | | | | | | | | |
|---|---|---|---|---|---|---|---|---|---|
| Listeria monocytogenes | Freshly cut salads, paté, soft cheeses | 48hrs–3wks | Slight | Slight | Often present | | Present | Pregnant women especially vulnerable | Few days |
| Norovirus | Contaminated water and food, especially shellfish | 24–48hrs | Moderate | Moderate | Not usually | | Present | Person-to-person spread common via contact with faeces and vomit | |
| Salmonella (infection) | Meat, poultry, eggs, dairy products | 6–36hrs usually 12–24hrs | Slight | Moderate | Often present | Possibly in later stages | Often present | Blood-stained faeces in up to 25% cases | 1–7 days |
| Staphylococcus aureus (toxin in food) | Cooked food (meat, poultry, fish) and dairy products (custards, creams, trifles) | 2–6hrs | Profuse | Slight | Often present | Often severe | Absent | | 6–24hrs |
| Vibrio parahaemolyticus (infection) | Seafood | 2–48hrs usually 12–18hrs | Moderate | Moderate | Often present | Slight | Absent | | 2–5 days |
| Vibrio cholerae | Water, seafood | 24–72hrs | Slight | Profuse | Often present | Often severe | Often present | | |

Note: cholera and food poisoning are statutorily notifiable diseases, Public Health (Control of Diseases) Act, 1984

# Human immunodeficiency virus

HIV is a retrovirus that infects immune system cells particularly the CD4 (T-helper cells) and over a number of years the CD4 cells malfunction and die to a point where they jeopardize immunity. Due to the advancement in treatments the term AIDS (acquired immune deficiency syndrome) is no longer used in diagnosis (although still used for epidemiological purposes). About 96,000 people living with HIV in the UK in 2011.

## Transmission

HIV is transmitted through body fluids: semen, vaginal fluids, including menstrual fluids, breast milk, and blood. In the UK most people with HIV are either MSM or people of sub-Saharan African origin. Injecting drug users are also at high risk. Transmission from mother to baby and through infected blood products is very rare in the UK.

## Prevention

- Safer sex practices, e.g. use of male and female condoms with lubricant.
- ↓ IV drug abuse and ↓ needle sharing.
- All donated blood screened for HIV.
- Risk ↓ of mother to child transmission by antiretroviral treatment given antenatally, during delivery, and to the baby 6wks, elective Caesarian delivery, and not breastfeeding.
- HIV positive individuals follow safer sex and safer drug use practice.
- PEP for occupational exposure, or following sexual assault, is a combination of antiretroviral medicines started as soon after possible exposure and taken for 4wks. Available through GUM clinics (genitourinary medicine), ED, and some GPs.

## Detection

HIV infection is detected by an HIV antibody test. It is available through GUM clinics and some GPs. Test 3mths after possible exposure to ensure true negatives. Early detection ensures treatment at the earliest stage. Pre and post-test information and psychological considerations are important, checklist given in MEDFASH guide.

## Disease progression

Normal CD4 count is >500 cells/mcL.

- *Primary HIV infection:* flu-like symptoms also fever, fatigue, diffuse rash, oral ulceration, diarrhoea. Known as seroconversion illness.
- *Asymptomatic HIV:* follows seroconversion, present for some years.
- *Symptomatic HIV:*
  - CD4 count <400 cells/mcL risk of serious opportunistic infection, e.g. *Pneumocystis* pneumonia (PCP), TB, toxoplasmosis, candida, herpes simplex, varicella zoster.
  - CD4 count <200 cells/mcL ↑ risk of more serious infections, e.g. mycobacterium avium intracellulare, cytomegalovirus and aggressive malignancies, e.g. Kaposi's sarcoma.
  - Untreated disease progression leads to wasting and malnutrition, multisystem failure and death.

## Management of HIV infection

Undertaken by specialist teams (and community nursing services when specialist services unavailable). Antiretroviral therapy (BNF 5.3.1) involves:

• Antiretroviral therapy (ART) limits HIV replication. Three or more antiretrovirals are used in combination. Adherence essential as HIV mutates easily and cross resistance irreversible. Decisions to start ART are based on CD4 counts and viral load. Side effects common and some are serious.

• Prophylactic antibiotics based on CD4 counts.

## Living with HIV infection

Specialist teams and services available to help address a wide range of psychological, emotional, social, as well as physical needs arising from the infection, treatments, and progression of the disease. Primary care services work in partnership as in any long-term condition. Also has health promotion role:

• Health promotion advice, e.g. safe sex practices even when both partners have HIV diagnosis as they are at risk of acquiring drug resistant strain.

• Screening, e.g. annual cervical smears as more at risk of malignancies.

• Immunization, e.g. annual influenza immunization, hepatitis A immunization for MSM.

## Palliative care

While ART has meant that death is much less common, there are still patients who progress through the stages and require all aspects of palliative care (📖 Palliative care in the home, p. 509).

## Further information

British HIV Association. Current HIV treatment clinical guidelines. Available at: ℘ www.bhiva.org/Guidelines.aspx

Children with AIDS charity (CWAC). Available at: ℘ www.cwac.org

Health protection Agency. HIV in the United Kingdom: 2012 Report. Available at: ℘ http://www.hpa.org.uk/Publications/InfectiousDiseases/HIVAndSTIs/1211HIVintheUK2012/

Madge S, Mathews P, Singh, S, et al. (2011). HIV in Primary Care, 2nd edn. Medical Foundation for Aids and Sexual Health (MEDFASH). Available at: ℘ www.medfash.org.uk/publications

National AIDS Trust (NAT). Available at: ℘ www.nat.org.uk/default.aspx

Terrence Higgins Trust. Available at: ℘ www.tht.org.uk

# Common musculoskeletal problems

## Sporting-related injuries

These can often be avoided with suitable equipment, e.g. good warm up routines, knowing your limitations, gradual buildup of activity, trainers, proper training and supervision. As a general principle remember 'RICE'.

- *Rest*: rest affected part.
- *Ice*: use straightaway to deal with injury (e.g. ice in towel, bag of frozen peas) for 10min max, and analgesia.
- *Compression* strapping and bandaging can be used to help reduce swelling and help prevent acute sprains and strains.
- *Elevation*.

Muscle and ligament injuries may need referral to GP and/or physiotherapist.

## Neck problems

Most neck pain is acute, but self-limiting within days or weeks. Patients with persistent pain should be referred to GP. Causes can be multifactorial, e.g. arthritis, infection.

> *Note:* any significant neck trauma requires neck immobilization with a hard collar and referral to ED.

- *Cervical spondylosis*: degenerative disease of the cervical spine, characterized by intermittent pain often related to exercise and decreased movement. Can cause nerve root pain. Will need diagnosis confirmed, usual treatment: analgesia.
- *Torticollis*: relatively common, can be triggered by poor posture, sleeping awkwardly. A sudden onset of pain due to muscle spasm that immobilizes neck. Self-limiting, treat with heat, gentle mobilization, and analgesia.
- *Whiplash injuries*: often after RTA—sudden extension of neck → stretches or tears cervical muscles. Pain may occur hours or days after injury, can radiate to head, shoulders, and arms. Medical assessment to exclude other causes. Treatment—analgesia, early mobilization, and a collar initially not long term. Recovery often slow.

**Back pain** See 📖 Low back pain, p. 560.

## Shoulder problems

Always consider the possibility of pain being referred from elsewhere, e.g. neck, cardiac ischaemia, PE, gallbladder problems, or subphrenic abcess.

- *Frozen shoulder (adhesive capulitis)*: affects patients often between 40–60yrs, cause unknown, more common in people with diabetes. Painful stiff shoulder with very restricted movement, pain often worse at night. Care—NSAIDs, referral to physiotherapist. May benefit from steroid injections. Recovery is often slow with uncertain outcome.
- *Dislocated shoulder*: usually because of a fall, referred to ED for reduction. Recurrent dislocation can occur in teenagers with no history of injury, but general joint laxity: referral to physiotherapy and/or GP.

### Elbow, wrist, and hand problems

- *Pulled elbow:* common in children <5yrs, a traction injury often occurs when child pulled up suddenly by the hand. Child stops using the arm. Refer to GP.
- *Golfer's elbow and tennis elbow:* characterized by pain and tenderness— tendon inflammation caused by repeated strain, advise patient to avoid trigger movements, take NSAIDs, often resolves with rest. Physiotherapy and/or local steroid injection may help.
- *Repetitive strain injury:* work related upper limb pain often in arm and wrist, e.g. related to computer keyboard use. Suggest patient review working posture and involve occupational health to review office equipment. Advise rest from aggravating activities and then gradually reintroduce, may help to have workstation and physiotherapy assessment.
- *Carpal tunnel syndrome:* pain, numbness, pins and needles in the fingers due to nerve compression, often worse at night. Symptoms are improved by shaking wrist. Can occur with pregnancy, hypothyroidism, obesity, and carpal arthritis. Symptoms can be helped with night splints and steroid injections. Surgery an option in moderate to severe pain.

### Growing pains and leg cramps

- *Growing pains:* term used for non-specific and diffuse pain in children. May involve child waking at night with leg or arm pain, rubbing the affected limb brings rapid relief. Resolves spontaneously.
- *Leg cramps:* transient involuntary episode of pain lasting for a few minutes (10min max.) cause unknown. Care and management— check not on drugs with side effects of cramps, reassure benign, advise passive stretching and massaging of affected muscle. If persist refer to GP.

### Ankle and foot problems

- *Ruptured Achilles tendon:* patient complain of sudden pain in back of ankle 'like a kick' during activity. Walks with a limp and cannot raise heel from floor or stand on tiptoe. Urgent orthopaedic referral.
- *Plantar fascitis (burstitis):* common cause of heel pain. Worst when person gets out of bed. Suggest shoes with soft padding and support, if pains persistent refer to GP for review.
- *Flat feet:* normal in young children, painless flat foot where arch is restored when standing on tiptoe does not need treatment. Needs referral if painful and/or not restored on tiptoe.
- *Hammer and claw toes:* if causing pain, footwear or mobility problems will need surgery.
- *Bunion (hallux valgas):* lateral deviation of the big toe exacerbated by wearing high heels and tight fitting shoes, arthritis pads can help, but severe deformation will need surgery.
- *In-growing toe nail:* most common in big toe caused by ill-fitting shoes and poor nail care. Nail grows into skin causing pain and inflammation. If infected will need antibiotics. Advise to cut nails straight and with edges beyond the flesh and refer to podiatry. Persistent problems may need referral to podiatrist for surgery.

**Related topics**

📖 Osteoarthritis, p. 553; 📖 Rheumatoid arthritis, p. 555.

**Further information**

NHS Choices. Sports injuries. Available at: ℘ www.nhs.uk/Conditions/Sports-injuries/Pages/Treatment.aspx

NICE. CKS Guidance on acute torticollis, carpel tunnel syndrome, leg cramps, neck pain, plantar fasciitis, shoulder pain, tennis elbow. Available at: ℘ http://cks.nice.org.uk/

# Bone and connective tissue disorders

## Paget's disease of bone

A metabolic disorder of unknown cause that can be asymptomatic. Affects bone growth, bone deformity, weakness, and risk of fracture. Present in 1:10 of older people. Many are asymptomatic and only a small proportion experience severe symptoms. Patients may experience:

- Pain or dull ache aggravated by weight bearing, but can persist at rest.
- Deformity of the bone, bowing of weight bearing bones, e.g. femur. Skull may increase in size and spine may curve.
- May have associated symptoms of nerve compression and pain, disturbed vision and dizziness.
- May have fractures as 2° complication and osteoarthritis.

Patient will need rheumatology referral for treatment and ongoing management. Pain managed with analgesia.

## Rickets/osteomalacia

Caused by vitamin D deficiency. Vitamin D is present in oil-rich, fish and margarine with D supplements (☐ Nutrition and healthy eating, p. 304) and sunshine. Rickets is the term used for children and osteomalacia for adults. Characterized by:

- Widespread bone pain, muscle weakness, and muscle cramps.
- *Deformity:* e.g. bow legs, pigeon chest, and pelvic deformities.
- Pathological fractures.
- Dental caries and delayed teeth formation.
- Impaired growth and short stature (may not be reversible).
- Low calcium → numbness of extremities—hands and feet.

People most at risk of rickets/osteomalacia:

- Older people especially >80yrs and those in residential care.
- People with deficient diet and/or little access to sunshine.
- Immigrants with pigmented skin.
- People with CrD, coeliac disease, and other absorption problems.

*Care and management:* following diagnosis by blood test, majority treated with vitamin supplements.

## Osteomyelitis

An infection of the bone requiring urgent referral to 2° care, *Staph. aureus* most common cause (also *E. coli, Proteus, Pseudomonas,* TB). May follow systemic infection and/or injury, children and people with DM most susceptible. Complications: septic arthritis, chronic osteomyelitis chronic infection, bone deformity, and pathological fracture. Characterized by:

- Pain and reluctance to move affected limbs.
- Warmth and effusion in affected joints.
- Fever and malaise.

Treatment is with IV and then po antibiotics and surgery to drain abscesses.

## Systemic lupus erythematosus

SLE is a rare autoimmune connective tissue disease 1:3000 >♀ onset 15–40yrs higher prevalence in African Caribbean and Far East Asian populations. No cure. It affects multiple systems. Majority of patients have skin and joint involvement and often complain of severe fatigue:

- *Joints:* e.g. arthritis, arthralgia.
- *Skin:* hypersensitivity, facial 'butterfly rash', vasculitis, hair loss.
- *Lungs:* pleurisy, pneumonitis, alveolitis.
- *Kidneys:* proteinuria, ↑ BP, glomerulonephritis, renal failure.
- *Heart:* pericarditis, endocarditis.
- *Central nervous system:* depression, psychosis, infarction, fits, psychosis.

Patients will need specialist rheumatology treatment and ongoing care. Steroids are used to control acute episodes (advise on side effects of steroids).

### Care and management
- Advise patients to avoid direct sunlight (can exacerbate rash).
- *Medications include:* NSAID, hydroxychloroquine, corticosteroids, immunosuppressants—advise on side effects.

*Note:* hormonal contraception/HRT may aggravate symptoms in ♀.

## Raynaud's syndrome

Approx. 10million sufferers in UK affecting mainly women. Intermittent ischaemia of the fingers, precipitated by cold and/or emotion. Cause unknown. Fingers are very painful, numb, tingle ache, and change colour becoming pale then blue and red on being warmed. 5% may go on to develop other rheumatic disease, e.g. SLE and scleroderma (rare disease in which the skin becomes tight shiny/fibrosed and can involve other organs).

### Care and management
- Advise on keeping warm. Patients with mild symptoms should use thermal gloves, avoid cold and draughts.
- Smoking cessation (📖 p. 315).
- More severe symptoms treated with medication, e.g. vasodilators and serotonin re-uptake inhibitors and specialist referral.

## Vibration induced white finger
- People who work with machinery that vibrates are prone to Raynaud's.
- Condition is permanent—an industrial disease eligible for compensation.

## Related topics
📖 Osteoarthritis, p. 553; 📖 Rheumatoid arthritis, p. 555.

## Further information
Lupus UK. Available at: 🖰 www.lupusuk.org.uk/home
National Association for the Relief of Paget's Disease. Available at: 🖰 www.paget.org.uk
Raynauds and Scleroderma Association. Available at: 🖰 www.raynauds.org.uk

# Seizures and epilepsy

A seizure or fit is when there is a sudden disturbance of neurological function associated with an abnormal neuronal discharge. All children, young people and adults with a recent onset suspected seizure should be seen urgently by a specialist (see 📖 Febrile convulsions, p. 272).

Fits may take many forms and a first fit has enormous consequences. The term 'seizure' is used to avoid the emotive term of epilepsy unless a specialist diagnosis has already been made.

## Epilepsy

Is recurrent seizures other than febrile convulsions. 60% of adult epilepsy starts in childhood. 456,000 people in the UK have a diagnosis of epilepsy. Suspected cases are referred to neurologists. Diagnosis made on history, clinical examination, and EEG (can be a prolonged process).

### Causes

Often none is found, but of the known causes:

- *Genetic:* (20%).
- *Physical:* trauma and injury, space-occupying lesions, raised BP, CVA.
- *Metabolic:* alcohol withdrawal, drug related, hyper/hypoglycaemia, hypoxia, electrolyte disturbance.
- *Infective:* e.g. encephalitis.

### Focal epilepsy

Involves one part of the body and may progress to other parts becoming generalized (Jacksonian epilepsy).

### Grand mal epilepsy

Generalized seizure with sudden onset of tonic contraction of the muscles, often associated with a cry or a moan, and falling to the ground. The tonic phase gives way to clonic convulsive movements occurring bilaterally and synchronously, slows and stops, followed by a variable period of unconsciousness and gradual recovery.

### Myoclonic epilepsy

A variant of petit mal epilepsy characterized by atonic drop attacks.

### Petit mal epilepsy

A pause in speech or other activity and patient is unaware of the episode.

### Temporal lobe epilepsy

A disorder with seizures originating from the temporal lobe with numerous, bizarre presentations can include altered perception and oral and auditory hallucinations.

### Status epilepticus

A generalized convulsion, lasting 30min or longer, or when successive convulsions occur that the patient does not recover consciousness between them.

## Management and support

Structured person-centred care plan is agreed in secondary and primary care and review undertaken at least annually with specialist.

### Medication

It is controlled by AED medication as per NICE guidance. In 80% of cases fits are controlled:

- Treatment individualized by seizure type, epilepsy syndrome, co-morbidity, lifestyle, and preference.
- Adherence to treatment is important, especially with teenagers.
- Usually started at a low dose, dose ↑ until fits are controlled or side effects occur.
- Buccal midazolam (first line treatment) or rectal diazepam prescribed for prolonged seizures and convulsive status epilepticus (see 📖 Working in schools, p. 38 for medicine administration in schools).
- Once stable and management straightforward, continuing AED therapy (BNF 4.8.1) is prescribed in primary care.
- Once seizure free for >2yrs specialist with person/parents may decide to gradually withdraw AED.

### Information and education

Epilepsy is a diagnosis that can cause alarm, fear, and stigma. People with epilepsy and their families need clear information on:

- Epilepsy in general, specifics of diagnosis, prognosis, AED, and side effects.
- Management, self-care, and risk management.
- Life should be as normal as possible, advice about avoiding risks, e.g. swimming or cycling alone—but not being overprotective.
- Possible triggers for seizures, e.g. stress, drugs, and alcohol, antidepressants, tiredness, flickering lights, menstruation, and illness.
- *Women:* information on AED side effects for contraception, pregnancy, childcare, menopause.
- Inform patient about counselling services (📖 Talking therapies, p. 429), voluntary organizations, and expert patient (📖 p. 303) programme.
- Need to ensure that school staff is aware of the diagnosis, but are careful not to stigmatize or over protect children.
- *DVLA restrictions apply:* patient to notify DVLA and insurer.
- Employer should be aware. Some occupations are precluded for people with epilepsy, e.g. pilot, train driver.
- Financial issues, see 📖 Benefits for illness, disability and carers, p. 795.

**Key principles for managing a seizure**
**keep the person safe from harm and stay with them as**
**they recover afterwards**

- Note the time.
- Are they in a safe place?– if so leave them, cushion their head if they have collapsed to the ground.
- *DO NOT* place anything in mouth, restrain person, or move person unless in immediate danger and let them lie down.
- *After the seizure has stopped:* place in recovery position, check breathing and ensure clear airway. Stay and reassure the person. Do not offer food or drink until fully recovered and oriented.

❶ If this is the person's first seizure or if seizure continues >5min or >3× in one hour call for an ambulance.

## Further information

Epilepsy Action: ☎ 0808 800 5050. Available at: ⅏ www.epilepsy.org.uk
Epilepsy Society: ☎ 01494 601 400. Available at: ⅏ www.epilepsysociety.org.uk/
NICE (2012). *Epilepsy (CG137)*. Available at: ⅏ http://guidance.nice.org.uk/CG137

# Migraine

Migraine is a syndrome characterized by periodic headaches with complete resolution between attacks. Most common cause of recurrent disabling headache in the population (*Note:* <1% patients with headaches have a brain tumour):

- *Trigger factors:*
  - Emotional and/or physical stress.
  - Diet/food, e.g. sugary foods or long breaks without food.
  - Environmental, e.g. bright lights.
  - Hormonal.
- Most patients can successfully manage the condition.

## Signs and symptoms

An attack can include all or some of the following stages:

- *Prodrome:* change in mood or appetite before migraine onset.
- 10% sufferers experience aura before onset of headache—visual disturbance; motor or sensory disturbance.
- *Headache (common migraine):* often pulsatile and unilateral, lasts 4–72hrs; moderate/severe intensity may be associated with symptoms of nausea and vomiting, photophobia, phonophobia, aggravated by movement.

## Management and health promotion advice

- Identify and avoid trigger factors. Foodstuffs trigger in 20% patients. Refer to GP to discuss use of prophylactic medications, e.g. beta-blockers, amitriptyline.
- Explanation and reassurance to patient, treatable, but not curable.
- Offer patient information:
  - Avoiding trigger factors can ↓ frequency by up to 50%.
  - Regular sleep pattern and dietary pattern.
  - ↓ caffeine and alcohol intake and drink 2L water a day.
  - Keep a migraine diary to help identify triggers.
  - Review possible environmental triggers, e.g. ↓ VDU use.
- ♀ who have focal aura are contraindicated for COC (🕮 Combined hormonal methods, p. 361).

### Management of acute attack

1st line treatments should be taken early in an attack, e.g. aspirin, ibuprofen, or paracetamol, see 🕮 Pain assessment and management, p. 513.

- Anti-emetics, e.g. metoclopramide, domperidone relieve nausea.
- If 1st line treatment inadequate then should consult GP for 2nd line treatments (triptans) and for patients with persistent symptoms referral to migraine clinic may be an option.

## Further information

Migraine Trust. Available at: ℘ www.MigraineTrust.org
NHS Choices. Migraine. Available at: ℘ www.nhs.uk/Conditions/Migraine/Pages/Introduction.aspx
NICE. CKS Migraine (2008). Available at: ℘ http://cks.nice.org.uk/migraine#!topicsummary

# Common problems affecting eyes

## Conjunctivitis

Inflammation of the conjunctiva cause can be infective irritant or allergic unilateral (often if infection present) or bilateral most common condition seen in primary care. Characterized by:

- Red sore eye.
- Discharge.
- Swollen eyelids.
- Eyes stuck together after sleep.
- Linked to seasonal changes (hayfever) or contact with allergen, e.g. cats (allergic).
- Close contact with another affected person (infective).
- Presence of upper respiratory infection (infective).
- In neonates <21 days old with purulent discharge possibility of STI related infection from mother. Take swabs for MC&S, chlamydia. If positive for *N. gonorrhoea* treated with topical antibiotics and referred to specialist.

### Care and management

- Most symptoms self-limiting and resolve in 2–5 days, maintain good eye hygiene. If symptoms persist may benefit from topical antibiotics e.g. chloramphenicol (OTC).
- If infective conjunctivitis advise on not sharing towels, pillows, or face-cloths, and good hand hygiene. School and group child care exclusion until treated (📖 Table 7.2, Infections diseases exclusion times, p. 286). Avoid contact lens until no symptoms.
- For people with allergic conjunctivitis treat with antihistamines or topical anti-inflammatory (BNF 11.4.2).

## Blepharitis

4.5% of all opthamological problems seen in primary care, cause are unknown, a chronic persistent condition, usually bilateral, may be characterized by:

- Sore inflamed eyelids, red rimmed eyes.
- Eyelids may stick together in the morning (consider possibility of infection).
- Eyes may feel gritty.
- May be scales on eyelashes.
- Complain of dry eyes, blurred vision.
- Unable to tolerate contact lens.

*Care and management*
- Good eye hygiene is the mainstay of treatment.
  - Warm compresses (clothes) to closed eyelids for 5–10mins 2x then 1x day.
  - Clean the eyelid with a wet cloth plus cleanser, e.g. dilute baby shampoo 1:warm water.
  - Gentle massage of the eyelids.
- Advise patients to avoid eye makeup or use water soluble eyeliner.
- Do not use contact lens.
- Avoid rubbing eyes.
- If eyes are persistently dry may benefit from artificial tears (BNF 11.8).
- If persists may need specialist referral.

## Floaters

Floaters are small shapes, e.g. spots, shadowy strands caused by debris floating in the eye's vitreous humour. Occur with ↑ age, but may be a sign of retinal detachment. If sudden onset or increases with white flashes the person should visit the optician immediately. Do not require treatment, but advise to have regular eye checks (2yrly).

## Subconjunctival haemorrhage

*Common in older people:* a painless localized haemorrhage in the eye that occurs spontaneously. Clears in 1–2wks, consider referral to specialist if history of trauma or edges of haemorrhage cannot be seen.

---

❶ Red eye symptoms that are potentially dangerous should have same day referral to doctor/specialist if one or more following are present:
- Moderate-to-severe eye pain (not surface irritation) and/or photophobia.
- Reduced visual acuity.
- Inability to move eye.
- Visibly dilated blood vessels seen between white of eye and iris. Loss and/or affected sight.
- Corneal damage (often only visible after fluroscein staining).
- Absent or sluggish pupil response.
- Eye involvement when patient has shingles (herpes zoster).
- History of trauma or post-operatively.

---

## Related topics

📖 Blindness and partial sight, p. 699; 📖 Allergies, p. 647; 📖 Eye trauma, p. 766.

## Further information

NHS Choices. Floaters. Available at: ℬ www.nhs.uk/conditions/floaters/Pages/Introduction.aspx
NICE. CKS: Conjunctivitis infective (2012) and blepharitis (2012). Available at: ℬ http://cks.nice.org.uk/

# Blindness and partial sight

Blindness is inability to perform any work where sight is essential. *Note:* blindness does not always mean total absence of sight. Blindness: <3/60 vision (although may be >3/60 if severe visual field defect). Partial blindness: no one definition, but implies vision in the range 3/60–6/60). It affects 2:1000 in UK. ❶ Sudden loss of vision is an emergency needing specialist attention via ED.

### Risk factors

*Include:* DM, smoking, FH, ↑ age, poor diet, hypertension (▢ Hypertension, p. 586), steroid treatments, alcohol (▢ Alcohol, p. 319) misuse, prolonged exposure to sunlight.

### Health promotion advice

- Protect eyes from bright sunlight with sunglasses.
- Eat fruits and green leafy vegetables (▢ Nutrition and healthy eating, p. 304).
- Monitor BP (▢ Hypertension, p. 586).
- Smoking cessation (▢ p. 315).
- Eye test every 2yrs.

### Age-related macular degeneration

Cause of blindness in 1:2 people registered blind. It is a bilateral disease affecting one eye more than the other. Characterized by deterioration of central vision affects reading, face recognition, and ability to see colour.

- Most common form of age related macular degeneration (AMD) macula cells decay and disintegrate.
- Emphasize that not all sight will be lost, should be possible to maintain independence, but reading, television, and driving will become impossible.

### Cataracts

Occurs when the lens of an eye becomes cloudy, develops gradually. Affects 1:3 people >65yrs. Experienced as blurred vision, spots, or halos around bright lights and dazzled by car lights. Affects distance judgement.

- Advise patients to have regular eye checks.
- Check patient does not have DM.
- *Treatment when interferes with everyday life:* routine surgery day case operation. Cloudy lens is removed and is replaced with an artificial plastic lens. Patient will need glasses to adjust for refractive changes.

### Chronic simple glaucoma

An increase in eye pressure causes damage to the optic nerve. The prevalence of glaucoma rises from 1–2% >40s to 5% >75s. African-Caribbeans have 4x greater risk than white people. Initially, asymptomatic as peripheral vision is the first to be affected, people often present late. Symptoms include visual loss and sausage-shaped blind spots. Patients will need lifelong follow-up, therefore important:

- All adults with a FH are regularly checked.
- All adults >35–40yrs should have regular eye (every 2–4yrs) checks to detect early glaucoma. >50yrs 1–2yrs.

- *Treatment:* aims to reduce eye pressure and prevent further damage to optic nerve. Achieved through:
  - *Eye drops:* these will either ↓ amount of aqueous humour or ↑ drainage of aqueous humour. Important that treatment maintained (BNF 11.6).
  - *Surgery:* trabeculectomy, creating channel between inside of eye to under conjunctiva.

## Retinal detachment

*Relatively rare condition:* painless loss of vision, like a curtain coming across the vision. 50% have some premonition with flashing lights, spots or floaters. ❶ Should attend optician immediately for eye assessment as may need to be referred for urgent treatment to secure retina (laser or freezing).

## Diabetic retinopathy

📖 Diabetes overview, p. 611.

## Registering as blind

Only 50% of those eligible to register actually do so. The majority of people eligible to register are likely to have low vision.
- Referred to consultant ophthalmologist for assessment to determine eligibility and for referral to LA social services.
- Eligible for support from LA social worker/rehabilitation officer and specific benefits including income support, training in Braille or typing, information about further education and leisure activities disabled parking badge see 📖 Benefits for illness, disability and carers, p. 795.
- Access to equipment and aids to support independent living, e.g. talking clocks and books, large button telephones (📖 Assistive technology, p. 779).
- A free radio from the Wireless for the Blind ℬ www.blind.org.uk.
- Free directory enquiries from BT.
- Concessionary travel (📖 Benefits support, p. 789).
- Free NHS sight tests, prescriptions, dental treatment, help with fares to hospital and with cost of glasses. See 📖 Benefits for illness, disability and carers, p. 795.
- Free postage on items marked 'articles for the blind'.

## Related topics

📖 Common problems affecting eyes, p. 697; 📖 Allergies, p. 647; 📖 Eye trauma, p. 766.

## Further information

Macular Disease Society. Available at: ℬ www.maculardisease.org
NHS Choices Visual impairment. Available at: ℬ www.nhs.uk/Conditions/Visual-impairment/Pages/Introduction.aspx
Royal National Institute for the Blind: ☎ 0303 123 9999. Available at: ℬ www.rnib.org.uk

# Pneumonia

Inflammation of the lungs is usually caused by infection, most commonly *Streptococcus*. Community acquired pneumonia (different from hospital acquired) is very common in the UK, annual incidence about 250,000 cases. Can affect any one, but more common and usually more serious in the very young, the very old, smokers, anyone with long-term illness, and those immune-compromised (e.g. those with 1° immunodeficiency, receiving chemotherapy, receiving immunosuppressant drugs, HIV+, or other conditions such as hyposplenism, malnutrition, nephrotic syndrome). Those less seriously affected are managed in the community, but about 20% need hospital admission, of these between 6–14% die.

## Symptoms

Acute illness characterized by:

- Flu-like symptoms, e.g. fevers, shivers, aches, raised temperature.
- Cough with usually purulent sputum.
- Dyspnoea.
- Some have pleural chest pain.
- Older people may have acute confusion and/or walking difficulties.

## Prevention

- Pneumococcal and influenza vaccination (☐ Targeted immunization for adults, p. 347).
- Smoking cessation (☐ p. 315).

## Treatment and management

Clinical assessment (may include investigations and pulse oximetry increasingly available in primary care), and decision made as to whether hospital admission required based on severity, social circumstances, and concomitant illness. If patient has one or more of following considered for hospital admission, if 3 or more then urgent admission required:

- Confusion.
- Respiratory rate ≥30 breaths/min.
- *BP*: systolic <90 mmHg; diastolic ≤60 mmHg.
- Age ≥65yrs.

### When managed at home

- Advised:
  - No smoking and other smokers in home to cease.
  - Get plenty of rest and drink plenty of fluids.
  - Simple analgesia as required, e.g. paracetamol.
- Commenced on antibiotics, usually amoxicillin 500mg tds (BNF 5.1).
- Should improve within 48hrs. Patient should be reviewed at this point and if deteriorating or not improving considered for hospital referral.

## Further information

British Lung Foundation. Available at: ℡ www.lunguk.org
British Thoracic Society (2009). *Guidelines for the management of community acquired pneumonia in adults.* Also for children (2011). Available at: ℡ www.brit-thoracic.org.uk

# Occupational lung disease

Inhaling gases, dust, vapours can lead to occupational lung disease. Occupations especially at risk are: coal miners, farmers, asbestos workers, workers with epoxy resins or isocyanates.

## Occupational asthma

>200 substances known to produce asthma (📖 Asthma in adults, p. 566) like symptoms and treated as such. Employers should seal off hazardous substances, fit extractor fans, and provide protective masks and clothing. Estimates of 3000 case a year. Vehicle spray painters, bakers, and flour confectioners have the highest estimated risk of occupational asthma.

## Pneumoconiosis

A lung disease caused by inhalation of mineral dust, results in fibrosis of the lungs. Current laws about working conditions should prevent workers from developing pneumoconiosis in the future. Types include:

- Coal worker's pneumoconiosis from coal dust.
- Asbestosis and related lung cancer, e.g. mesothelioma from asbestos fibres (3500 asbestos related deaths in 2003).
- Silicosis from silica dust in iron foundries, potteries, and ceramics.

There is no treatment, but patient should not be further exposed to substance, stop smoking, and symptoms managed as COPD (📖 Chronic obstructive pulmonary disease, p. 574), lung cancer (📖 p. 704), and palliative care (📖 Symptom control in palliative care: breathlessness, p. 518).

## Alveolitis

Inflammation of alveolar wall, referred to specialist and treated with oral steroids. Two types:

- *Fibrosing alveolitis*: associated with occupational exposure wood or metal (also non-occupational causes linked to other diseases, drug use, e.g. cytotoxic drugs).
- *Extrinsic allergic alveolitis*: (farmers—lung-inhaled fungal spores, bird fanciers—lung-inhaled avian protein) is an allergic reaction to inhaled substances.

## Notification of prescribed occupational disease

GP, with patient's permission, informs employer in writing of any legally notifiable occupational illness and the employer (or patient if self-employed) must report it to RIDDOR.

## Benefits and compensation

The patient may be eligible for government industrial injuries benefit scheme. Information leaflets and claim forms available online at Job Centre Plus and Social Security Offices. 📖 Benefits for illness, disability and carers, p. 795.

Affected individuals can also make a personal injury claim against employers. Advice available from Trade Unions, CABs, and solicitors. See 📖 Benefits and support, p. 789.

Government scheme for compensation Under the Pneumoconiosis, etc. (Workers' Compensation) Act 1979 if unable to get damages from employer (e.g. out of business). See UK GOV or TUC website.

## Related topic

📖 Health and safety at work, p. 88.

## Further information

Benefit Enquiry Line: ☎ 0800 882 200: People using a textphone ☎ 0800 243 355

British Lung Foundation. Available at: ℘ www.lunguk.org

RIDDOR: ☎ 0870 1545500. Available at: ℘ www.riddor.gov.uk email: hseinformationservices@natbrit.com

TUC guide to work related injuries and personal injury claims. Available at: ℘ www.worksmart.org.uk

UK. Gov Online guides to all benefits and compensation claims. Available at: ℘ www.gov.uk/browse/benefits

# Lung cancer

Lung cancer is the second commonest cancer after breast cancer. >40,000 people in the UK are diagnosed annually. It is the leading cause of cancer death. Affects more ♂ than ♀, second leading cause of death in men, after CHD. Smoking and passive smoking cause 90% lung cancers.

- *Incidence ↑ with age:* 80% aged >60yrs and 1% <40yrs at presentation.
- 20% are small cell lung cancer, the rest are non-small cell mainly SCC or adenocarcinoma.
- 80% of people diagnosed with lung cancer die within the year as at diagnosis majority have advanced disease.

Prevention: 📖 Smoking cessation, p. 315.

## Signs and symptoms

- Persistent cough.
- Dyspnoea.
- Haemoptysis.
- Chest/shoulder pain.
- Finger clubbing.
- Unexplained weight and appetite loss.

Referred for urgent X-ray and to specialist. Investigations may include bronchoscopy, lung biopsy, CT, PET or other scans.

## Stages of lung cancer

Non-small cell lung cancer—4 stages:
- Stage 1. Localized cancer.
- Stage 2. Cancer in lymph nodes at top of lung.
- Stage 3. Cancer spread to chest wall.
- Stage 4. Metastases.

Small cell lung cancer stages—2 stages:
- Stage 1. Limited (to nearby lymph nodes).
- Stage 2. Extensive (metastases).

## Treatment and management

Depends on type of cancer. It may include:
- *Surgery:* rarely suitable for small cell lung cancer.
- Radiotherapy.
- *Chemotherapy:* standard for small cell lung cancer.

If in advanced stage palliative care offered with full involvement of primary care professionals and palliative care services.

## Related topics

📖 Palliative care in the home, p. 509; 📖 Symptom control in palliative care: breathlessness, p. 518.

## Further information

Cancer Research UK (2013), Lung cancer: key facts. Available at: ℔ www.cancerresearchuk.org
Macmillan Cancer Support: ☏ 0808 808 00 00. Available at: ℔ www.macmillan.org.uk/
NICE (2011). *The diagnosis and treatment of lung cancer (CG121).* Available at: ℔ http://guidance.nice.org.uk/cg121

# Renal problems

See 📖 Urinary tract infection, p. 707.

## Glomerulonephritis
Inflammation of both kidneys that can affect all or part of the kidney's glomeruli. It is most common in children, young adults, and men. Can be acute or chronic, but can cause renal damage with long-term consequences. Patient may be initially asymptomatic or have vague symptoms, e.g. tiredness, more acute symptoms include proteinuria, oliguria, haematuria, oedema, anorexia, and hypertension. Suspected cases need urgent referral to specialist.

## Nephrotic syndrome
Proteinuria that leads to oedema and hypoalbuminaemia. Patients have ascites, swelling of the face, peripheral oedema fatigue, anorexia due to kidney damage arising from:
- Minimal change glomerulonephritis (90% children, 30% adults).
- *Nephropathy:* caused by thickening of glomeruli.
- Glomerulonephritis.
- Scarring of glomeruli (focal segmental glomerulopnephritis).
- DM.

Suspected cases referred to specialist. Prognosis depends on cause, e.g. children with minimal change disease respond well to treatment.

## Renal stones
Passage of a stone in the ureter or kidney or bladder that causes acute, severe pain that comes in waves (renal colic). Patients may have haematuria and appear pale and sweaty. Occurs in 0.2% of population, ♂>♀. Believed incidence of stones ↑ because of western diet and obesity, often no underlying cause. Severity of pain unrelated to size of stone. Risk factors:
- People with recurrent UTI.
- People with neuropathic bladder dysfunction, e.g. paraplegia.
- People on certain medication, e.g. loop diuretics, thiazides, antacids, aspirin, calcium, vitamin D, steroids.
- People with congenital kidney abnormalities that cause urinary stasis.
- Dehydration.
- Patient with ileostomy → increased alkali loss from gut.
- FH.

### Care and management
Stones usually pass spontaneously, priority is good pain control. Patient will need an emergency hospital admission if fever, pain uncontrolled, has not passed urine, lives alone and/or symptoms persist for >24hrs.
- *Pain relief:* diclofenac IM (BNF 7.4).
- ↑ fluid intake, and encourage high fluid intake to ↓ risk of recurrence.
- Sieve urine to catch stone for future analysis; composition of stone will guide future dietary advice and interventions to prevent recurrence.

## Chronic kidney disease/chronic renal failure

CKD is progressive loss of renal function over time. Prevalence of CKD: ↑ age, ♂, South Asian, and African Caribbean ethnicity. The causes are: hypertension (📖 p. 589), vascular disease, diabetes (📖 p. 611), glomerulonephritis, chronic infection and recurrent UTIs (📖 p. 707), obstruction, possibly from renal stones, polycystic kidneys, hyperlipdae-mia. The aim is to treat causes early to prevent chronic renal failure (CRF):

- Early identification important to ↓ progression and risk of CVD and other health problems.
- 5 stages of CKD are based on estimated glomerular filtration rate (eGFR). eGFR is a sensitive measure of renal function.
- A minority of those with CKD stage 1 or 2 develop more advanced disease.
- CKD stage 3–5 = eGFR <60mL/min/1.73m$^2$ for >3mths), these people have <60% kidney function. 5% population have CKD stage 3–5.

### Care and management

- GP treats reversible causes, e.g. stops nephrotoxic drugs like NSAIDs.
- Monitors creatinine/eGRF levels and those patients with CKD stage 4 or 5 referred to specialist (see 📖 Quality and outcomes framework, p. 66).
- Monitors and reduces CVD risk, e.g. hypertension (📖 p. 589), smoking cessation (📖 p. 315) and other effects, e.g. bone disease, low vitamin D, anaemia, oedema. Depression (📖 People with depression, p. 435) is common.
- Patient advised:
  - Smoking cessation (📖 p. 315), regular exercise (📖 Exercise, p. 313), moderate alcohol (📖 p. 319) intake, no OTC NSAIDs.
  - Healthy low fat diet (📖 Nutrition and healthy eating, p. 304).
  - ↓ salt intake <6g (0.2oz) a day.
  - To have influenza immunizations (📖 Targeted immunization for adults, p. 347).

### End-stage renal failure

When kidney function is <5% of normal function and damage is irrevers-ible. Dialysis is used when GFR 10–15% of normal. It is needed for the rest of the patient's life or until kidney transplant. Two types:

- *Haemodialysis:* blood flows through dialysis machine, waste products cleared along a concentration gradient across a semi permeable membrane. Occurs 3x a week in hospital, a session takes 3–5hrs.
- *Continuous ambulatory peritoneal dialysis* (CAPD): a permanent catheter inserted into peritoneum and dialysis fluid is introduced and kept there. Changed for fresh fluid up to 5x a day. Process takes approx. 30mins, can be done at home. Automated peritoneal dialysis: uses a machine, and can be performed overnight. Possible problems include: peritonitis, catheter blockage (requires admission to hospital as emergency), weight gain, pleural effusion, leakage, and poor diabetic control.

### Further information

Kidney Research UK. Available at: ℘ www.kidneyresearchuk.org/
National Kidney Federation. Available at: ℘ www.kidney.org.uk

# Urinary tract infection

UTI may be asymptomatic occurring at any site of the urinary tract. is the commonest bacterial cause in the community >70%. Up to ½ with symptoms do not have bacteriuria. (See Table 12.3 for risk factors.)

## Types and symptoms

- *Cystitis* (infection of bladder): frequency, urgency, dysuria, polyuria, supra-pubic pain, fever, flank or back pain.
- *Pyelonephritis* (infection of kidney): fever, rigor, vomiting, loin pain and tenderness, acute renal failure.

Patients who are catheterized may complain of suprapubic pain and discomfort and have cloudy and foul smelling urine.

*Note:* older people who appear confused and disoriented may have UTI.

**Table 12.3** Risk factors for UTI

| ♀ | ♀ and ♂ |
|---|---|
| • Sexual intercourse. | • Urinary tract obstruction or malformation. |
| • Diaphragm contraceptive. | • Dehydration. |
| • Pregnancy. | • Delayed micturition (e.g. due to long journeys). |
| • Menopause (decreased oestrogen). | • Renal stones. |
| | • DM. |
| | • Catheterization. |

## Management

Majority of untreated, acute, uncomplicated cystitis will resolve in 3 days. SIGN[1] advises antibiotics should only be used when evidence that eradicating a bacterial infection will result in health gains, e.g. symptom relief. *Note:* bacteriuria common in asymptomatic older patients and treating = more harm than good.

- In non-pregnant ♀ <65yrs with <2 symptoms of UTI, use a dipstick. If positive commence empirical antibiotics as per local guidelines, e.g. trimetheoprim 3-day course.
- In non-pregnant ♀ <65yrs with ≥3 symptoms, including systemic signs, requires medical assessment as could have bacteraemia or other problems. Midstream urine taken and antibiotics commenced as per local guidelines ciprofloxacin 7day course.
- Pregnant women with symptoms of UTI, midstream urine taken, and commenced on antibiotics as per local guidelines.
- ♂ with signs and symptoms of UTI, urine sample taken for culture, if uncomplicated (no fever or back pain) treated as per local guidelines, e.g. trimethoprim 7-day course, if fever, back pain, fails to respond to treatment or recurrent UTI, it requires medical assessment (see 📖 UTI, p. 707).

- *Older people:* check no other symptoms suggestive of infection outside urinary tract, DO NOT use dipstick, obtain urine for culture, commence antibiotics as per local guidelines.

## Prevention and care
- *Pain relief:* paracetamol or ibuprofen (BNF 10.1, 4.7.1).
- Drink plenty of fluid (especially if patient is catheterized).
- *Double voiding:* go to the toilet and repeat 5min later.
- Voiding after intercourse (if UTI persist may need prophylactic antibiotics post-coitally).
- Wipe from front to back after going to the toilet (♀).
- *Limited evidence cranberry juice:* some evidence to suggest ↓2° bacteruria.
- ♀ with recurrent UTI may need prophylactic antibiotics or have a prescription in readiness for prompt treatment when first have symptoms.
- Menopausal ♀ with recurrent symptoms may benefit from topical or oral HRT (📖 Menopause, p. 323).
- Pregnant ♀ should be monitored carefully.

The patient is referred to specialist 2° care if symptoms unresolved.

## Related topics
📖 Urinary continence in women, p. 448; 📖 Urinary catheter care, p. 454; 📖 Sexual health: general issues, p. 711.

## Reference
[1]Scottish Intercollegiate Guidelines Network (SIGN) (2012). *SIGN 88 Management of suspected bacterial urinary tract infection in adults.* Available at: ⌖ www.sign.ac.uk

## Further information
Bladder and Bowel Foundation. Available at: ⌖ http://www.bladderandbowelfoundation.org/
NICE. CKS Urinary tract infection (lower) –men and women: Available at: ⌖ http://cks.nice.org.uk/
NICE (2010). *The management of lower urinary tract symptoms in men (CG97).* Available at: ⌖ http://guidance.nice.org.uk/CG97

# Prostate problems

## Benign prostatic hypertrophy

Benign prostatic hypertrophy (BPH) is also known as benign prostatic hyperplasia. It affects 10–30% ♂ >70yrs. The prostate enlarges with ageing → narrowing of urethra and partially obstructs the flow of urine. Symptoms often initially mild, but may interfere with QoL and become more severe, patients may complain of:

- *Poor and reduced stream:* taking longer to empty their bladder.
- *Hesitancy:* have to wait before urine flows.
- Dribbling of urine soon after finishing micturition causing staining and leakage.
- Feeling of incomplete emptying.
- Frequency, urgency, and nocturia.

### Complications

- Recurrent UTI (📖 UTI, p. 707).
- Acute urinary retention (1–2% develop urinary retention).
- Chronic obstruction.
- Overflow incontinence.
- Haematuria.
- Affect sexual function (erectile dysfunction, pain on ejaculation).

### Care and management

- Patient completing the International Prostate Symptom Score (IPSS) provides a useful baseline measure of severity and impact on QoL.
- Address any concerns about possibilities of cancer.
- *Patients with mild-to-moderate symptoms:* strategy of 'watchful waiting', reassurance, education, and advice on reducing caffeine and alcohol (📖 p. 319) intake, avoiding constipation (📖 Constipation in adults, p. 457), reducing fat intake in diet (📖 Nutrition and healthy eating, p. 304), bladder retraining (📖 Urinary incontinence in men, p. 453).
- Planning ahead and reducing fluid intake before important events, but important to maintain good fluid intake of minimum 1.5L per day.
- Control urgency with distraction and relaxation techniques.
- ♂ with mild-to-moderate symptoms and/or who experience ↓ QoL may benefit from drug treatment—alpha blockers, 5-alpha reductase inhibitors, or combination of both (BNF 2.5).
- Referred for surgery if other treatment failed or there are complications.

## Prostatitis

Considered a possibility for all men with UTI (📖 p. 707) treated with antibiotics.

## Prostate cancer

- Prostate cancer is the most common cancer in ♂, 90% >65yrs, and kills 10,000/yr in the UK.
- Incidence rising.
- Early cancer is symptomless. ♂ may present with:
  - Haematuria.

- Urinary retention/obstruction.
- Erectile dysfunction.
- Lower back pain and or bone pain (from metastases).
- Weight loss.

*Risk factors*
- ↑ Age >65yrs.
- FH.
- *Ethnic group:* highest rates in black men, lowest in Chinese men.
- Diet some evidence to suggest low fruit intake and high fat, high meat diet predisposes to prostate cancer.

England has introduced an informed choice risk management programme to provide information on prostate cancer and use of prostate specific antigen test (PSA test). PSA test has poor sensitivity and specificity so about 2 out of 3 with a raised PSA level will not have cancer. If PSA level is slightly raised GP undertakes further clinical assessment, e.g. digital rectal examination (DRE). On the basis of this or higher levels of PSA GP refers to urology specialist.

*Care and management*
*Note:* if asymptomatic then opinion divided about treatment options, i.e. no intervention vs. aggressive treatment.
- *Watchful waiting and careful monitoring PSA:*↑ PSA or DRE or ↑ nodule size then active treatment.
- *Radical prostatectomy:* potential for cure, but risks and complications associated with surgery in older patients as well as impotence and incontinence.
- *Radiotherapy:* evidence on effectiveness unclear.
- *Hormone therapy:* evidence on effectiveness unclear in early disease.

*For patients with symptoms*
Hormone manipulation is the main treatment approach to help ↓ PSA, bone pain, and incidence of complications such as spinal cord compression.
- *Luteinizing hormone releasing hormone (LHRH) analogues:* a SC injection every 4–12wks to ↓ testosterone levels equivalent to those of a castrated man (BNF 8.3.4.2) (☐ Injection techniques, p. 532). Side effects—impotence, hot flushes, gynaecomastia, local bruising around injection site.
- Anti-androgens either in combination with LHRH or as monotherapy.
- Surgical castration.
- *Bony metastases:* corticosteroids and radiotherapy.

**Further information**
Cancer Research UK (2013). Prostate Cancer Key Facts. Available at: ℬ www.cancerresearchuk. org/cancer-help/type/prostate-cancer/
NICE (2008). *Prostate cancer: diagnosis and treatment (CG58).* Available at: ℬ http://guidance.nice. org.uk/CG58
NICE (2010). *The management of lower urinary tract symptoms in men (CG97).* Available at: ℬ http:// guidance.nice.org.uk/CG97NICE:
NICE (2010). The management of lower urinary tract symptoms in men Appendix H (CG97). Available at: ℬ http://guidance.nice.org.uk/CG97
Prostate Cancer Risk Management Programme (England). Available at: ℬ www.cancerscreening. nhs.uk/prostate/
Prostate Research Campaign UK. Available at: ℬ www.prostate-research.org.uk

# Sexual health: general issues

Continued increases in sexual risk behaviour, and diagnoses of HIV and sexually transmitted infections (STIs) highlight the need to provide access to a range of prevention, diagnostic, and treatment opportunities. Target groups include young adults (<25yrs), MSM, and black African and Caribbean communities. Treatment of STIs should be in accordance with national clinical effectiveness guidelines and free of prescription charges. People at risk of STIs should have their care managed by appropriately trained staff in a range of 'open access' services, including primary care. If in doubt, refer suspected cases of STIs and HIV to local GUM clinic (📖 Sexual health consultations, p. 713).

## Confidentiality

People have the right to confidentiality regardless of where they access care. Concerns over confidentiality can be overcome by developing a sensitive and non-judgemental culture (📖 Anti-discriminatory health care, p. 76). Non-discrimination and confidentiality statements should be displayed for patients to see. NHS organizations have an obligation to keep secure any information about STIs obtained by health care workers. Information should be regarded as confidential and not communicated except to other health care practitioners for the purposes of treatment or prevention. In exceptional circumstances, information may need to be shared in the interest of the patient or public as set out in guidance documents, e.g. local safeguarding policies.

*Confidentiality and <16yrs*
See Fraser guidelines, 📖 Contraception: general, p. 359.

## Partner notification

- All services should instigate partner notification (PN) as part of STI management.
- Explain to patient that PN is essential (except for candida and bacterial vaginosis (BV)) to reduce risk of re-infection to self, and to stop the spread of infection to other sexual partners.
- Encourage patient to notify recent sexual partner(s) of their STI, and advise them to seek treatment.
- For complex cases, seek advice or refer to health advisers or other GUM staff. Health advisers can perform provider referral PN, whereby the index patient provides information on partner(s) to a health adviser, who then confidentially traces and notifies the partner(s) directly.

## Sexual assault

Disclosure of non-consenting sex should never be ignored. People who have been sexually assaulted or raped can be referred as urgent cases to GUM services, or to designated sexual assault referral centres (SARCs) that can provide medical care, forensic examination and liaison with the police, as and if requested by the patient. Patients can self-refer to SARCs.

Non-consenting sex in <16yrs requires local child protection procedures to be followed (📖 Child protection, p. 230).

## Health promotion

Sexual health should be proactively and positively promoted as an important aspect of an individual's overall health and wellbeing. Specific interventions should focus on safer sex skill acquisition, enhancing communication skills and increasing motivation to adopt safer sex behaviours.

- Promote consistent condom use for vaginal and anal sex, plus water-based lubricant (lube) for anal sex.
- Provide free condoms and lube, or suggest where client can access these. Demonstrate condom use as required.
- Discuss regular contraception and promote awareness of emergency contraception and long-acting reversible contraception (LARC).
- Awareness of sexually transmitted infection signs and symptoms.
- Provide sexual health leaflets, web-links, and helpline numbers.
- Where there is an ongoing risk of HIV transmission (e.g. HIV sero-discordant couple), discuss HIV PEP.
- Refer to sexual health services for specialist intervention on risk reduction.

## Related topics

📖 Sexually transmitted infections, p. 715.

## Further information

British Association for Sexual Health & HIV (BASHH) STI management guidelines. Available at: 🖱 www.bashh.org

British HIV Association HIV testing and management guidelines. Available at: 🖱 www.bhiva.org

Brook provides free & confidential advice for under 25s: 📞 Helpline: 0808 802 1234. Available at: 🖱 www.brook.org.uk

FPA provides information, advice and support on sexual health, sex and relationships for everyone in the UK. 📞 Helpline: 0845 122 8690 (England) 0845 122 8687 (Northern Ireland). Available at: 🖱 www.fpa.org.uk

Government policies on reducing STIs in each country of UK see 📖 Useful websites, p. 800.

HPA STI/HIV epidemiological data: Available at: 🖱 www.hpa.org.uk/Topics/InfectiousDiseases/InfectionsAZ/STIs/

NAM Comprehensive prevention, treatment and support information about HIV: Available at: 🖱 www.aidsmap.com

RCGP and BASHH (2013). Sexually Transmitted Infections in Primary Care (2nd edition) Available at: 🖱 www.bashh.org and www.rcgp.org

Sexual Health Symptom Checker. 📞 Sexual Health Helpline (any age) 0800 567 123. Available at: 🖱 www.nhs.uk/NHSdirect/pages/symptoms.aspx?sat=DHASMaleSexualHealth

Sexual health information and advice for young people: 📞 Helpline: 0800 28 29 30 (under 20s). Available at: 🖱 www.nhs.uk/worthtalkingabout

# Sexual health consultations

See 📖 Sexual health: general issues, p. 711.

Practitioners should ensure that the consultation is under taken in a sensitive and non-judgemental manner. Reassure confidentiality and ensure privacy. When undertaking care of under-18s, follow local and national guidance on safeguarding children.

## Sexual history assessment

Degree of assessment depends on practitioner skill and competence. Good practice suggests:
- Ask about symptoms (location, type, severity, duration, aggravation/alleviating factors, self-treatment).
- Recent sexual partner(s) (gender, type of sex, condom use).
- Contraception use.
- Past STIs, HIV status and testing history, and cervical cancer screening in ♀.

## Physical examination

Degree of examination is dependent on practitioner competence. Referral to medical colleagues or GUM service may be required if not competent, equipment not available, or history indicates complex problems. If performing an examination, offer a chaperone (📖 Chaperones, p. 79). Good practice suggests an examination should include:
- Observe external genital area for ulceration, rashes, warts, and other abnormal lesions/growths, other dermatoses, pubic lice, scabies, palpate for lymphadenopathy.
- ♂: observe for urethral discharge (colour, consistency), palpate testicles for irregularities, pain, epididymal tenderness, other abnormalities.
- ♀: speculum examination for abnormal discharge (colour, consistency, odour, pH), internal warts or ulcers, cervical erosion or contact bleeding. Palpate for lower abdominal tenderness. Bimanual examination for adnexal tenderness and cervical excitation (*note*: if competent).

## STI testing

- Undertaken in primary care according to commissioned pathway, availability of skilled staff, equipment, and diagnostic capability.
- Practices and clinics preparing to undertake testing should confirm with local laboratory the testing methods available, required samples, transport medium and how soon these should reach the laboratory as these often differ between services.
- Local treatment and referral pathways determined by local sexual health clinical networks.
- Opportunistic chlamydia self-taken swab or urine screening widely available for <25yrs in GP, family planning clinics, high street pharmacies, youth centres.
- Other STI tests performed according to signs and symptoms (📖 Sexually transmitted infections, p. 715).

- Genital sites for STI testing dependent on signs and symptoms, and sexual behaviour/orientation.

## HIV testing

- All nurses have the communication skills required to engage patients in a pre-HIV test discussion, supported with leaflets and information on availability of testing.
- Local policies will determine if practice or clinic provides HIV antibody tests, including rapid point of care tests.
- Where high risk of HIV infection, the patient may require support before or after testing, which can be provided in GUM clinics.

## Referral to GUM clinics

- Patients should be referred if equipment and/or diagnostic technology not available, diagnosis unclear, specialist investigation or treatment required, or according to local care pathways.
- Complex partner notification should be managed by GUM specialists.
- Referral letter useful if investigations have already been performed and treatment commenced.
- Patients can self-refer to GUM clinics and SARCs.

## Confidentiality and partner notification

See 📖 Sexual health: general issues, p. 711.

## Sexual health promotion

See 📖 Sexual health: general issues, p. 711.

## Related topic

📖 Sexually transmitted infections, p. 715.

## Further information

British Association for Sexual Health & HIV (BASHH) STI management guidelines. Available at: ℅ www.bashh.org

British HIV Association HIV testing and management guidelines. Available at: ℅ www.bhiva.org

Government policies on reducing STIs in each country of UK see 📖 Useful websites, p. 800.

HPA STI/HIV epidemiological data. Available at: ℅ www.hpa.org.uk/Topics/InfectiousDiseases/InfectionsAZ/STIs/

RCGP and BASHH (2013). Sexually Transmitted Infections in Primary Care (2nd edition). Available at: ℅ www.bashh.org and www.rcgp.org

### Patient information and support

Brook provides free & confidential advice for under 25s: ☎ Helpline: 0808 802 1234. Available at: ℅ www.brook.org.uk

FPA provides information, advice and support on sexual health, sex and relationships for everyone in the UK: ☎ Helpline: 0845 122 8690 (England) 0845 122 8687 (Northern Ireland). Available at: ℅ www.fpa.org.uk

NAM Comprehensive prevention, treatment and support information about HIV. Available at: ℅ www.aidsmap.com

Sexual Health Symptom Checker: ☎ Sexual Health Helpline (any age) 0800 567 123. Available at: ℅ www.nhs.uk/NHSdirect/pages/symptoms.aspx?sat=DHASMaleSexualHealth

Sexual health information and advice for young people: ☎ Helpline: 0800 28 29 30 (under 20s). Available at: ℅ www.nhs.uk/worthtalkingabout

# Sexually transmitted infections

## Bacterial vaginosis
(See 📖 Vaginal and vulval problems, p. 737.)

## Candidiasis (thrush)
(See 📖 Fungal infections, p. 638; ♀ see 📖 Vaginal and vulval problems, p. 737.)

## Chlamydia
- ♀: mostly asymptomatic or ↑ vaginal discharge, post-coital or intermenstrual bleeding, dysuria, lower abdominal pain, dyspareunia.
- ♂: often asymptomatic or mild to moderate clear or whitish urethral discharge, dysuria.
- *Rectal:*↑ MSM. Mucopurulent blood stained rectal discharge, rectal pain and tenesmus. GUM referral essential for management of potential lymphogranuloma venereum.
- *Pharyngeal:*↑ MSM, although incidence and natural history unclear.

*Investigations*
- ♀: endocervical, vaginal self-swab or urine for nucleic acid amplification test (NAAT).
- ♂: urethral swab or urine for NAAT.

*Treatment*
- Azithromycin 1g po as a single dose (BNF 5.1.5).
- Doxycycline 100mg/12h po for 7 days (contraindicated in pregnancy) (BNF 5.1.3).
- Erythromycin 500mg/12h po for 14 days (BNF 5.1.5).

## Genital herpes
Presents as blistering and ulceration, usually painful, multiple, and clustered. Systemic flu-like symptoms may be present. ❶ Specialist advice required if in third trimester of pregnancy.

*Investigations*
Swab base of lesion(s) and place in appropriate viral transport medium.

*Treatment*
Advise saline bathing and analgesia for symptom relief. Oral antiviral drugs indicated within 5 days of the start of the episode and while new lesions are still forming. Aciclovir, famciclovir, or valaciclovir (BNF 5.3.2).

## Genital warts
External ano-genital skin lesions. Also found on vagina, cervix, urethral meatus, and anal canal. Soft and fleshy, or firm and irregular growths. Single or multiple, raised or flat. Usually non-painful, sometimes itchy.

*Diagnosis*
Clinical observation in most cases. Refer to GUM if in doubt.

*Treatment*
Podophyllotoxin solution or cream (BNF 13.7) suitable for home treatment. Other treatments are available in GUM clinic.

## Gonorrhoea

- ♀: ~50% asymptomatic or ↑ vaginal discharge, dysuria, intermenstrual bleeding.
- ♂: almost always yellow/green purulent discharge, dysuria within 2–5 days of sexual contact.
- *Rectal:*↑ MSM. Often asymptomatic. Mucopurulent discharge, pain, tenesmus, bleeding, constipation, anal pruritus.
- *Pharyngeal:*↑ MSM. Usually asymptomatic, occasionally pharyngitis.

*Investigations*
Exposed sites (endocervical, urethral, pharyngeal, rectal) swabbed and sent for culture or NAAT. Rapid diagnosis is available in GUM.

*Treatment*
Ceftriaxone 500mg IM as a single dose (BNF 5.1.2) plus azithromycin 1g po as a single dose (BNF 5.1.5).

## HIV

📖 Human immunodeficiency virus, p. 686.

## Hepatitis A/B/C

📖 Viral hepatitis, p. 676.

## Lymphogranuloma venereum (LGV)

UK outbreaks in MSM since 2004. Ano-rectal syndrome presents with anal discharge, pain, and tenesmus. Inguinal syndrome presents with genital ulceration, painful inguinal adenopathy.

*Investigation and treatment*
Refer MSM with ano-rectal symptoms to GUM for management.

## Non-gonococcal urethritis (NGU)

♂ only: mild to moderate clear or whitish urethral discharge ± dysuria. Chlamydia is the cause in 30–50% of cases.

*Investigations*
Diagnosis relies on microscopy, usually only available in GUM clinics. Urethral swab for gonorrhoea and chlamydia. Can be treated on clinical signs and symptoms if other STIs excluded.

*Treatment*
- Azithromycin 1g stat po (BNF 5.1.5).
- Doxycycline 100mg/12h po for 7 days (BNF 5.1.3).

## Pubic lice

See (📖 Insects and infestations, p. 287). Treated with permethrin, phenothrin or malathion (BNF 13.10.4).

## Syphilis

Resurgence in UK since 1999; substantial increases in MSM. Incubation 9–90 days. Refer to GUM for investigation, treatment, and PN. Presents in 4 stages:

- *Primary syphilis:* usually a solitary, painless, indurated ulcer (chancre) at point of sexual contact (genital, oral, rectal).
- *Secondary syphilis:* 2–4wks after chancre. Non-itchy, macular or papular rash, may affect palms and soles. Systemic symptoms: fever, malaise, generalized lymphadenopathy.
- *Latent syphilis:* asymptomatic period between untreated secondary and tertiary stages.
- *Tertiary syphilis:* very rare in UK. Cardiovascular or neurological manifestations up to 30yrs after untreated infection.

### Treatment
Dependent on stage. Refer to GUM for management.

## Trichomonas vaginalis (TV)

- ♀: ↑ vaginal discharge (discoloured, offensive, frothy), vulval soreness, dyspareunia, dysuria. Can be asymptomatic.
- ♂: rarely diagnosed in men, but should always treat if a sexual contact.

### Investigations
Usually swab from posterior vaginal fornix sent in transport media (e.g. Amies, Stuarts) to laboratory within 6hrs. Refrigerate while awaiting transportation. Rapid diagnosis is available in GUM clinics.

### Treatment
- Metronidazole 2g po as a single dose (BNF 5.1.11).
- Metronidazole 400mg/12h po for 5 days (preferred in pregnant women).

## Further information

British Association for Sexual Health & HIV (BASHH) STI management guidelines. Available at: ℘ www.bashh.org

RCGP and BASHH (2013). Sexually Transmitted Infections in Primary Care (2nd edition) Available at: ℘ www.bashh.org and www.rcgp.org

### Patient information and support

Brook provides free & confidential advice for under 25s: ☎ Helpline: 0808 802 1234. Available at: ℘ www.brook.org.uk

FPA provides information, advice and support on sexual health, sex and relationships for everyone in the UK: ☎ Helpline: 0845 122 8690 (England) 0845 122 8687 (Northern Ireland). Available at: ℘ www.fpa.org.uk

Sexual Health Symptom Checker: ☎ Sexual Health Helpline (any age) 0800 567 123. Available at: ℘ www.nhsdirect.nhs.uk/checksymptoms/topics/sexualhealth

Sexual health information and advice for young people: ☎ Helpline: 0800 28 29 30 (under 20s). Available at: ℘ www.nhs.uk/worthtalkingabout

# Sexual problems

Sexual problems can be physical or psychogenic in origin, or a mix of both. Careful, non-judgemental history taking can ascertain whether referral to practitioners specializing in psychosexual counselling or pharmacotherapy is warranted. General counselling (📖 Counselling skills, p. 123; 📖 Talking therapies, p. 429) can help resolve hidden conflicts, deal with various emotions, and explore relationship issues. Psychosexual therapy provides more specialist intervention. Local GUM, urology, and contraception services offer various degrees of assessment and management. In all problems it is useful to provide patient with accurate and relevant information. Various self-help books and videos are available.

## History taking

Define the exact nature of the problem and consider key clues as to its origin. Explore associated factors:

- Why is the patient seeking treatment now?
- What does the patient think is the cause?
- What has the patient tried?
- Does the patient's partner know?
- What is the partner's attitude?
- What does the patient hope to achieve?
- Past/current medical and psychiatric history.
- Social and relationship history including life events associated with problem.

## Loss of libido

Poorly understood and often difficult to treat. May be a result of physical illness, hormonal changes, medication side effects, psychological problems, relationship difficulties, partner attraction issues, or life changes. Identify and treat physical cause and/or refer for counselling.

## Dyspareunia

Dyspareunia is recurrent genital or pelvic pain associated with sexual activity. Repeated sexual pain can set up a cycle, in which fear of pain leads to avoidance of the sexual activity that produces it, in turn leading to lack of arousal, failure to achieve orgasm, and loss of sexual desire.

- ♂ may be anatomical problem, e.g. phimosis, or infection.
- ♀ may be physical causes, e.g. scarring from childbirth, genital circumcision, lack of lubrication, or psychosexual problems.

Abdominal and vaginal examination ± STI screening and treatment as required excludes physical causes. Referred to GUM as necessary. Psychosexual: similar treatment approaches used for vaginismus can be effective.

## Vaginismus

Vaginismus is an involuntary reflex spasm of the muscles surrounding the entrance to the vagina that may be severe enough to prevent any form of vaginal penetration. Vaginal examination may exclude physical cause. A penetration desensitization programme may be helpful, in which patient is encouraged to insert 1 finger, then 2, then 3 into her vagina, while relaxing the lower vaginal muscles. Clear instructions and regular follow-up are vital for success. If problems persist, refer to psychosexual therapist or sexual problems clinic. Partner involvement may be helpful.

## Erectile dysfunction

Failure to achieve or maintain satisfactory erection. History may denote physical or psychogenic cause. ↑ association with CVD or diabetes. May be the adverse effect of medication (e.g. some antidepressants, anti-hypertensives). Hormonal evaluation is often requested, although erectile dysfunction is seldom due to hormonal problems. Mainstay of treatment includes oral pharmacological agents taken prior to sex (e.g. sildenafil, BNF 7.4.5). Counselling may be of benefit for psychogenic causes.

## Premature ejaculation

Ejaculation with minimal sexual stimulation before the person or partner wishes. Clinical and psychosocial history may identify cause (e.g. anxiety/ depression, relationship difficulties). Squeeze/stop-start technique common approach to controlling ejaculation—intercourse is halted and penis is firmly squeezed at base of glans when man feels close to ejaculation/ orgasm. Sex can then resume until point of ejaculation is reached again, squeeze/stop-start repeated, and so on. Other treatments include formal psychosexual counselling and pharmacotherapy prescribed by sexual dysfunction specialist.

## Further information

BASHH Sexual dysfunction management guidelines. Available at: ℘ www.bashh.org

Sexual Advice Association provides public and professionals with information about sexual problems. Available at: ℘ www.sda.uk.net

## Patient information and support

College of Sexual and Relationship Therapists provides a list of UK therapists. Available at: ℘ www.cosrt.org.uk

PACE provides sexual and relationship counselling for lesbians and gay men. Available at: ℘ www. pacehealth.org.uk

Relate provides therapy for sex problems. Available at: ℘ www.relate.org.uk

# Sexual health and adults with a learning disability

See 📖 People with learning disabilities, p. 408. Most people with are seen in a primary care setting at least once per year due to concomitant health needs. Sexual health needs of people with LDs will vary, but frequently include the following:

- Relationship guidance and counselling (boundary setting, giving and withholding consent, keeping safe, emotional health and issues such as love, friendship, etc.).
- Bodily awareness and information on sexual functioning and management, e.g. menstruation, erection, sexual intercourse, etc.
- Contraception and family planning, e.g. the use and application of barrier and chemical contraceptives.
- Pregnancy and childbirth.
- Information on and access to screening services, e.g. cervical and breast screening.
- Information on and access to GU services when needed.

## Fundamental elements in service provision

- Liaise with the community learning disability team to acquire background knowledge.
- Involve family and carers when appropriate. ❶ *But* maintain confidentiality wherever possible.
- Communicate directly with the client. 48% of people with a LD has impairment in one sensory domain and 18% are doubly impaired ∴ informed consent is hard to achieve.
  - Assess on an individual basis, check understanding, e.g. asking client to outline what has just been explained to them.
  - Speak clearly and directly to the client.
  - Treat clients with the same dignity and respect given to any other client.
  - Use pictures, signs, and large clear print to get your message across. For resources contact the local community LD team.
  - Use models to demonstrate techniques where appropriate, and allow return demonstration and follow-up when necessary.
  - People with LD may be limited in terms of conceptual thinking, where possible try to demonstrate on life like equipment.
- Many women smoke cigarettes, combined with unprotected sexual intercourse ↑ vulnerable to cervical cancer (📖 Cervical cancer screening, p. 337).

### Attitudes of professionals and carers

Many people with LD are sexually active, and their carers may not know or acknowledge this.

- Assumptions regarding health need and negative attitudes are related to the degree of physical evidence of a disability, but may bear little resemblance to reality.
- Be extra vigilant for signs of abuse and look out for warning signs and listen to the client.

*Note:* some women with LD may have been sexually abused. Studies show this often starts at an early age, and is unrelated to the severity of LD.

### Consent vs. cooperation
Ethical dilemmas arise when client cannot give verbal consent, and the difficulty is in determining whether the treatment is in the client's best interest. Where verbal consent is not possible, and there is reason to believe that the client is sexually active or has been exposed involuntarily to sexual activity.

Co-operation may be all that is achievable. Consider the consequences to the client of withholding the treatment/service when making a decision.

### Time and place
*People with LDs will need more time:* plan visit/try to allocate a double appointment accordingly.
- Try to allocate the first or last appointment.
- Try to avoid crowded rushed or noisy situations.
- Ensure that access to your service is physically possible, some people with LD are also physically disabled.

### Related topics
📖 Models and approaches to health promotion, p. 298; 📖 Contraception: general, p. 359; 📖 Mental capacity, p. 424.

### Further information
Family Planning Association Projects supporting people with learning disabilities. Available at: ℘ www.fpa.org.uk/advice-parents-and-carers/if-your-child-has-learning-disability

National Health Service Cancer Screening Programmes (2006). Equal Access to Breast and Cervical Screening for Women With Disabilities. Available at: ℘ www.cancerscreening.nhs.uk/publications/cs2.html

# Breast problems

❶ Women should consult or be referred to GP if they report:
- *Lump:* new, discrete lump; breast abscess; refilling/recurrent cyst.
- *Pain:* associated with a lump; persistent pain.
- Nipple discharge.
- Nipple retraction, distortion, or nipple eczema.
- Change in skin contour.
- FH of breast cancer.
- GP assessment includes need for referral to specialist.

**Breast cysts** Firm, rounded lump of any size, single or multiple, occurs pre-menopause, not associated with skin changes. Refer to GP.

**Fibro-adenoma** Majority of all benign breast neoplasms. Common in women <35yrs. Giant fibro-adenomas may occur in older women. Presents with painless, hard, extremely mobile lump. It is usually removed.

**Breast problems associated with breastfeeding** Mastitis, breast abscess, see 📖 Breastfeeding, p. 176.

*Breast pain (mastalgia)* Many ♀ experience breast pain. Most common in ♀ 30–50yrs. Cause is unknown. In many women it is mild, but in some women it becomes more severe and can affect day-to-day life. It can present as cyclical pain associated with menstruation or non-cyclical. For some it is also associated with a lump or diffuse lumpiness that changes size through the cycle (known as benign mammary dysplasia). Refer to GP for assessment.

*Management of mastalgia*
Once other serious problems ruled out includes:
- *Mild:* no treatment, simple analgesics, advise on well-supporting bra.
- *More severe:*
- Wear a well-supporting bra 24hrs especially approaching period.
  - Some ♀ find caffeine ↑ pain so stop tea, coffee, and cola, although evidence limited to support this.
  - Some ♀ find low fat, high carbohydrate diet helps.
  - Take painkillers, e.g. ibuprofen regularly when breasts are painful.
  - COC or HRT can make pain worse in some ♀. Review by GP.
  - Topical NSAID, e.g. ibuprofen (BNF 10.1.1) is effective and well tolerated, available OTC.
  - Oestrogen reducing medication (e.g. danazol BNF 6.7.2) used for severe, cyclical, persistent pain, but side effects, e.g. weight gain, menorrhagia. Effective in about 80% ♀.

## Related topics
📖 Breast cancer awareness and screening, p. 335; 📖 Breast cancer, p. 723.

## Further information
NICE. CKS Breast Pain-cyclical: Available at: ℛ www.clinicalevidence.com http://cks.nice.org.uk/breast-pain-cyclical#!topicsummary

# Breast cancer

Breast is the commonest cancer in the UK. Accounts for 18% of all female cancers—British women have a 1:8 lifetime risk of developing the disease. Although mortality is falling, breast cancer is the 3rd most common cause of cancer death in the UK accounting for ~12,000 deaths/yr.

## Risk factors

- *Age:*↑ with age—80% in women >50yrs.
- *Reproductive history:*↑ risk if early menarche or late menopause; late age at 1st birth ↑ risk; ↑ parity →↓ risk; breastfeeding ↓ risk.
- *Hormones:* slight ↑ risk in current and recent users of combined oral contraceptives—excess risk disappears >10yrs after stopping; in users of combined HRT risk ↑ by 6 cases/1000 after 5yrs and 19 cases/1000 after 10yrs use.
- *Lifestyle:* obesity ↑ risk post menopause; 30% ↓ risk if taking regular physical activity; high fat diet is probably associated with ↑ risk; alcohol ↑ risk by 7%/unit consumed/day.
- *Physical characteristics:* taller women have ↑ risk; women with denser breasts have 2–6x ↑ risk.
- *Ionizing radiation:* exposure ↑ risk.
- *Previous breast disease:* past history of either benign or malignant breast disease ↑ risk.
- *Family history:* 1 first degree relative with breast cancer (mother or sister) ↑ risk x 2—but 85% of women with breast cancer have no FH. If several family members with early onset breast cancer referred for genetic screening—BRCA1 and BRCA2 genes account for 2–5% all breast cancers.

## Prevention

- *Lifestyle measures:* ↓ alcohol intake; ↓ weight; avoid exogenous sex hormones (e.g. HRT); breast feed.
- *Chemoprophylaxis:* tamoxifen ↓ risk of breast cancer by 40% in high-risk women, but limited by side effects (thromboembolism and endometrial carcinoma)—other drug trials in progress.
- *Prophylactic surgery:* ↓ risk by 90% in very high-risk women.

## Presentation

- Found at breast screening (📖 Breast cancer awareness, p. 335).
- *Clinical presentation:* breast lump (90%); breast pain (21% present with painful lump; pain alone <1%); nipple skin change; FH (6%); skin contour change (5%); nipple discharge (3%). In the older people breast cancer may grow slowly and present with extensive local lesions.
- *Paget's disease of the breast:* intra-epidermal, intraductal cancer. Any red, scaly lesion or eczema around the nipple suggests Paget's disease.

### Management
Referred for urgent assessment to a breast surgeon. Specialist investigation includes USS; mammography ± fine needle aspiration or biopsy; investigations to evaluate spread (e.g. CT, liver USS, bone scan).

### Classification
Virtually all breast cancers are adenocarcinomas.
- *In situ* (non-invasive) *Stage I:* ≤2cm diameter; no LNs (lymph nodes) affected; no spread beyond breast.
- *Stage II and III:* 2–5cm or >5cm diameter and/or LNs armpit affected; no evidence of spread beyond armpit.
- *Stage IV:* any sized tumour; LNs armpit affected; spread to other parts of the body.

### Treatment
Treatment includes surgery (lumpectomy ± axillary clearance, mastectomy) and other treatments: radiotherapy, hormonal therapy, biological therapy and/or chemotherapy. Tamoxifen ↑ survival of patients with oestrogen receptor +ve tumours (60% tumours) of any age but rare risk of endometrial carcinoma—warn to report any untoward vaginal bleeding. Tamoxifen for ≥5yrs (BNF 8.3.4.1). Anastrozole blocks oestrogen synthesis. Higher efficacy than tamoxifen in hormone sensitive early cancer in post-menopausal ♀ and first choice for post-menopausal ♀ with advanced cancer. Used for ≥5yrs. In ♀ who are HER2 positive (i.e. the 1.5 ♀ whose breast cancer cells have a large number of the HER2 receptors on surface), Trastuzumab (Herceptin®) is used when at high risk of recurrence or at advanced stage. Given IV 3 weekly for 1yr.

### Lymphoedema
All patients who have breast surgery are at risk. Injury to the arm on the surgery side may precipitate/worsen lymphoedema. *Do not* take blood from that limb or BP measurement; use it for IV access or vaccination (see 📖 Lymphoedema, p. 505).

### Post surgery
- Pain: some women find that their breast and arm are sore for up to a year after the treatment, encourage appropriate pain relief.
- Arm and shoulder stiffness, tingling: encourage exercises.
- Pins and needles, burning, numbness or darting sensations in the chest area and down the arm quite common. Can go on for weeks.
- Cording feels like a tight cord running from armpit, down arm through to the back of hand. Can appear 6–8wks after surgery. Thought to be hardening of lymph vessels. May resolve or may need physiotherapy.
- A lightweight foam prosthesis (sometimes called a cumfie or softie), given to be worn inside bra post-surgery. When wound healed (6–8wks), can be fitted with silicone prosthesis. Breast care nurse (usually linked to local acute hospital) provides advice on type and care. Several types available from the NHS.
- Possibilities of reconstructive surgery discussed with specialists.

## Psychological impact of breast cancer
Depression, anxiety, marital, and sexual problems are common. Psychological support should be offered.

## Related topics
📖 Breast cancer awareness, p. 335; 📖 Palliative care in the home, p. 509; 📖 Post-operative wound care, p. 478.

## Further information
Breast Cancer Care. ☎ 0808 800 6000. Available at: 🖰 www.breastcancercare.org.uk

Cancer Research UK Breast Cancer Key Facts. Available at: 🖰 www.cancerresearchuk.org/cancer-info/cancerstats/keyfacts/breast-cancer/

Macmillan Cancer Support Cancer Research UK. Available at: 🖰 www.macmillan.org.uk/Home.aspx

# Gynaecological cancers

The possibility, as well as the diagnosis of cancer provokes fear and anxiety in everyone. Most women feel shocked and upset by the idea of having treatment to the most intimate and private parts of their body. Psychological support is important as well as clear information about investigations, treatments, effects including on sex life. Treatment may involve surgical removal of part or whole organs that many women feel are important parts of their female identity. This is often an important area of grieving and loss to address. The most common cancers are ovarian (4th most common cancer in ♀), cervical, and uterine.

## Cervical cancer

Incidence dropping due to screening programme (📖 Cervical cancer screening, p. 337).

### Symptoms

Abnormal smear test, post-coital bleeding, vaginal bleeding and/or discharge. Referred to gynaecologist. Diagnosis is by colposcopy or cone biopsy.

### Treatment

Dependent on stage. Localized early cancerous changes destroyed by electrocoagulation, diathermy, laser treatment or cryosurgery, cone biopsy. Later stage cancer requires surgery and radiotherapy (if cancer confined to cervix 5-yr survival rate >90%).

## Ovarian cancer

Most common cancer affecting the pelvic organs. 5000 ♀ are diagnosed in UK each year. Average age 63yrs.

### Risk factors

Increasing age, family history, nulliparity.

### Symptoms

Vaginal bleeding, abdominal discomfort and bloating, ascites.

### Treatment

Surgery—extent depends on stage (📖 Hysterectomy, p. 733) and sometimes adjuvant chemotherapy. May also have chemotherapy prior to surgery. If disease is confined to the ovaries/pelvis 5-yr survival is 50–90%.

## Uterine cancer

Endometrial is the most common form. Peak incidence is between 55–70yrs.

### Risk factors

Age, obesity, nulliparity, late menopause, DM, family history of breast, ovary, or colon cancer.

### Symptoms

Abnormal vaginal bleeding, dysparunia, post-menopausal bleeding.

*Treatment*

Surgery, usually hysterectomy (📖 p. 733), radiotherapy, progesterone treatment and/or chemotherapy. Radiotherapy in pelvic area can cause diarrhoea and cystitis.

## Vaginal cancer

Rare, <300 ♀ diagnosed/yr in UK. More common as a 2° cancer. SCC most common, develops in ♀ 60–80yrs. Adenocarcinoma rare, mainly in ♀ <20yrs.

*Symptoms*

Vaginal bleeding, dysparunia, problems with micturition.

*Treatment*

- *Surgery:* type depends on the position and size of cancer. May be part (remaining tissue stretched so vagina intact) or whole vagina (vaginectomy). Sometimes possible for vaginal reconstruction using tissue from other parts of the body. May also need hysterectomy (📖 p. 733).
- *Radiotherapy:* may be external or internal. In pre-menopausal ♀, radiotherapy likely to produce menopause about 3mths after treatment, also can cause diarrhoea and cystitis. Radiotherapy causes shortening and narrowing of the vagina, and to prevent this advised to use a vaginal dilator each day during and for some time after the treatment.
- Chemotherapy.

Affect on sex life depends on the type of surgery as well as woman's emotional response to the experience. Clitoris is not affected by surgery and orgasms can still be achieved through clitoral stimulation. Vaginal orgasm is not possible after vaginal reconstruction.

## Vulval cancer

Rare. 90% SCC, usually grow very slowly. 4% melanoma. ⅔ develop in ♀ who have vulval intraepithelial neoplasia linked to some types of HPV.

*Symptoms*

Skin colour or texture change, itching, burning, lump, or swelling.

*Treatment*

Surgery, extent depends on size and position of cancer—may involve removal of labia and clitoris (vulvectomy), radiotherapy, and chemotherapy. Radiotherapy in pelvic area can cause diarrhoea and cystitis. Vulvectomy alters the outward appearance of the body. It is a change that shocks many and they find hard to accept. Often has a profound effect on attitude to sex. Orgasms still achievable, but may need to explore different ways of achieving them.

## Related topics

📖 Hysterectomy, p. 733.

## Further information

Cancer Research UK: ☏ Helpline 0808 800 4040. Available at: ✍ www.cancerresearchuk.org
Macmillan Cancer Support Cancer Research UK: ☏ Helpline: 0808 808 00 00. Available at: ✍ www.macmillan.org.uk/Home.aspx

# Menstrual problems

## Menstruation

This is the periodic shedding of the endometrium. Day 1 of bleeding is the start of the menstrual cycle. FSH stimulates the egg follicle to mature, secreting oestrogen which thickens the endometrium. LH causes egg release (ovulation). Some ♀ feel a pain (known as mittelschmerz). The egg is viable for about 2 days in the fallopian tube. Empty egg follicle produces progesterone. If egg is not fertilized, oestrogen and progesterone production stops. This causes the endometrium lining to shed, about 14 days after ovulation. Normal cycle length 21–40 days, average 28 days. Normal bleeding is for 2–8 days, average 4–5 days. In cycle, changes in consistency of cervical mucus, cervix position, body temperature, breasts, abdominal pain and mood.

*Menstrual loss* is about 80mL a month. ♀ use internal tampons or external pads for containment. Mooncup (see ᛞ http://www.mooncup.co.uk/) is a reusable silicone menstrual cup used internally. It addresses environmental concerns, financial issues, and concerns about bleaches, etc. in internal tampons.

## Toxic shock syndrome

Very rare, acute illness caused by toxins from staphylococci or streptococci. Association with tampons unclear, but tampon absorbency thought to be a factor. Preventative advice includes frequent changes, occasional use of pads, not to use 2 tampons at once.

## Premenstrual tension and syndrome

These are a collection of symptoms and bodily changes that occur on a regular basis. It lasts for anything from a few days to weeks before a woman's period and cease with its arrival. >95% women have some symptoms—debilitating symptoms occur in 5%. Commonest are nervous tension, mood swings, irritability, ↑ weight and abdominal bloating, breast tenderness and headache, cramping and pain. Advice:

- Keep diary of symptoms to establish cyclical symptoms.
- Beneficial effect of good nutrition, weight management, and exercise.
- Treatment may be by trial and error as poorly understood condition, much conflicting evidence and variety in symptoms experienced.

### Treatments

- Conflicting evidence on Oil of Evening Primrose, vitamin B6 and magnesium supplements, relaxation, reflexology, but may help some ♀.
- Calcium supplements improve breast tenderness, headaches, and abdominal cramps.
- Cognitive therapy improves severe symptoms.
- NSAIDs (BNF 10.1.1) for cramping and pain.
- Effective medical treatments according to symptoms include COC, danazol (BNF 6.7.2), SSRIs (BNF 4.3.3), anxiolytics (BNF 4.1.2).

## Menorrhagia/heavy periods

Bleeding >7 days and >80mL. In 50% cause unexplained. Other causes: IUD, fibroids, endometriosis, cancer, blood clotting disorder. Following examination and investigations, if does not require or wish hormonal contraception treated with mefenamic acid (BNF 10.1.1) or tranexamic acid (BNF 2.11). If requires contraception as well offered COC or long-acting progesterone or IUS. If has an IUD, this is changed to IUS. Patient is referred to gynecologist if symptoms indicate or treatment failure.

## Dysmenorrhoea/painful periods

Tends to start 6–12mths after menarche when ovulatory cycles are established. Tends to improve after adolescence and after child birth. Uterine hypercontractility (associated with prostaglandin production) and ischaemia of the uterine wall causes pain. It occurs in the first 1–2 days of each period. Lower abdominal cramps ± back ache. It may be associated with gastrointestinal disturbance (e.g. constipation, diarrhoea/vomiting). In about 15% ♀ interferes with ability to go about daily life, attend school, work.

## Self-help advice

• OTC painkillers paracetamol, ibuprofen.
• Exercise relieves cramps.
• Hot water bottles or self-heating patches or pack (microwaved) comforting.

If pain still a problem may need POM to address pain, e.g. mefenamic acid. TENS machines may help some ♀. It can be treated by COC, IUS insertion. Some ♀ report acupuncture helps.

Pain that still doesn't respond may have underlying pathology and requires medical investigation.

## Amenorrhea

### Primary amenorrhea
Menstruation delayed (📖 Growth 12–18yrs, p. 221).

### Secondary amenorrhea
Absence of menses ≥6mths in a previously menstruating woman. Causes may be pregnancy, menopause, stress, low nutritional intake (e.g. anorexia), high levels of exercise, disease of the brain, thyroid, adrenal glands, ovaries. Treatment or action based on cause.

## Further information

National Association for Premenstrual Syndrome. Available at: ℜ www.pms.org.uk/
NHS Choices. Pre-menstrual syndrome. Available at: ℜ www.nhs.uk/conditions/Premenstrual-syndrome/Pages/Introduction.aspx
NICE (2007). Heavy menstrual bleeding: CG44. Available at: ℜ www.nice.org.uk/CG044
NICE CKS (2009). Premenstrual Syndrome. Available at: ℜ cks.nice.org.uk/premenstrual-syndrome

# Problems of the ovaries and uterus

## Ovarian problems

### Ovarian cysts

A growth on, or inside, the ovary. These are very common. Functional cysts are the most common type. Many ♀ experience no symptoms. Dependent on size and position may cause discomfort and pain. If <5cm diameter usually resolve spontaneously. >5cm referred to gynaecologist. Acute severe pain and vomiting caused by bleeding into the cyst, rupture or torsion and needs medical assessment urgently.

*Treatment*

Depends on size, position, and possibility of rupture. Laparoscopic fenestration can be used to drain contents, or laporotomy for removal.

### Polycystic ovary syndrome

A polycystic ovary is larger than normal with multiple cysts around the edge, disrupting hormonal cycle and inhibiting release eggs. It is common in 5–20% pre-menopausal women. Cause unknown. Associated with ↑ risk of cardiovascular disease and endometrial cancer. Women may be asymptomatic or have any or all symptoms of: acne, obesity, infertility, irregular periods, insulin resistance, hirsutism (because excess testosterone produced). It is diagnosed on history, pelvic USS, and blood tests.

*Treatment*

Dependent on symptoms, encouraged to maintain weight in BMI range 19–25. Oligomenorrhoea may be treated with progestogens. Clomifene may be used to induce ovulation. Hirsutism may be treated with COC and anti-androgen.

## Uterine problems

### Endometriosis

Fragments of the endometrium (lining of the uterus) located in other areas of the body, usually pelvic cavity. Fragments under hormonal control so breaks down and bleeds each month. It leads to inflammation, pain, and scar tissue. Most common in ♀ 25–40yrs, Cause unclear. It may cause infertility.

*Symptoms*

May cause heavy menstrual bleeding, severe abdominal pain, dyspareunia, bowel and bladder symptoms. Patient is referred to gynaecologist and diagnosis confirmed on laparoscopy.

*Treatment*

Either hormonal treatment to stop ovulation and allow the endometrial deposits to regress or surgical, e.g. local ablation using laser during laparoscopy, or more radical surgery dependent on symptoms.

### Fibroids

Benign, often multiple, tumours of the uterus. Affect ~20% women. Fibroids are oestrogen dependent so more common in pre-menopausal women and then shrink post-menopause.

*Symptoms*
Usually asymptomatic but may cause heavy periods (in turn cause anaemia), pelvic discomfort, back ache, pressure on bladder. It is diagnosed by pelvic USS. Referred to gynecologist if symptomatic.

*Medical treatment*
COC ↓ menses, GnRH analogues—tranexamic acid, mefanamic acid may shrink up to 50% can only be used for 6mths, or insertion of IUS.

*Surgical treatment*
Myomectomy (removing fibroids individually), hysterectomy, or uterine artery embolization (blocking blood supply).

**Pelvic organ prolapse**
Very common, particularly in older women. It is caused by poor pelvic muscle tone and weakness of pelvic ligaments.

*Risk factors*
Childbirth, menopause. It is aggravated by obesity.

*Prevention*
Includes pelvic floor exercises weight maintenance in normal BMI range (📖 Nutrition and healthy eating, p. 304) and avoiding constipation. Types of prolapse:
- Bladder and anterior vaginal wall (cystocoele).
- Urethra (urethrocoele).
- Rectum and posterior vaginal wall (rectocoele).
- Herniation of the top of the vagina (enterocoele).
- Uterine prolapse.

*Treatment*
According to severity and symptoms.

**Uterine prolapse**
Most common type. Uterus descends into the vagina. Classified by degree:
- *1st degree:* cervix remains in the vagina.
- *2nd degree:* cervix protrudes from vagina on coughing/straining.
- *3rd degree* (procidentia): uterus lies outside the vagina and may ulcerate).

*Signs and symptoms*
Dragging sensation. Often gets worse if standing for a long time, coughing or straining. May be associated with bowel and bladder problems, e.g. stress incontinence.

*Treatment*
Depends on severity. In primary care, pelvic floor exercises (📖 Urinary incontinence in women, p. 448) and weight reduction are encouraged plus treatment of co-existing problems, e.g. constipation. Referred to gynecologist. Sometimes HRT prescribed to help, 2nd and 3rd degree prolapse may be treated with surgical repair or hysterectomy.

*Vaginal ring pessaries*
Used to hold uterus in place while waiting for surgery or if surgery not appropriate. Made of latex or PVC, similar to a diaphragm, measured in mm. Fits under pubic bone at the front and to the posterior fornix at the back so the cervix lies within the ring. Ring softens when immersed in warm water to aid fitting. ♀ asked to bear down after fitting to check not expelled. ♀ should not feel it. Oestrogen cream may be used 1 or 2x wk. At 3mths ring removed and cervix and vaginal vault checked, ring washed in soapy water before re-inserted. Checked and replaced every 4–6mths thereafter. Complications include ulceration of vaginal walls, vaginitis, and discharge.

## Related topics
📖 Menstrual problems, p. 728; 📖 Vaginal and vulval problems, p. 737; 📖 Urinary incontinence in women, p. 448; 📖 Problems with fertility, p. 735.

## Further information
National Endometriosis Society: ☏ Helpline: 0808 808 2227. Available at: ℅ www.endometriosis-uk. org/
Royal College of Obstetricians and Gynecology information sheets. Available at: ℅ www.rcog. org.uk
Verity for women with polycystic ovary syndrome. Available at: ℅ www.verity-pcos.org.uk

# Hysterectomy

One of the most common operations for women. Over 60,000 hysterectomies are carried out in the UK annually. Majority are in ♀ 40–50yrs. Most commonly undertaken for:

- Electively for painful menorrhagia, endometriosis, fibroids causing pain and bleeding, prolapsed uterus, or pelvic inflammatory disease (PID) or adhesions which cause pain that is not controlled by other means.
- Cancer of the uterus, ovaries, fallopian tube/s or cervix (🕮 Gynaecological cancers, p. 726).
- Also in emergencies such as rupture/puncture of the uterus during other surgery.

In elective situations, women should have counselling to help make informed choice, based on understanding alternatives, benefits, risks, long-term consequences including:

- Loss of menstruation and ability to have a child.
- Immediate menopause if surgery also removes ovaries regardless of age. 50% who have ovaries intact post-surgery experience menopause within 5yrs of operation regardless of age.
- Some women have strong emotional response to the loss of this organ, and experience mourning, loss, and an altered sense of self, but others feel liberated and relieved after years of severe pain and heavy bleeding.

Endometrial ablation and resection is a surgical alternative with less consequences used to treat heavy bleeding and remove fibroids and polyps. Techniques include lasers, microwaves, electricity, balloons filled with hot water, freezing, and heated loops.

## Types of hysterectomy

- Subtotal hysterectomy removes the uterus leaving the cervix in place (cervical smears still required, see 🕮 Cervical cancer screening, p. 337).
- Total hysterectomy (most common) removes uterus and cervix.
- Total hysterectomy with bilateral or unilateral salpingo-oophorectomy removes body of uterus, cervix, fallopian tube(s), and ovary/ies.
- A radical hysterectomy removes the uterus, cervix, part of the vagina, fallopian tubes, peritoneum, the lymph glands and fatty tissue of the pelvis, and possibly one or both ovaries.

Performed either through an incision in the lower abdomen (clips or stitches removed after 5 days), or through an incision in the top of the vagina, or vaginal surgery with laporoscope (key hole surgery). Decisions about type of surgery are influenced by individual circumstances.

**Post-hysterectomy**

- Takes about 6–8wks for abdominal muscles and tissues to heal. Advice to remain off work for this period, take gentle exercise, avoid strenuous exercise or lifting.
- Vaginal discharge for up to 6wks. Sanitary pads rather than tampons used to reduce risk of infection.
- Sex can be resumed after a minimum of 6wks, post-surgery check. Many have no problems with sex, but some find the surgery has shortened their vagina and slightly changed its angle. They experience different sensations and responses during sex. This can be very distressing and takes time to come to terms with. May also find their vagina is dry and would benefit from a lubricant.
- HRT often prescribed for those whose ovaries removed (☐ Menopause, p. 323).
- More general advice:
  - Avoid any lifting or housework for the first few weeks.
  - Avoid heavy lifting for about 3mths.
  - Avoid standing for long periods.
  - Do some form of gentle exercise every day, e.g. walking a short distance, slowly increasing.
  - Do the exercises recommended by hospital physiotherapist for Pelvic floor and abdominal muscle strengthening (☐ Stress urinary incontinence, p. 451).
  - After vaginal discharge has disappeared exercise like swimming is beneficial.
  - Ensure a balanced diet and fluids to help avoid constipation.
  - Feeling low after an anesthetic is common, but should recede.

**Further information**

Hysterectomy Association. Available at: ℘ www.hysterectomy-association.org.uk
NHS Choices. Hysterectomy. Available at: ℘ www.nhs.uk/Conditions/Hysterectomy/Pages/Introduction.aspx

# Problems with fertility

Many couples trying to conceive are aided by additional information on the most fertile time in the menstrual cycle, but should be encouraged to have sex 2 or 3 times a week throughout the cycle. Timing of intercourse using temperature charts or hormone detection kits causes stress and does not improve conception rates, so not recommended. Couple should also be given lifestyle advice on alcohol intake, weight management, smoking as well as preconception care. Female fertility declines significantly after 35yrs. Sperm function also declines past 55yrs, but less markedly.

## Infertility

Affects ~1:7 couples and is a cause of considerable psychological distress. Infertility is defined as absence of pregnancy after 1yr of regular unprotected intercourse. Infertility is classed as 1° in couples who have never conceived and 2° in couples who have previously conceived. Investigated earlier if other factors present, e.g. woman's age, previous surgery, or irregular menstrual cycles. Usually health consultations and investigations dealt with as a couple. This may be in 1° care by GP or referred to specialists. Investigations follow the same pathway:

- Checking ♀ partner is ovulating normally.
- Checking ♂ partner has a normal semen analysis.
- Confirming normality of the female genital tract.

Infertility may be unexplained (30%), or 2° to ovulatory failure (27%), male factors (19%), tubal factors (14%), or endometriosis (5%).

### Treatment

Types of treatment dependent on problems identified:

- Medicines to assist with ovulation, e.g. clomifene.
- Surgical treatment, e.g. tubal surgery to remove obstruction.
- Assisted conception:
  - Intra-uterine insemination (IUI) sperm placed in woman's uterus.
  - Donor insemination (DI) insemination of sperm from a donor into a woman, via her vagina (IUI).
  - In vitro fertilization (IVF) retrieval of the egg(s) mixed with sperm and incubated for 2–3 days; the resultant embryo(s) then injected into the uterus via the cervix.
  - Intracytoplasmic sperm injection (ICSI) an individual sperm injected directly into the egg.
  - Oocyte donation stimulation of the donor's ovaries and collection of eggs, then fertilized by the recipient's partner's sperm, embryos transferred to the uterus of the recipient following hormonal preparation of the endometrium.
  - Embryo donation. Couples who have had successful IVF or ICSI decide to donate their spare embryos to help other infertile couples.

Many 2° care centres carry out a range of infertility treatments, but usually only specialist infertility clinics offer IVF, ICSI, and DI. National and local guidelines apply in terms of what NHS treatments are available and to whom. NICE recommend that three full cycles of IVF or ICSI be made available to people where the female is <39yrs with a clinical diagnosis requiring IVF or unexplained infertility for 2yrs duration. Many couples may need counselling (🕮 Talking therapies, p. 429) at the same time as investigations and treatments.

## Repeated miscarriages

Recurrent miscarriage is defined as 3 times, before 20wks gestation. 1 in 100 women miscarry 3 or more times consecutively. Maternal age and previous miscarriages are independent risk factors. All couples with recurrent miscarriages tested for chromosome abnormalities (referred to clinical geneticist if positive). At subsequent pregnancy, ♀ is referred to early pregnancy clinic at hospital.

## Further information

Human Fertilization and Embryology Authority. Available at: ℘ www.hfea.gov.uk
Infertility Network UK (INUK): ☎ 0800 008 7464. Available at: ℘ www.infertilitynetworkuk.com
Miscarriage Association: Available at: ℘ www.miscarriageassociation.org.uk
NHS Choices. Infertility. Available at: ℘ www.nhs.uk/Conditions/Infertility/Pages/Introduction.aspx
NICE (2013). Fertility (CG156). Available at: ℘ guidance.nice.org.uk/CG156
NICE CKS (2010). Miscarriage. Available at: ℘ cks.nice.org.uk/miscarriage

# Vaginal and vulval problems

## Vaginal discharge

All women produce vaginal discharge. It is part of the physiological changes in sexual activity, pregnancy, and menstrual cycle. It is affected by age and stress and use of COC. In the menstrual cycle secretions change in texture and colour. At the fertile part of the month (luteal phase) secretions are thinner, colourless, and slippery. In the infertile part the secretions become whiter, thicker, and stickier. It may become yellow on contact with air. The amounts of discharge vary between women and over the month.

## Abnormal discharge

Only abnormal when it is different from individual woman's normal discharge. Abnormal discharge mostly caused by *Candida albicans* (thrush), bacterial vaginosis, *Tricomonas vaginalis*, and cervicitis. See 📖 Sexually transmitted infections, p. 715.

### Bacterial vaginosis

Commonest cause of abnormal discharge. BV is an offensive fishy smelling, thin, white, homogeneous vaginal discharge. Not usually associated with soreness, itching, or irritation. ~50% are asymptomatic, but may be found to have BV when vaginal swab taken for other indications. BV can be recurrent and generally not sexually transmissible.

*Investigations*

Can be diagnosed by clinical signs/symptoms alone plus ↑ pH of vaginal fluid >4.5. No culture available. Diagnosis by use of microscopy.

*Treatment*

Advise to avoid vaginal douching, use of shower gels and soaps, and use of antiseptic agents in the bath.

Metronidazole 2g stat po (BNF 5.1.11) or metronidazole 400mg/bd po for 5–7 days (preferred in pregnancy).

Alternative treatment regimens advised for lactating women.

### Candida albicans (thrush)

Vulval pruritis and soreness, curdy white discharge, superficial dyspareunia, superficial dysuria. It can be recurrent, generally not sexually transmissible. OTC treatments.

*Investigations*

Clinical observation in most cases. High-vaginal swab for MC&S. Diagnosis using microscopy.

*Treatment*

Advise to avoid vaginal douching, use of shower gels, soaps, and use of antiseptic agents in the bath. ❶ Topical treatments may cause condoms to split.
• 1% clotrimazole cream to externally affected genitalia (OTC).
• Clotrimazole 500 mg PV stat (OTC) (BNF 7.2.2).
• Fluconazole 150mg po stat (OTC).

*Atrophic vaginitis* Post-menopausal changes create dryness that presents as vaginal soreness and dysparareunia. Treated short term with topical oestrogen as pessaries or vaginal ring (BNF 7.2.1) and advise on lubricants during sexual intercourse.

*Bartholins gland swellings* Two glands with ducts opening into vulva, in sexual arousal these secrete lubricant. Obstruction of the ducts leads to vulval swelling and cyst formation. Cysts resolve spontaneously. If infected an abscess results that may respond to antibiotics or need surgical drainage.

*Genital warts and herpes* See 📖 Sexually transmitted infections, p. 715.

## Vulval swelling

Can be due to venous or lymphatic obstruction, causes include:
- Secondary to malignancy in the pelvis (📖 Gynaecological cancers, p. 726).
- Dependent oedema with prolonged sitting in bed, addressing positioning and movement.
- Pregnancy, where varicosities may appear, resolves at end of pregnancy.
- With bruising may be trauma of a sexual nature (📖 Victims of crime, p. 404).

## Vulval itching (pruritis)

May be caused by infection, infestations, vulval atrophy, dystrophy, carcinoma, allergic response to perfumed soaps, etc. Aim of care is to identify cause and treat.

## Vulval dystrophy

Changes in appearance of the skin, sometimes with white plaques, and itching, sometimes dysparunia. It occurs mostly in post-menopausal women. Correct term: squamous cell hyperplasia. Lichen sclerosis is uncommon. Skin appears thin, white, and crinkly. Squamous cell hyperplasia is uncommon, found in older women. There are thickened, asymmetrical, white or grey areas. It is treated with clobetasol propionate 0.05% ointment (BNF 13.4).

**Psychosexual problems** Women who have any chronic genital disorders may lose interest in sexual activity and have psychosexual problems. Important to give patients the opportunity to express concerns on their sexual function and to offer referral or information on psychosexual counselling (often via community family planning service, sexual health services or RELATE[1]).

## Related topics

📖 Gynaecological cancers, p. 726.

## Reference

[1]RELATE Relationship and psychosexual counselling. Available at: 🔗 www.relate.org.uk

## Further information

RCGP and BASHH (2013). Sexually Transmitted Infections in Primary Care (2nd edition). Available at: 🔗 www.bashh.org and www.rcgp.org

Royal College of Obstetricians and Gynecology. Information sheets. Available at: 🔗 www.rcog.org.uk/

# Termination of pregnancy

## UK Law

### England, Wales, and Scotland (not Northern Ireland)

The 1967 Abortion Act and 1990 Human Fertilization/Embryology Acts govern abortion also known as termination of pregnancy (TOP). TOP allowed up to 24wks of pregnancy if 2 doctors agree that it is necessary because of one or more of the following:

- Continuation of pregnancy involves ↑ risk to the life of the woman.
- Continuation would cause injury to the mother's physical or mental health (90% TOPs are carried out under this clause).
- Continuation would cause injury to the physical or mental health of the mother's existing children.
- The baby is at substantial risk of being physically or mentally handicapped.

Note: upper gestation limit does not apply if mother's life threatened or serious injury or fetal handicap.

## Consultations in primary care

### Women with an unplanned and unwanted pregnancy

These women need to talk through with partners, and/or relatives and/or close friends, their emotions, and choices. Primary care and contraceptive services are often the first health services consulted to confirm pregnancy and advise on options and processes for TOP.

### Prenatal diagnosis of abnormality

♀ undergoing routine antenatal screening (📖 Antenatal care and screening, p. 380) may also be told that their baby has a serious risk of physical and mental impairment and TOP could be considered. Requires specialist support in counselling on options.

### Role of health professionals

All health professionals should ensure ♀ are treated non-judgementally and has access to full information, irrespective of their own personal views (📖 Professional conduct, p. 74). This may mean offering another professional for that consultation or referring the woman elsewhere to receive counselling of options and full information to make an informed choice.

## Main areas of information

- ♀ has right to confidentiality irrespective of age (📖 Confidentiality, p. 86).
- ♀ alone gives consent, does not need agreement of partner or parents (informed Consent (📖 p. 77) and <16yrs).
- TOPs safer earlier in pregnancy.
- TOPs available through the NHS (local services may have self-referral process) and private organizations (self-referral and payment). All carried out in NHS hospitals or special licensed clinics.
- Process in all organizations ensures a counselling/assessment visit to help ♀ reach the decision right for her and then time before the TOP visit to change mind.
- Types of TOP.
  - <9wks pregnancy early medical abortion. Involves 2 appointments. Oral mifepristone given at first followed 2 days later by oral or vaginal prostaglandin to expel pregnancy in next 4–6hrs.
  - >7–12 or 15wks vacuum aspiration usually under sedation and local anesthetic.
  - >9–20 wks late medical abortion undertaken as early medical abortion, but may take longer and often requires overnight stay.
  - >15wks surgical dilation and evacuation under general anesthetic.
  - Late abortion 20–24wks either 2 stage surgical procedure under general anesthetic or medically induced labour followed often by surgical procedure to ensure uterus is empty.
- *Risks of procedures include:* haemorrhage, failure and on-going pregnancy, infection, psychological impact. No association between TOP and subsequent infertility or miscarriage.
- All TOP have a follow-up visit to clinic or GP 2wks later.
- ♀ experience a range of emotions afterwards from relief to sadness and loss, depending on circumstances, reasons for TOP, and decision-making process.
- After TOP menstrual cycle returns to normal and can conceive again within 2wks. Contraception options to be considered as part of pre-TOP counselling (📖 Contraception: general, p. 359).

## Further information

Antenatal results and choices (ARC): supports parents faced with prenatal diagnosis of foetal abnormality and those that have had terminations. ☎ 0845 077 2290 or 0207 713 7486 from a mobile phone. Available at: 🖱 www.arc-uk.org

British Pregnancy Advisory Service (England, Wales, Scotland): ☎ 08457 30 40 30. Available at: 🖱 www.bpas.org/

FPA Northern Ireland: ☎ 028 9032 5488.

FPA UK: ☎ 0845 122 8690. Available at: 🖱 www.fpa.org.uk

Marie Stopes UK: ☎ 0845 300 8090. Available at: 🖱 www.mariestopes.org.uk

NHS Choices. Abortion. Available at: 🖱 www.nhs.uk/Conditions/Abortion/Pages/Introduction.aspx

# First aid and emergencies

# Adult basic life support

Basic life support (BLS) implies that no special equipment is used by the rescuer other than a protective device.

Effective chest compressions, and reducing the number and duration of pauses are the key to improving victim's chance of survival.

## Cardiac arrest: diagnosis

If the victim is unresponsive and not breathing normally, make a diagnosis of cardiac arrest (see Fig. 13.1).

## Adult basic life support sequence of actions 1–7

*Step 1* Make sure victim, bystanders, and you are safe.

*Step 2* Check victim for response. Gently shake shoulders and ask loudly, 'Are you all right?'.

*Step 3a* If there is a response:
- If no further danger leave in position found.
- Try to find out what is wrong, obtain help, offer reassurance.

*Step 3b* If there is *no* response:
- Shout for help.
- Turn the victim onto their back.
- Place your hand on their forehead and gently tilt their head back.
- With your fingertips under point of victim's chin, lift chin to open airway.

*Step 4* Keeping airway open, look, listen, and feel for normal breathing.
- Look for chest movement.
- Listen at the victim's mouth for breath sounds.
- Feel for air on your cheek.

The first few minutes after cardiac arrest, the victim may be barely breathing or taking infrequent, noisy gasps. Do not confuse with normal breathing. Look, listen, and feel for *no more than 10s* to determine if breathing normally. If in doubt act as if it is *not* normal.

*Step 5a* If they *are* breathing normally:
- Turn them into the recovery position (see 📖 Recovery position, p. 746).
- Send or go for help, or summon an ambulance.
- Check for continued breathing.

*Step 5b* If they are *not* breathing normally:
- Ask someone to call an ambulance; if alone, do this yourself (note: you may need to leave the victim temporarily) and ask for an automated external defibrillation (AED), one may be available.
- *Start chest compression:*
  - Kneel by side of victim.
  - Place heel of one hand in centre of victim's chest.
  - Place heel of other hand on top of first hand.

- Interlock fingers of hands and ensure that pressure is not applied over victim's ribs.
- Do *not* apply any pressure over upper abdomen or bottom end of the bony sternum (breastbone).
- Position yourself vertically above the victim's chest, and with your arms straight, press down to depress sternum 5–6cm.
- After each compression, release all pressure on the chest without losing contact between your hands and the sternum.
- Repeat at a rate of 100–120 times/min (2/s).
- Compression and release should take an equal amount of time.

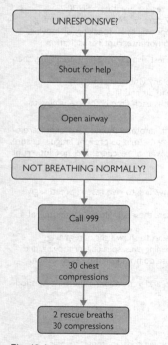

**Fig. 13.1** Adult basic life support algorithm.
Reproduced with permission of the Resuscitation Council UK)

***Step 6a*** Combine chest compressions with rescue breaths.
- After 30 compressions, open airway again (as described in Step 3b).
- Pinch closed soft part of nose, using index finger and thumb of hand placed on victim's forehead.
- Allow mouth to open, but maintain chin lift.

- Take a normal breath and place lips around mouth, ensuring a good seal.
- Blow steadily into mouth while watching for chest to rise. It takes about 1s to make chest rise as in normal breathing.
- Maintaining head tilt and chin lift, take mouth away from victim and watch for chest to fall as air is expelled.
- Take another normal breath and blow into victim's mouth once more to give a total of two effective rescue breaths. This should not take more than 5s.
- *Without delay*, return hands to correct position on sternum and give a further 30 chest compressions.
- Continue chest compressions and rescue breaths, ratio 30:2.
- Stop to recheck victim only if they start to show signs of regaining consciousness, such as coughing, opening eyes, speaking, or moving, *and* starts to breathe normally. **Do not interrupt resuscitation**.

If rescue breaths do not make the chest rise as in normal breathing, then before next attempt:
- Check victim's mouth and remove any visible obstruction.
- Recheck that there is adequate head tilt and lift.
- Do not attempt more than 2 breaths each time before returning to chest compressions.

If more than one rescuer is present, another should take over cardio-pulmonary resuscitation (CPR) ~every 1–2min to prevent fatigue. Ensure minimum delay during each changeover of rescuers. **Do not interrupt resuscitation**.

### Step 6b Compression-only CPR.
- If you are not trained to, or are unwilling to give rescue breaths, give chest compressions only.
- If chest compressions only are given, these should be continuous at a rate of 100–120/min.
- Stop to recheck victim only if they start to show signs of regaining consciousness, such as coughing, opening eyes, speaking, or moving, *and* starts to breathe normally. Otherwise **do not interrupt resuscitation**.

*Note*: combined chest compression and ventilation is the best method of CPR.

### Step 7 Continue resuscitation until:
- Qualified help arrives and takes over.
- Victim starts to show signs of regaining consciousness, such as coughing, opening his eyes, speaking, or moving, *and* starts to breathe normally, *or* you become exhausted.

#### Mouth-to-nose ventilation
Mouth-to-nose ventilation is an effective alternative to mouth-to-mouth ventilation. Consider if:
- Victim's mouth is seriously injured or cannot be opened.
- Rescuer is assisting a victim in water.
- Mouth-to-mouth seal is difficult to achieve.

*Mouth-tracheostomy ventilation* May be used for a victim with a tracheostomy tube or tracheal stoma.

## Recovery position

See 📖 The recovery position, p. 746; Fig. 13.2.

There are several variations of the recovery position, no single position perfect for all victims. The position should be:
• Stable.
• Near a true lateral position with the head dependent.
• With no pressure on the chest to impair breathing.
• Check breathing regularly.
• If victim is in recovery position for more than 30min, turn them to opposite side to relieve pressure on lower arm.

## Related topics

📖 Child BLS, p. 748; 📖 Anaphylaxis, p. 751; 📖 Child choking, p. 762; 📖 Adult choking, p. 760; 📖 Poisoning and overdose, p. 770.

## Reference

Resuscitation Council (UK). Resuscitation guidelines. Available at: 🔗 www.resus.org.uk

# The recovery position

When circulation and breathing have been restored, it is important to:
- Maintain a good airway.
- Ensure tongue does not cause obstruction.
- Minimize risk of inhalation of gastric contents.

For this reason the victim should be placed in the recovery position (Fig. 13.2). This allows the tongue to fall forward, keeping the airway clear.

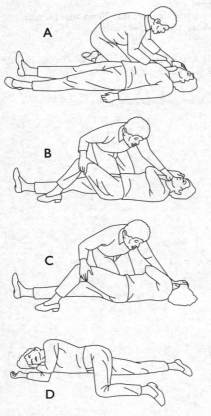

**Fig. 13.2** The recovery position.

Reproduced from Simon C, Everitt H, Van Dorp F. (2010). *Oxford Handbook of General Practice*, 3rd edn. Oxford: Oxford University Press. By permission of Oxford University Press.

## Putting a patient in the recovery position

- Remove patient's glasses.
- Kneel beside patient and make sure that both legs are straight (A).
- Place arm nearest to you out at right angles to body, elbow bent with hand palm uppermost (A).
- Bring far arm across chest, and hold back of hand against patient's cheek nearest to you (B).
- With other hand, grasp far leg just above knee and pull it up, keeping foot on ground (B).
- Keeping patient's hand pressed against his cheek, pull on leg to roll patient towards you onto his side (C).
- Adjust upper leg so that both hip and knee are bent at right angles (D).
- Tilt head back to make sure airway remains open (D).
- Adjust hand under cheek, if necessary, to keep head tilted.
- Check breathing regularly.

**❶** Monitor the peripheral circulation of the lower arm. If the patient has to be kept in the recovery position for >30min, turn the patient onto the opposite side.

## The unconscious child

- The child should be in as near a true lateral position as possible with his mouth dependent to allow free drainage of fluid
- The position should be stable. In an infant this may require the support of a small pillow or rolled up blanket placed behind the infant's back to maintain the position.

## Cervical spine injury

- If spinal cord injury is suspected (e.g. if victim has sustained a fall, been struck on head or neck, or has been rescued after diving into shallow water) take particular care during handling and resuscitation to maintain alignment of head, neck, and chest in neutral position.
- A spinal board and/or cervical collar should be used if available.

# Child basic life support

Child basic life support follows an algorithm (Fig. 13.3).

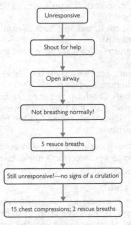

**Fig. 13.3** Child basic life support algorithm.
Reproduced from *Resuscitation Guidelines* (2010) with permission of the Resuscitation Council UK.

## Check responsiveness
- *Step 1.* Ensure safety of both rescuer and child.
- *Step 2.* Check responsiveness, ask loudly 'are you alright?', stimulate child. **Do not shake those who may have a neck injury.**
- *Step 3.* If child responsive, leave in position found, reassure them and check their condition, and if required seek further help.

## If *no* response
- Shout for help.
- Place child on back and open airway by gently tilting head and lifting chin (Fig. 13.4), avoiding pushing on soft tissue under chin as this may block airway. If this is does not open airway, try to lift jaw by placing first two fingers of each hand at side of jaw and gently lift jaw upwards.

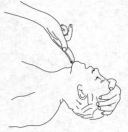

**Fig. 13.4** Lifting the chin.

- Keeping airway open, place face close to child's face. Assess for normal breathing:
  - *Look* for chest movement.
  - *Listen* for breath sounds over the mouth and nose.
  - *Feel* for air on your cheek.

Sometimes when cardiac arrest first occurs, the child may appear to gasp for air infrequently, this is *not* normal breathing.

## Start infant and child BLS sequence

- Give 5 initial *rescue breaths*.
- After the 5 breaths, take no more than 10s to check response before starting *chest compression*.
- If you are on your own, perform *CPR*—30 chest compressions to 2 rescue breaths for 1min before seeking help.

### Rescue breaths for a child >1yr

- Ensure head tilt and chin lift.
- Pinch closed soft part of child's nose with index finger and thumb of hand placed on their forehead.
- Open mouth a little, but keep supporting chin/jaw.
- Take a breath and place your lips around their mouth, ensuring a good seal:
  - Blow steadily into child's mouth for about 1–1.5s, watching for chest to rise then take mouth away, watching for chest to fall as air comes out.
  - Take another breath and repeat sequence 5×.
- If there appears to be airway obstruction, open child's mouth and remove any visible obstruction. Do *not* do blind finger sweep of mouth.

### Rescue breaths for an infant

As for >1yr, only ensure a neutral position of the head and apply the chin lift, and cover the mouth and nose of the infant with your mouth, ensuring you have a good seal.

## Checking response to rescue breaths in <10s

Look for signs of circulation. Movement, coughing, breathing. Check pulse of child >1yr, feel for carotid pulse in the neck. In an infant, feel for a brachial pulse on the inner aspect of the upper arm. If the pulse rate is slower than 60/min they will need chest compressions.

- If signs of a circulation within 10s, continue rescue breathing, until the child starts breathing on their own.
- If no signs of a circulation or no pulse, or uncertainty. **Start chest compression and combine with rescue breathing.**

*Chest compressions*
- For all children, compress lower half of sternum. Locate xiphisternum by finding where lowest ribs join in middle, compress sternum one finger's breadth above this.
- Compress chest by ~⅓ of its depth, but do not be afraid to push too hard.
- For infants <1 yr (with a lone rescuer) use tips of 2 fingers. If there are 2 or more rescuers use the encircling technique (see Fig. 13.5). Place both thumbs flat on the lower third of the sternum with tips pointing towards the infant's head and encircle the lower part of the infant's rib cage with the tips of the fingers supporting the infant's back. Press down with both thumbs.
- For child >1yr use one hand over the lower half of the sternum.
- For larger children you may use two hands.
- Repeat at a rate of 100–120 compressions/min.
- After 15 (30 if alone) compressions, give two effective breaths.

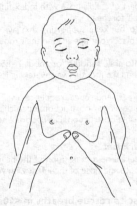

**Fig. 13.5** Encircling technique.

*Continue resuscitation until* the child shows signs of life (spontaneous respiration, pulse, movement), or further qualified help arrives and takes over.

*It is vital for rescuers to get help quickly when a child collapses* If alone and *witness sudden collapse* in child, it is likely to be a cardiac arrest through arrhythmia and the child may need defibrillation. Seek help immediately, rather than perform 1min CPR.

*Automated external defibrillators (AEDs)*
An unmodified AED may be used in children >1yr. Insufficient evidence to support a recommendation for or against the use of AEDs in infants <1yr.

## Reference
Resuscitation Council. Available at: ℘ www.resus.org.uk

# Anaphylaxis

No universally-accepted definitions of anaphylactic and anaphylactoid reactions. Anaphylaxis is a severe systemic hypersensitivity/allergic reaction typically mediated by immunoglobulin E (IgE).

## Common causes

See also 📖 Allergies, p. 647.
- *Foods:* nuts, shellfish, sesame seeds and oil, milk eggs, pulses, strawberries.
- *Stings:* wasp or bee.
- *Drugs:* antibiotics, especially penicillins, muscle relaxants, contrast media aspirin, and other NSAIDs.
- *Complement mediated:* human proteins, e.g. γ-globulin, blood products.
- Latex.
- Unknown ('idiopathic').
- Vaccines.
- Anaesthetic agents (important causes of anaphylactoid reactions).

**Clinical features** Reactions vary in severity, according to the nature and amount of the stimulus, progress may be rapid, slow, or (unusually) biphasic. Onset is usually within minutes or hours.

## Clinical presentations

### Respiratory system

Respiratory difficulty dyspnoea, swelling of the lips, tongue, larynx, pharxnx, and epiglottis may lead to complete upper airway occlusion. Lower airway involvement—dyspnoea, wheeze, chest tightness, hypoxia, hypercapnoea, stridor. Patients can die from acute, irreversible asthma, or laryngeal oedema.

### Cardiovascular system

Hypotension can present as fainting and loss of consciousness. Cardiovascular collapse is a common manifestation, especially in response to IV drugs or stings, and any cardiac dysfunction is due primarily to hypotension. Arrhythmias, ischaemic chest pain, and ECG changes may be present. Beta-blockers may increase the severity of an allergic reaction and antagonize the response to adrenaline.

### Skin

The skin colour usually changes and the patient may appear either flushed or pale. Urticaria and rhinitis, conjunctivitis, pruritus, erythema, urticaria, and angio-oedema may occur.

### GI tract

- Abdominal pain, nausea, vomiting, diarrhoea.
- Often reported that patients have a sense of impending doom.

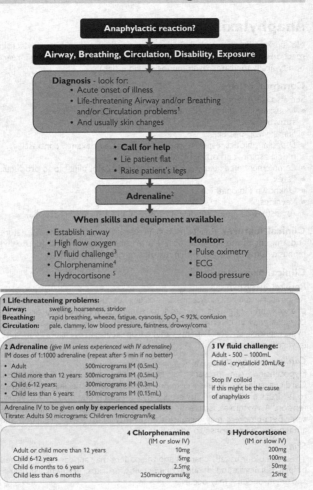

**Fig. 13.6** Anaphylactic reactions: treatment algorithm by first medical responders.
Reproduced with permission of the Resuscitation Council UK (2012).

All nurses involved in the administration of injections and other procedures in the home and/or clinics should carry/have direct access to an emergency adrenaline pack and be aware of local policy guidelines on the treatment of anaphylaxis.

## Treatment

See treatment algorithm, Fig. 13.6.

- If anaphylaxis suspected, call for emergency help immediately and rapidly assess Airway, Breathing, Circulation, Disability, Exposure (ABCDE).
- Make patient comfortable. If having difficulty breathing sit up, if hypotensive lie flat and elevate legs.
- Ask if patient has had similar reaction before and if they have an EpiPen®. If yes, use it.
- If having life-threatening difficulty in breathing, and/or signs of shock/skin changes administer adrenaline immediately.
- Adrenaline 1:1000 is available for use by UK community nurses. It reverses peripheral vasodilatation and ↓ oedema, dilates airways, ↑ force of myocardial contraction, and suppresses histamine and leukotriene release. IM adrenaline 1:1000 (IM dose) should be given immediately to all patients with clinical signs of shock, airway swelling, or breathing difficulty.
- **Do not** delay administration of adrenaline. Preferable injection site—mid-point anterolateral thigh.
- If $O_2$ available give at high flow rates 10–15L/min.

## Care and management

- Warn patients of possibility of recurrence.
- Advise sufferers to wear a medic alert or equivalent (☎ 0207 833 3034).
- Refer to GP to consider prescribing EpiPen® and provide training on its use.
- Encourage patients with known allergies to minimize risk—be vigilant for hidden allergens in foods, e.g. peanuts = groundnuts = arachis oil.
- Emphasize to patients that they should not be afraid of administering adrenaline and should not delay administration.
- *Write out a crisis plan:* ensure training available for friends, family, and school on how to handle an emergency and, if appropriate, where to locate adrenaline.

## Related topics

📖 Adult basic life support, p. 742; 📖 Child basic life support, p. 748; 📖 Allergies, p. 647; 📖 Immunization administration, p. 345.

## References

Anaphylaxis campaign. Available at: ✍ www.anaphylaxis.org.uk

British Red Cross Everyday First Aid online training to learn skills for an emergency. Available at: ✍ www.redcross.org.uk

Medic Alert British Isles & Ireland, 1 Bridge Wharf, 156 Caledonian Road, London N1 9UU UK. ☎ 0207 833 3034. Available at: ✍ www.medicalert.org.uk/

# External bleeding

There are three types of external bleeding:
- *Capillary:* most common type of external bleeding when blood oozes from capillaries. Usually not serious and easiest to control.
- *Venous:* occurs when a vein severed and blood flows steadily. Most veins collapse when cut, which aids control of this type of bleeding.
- *Arterial:* most severe type of external bleeding requiring urgent attention. Blood spurts with each heartbeat, often hard to control.

### First aid for external bleeding—key principles
- Stop or slow down bleeding using direct pressure.
- Preserve existing blood volume.
- Prevent infection using dressings.
- Prevent shock by reassurance and careful patient positioning.
- Prevent cross-infection between the person and yourself.

### Controlling blood loss
- Stay calm and reassure victim.
- *Superficial wounds:* wash with soap and warm water, remove any obvious loose debris or dirt, dry, and apply a sterile dressing.
- Apply direct pressure to the wound with thumb and/or fingers over a dressing if available. If a dressing unavailable, use a clean handkerchief, towel, piece of clothing, or your hand alone. If the wound is large, squeeze sides of wound together gently, but firmly. Patients are often able to apply direct pressure to their own wounds.
- Place a sterile, unmedicated dressing over the wound, ensuring it fully covers injury, and secure with bandage applied firmly enough to control bleeding, but not to impede the circulation.

If bleeding continues through original dressing, apply further dressings on top, and bandage firmly. Do not remove original dressing as this may disturb clots and restart the bleeding.

- If bleeding continues, and you have no reason to suspect a fracture, elevate wound above level of the heart if possible.
- *As a last resort to control arterial bleeding:* apply indirect pressure at a pressure point (e.g. brachial or femoral arteries), for timed periods of 15min only.
- Lay victim down if fainting is a possibility.
- If a foreign body, such as a knife, arrow, bullet, or stick becomes embedded in the body, **do not remove it**. Place pads and bandages around foreign body and use tape to stabilize it. Seek emergency medical attention immediately.

**General precautions** Some diseases such as AIDS and hepatitis B are transmitted through the exchange of body fluids. To minimize the risk of infection, wear disposable gloves and plastic goggles and, where appropriate, a surgical mask (📖 Personal protective equipment, p. 98).

## Internal bleeding

Signs and symptoms of internal bleeding are:
• Deteriorating conscious level.
• Cool, moist skin.
• Abnormal pulse and breathing difficulties.
• Slow capillary refill time (following cutaneous pressure on a digit, or preferably on centre of sternum for 5s, capillary refill should occur within 2s. A slower refill time indicates poor skin perfusion).
• Haemoptysis and haematemesis.
• Bruises on chest or signs of fractured ribs.
• Penetrating wounds to chest or abdomen.
• Bruised, swollen, tender, or rigid abdomen.
• Bleeding from vagina or rectum.

First aid for internal bleeding is limited:
• For simple bruising, apply cold compresses to slow bleeding, relieve pain, and reduce swelling.
• Monitor patient and be prepared to administer CPR if required.
• Referred to hospital/ED for specialist investigations and treatment.

## Bleeding disorders

Suspect a bleeding disorder if:
• Spontaneous or excess haemorrhage occurs from multiple or uninjured sites into deep tissues.
• Delayed bleeding occurs after hours or days.

Ask about previous history of bleeding following trauma, surgery, etc., current medication, and recent medical history.

### Congenital disorders

Most adults with a congenital disorder carry a National Haemophilia card or a Medic-Alert bracelet. Many haemophiliacs are the experts about required treatment and will be registered at a haemophilia centre, which should be contacted for advice.

### Acquired disorders

May be due to liver disease, uraemia, drug use (specifically aspirin, NSAIDs, warfarin/anticoagulants, alcohol (🕮 Alcohol, p. 319)) or unrecognized conditions, such as haematological malignancy.

Routine wound management of patients with bleeding disorders follows standard procedures as described, accompanied by prior or simultaneous administration of factor concentrates and platelets under haematological advice.

## Related topics

🕮 Child BLS, p. 748; 🕮 Adult basic life support, p. 742; 🕮 HIV, p. 686; 🕮 Viral hepatitis, p. 676; 🕮 Sickle cell disorders, p. 292; 🕮 Patients on anticoagulant therapies, p. 600.

## References

Resuscitation Council (UK) Resuscitation guidelines. Available at: 🖰 www.resus.org.uk
St John's Ambulance. Available at: 🖰 www.sja.org.uk

# Burns and scalds

The highest rates of burns occur in children <5yrs and people >75yrs. Most burns occur at home. Younger children suffer more scalds, older children more flame burns. Most fatal burns occur in house fires where smoke inhalation is the usual cause of death.

- All flame burns involve high temperatures → most serious injuries.
- Scalds commonly caused by hot drinks, bath water, or cooking oil. Scalds generally involve water below boiling point and contact for <4s, those involving hot fat or steam at much higher temperatures, → more serious injury.
- Strong association between burns to children and low socio-economic status. Always consider non-accidental injury in children (🕮 Child protection, p. 230).

Two main factors determine the severity of burns and scalds:

- Temperature of the heat source.
- Duration of contact.

Epidermal injury occurs after 30s at 54°C and within 1s at 70°C.

*Note:* ask about detailed circumstances of the burn to establish cause (thermal, chemical, electrical, radiation) and the possibility of other injury (e.g. injuries from escaping fire, inhalation of poisonous fumes, etc.).

## Assessing depth and extent

Consider cause, appearance, size, and thickness of burn, and the level of pain/sensation at the burn site. Burns that blister are generally superficial.

- *Superficial (epidermal burn):* tissue damage to the epidermis only. Commonly seen in sunburn. May only require only symptomatic relief.
- *Superficial/dermal:* tissue damage extends through epidermis into upper layers of dermis. Pale pink or mottled appearance. These heal in 2–3wks with minimal scarring and full functional recovery.
- *Deep dermal (partial):* tissue damage extends into deeper layers of dermis (normal healing associated with contraction and scarring).
- *Full thickness:* tissue damage extends through dermis (sometimes down to fat (SC layer), or muscle and bone. The skin is white or charred, painless, and leathery to touch. Healing occurs from edges of wound with contraction and scarring. These injuries may need surgical debridement and skin grafting.

The 'Rule of Nines' is a standardized method used to assess how much body surface area (BSA) has been burned. It does not apply to children <10yrs. Applies to partial thickness and full thickness burns in adults (Table 13.1).

**Table 13.1** Percentage of BSA

| Anatomic surface | % total body surface |
| --- | --- |
| Head and neck | 9% |
| Arms, including hands | 9% |
| Legs, including feet | 18% each (14% children >10yrs) |
| Genitalia | 1% |
| Head all over | 9% ( 14% children >10yrs) |
| Front | 18% |
| Back | 18% |

**Minor burns**

Partial thickness burns involving <15% body surface area (BSA) in low-risk patients *or* 10% high-risk patients.

• *Cool the burn:* hold burnt area under cold, running water for 15min (timed). If impractical, immerse in cold water or cool with cold compresses. Cooling burn ↓ swelling. Do not put ice directly onto burn—may cause tissue damage. If water unavailable, use cold, harmless liquid such as beer, lemonade, milk, or bag of frozen peas.

• *Remove gently any potential constrictions:* e.g. rings, watches, belts, shoes, before injured area begins to swell.

• *Dress the burn:* with a clean, preferably sterile, non-fluffy material, and bandage. This restricts air to the injured area, ↓ pain and protects blistered skin. Cling film ideal *for the immediate treatment* of superficial and partial thickness burns, if there are low levels of exudate.

• Offer pain relief.

• Do not use adhesive dressings.

• Do not break blisters (which protect against infection).

• Do not apply lotions, ointments, or fat to the injury.

• Minor burns usually heal in 1–2wks without further treatment.

• Monitor burns for signs of infection.

• Advise patients to use high factor sunscreens for 1yr.

**Sunburn** Can cause pain, blistering, and systemic upset. Treat with calamine lotion and paracetamol. Hospitalization in severe cases for fluid management.

**Partial and full-thickness burns (moderate and major) burns**

For children and people at risk (e.g. frail, older people) refer to specialist services for full-thickness burns exceeding 5% of BSA, partial thickness exceeding 10%.

Consider referral of all but the smallest burns for assessment. Includes burns involving hands, face, feet, perineum, or crossing major joints or circumferential of an extremity, plus burns complicated by fractures, other trauma, inhalation, or electrical burns.

*Common causes*
- Clothing on fire.
- Hot water immersion.
- Contact with flames, hot objects, electricity.
- Corrosive chemicals.

*Flame burns*
*Clothing on fire*
- Lay the casualty down immediately to prevent flames burning face.
- Douse flames with water or other non-flammable liquid.
- Smother flames with a blanket or jacket, while rolling casualty on ground.
- Remove jewellery and tight clothing from burnt area.
- Do not remove clothing adherent to burn.
- Do not apply ice, lotion, ointments, or home remedies.
- Immerse burnt area in cold water or apply cold compresses briefly.
- Children should never be transported with cold soaks in place.
- Wrap patient loosely in clean sheet and transport to hospital.
- If patient is conscious, not vomiting, and if medical help is more than 2hrs away, give small sips of water.
- Treat for shock.

*Chemical burns*
- Usually caused by strong acids or alkalis.
- Wear gloves to remove contaminated clothing.
- Irrigate with cold running water for at least 20min.
- *Do not attempt to neutralize chemical:* can exacerbate injury by causing heat.
- Dress burn with clean, sterile, non-fluffy material, and bandage.
- Remove to hospital immediately unless minimal and pain free.
- Alert hospital to ensure containment of any chemical hazard and safe disposal of contaminated materials.
- OH department and Health Protection Agency may need to follow-up.

*Electric shock and burns*
- If person in contact with electrical source, if possible turn off electricity. If not, move away from source using a dry, non-conducting object made of cardboard, plastic, or wood.
- If signs of circulation absent, begin BLS (📖 Adult Basic Life Support, p. 742).
- Skin burns may be seen at entry and exit point of current, internal damage may be severe despite minimal skin injury.
- Cover affected areas with a sterile gauze. Refer to A&E.

*Radiation burns*
- In the UK, 24-hr advice and assistance via NAIR (National Arrangements for Incidents involving Radioactivity) on ☎ 0800 834153 or via police.
- In an emergency, patients may be taken to any ED for radioactive decontamination treatment.
- Advice and help should be sought urgently from the duty ED consultant and a radiation physicist (medical physics or radiotherapy departments).
- Treatment must take place in a designated decontamination room.
- All staff must be decontaminated and checked before leaving this area.

*Smoke inhalation*
- If smoke inhalation suspected, refer to A&E patient may deteriorate later.
- Thermal or chemical damage can cause oedema and airway problems, suspect if singed nasal hairs or hoarse voice.

## Related topics
📖 Wound assessment, p. 475; 📖 Wound dressings, p. 492.

## References
NHS Choices. Available at: ℡ www.nhs.uk/Conditions/Burns-and-scalds/Pages/Treatment.aspx
NAIR. Available at: ℡ www.hpa.org.uk/webc/HPAwebFile/HPAweb_C/1194947334572
PatientPlus Burns—assessment and management. Available at: ℡ www.patient.co.uk
Health Protection Agency. Available at: ℡ www.hpa.org.uk

# Adult choking

## Foreign body airway obstruction (FBAO)

Choking usually results from airway obstruction by a foreign body. Early recognition is key, important not to confuse this emergency with fainting, heart attack, stroke, or other conditions, which may cause sudden respiratory distress, cyanosis, or loss of consciousness. Older people are a vulnerable group and FBAO because of ill-fitting or absent dentures, neurological impairment and risk associated with soft/slick foods.

## General signs of choking

- Attack occurs while eating.
- Victim may clutch his neck.

Foreign bodies may cause either mild or severe airway obstruction (Table 13.2).

Vital to ask the conscious victim, 'Are you choking?'.

**Table 13.2** Signs of airway obstruction

| Signs of mild airway obstruction | Signs of severe airway obstruction |
|---|---|
| Response to the question, 'Are you choking?' | Response to the question, 'Are you choking?' |
| • Victim speaks and answers, 'yes' | • Victim unable to speak<br>• Victim may respond by nodding |
| • Other signs | • Other signs |
| • Victim unable to speak, cough, and breathe | • Victim is unable to breathe<br>• Breathing sounds wheezy<br>• Attempts at coughing are silent<br>• Victim may be unconscious |

## Adult choking treatment sequence (Fig. 13.7)

*If victim shows signs of mild airway obstruction*

Encourage them to continue coughing, but do nothing else.

*If victim shows signs of severe airway obstruction and is conscious*

- Stand to the side and slightly behind the victim.
- Support chest with one hand and lean victim well forwards so that head is lower than chest, so that when obstruction is dislodged, it comes out of mouth and not further down airway.
- Give *up to* five sharp blows between shoulder blades with heel of other hand.
- Check to see if each back blow has relieved airway obstruction, aim is to relieve obstruction with each blow, rather than necessarily to give all five.

- If this fails, give up to five abdominal thrusts.
- Stand behind victim and put both arms round upper part of their abdomen.
- Lean victim forwards.
- Clench your fist and place it between umbilicus (navel) and bottom end of sternum (breastbone).
- Grasp this hand with your other hand, and pull sharply inwards and upwards.
- Repeat up to five times.
- If obstruction is still not relieved, continue alternating five back blows with five abdominal thrusts.

*If the victim becomes unconscious*
- Support victim carefully to the ground.
- Call ambulance immediately.
- Begin CPR (📖 Adult basic life support, p. 742). Initiate chest compressions even if a pulse is present in the unconscious, choking victim.

❶ Following successful treatment for choking, foreign material may remain in the upper or lower respiratory tract causing complications later.
- Victims with a persistent cough, swallowing difficulties, or with a sensation of an object still lodged in the throat must be referred for an expert medical opinion.
- Abdominal thrusts may cause serious internal injuries and all victims receiving abdominal thrusts must be examined for injury by a doctor.

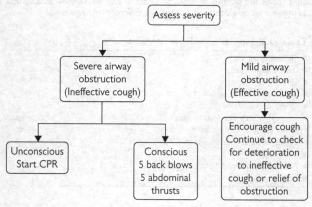

**Fig. 13.7** Adult choking treatment.
Reproduced from Resuscitation Guidelines (2010) with permission of the Resuscitation Council UK.

### References

Choking and Foreign Body Airway Obstruction (FBAO). Available at: ✍ www.patient.co.uk
Resuscitation Council UK. Available at: ✍ www.resus.org.uk/

# Child choking

## FBAO in a child

About 16,000 cases of choking occur every year; if a blockage completely prevents airflow → permanent brain damage in 2min and death in 3min (see also (📖 Adult choking, p. 760). Babies and toddlers frequently put objects in their mouths. The majority of choking events in children occur either during play or while eating with carer.

## Recognition of foreign body airway obstruction

When a foreign body enters airway, a child will react immediately by coughing (Table 13.3). A spontaneous cough is likely to be more effective than any manoeuvre a rescuer might perform. If coughing absent or ineffective and airway obstructed, the child will rapidly become asphyxiated. FBAO is characterized by:

- Coughing or choking, gagging or stridor (high pitched, noisy respirations like blowing of the wind).
- Sudden onset.
- Recent history of playing with or eating small objects.

Suspect FBAO if:

- There are no other signs of illness.
- History of eating or playing with small items immediately prior to onset of symptoms.

Similar signs and symptoms may also be associated with other causes, such as laryngitis or epiglottitis, which require different management.

---

**Table 13.3** Types of coughing in FBAO

*Ineffective cough*
- Unable to vocalize.
- Quiet or silent cough.
- Unable to breathe.
- Cyanosis.
- Decreasing level of consciousness.

*Effective cough*
- Crying or verbal response to questions.
- Loud cough.
- Able to take a breath before coughing.
- Fully responsive.

---

## Relief of FBAO

See Fig. 13.8 for treatment algorithm.
- If child is coughing effectively, no external manoeuvre is necessary. Encourage child to cough and monitor continuously.
- If child's cough is, or is becoming, ineffective shout for help immediately, and determine child's consciousness level.

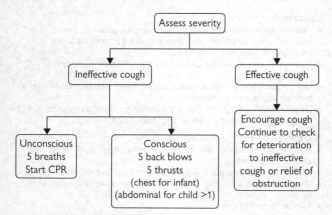

**Fig. 13.8** Paediatric FBAO treatment algorithm.
Reproduced from Resuscitation Guidelines (2010) with permission of the Resuscitation Council UK.

### Conscious child with FBAO
With absent or ineffective coughing.

*Back blows in an infant*
- Support infant in a head-downwards, prone position, to enable gravity to assist removal of foreign body.
- A seated or kneeling rescuer should be able to support infant safely across lap.
- Support infant's head by placing thumb of one hand at angle of lower jaw, and one or two fingers from same hand at same point on other side of jaw.
- Do not compress soft tissues under infant's jaw as this will exacerbate airway obstruction.
- Deliver up to 5 sharp back blows with heel of one hand in middle of back between shoulder blades.
- Aim is to relieve obstruction with each blow, rather than to give all five.

*In a child over 1yr*
- Back blows are more effective if child is positioned head down.
- A small child may be placed across rescuer's lap as with an infant.
- If this is not possible, support child in a forward-leaning position and deliver back blows from behind.

If back blows fail to dislodge the object, and the child is still conscious, use chest thrusts for infants or abdominal thrusts for children. Do NOT use abdominal thrusts (Heimlich manoeuvre) for infants.

*Chest thrusts for infants*
- Turn the infant into a head-downwards supine position. This is achieved safely by placing your free arm along infant's back and encircling occiput with your hand.
- Support infant down your arm, which is placed down (or across) your thigh.
- Identify landmark for chest compression (lower sternum ~one finger's breadth above xiphisternum).
- Deliver five chest thrusts. These are similar to chest compressions, but sharper in nature, and delivered at a slower rate.

*Abdominal thrusts for children over 1yr*
- Stand or kneel behind child. Place your arms under child's arms and encircle their torso.
- Clench your fist and place it between umbilicus and xiphisternum.
- Grasp this hand with your other hand, and pull sharply inwards and upwards.
- Repeat up to five times.
- Ensure that pressure is not applied to xiphoid process or lower rib cage, as this may cause abdominal trauma.

*Following chest or abdominal thrusts reassess the child*
- If object has not been expelled and child is still conscious, continue sequence of back blows and chest (for infant) or abdominal (for children) thrusts.
- Call out or send for help if it is still not available.
- Do not leave child at this stage.

If the object is expelled successfully, assess child's clinical condition. Any doubt that part of the object may remain in the respiratory tract seek medical assistance. Abdominal thrusts may cause internal injuries. Children should be examined by a medical practitioner.

### Unconscious child with FBAO
- If child with FBAO is, or becomes unconscious, place them on a firm, flat surface.
- Call out or send for help if it is still not available.

**Do not leave the child at this stage.**

*Airway opening*
- Open the mouth and look for any obvious object.
- If anything is seen, make an attempt to remove it with a single finger sweep.
- Do not attempt blind/repeated finger sweeps in children because these can impact the object more deeply into pharynx and cause injury.

*Rescue breaths*
- Open the airway and attempt five rescue breaths.
- *Assess effectiveness of each breath:* if a breath does not make chest rise, reposition head before making next attempt.

*Chest compression and CPR*
- Attempt five rescue breaths and if no response, proceed immediately to chest compression.
- Follow sequence for single rescuer ~1min before summoning emergency medical services (if not done already by someone else).
- If child regains consciousness and is breathing effectively, place in a safe side-lying (recovery) position, and monitor till help arrives.

## Related topics

&#x1F4D6; Adult basic life support, p. 742; &#x1F4D6; child basic life support, p. 748; &#x1F4D6; Child injury prevention, p. 162.

## References

First aid for choking: An illustrated guide. Available at: &#x1F50D; www.babycentre.co.uk/baby/safety/chokingguide

BBC online and interactive tests for first aid. Available at: &#x1F50D; www.bbc.co.uk/health/first_aid_action

Resuscitation Council UK. Available at: &#x1F50D; www.resus.org.uk/

# Eye trauma

There are more than >120,000 accidents in England involving eye injuries every year. The most urgent eye injuries are chemical burns, retrobulbar haemorrhage (RH), and open globe injuries including intraocular foreign bodies (FBs).

## Assessment

- *Examine eye in a well-lit area:* to find the object, ask person look up and down, then side-to-side.
- *Time and mode of injury:* physical/chemical, superficial blunt, or penetrating trauma, speed of impact size of object.
- *What was patient doing:* were glasses or goggles worn?
- Possibility of foreign body.
- *Possible high-velocity injury:* e.g. if injury involved power tools, metal on metal work, hammer and chisel, lawn mowing, glass injuries.
- *Previous and current acuity:* tenderness, bruising, conjunctival haemmorhage.
- *Abnormal pupil reactivity, size, or shape:* refer for medical assessment immediately.
- Other injuries sustained.
- *Current symptoms:* pain, reduced vision, diplopia, flashes/floaters, foreign body sensation.
- An emergency if there is severe eye pain with progressive visual loss, proptosis, possible RH.
- Past medical history, tetanus immunization, medication, and allergies.

## Prevention of injury and/or further damage

- *Wear protective goggles:* e.g. during construction work, and high-risk sports, e.g. squash.
- *UV protection glasses:* for sailing, skiing, and sunbed use.
- Tell patient not to rub eyes if trauma suspected.
- Stop wearing contact lens until symptom free.
- If in need of further care to reduce eye movement and risk of further infection cover with sterile dressing.

## Common injuries

- *Corneal abrasion:* often caused by small sharp objects, e.g. finger nail, characterized by intense pain, irritation, and photophobia. Drops of local anaesthetic (e.g. amethocaine BNF 11.7) and fluroscein used (if not available refer to ED) to check no foreign objects in eye, abrasion should heal within 48hrs. Antibiotic drops for healing and dressing only needed to protect eye following anaesthetic.
- *Foreign bodies in the eye:* e.g. small pieces of grit, eyelashes; usually move to lower part of eye, can be washed out or lifted out with a sterile cotton bud tip. If irritant not obvious, grasp lower eyelid and gently pull down on it to look under lower eyelid. To look under the upper lid, place a cotton-tipped swab on the outside of the upper lid and gently flip the lid over the cotton swab. If the object is embedded **do not try to remove or apply any pressure**. To reduce eye

movement and risk of further infection cover with sterile dressing and refer for immediate specialist care.

- *Chemical injuries:* treat chemical burns *immediately*; hold eyelids open and bathe eyes with copious amounts of water (may be painful to keep eyes open so use anaesthetic drops). Chemical burns often have serious consequences refer urgently to specialist.
- *Arc eye:* welders, skiers, and sunbed users with no eye protection against UV light may damage corneal epithelium. Severe eye pain, watering, and blepharospasm. Give oral analgesic (paracetamol, ibuprofen (BNF 4.7.1)) and pad eye, should recover in 24h, if not refer to specialist. Advise on eye protection in the future.

### Serious signs and symptoms and injuries that require urgent referral to an ophthalmologist

Eye trauma that should have **immediate** referral for emergency specialist treatment include:

- Penetrating injury to eye.
- All high-velocity injuries, e.g. arising from hammering, lawn mowing, should be assumed to be penetrating injuries until proven not to be.
- All strongly adherent foreign bodies, especially those that lie near centre of cornea as there is increased risk of visual loss.
- Pain not relieved by anaesthetic.
- Diplopia.
- *Flashes and (new) floaters:* can indicate retinal injury.
- Reduction in visual acuity particularly if progressive.
- Large abrasions (covering >60% eye).
- *Hyphaema:* blood in anterior chamber of the eye.
- Any pupil, iris, or fundal abnormality:
  - Abnormalities of eye movements.
  - Chemical burn.
  - Unclear history, lid swelling, a young child, or reduced conscious level.
  - Corneal foreign body which cannot be removed.
  - Corneal abrasions opacities, rust rings.
  - *Deep lid laceration*—there may be damage underneath.
  - Marginal lacerations as lacrimal ducts may be affected.

- *Corneal ulceration:* presents with pain and photophobia, watering of eye and blurred vision. Causes include contact lens, trauma, previous disease. Refer for same day specialist appointment.

### Related topics

📖 Common problems affecting eyes, p. 697; 📖 Blindness and partial sight, p. 699.

### References

BBC online and interactive tests for first aid. Available at: 🔎 www.bbc.co.uk/health/first_aid_action/
Eye Trauma. Available at: 🔎 www.patient.co.uk

# Hypothermia

Under most conditions, the body maintains a healthy temperature. Exposure to cold temperatures or a cool, damp environment for prolonged periods → body's control mechanisms may fail to maintain normal temperature. When more heat is lost than the body can generate = hypothermia. Hypothermia is defined as a core (rectal) temperature of <35°C, and designated mild (32–35°C), moderate (30–32°C), or severe (<30°C).

## Risk factors

- Infants, young children, and the very lean.
- *Older people:* with ↑ age there is impaired thermoregulation, ↓ metabolism often of multifactorial origin, including immobility (e.g. Parkinson's, following a fall), lack of cold awareness, unsatisfactory housing, and those whose judgement may be impaired by mental illness.
- *In young adults:* hypothermia is usually due to environmental exposure (e.g. cold water immersion, hill walking), or to immobility, and/or impaired conscious level from alcohol or drugs.
- Abnormal mental state.
- *Drugs:* alcohol, barbiturate, major tranquillizers, antidepressants.
- *Endocrine:* hypothyroidism, hypoglycaemia, adrenal insufficiency, hypopituitarism.
- *Autonomic neuropathy:* diabetes mellitus.
- 📖 Weight management: malnutrition, p. 309.
- 📖 Renal problems, p. 705.
- *Sepsis:* excessive heat loss from vasodilatation.
- *Exposure:* inadequate clothing, heating, near-drowning.

## Clinical features

The following signs and symptoms may occur, not in any particular order:
- Shivering.
- Slurred speech.
- Visual abnormalities.
- Abnormally slow breathing.
- Cold pale skin.
- Loss of coordination.
- Fatigue, lethargy, or apathy.

Although wide variations occur, as core T°, cerebral and cardiovascular functions deteriorate.
- Mild hypothermia presents as shivering, which is maximal at 35°C and decreases, being absent at 32°C.
- At 32–35°C, apathy, amnesia ataxia, and dysarthria are common.
- At <32°C, consciousness falls progressively leading to coma, ↓ BP, arrhythmias, respiratory depression, and muscular rigidity. Progressive hypothermia is associated with delirium, coma, bradycardia, and low respiratory rate, cardiac arrhythmias, dilated pupils, and loss of reflexes.

*Severe hypothermia may mimic death* Ventricular fibrillation (VF) may occur spontaneously when T° <28°C and may be provoked by excessive movement or invasive procedures. VF is refractory at temperatures below 30°C and resuscitation must be continued until the temperature reaches 32°C.

## Hypothermia first aid

- *Move patient out of cold:* if not feasible, protect patient from wind and rain, cover his head and insulate him from cold ground.
- Handle patient gently.
- Remove wet clothing and replace with a warm, dry covering.
- Call 999 for emergency medical assistance.
- If breathing ceases or seems dangerously slow or shallow, begin BLS ( Adult basic life support, p. 742) immediately.
- Do *not* apply direct heat to warm victim. Direct heat (e.g. hot water bottle) can cause rapid fluid shifts and potentially pulmonary oedema.
- Apply warm compresses to the neck, chest wall, and groin.
- Do not attempt to warm the arms and legs.
- Do not offer alcohol. Give conscious patient warm drinks unless vomiting.
- Treat the patient in a warm room (>21°C).
- Do not massage or rub the patient, and treat very gently.

## Rewarming methods

External rewarming is usually sufficient if the core temperature is >32°C. Endogenous metabolism and shivering generate heat allowing spontaneous rewarming. Easy, non-invasive process involving removing cold, wet clothing, and wrapping in warm blankets.

*In hospital*

- Infrared radiant lamps and heating blankets may be used for children.
- Aim to rewarm adults at a rate of 0.5–2°C/h, but do not rewarm older people with prolonged hypothermia too rapidly (>0.6°C/h) danger of cerebral/pulmonary oedema.

Active rewarming and core rewarming are available in hospital:
- Water bath at 37–41°C.
- Hot air blanket.
- Warm IV fluids to 39°C.
- Gastric or bladder lavage with normal saline at 42°C.
- Airway warming in self-ventilating patients.
- Peritoneal lavage.
- *Extracorporeal:* cardiopulmonary bypass maintains brain and vital organ perfusion, in patients with severe hypothermia or those in cardiac arrest.

## Related topics

 Adult basic life support, p. 742;  Child basic life support, p. 748.

## References

BBC First aid action. Available at: ℬ www.bbc.co.uk/health/first_aid_action
Hypothermia. Available at: ℬ www.patient.co.uk/health

# Poisoning and overdoses

## Deliberate self-poisoning

Commonest form of self-harm in adults, one of the top five causes of acute medical admissions. The most at-risk groups are children under the age of 5yrs and females aged 35–54yrs (4.4 deaths per 100,000 UK population in 2009). Most commonly ingested overdose substances are prescribed medication and analgesics, particularly paracetamol. Drugs or poisons may be taken impulsively. ~25% of all suicides attend a general hospital after a non-fatal act of self-harm within year before death.

## Unintentional or 'accidental' poisoning

- Peak incidence is 2yrs, involving household substances or medicines. (*Note:* many plants are poisonous, e.g. privet, laburnum seeds, laurel and yew berries.) Always consider non-accidental injury in children (📖 Child protection, p. 230).
- Adult poisoning may result from miscalculation or confusion of doses, or by taking the same medications under different names.
- Drug smugglers, who ingest multiple packages of drugs, are at serious risk of poisoning.

## Overdoses

- 65% of drugs involved belong to the patient, a relative, or friend.
- 30% of self-poisonings involve multiple drugs.
- 50% of patients will also have consumed alcohol.
- The history may be unreliable.
- People who deliberately self-harmed are entitled to same privacy, care, and respect of patient information.
- This may be unreliable but if it is possible ask:
  - What was taken, how much, when, and by what route?
  - Route of exposure: swallowed, inhaled, injected, etc.
  - Was alcohol consumed too?
  - Any vomiting since ingestion?
  - Establish past medical history, current medications, and allergies.
  - Was a suicide note left?
  - Is the patient pregnant?
  - *Take histories from others:* family, friends, and observers.
  - Note down information about exposure for specialist services.

## Emergency treatment

- Reduce absorption of the poison if possible.
- Give a specific antidote if available.
- Clear and maintain airway.
- If breathing appears inadequate, ventilate with $O_2$ using a bag and mask or endotracheal tube. (**Do not give mouth to mouth resuscitation in poisoned patients**).
- *Check pulse:* if unconscious and pulseless, start adult BLS.
- Monitor and record vital signs.
- If breathing, place in recovery position in case of vomiting.
- Call 999 for transport to hospital for specialist care.

## Information about poisons

UK National Poisons Information Centres. ☎ 087 0600 626611 (automatically routed to nearest centre).

TOXBASE. Available at: ℘ www.toxbase.org NHS intranet and internet-based information from the National Poisons Information Centre (registration free to NHS GPs and hospitals).

Mims Colour index or TICTAC to aid pill identification (a computer-aided tablet and capsule identification system available to authorized users, including Regional Drug Information Centres and Poisons Information Centres).

British National Formulary (BNF)/Data Sheet Compendium.

## Related topics

📖 Adult basic life support, p. 742; 📖 Child basic life support, p. 748; 📖 Child injury prevention, p. 162.

## References

Acute Poisoning. Available at: ℘ www.patient.co.uk

BBC online and interactive tests for first aid. Available at: ℘: www.bbc.co.uk/health/first_aid

Wyatt JP. (2006). *Oxford Handbook of Emergency Medicine.*. Oxford: Oxford University Press.

# Fractures

A fracture is a broken or cracked bone, most common are classified as:
- *Closed fracture:* there is no open wound associated with this fracture.
- *Open fracture:* there is an open wound associated with this fracture.
- *Complicated fracture:* end of fractured bone penetrates adjacent organs or causes damage to nerves or blood vessels.
- *Stress fracture:* occurs in foot and toes. Can occur following prolonged or excessive exercise.
- *Greenstick fracture:* a type of incomplete fracture occurring in children, where one cortical surface of a bone breaks and other side bends.
- *Torus ('buckle') fracture:* incomplete fracture in childhood characterized by buckling of the cortex.

All fractures have soft tissue injury with consequent bleeding and tissue swelling. Bony fragments may penetrate adjacent organs causing additional bleeding and, occasionally, major blood vessels and nerve damage. Open fractures ↑ risk infection. Fractures are often painful because of the extensive sensory nerve supply to the periosteum. Always consider non-accidental injury in children (⩗ Child protection, p. 230).

## Sprains and strains

Strains are injuries to the muscles moving the bones (often caused by overstretching). Often characterized by pain, tenderness, swelling, bruising, and difficulty moving the affected part.

### RICE procedure
- R: rest and support affected limb.
- I: apply ice or a cold compress to reduce swelling.
- C: comfortably support using effective support bandaging.
- E: elevate limb to reduce blood flow to affected area.

This treatment may relieve symptoms, but if in doubt treat as a fracture.

## Fractures: signs and symptoms
- Pain at or near the site of injury exacerbated by movement.
- Tenderness at fracture site on application of gentle pressure, with subsequent swelling and bruising.
- Restricted movement, immobility, or deformity (shortening, angulation, or rotation) of affected limb.
- Patient may report sound of a breaking bone.
- Limb movement may cause crepitus.
- If fracture involves a large or multiple bones, blood loss may be severe and life-threatening.
- Open fracture causes twice the blood loss of corresponding closed fracture, e.g. a single, open, femoral shaft fracture in a child may result in significant loss of circulating volume. This could be life-threatening.
- Trauma may also lead to partial loss (subluxation) or complete loss (dislocation) of congruity between articulating surfaces of a joint and may also be associated with fractures of one or more bones.

## General management of fractures

All patients with suspected fractures should be referred for X-ray and specialist assessment in A&E.

- Ensure personal safety. Assess patient's airway, breathing, and circulation.
- Recognize and treat life-threatening injuries *before* assessing and managing skeletal trauma.
- Haemorrhage must be controlled in first instance.
- Apply sterile dressings to all open wounds.
- Unless absolutely necessary, casualties with fractures should not be moved until skilled help arrives.
- Treat all fractures in position in which casualty is found, unless there is further immediate danger to life.
- Place soft padding around broken bones and splint injury with something rigid, e.g. rolled up newspapers or magazines to immobilize affected part.
- Splints should be long enough to extend beyond joints above and below the fracture.
- If there is an open fracture, cover with sterile gauze pad and apply pressure to control bleeding. **Under no circumstances attempt to push the bone back into the wound nor clean it**.
- Frequently check perfusion, including pulses, skin colour, and temperature. If appropriate, record an extremity assessment based on the five Ps: pain, pallor, pulses, paraesthesia, paralysis.
- Monitor and treat for shock.
- Do not give patients anything to eat or drink in case surgery is required.

## Immobilization

Severely angulated fractures aligned *only* by emergency medical services before transport to hospital, requires analgesia.

Fractures (or suspected fractures) should be immobilized to control pain and further injury. Emergency splinting techniques are summarized:
- *Hand:* this should be elevated and kept comfortable.
- *Forearm and wrist:* splinted flat on padded pillows or splints.
- *Elbow:* immobilize in a flexed position with a sling, which may be strapped to the body.
- *Arm and shoulder:* immobilize by sling, secured for additional support, across patient's chest. Circumferential bandages should be avoided as they may cause constriction, particularly when swelling occurs.
- *Femoral fractures:* should be treated in traction splints, but avoid in patients with suspected pelvic fractures.
- *Tibia and ankle fractures:* immobilized in padded box splints and foot perfusion, assessed before and after application.

## Traumatic amputation

Traumatic amputation of an extremity may be partial or complete, the former is the greater initial threat to life as completely transected blood vessels go into spasm. Exsanguinating haemorrhage must be controlled with sterile dressings, elasticated compression bandaging, and elevation wherever possible.

• Retain the amputated part for possible urgent re-implantation at a specialist centre, particularly if a child is involved.
• Amputated parts are viable for 8hrs at room temp, 18hrs if cooled.
• Amputated tissue should be wrapped in moist, sterile towel, Emergency services place in sterile bag in an insulated box, filled with crushed ice and water, and in same vehicle as patient.

At all costs, avoid direct contact between ice and the severed tissue.

## Related topics

📖 Bleeding, p. 745; 📖 Adult basic life support, p. 742; 📖 Child basic child support, p. 748; 📖 Child injury prevention, p. 162.

## Reference

BBC online. Available at: 🔊 www.bbc.co.uk/health/first_aid

# Useful information

# Assistive technology

Assistive technology refers to 'any device or system that allows an individual to perform a task that they would otherwise be unable to do, or increases the ease and safety with which the task can be performed'. Information about the range of assistive technology currently available for specific disabilities is provide by the network of disabled living centres, charities (e.g. Alzheimer's Society), and through therapists and specialist advisors (see 📖 Further information, p. 777).

## Provision

Equipment, home adaptations, and aids to nursing are provided through various public services (NHS, social services, housing, education, employment), the private, and voluntary sectors. The system for public provision and public funding is complex and grey areas exist. Individuals may be eligible for direct payment (📖 Social services, p. 26) to purchase their own equipment. Publicly-funded provision may not cover all types of equipment, or there may be a financial ceiling. Some charities provide individual grants, usually on application from a professional (see 📖 Benefits and support, p. 789). The Equality Act 2010 states that employers must make 'reasonable adjustments which includes modified equipment to accommodate the needs of disabled employees'.

## Public funding

Authorities divide up responsibilities by:
- The purpose for which equipment is required (e.g. NHS, health need; LA, social care need).
- By type of equipment (e.g. incontinence equipment as health care, NHS responsibility).

*LA responsibilities* Aids, adaptations, and equipment provided following an assessment that includes financial assessment. LAs will have charges.

### NHS responsibilities

Medical, nursing, or therapy equipment are usually free, but there exist variable and changing eligibility criteria for some items, e.g. continence pads and nebulizers. Some can be charged for, e.g. spinal supports. Equipment on the medical or nursing drug tariff, e.g. catheters, attracts prescription charges, except for those that are exempt (📖 Prescribing, p. 130).

## Therapists and specialists

Professionals most commonly involved in provision and advice on aids and equipment are:
- *OTs*: assess and find problems with daily living activities. Community OTs are part of social service departments or in specialist teams, e.g. reablement teams or special needs children teams.
- Rehabilitation officers for visually impaired people.
- Social workers for deaf people.
- *SALTs*: help with communication aids and eating/drinking.
- *Physiotherapists*: assess for mobility aids.

- *Orthotists:* who make and fit orthoses (externally applied devices, e.g. calipers, collars, splints, footwear, trusses); usually working to the prescription of consultants.
- *Podiatrists/chiropodists:* make and supply orthotic footwear.
- *Specialist nurses:* e.g. continence advisers, stoma care specialist.
- *Disability employment advisors:* in local Job Centres identify equipment and adaptations required by disabled people for the workplace and provide information on access to work grants for specialist equipment.

## Joint (NHS and LA) equipment stores

Most areas have a community or joint equipment store funded by the NHS and LA for the loan of some aids to independent living and nursing in the home, on the request of a professional, most commonly DNs, physiotherapists, and OTs. Each store has its own catalogue, ordering, delivery, and return system. In some areas, 'prescriptions' are issued for simple aids to daily living, e.g. raised toilet seats, so that people can have more choice by exchanging them at an accredited retailer.

## Other public service providers

- LA housing departments provide some home adaptations.
- Local education authorities and schools provide equipment and adaptations for special educational needs (📖 Children with special educational needs, p. 227).

## Other sources for the public

- *Retail outlets:* pharmacies, specialist shops, superstores, mail order catalogues/on-line shops, e.g. AgeUK, AssistUK.
- *Local voluntary organizations:* e.g. Red Cross, loan equipment generally for short-term needs, including wheelchairs, walking aids, commodes, bath seats.
- *Disabled living centres:* there is a network of 40 of these self-funding charities in the UK. They have permanent displays of equipment, and provide advice and online/mail order shops.
- Promocon provides information about continence products, has a permanent display and a mail order service.

## Related topics

📖 Assistive technology, p. 778; 📖 Benefits for illness, disability and carers, p. 795.

## Further information

Assist UK (formerly Disabled Living Centres Council) lists disabled living centres. Available at: 🔊 www.assist-uk.org/

British Red Cross lists local branches loaning medical equipment. Available at: 🔊 www.redcross. co.uk

Department of Health (1999). *With Respect to Old Age: long term care- rights and responsibilities.* Cm4192-1. London: Stationary Office.

Disabled Living Foundation. Provides a wide range of factsheets and advice. Available at: 🔊 www. dlf.org.uk

Promocon for equipment and aids for bladder and bowel problems. Available at: 🔊 www. disabledliving.co.uk/PromoCon/About

# Assistive technology and equipment for home nursing

### Aids to daily living and home adaptation

Social service departments (📖 Social services, p. 26) provide daily living equipment and home adaptations (following an OT assessment), usually as part of community care assessment (📖 Social services, p. 26). Some people will receive direct payments (📖 Benefits and support, p. 789) for equipment. Equipment is either loaned through joint equipment stores (📖 Assistive technology, p. 776), but may incur a charge, including for maintenance, or simple aids to living, e.g. trolleys are chosen from an accredited retailers using a 'prescription' from the joint equipment store. Types of equipment include:

- Aids for toilets, baths, beds, chairs, dressing, feeding and drinking, communication.
- Transfer aids, e.g. turntables, hoists.
- Household gadgets.
- Community alarms.

LAs may provide and fund (following financial assessment) home adaptations to allow a disabled person access to essential parts of the home. These may be minor, e.g. stair rails, or major, e.g. structural work to permit fixed hoists.

### Assistive technology and memory loss

For people with memory loss, there are a range of types of devices, AT Dementia provides information, including:

- *Memory aids:* such as reminder devices, automatic calendar clocks, locator devices, e.g. for keys.
- *Smart household devices:* e.g. lights with motion sensors, adapted plugs that respond to running taps to avoid floods.
- *Telecare:* monitors sensors remotely for real time emergencies via sensors, and calls a nominated person, e.g. sensors for floods, extreme heat, gas, lack of movement, or failure to return to the home after specified periods.
- *Global positioning technologies:* to help find someone who has gone missing.

## Home nursing equipment

This overlaps with aids to independent living and, in some areas, may be clearly defined when it is an NHS responsibility. Equipment that is the responsibility of the NHS is free at the point of care. Types of equipment that community nurses can usually obtain through an equipment store, to support nursing in the home, include:

- *Pressure relief equipment:* e.g. some types of beds, cushions, mattresses (alternating pressure, fluidized bead flotation, foam, low air loss, ripple, water) (📖 Pressure ulcer prevention, p. 473).
- Beds that change position and height (📖 Patient moving and handling, p. 92).
- *Raising aids:* e.g. monkey poles, chair raisers.
- *Transfer aids:* e.g. hoists, slide sheets, turntables.
- *Toilet aids:* e.g. urinals, commodes.
- *Incontinence aids* (📖 Continence products, p. 468).
- *Bathing aids:* often a LA responsibility.

Some local Red Cross branches provide the public with short-term loans of medical equipment, such as commodes.

## Mobility aids

- *Walking aids, e.g. sticks, frames:* usually assessed and provided by NHS physiotherapists (sometimes community nurses) from joint equipment stores.
- *Wheelchairs (manual and electric) and buggies:* provided for long-term disabled adults and children through NHS wheelchair clinics.
- *Wheelchairs for short-term use:* can be hired commercially or loaned from some local Red Cross branches.

## Other therapy-related NHS equipment for home use

The NHS supplies health-related equipment for medical, nursing, and therapy purposes in the home. Provision and maintenance may be from a commercial company or local hospital. Types include:

- Respiratory equipment, e.g. oxygen cylinders and concentrators, powered nebulizers (📖 Oxygen therapy in the community, p. 581).
- TENS machines (📖 Pain assessment and management, p. 513).
- Dialysis equipment (📖 Renal problems, p. 507).

## Further information

British Red Cross lists local branches loaning medical equipment. Available at: ℘ www.redcross. co.uk

Disabled Living Centres Council (lists disabled living centres). Available at: ℘ www.dlcc.co.uk

Disabled Living Foundation provides a wide range of fact sheets and advice. Available at: ℘ www. dlf.org.uk

AT Dementia provides information on assistive technology for people with dementia. Available at: ℘ www.atdementia.org.uk/

# Biochemical and haematological values

Table 14.1 is guide of the normal range for adults (excluding pregnant women). *Note:* some laboratories use slightly different ranges.

**Table 14.1** Guide to normal range for adults

| Haematology | |
| --- | --- |
| Measurement | Reference interval |
| Haemoglobin | ♂: 13.0–17g/L |
| | ♀: 12–15.0g/L |
| Red cell count (RCC) | ♂: 4.5–5.5 × 10$^{12}$/L |
| Erythrocytes | ♀: 3.8–4.8 × 10$^{12}$/L |
| Packed cell volume or haematocrit | ♂: 0.4–0.50L/L |
| | ♀: 0.36–0.46L/L |
| Mean cell volume | 80–100fl |
| Mean cell haemoglobin | 32–36.0g/dL |
| White cell count (WCC) | 4.0–11.0 × 10$^9$/L |
| Neutrophils | 2.0–7.5 × 10$^9$/L, 40–75% WCC |
| Lymphocytes | 1.5–4.0 × 10$^9$/L, 20–45% WCC |
| Eosinophils | 0.04–0.50 × 10$^9$/L, 1–6% WCC |
| Basophils | 0.02–0.1 × 10$^9$/L, 0–1% WCC |
| Monocytes | 0.2–1.0 × 10$^9$/L, 2–10% WCC |
| Platelet count | 150–400 × 10$^9$/L |
| Reticulocyte count | ♂: 25–100 × 10$^9$/L |
| | ♀: 20–1200 × 10$^9$/L |
| | 0.5–2.5% RCC* |
| Erythrocyte sedimentation rate | <50yrs: ♂ 10mm, ♀ 19mm |
| | 51–60yrs: ♂ 12mm, ♀ 19mm |
| | 61–70yrs: ♂ 14mm, ♀ 20mm |
| | >71yrs: ♂ 30mm, ♀ 35mm |
| | <50yrs: ♂ 10mm, ♀ 19mm |
| INR | 1 (Therapeutic ranges for warfarin initiation as per local protocol) |
| **Biochemistry** | |
| *Substance* | *Reference interval* |
| ALT | P | 5–42IU/L |
| Albumin | P | 32–47g/L |
| Alkaline phosphatase | P | 100–300u/L |
| Aspartate transaminase | P | 5–42IU/L |

**Table 14.1** (Continued)

| Substance | | Reference interval |
|---|---|---|
| Bicarbonate | P | 24–31mmol/L |
| Bilirubin | P | 0–17µmol/L |
| Calcium (total) | P | 2.15–255mmol/L |
| Cholesterol | P | Ideally <5.0mmol/L |
| Creatinine | P | 60–125µmol/L |
| Creatinine kinase | P | Men: 25–195IU/L |
| | | Women: 25–170IU/L |
| eGFR | P | >90mL is normal |
| Ferritin | P | 10–120 micrograms/L pre-menopausal ♀ |
| | | 14–200 micrograms/L post-menopausal ♀,♂ |
| Folate | S/P | 3–17 micrograms/L |
| Follicle stimulating hormone | P/S | 0.8–11.5u/L |
| | | >30u/L post-menopause |
| Gamma-glutamyl transpeptidase | P | Men: 10–46IU/L |
| | P | Women: 6–2IU/L |
| Glucose (fasting) | P | 4.0–6.0mmol/L |
| HbA1c | P | 5–8% |
| Iron | S | Men: 14–33µmol/L |
| | P | Women: 11–28µmol/L |
| Luteinizing hormone | P | 0.8–12u/L |
| Osmolality | P | 280–295mosmol/kg |
| Phosphate (inorganic) | P | 0.7–1.5mmol/L |
| Potassium | P | 3.5–5.0mmol/L |
| Prolactin | P | Men: <450u/L |
| | P | Women: <600u/L |
| Prostate specific antigen | P | <50yrs: 0–2.5 micrograms/L |
| | | 51–60yrs: 0–3.5 micrograms/L |
| | | 61–70yrs: 0–4.5 micrograms/L |
| | | >71yrs: 0–6.5 micrograms/L |
| Protein (total) | P | 63–80g/L |
| Sodium | P | 135–145mmol/L |
| Thyroxine ($T_4$) | P | 8–22pmol/L |
| Triglyceride | P | <2.1mmol/L |
| Urea | | 3.0–6.5mmol/L |
| Uric acid | P | Men: 0.15–0.45µmol/L |
| | | Women: 0.12–0.36µmol/L |

* Only use percentages as reference interval if RCC is normal.

P = plasma (e.g. heparin bottle); S = serum (clotted—no anticoagulant).

Adapted with permission from Simon C, Everitt H, van Dorp F. (2010). *Oxford Handbook of General Practice*, 3rd edn. Oxford: Oxford University Press.

# Complementary and alternative therapies

These are a wide range of health care practices, products, and therapies that are used by the public as an alternative or complementary to evidence-based health care and medicine. Key issues to be aware of are the lack of evidence for efficacy as follows, lack of regulation of practitioners (except osteopaths and chiropractors see 📖 Complementary and alternative therapies, p. 782) and substances. The following are examples of some, but not all types of complementary and alternative therapies.

## Acupuncture

The use of needles to alleviate symptoms or cure disease. The mechanism of action remains unclear. Broadly, two forms exist—Chinese and Western. Acupuncture is most commonly used to treat musculoskeletal problems and chronic disease. There is some evidence of effectiveness in dental pain, low back pain, migraine and headache, nausea and vomiting, neck pain, substance abuse, and stroke.

*Further information*

British Medical Acupuncture Society. Available at: ℘ www.medical-acupuncture.co.uk
British Acupuncture Council. Available at: ℘ www.acupuncture.org.uk

## Aromatherapy

Inhaling aromatic plant oils or applying them to the skin for physical or emotional benefit. No evidence of effectiveness. Aromatherapy oils are very strong, may cause skin irritation, and can be poisonous if ingested. They are volatile oils readily absorbed through mucus membranes and may be as potent as any other drug. Their safety and interactions with other medications are unknown.

*Further information*

International Federation of Professional Aromatherapists. Available at: ℘ www.ifparoma.org.

## Faith healing

Founded on the belief that people and places have the power to heal through a connection to a supreme being. There are many types of 'healers', but no evidence of effectiveness.

*Further information*

The Healing Trust (formerly the National Federation of Spiritual Healers). Available at: ℘ www.thehealingtrust.org.uk/.

## Herbal medicine

Use of plants for medicinal purposes, but not regulated. Some herbal compounds have some evidence of effectiveness, e.g. St John's wort (for depression), echinacea (common cold), feverfew (migraine prophylaxis), Herbal remedies may have potent side effects and interactions with other drugs.

## Further information

National Institute of Medical Herbalists. Available at: ℘ www.nimh.org.uk
Register of Chinese Herbal Medicine. Available at: ℘ www.rchm.co.uk.

## Homeopathy

Practitioners 'treat' using extremely dilute substances. There is no evidence that it works better than placebos and it is considered scientifically implausible.

### Further information

The Society of Homeopaths. Available at: ℜ www.homeopathy-soh.org/

## Hypnotherapy

Consists of training the patient to relax very deeply. Evidence is weak and may be no better than a placebo. May have some value in managing anxiety, symptom control in IBS, and smoking cessation.

### Further information

The Association for Professional Hypnosis and Psychotherapy. Available at: ℜ www.aphp.co.uk.

## Osteopathy and chiropractic

Physical treatments aimed at restoring alignment of the joints and improving functioning of the body. In the UK, they are distinguished from each other by being under statutory regulation. All osteopaths and chiropractors have to undergo training, and after that time are registered with their governing body that enforces a code of standards and discipline. They must have professional indemnity insurance. They are best known for treating musculoskeletal problems, particularly bad backs. Other conditions (e.g. headaches, stress) can respond well too. There is good evidence of effectiveness for back pain.

### Further information

The General Osteopathic Council. Available at: ℜ www.osteopathy.org.uk
The British Chiropractic Association. Available at: ℜ www.chiropractic-uk.co.uk.

## Reflexology

Considers that a representation of the body is found on the foot. Treatment consists of massaging points on the foot or applying acupressure to relieve symptoms. There is no evidence of effectiveness.

### Further information

Association of Reflexologists. Available at: ℜ www.aor.org.uk.

## Reference

House of Commons Science and Technology Committee (2010). Evidence Check 2: Homeopathy. Available at: ℜ www.publications.parliament.uk/pa/cm200910/cmselect/cmsctech/45/4502.htm

# Death confirmation and certification

Approximately one-quarter of deaths occur at home. The GP is often the first to be contacted. A doctor is not required to verify death or view the body of a deceased person or report that a death has occurred. The doctor who attended the deceased during their last illness is required to issue a certificate detailing the cause of death.

## Verification of the fact of death

### Expected deaths

In many organizations there are protocols and agreements for registered nurses, with specific training, to verify expected and inevitable deaths of patients to whom they had provided palliative care. These will usually also state the circumstances in which nurses cannot verify death, e.g. death of a child. The GP and nursing team, in discussion with the family, will have made a prior agreement that the nurse verifies death (using a locally agreed form) and informs the GP (usually via the form). The GP then issues a medical certificate of death for collection by relatives (see 🕮 Death confirmation and certification, p. 784). Some GP practices provide written authorization for a category of patients, rather than individual patients. Following verification, the family can arrange for undertakers to remove the body.

The recognized clinical signs when verifying death are:

- *Absence:*
  - Of a carotid pulse over 1min.
  - Of heart sounds over 1min.
  - Of respiratory movements and breath sounds over 1min.
- Fixed, dilated pupils (unresponsive to bright lights).
- No response to painful stimuli (e.g. sternal rub).

Parenteral drug administration or any life-prolonging equipment should not be removed prior to verification.

### Unexpected and/or sudden deaths

Practitioners visiting in the home finding someone unexpectedly dead should:

- *Initiate life support:* if appropriate, including calling 999 (🕮 Adult basic life support, p. 742).
- *In unequivocal death:* e.g. hypostasis, rigor mortis, massive cranial damage, decomposition, either call 999 or the GP, depending on circumstances and knowledge of deceased person and do not move the body.

Some organizations have developed protocols for first-contact practitioners, working in OOH services, to verify unexpected deaths at home.

## Certification of death

The process of completing the 'Medical Certificate of Cause of Death'. By law, this must be completed by a medical practitioner who attended the deceased person during the last illness. The certificate is usually issued in a sealed envelope, addressed to the registrar (📖 Registration of births, marriages, and deaths, p. 786), and given to next of kin to take to register the death.

Medical practitioners report the death to the coroner (procurator fiscal in Scotland) if:

- A doctor had not seen the patient in the preceding 14 days (28 in Northern Ireland).
- Within 24h of admission to hospital.
- The death was sudden, violent, unnatural, or suspicious in any way.
- The cause is unknown or uncertain.
- The death occurred during surgery or recovery from anaesthetic.
- The death occurred in prison or policy custody.
- The cause was an industrial disease.

The coroner will decide whether a post-mortem and further investigation are required in order to determine the cause of death.

It is good practice for general practices and primary care nurses to inform other care services (e.g. hospitals, social services involved with the deceased person) of their death to avoid ongoing appointments, etc. Some general practices keep registers of deaths.

### Related topic

📖 Bereavement, grief, and coping with loss, p. 528.

### References

Home Office (2003). *Death Certification and in England, Wales and NI. A fundamental review Cm 5831*. Available at: ℘ www.archive2.official-documents.co.uk/document/cm58/5831/5831.pdf

NMC Confirmation of death for registered nurses. Available at: ℘ www.nmc-uk.org/Nurses-and-midwives/Regulation-in-practice/Regulation-in-Practice-Topics/Confirmation-of-death-for-registered-nurses-/

# Registration of births, marriages, and deaths

It has been a legal requirement since the mid-1800s for UK residents to register births, marriages, and deaths with the civil authorities. It is a criminal offence not to register births and deaths within specified time periods. Birth, marriage, and death certificates are copies of the entries made in the register for that district. The Registrar of births, marriages, and deaths is an official position in each LA and is responsible for the registers for that district. Details of how to find the Registrar are on every council website, in libraries, and the telephone book.

## Births

All births (including stillbirths) must be registered within 42 days in the district in which the birth occurred. This can be done by either parent or both if married. A father not married to the mother can register the birth jointly with her to ensure parental responsibility (*Note:* In the case of unmarried parents, only the mother has automatic right of parental responsibility). If neither the mother nor the father can register the birth, someone present at the birth, or with responsibility for the child, can do so. See also 📖 Postnatal care, p. 391; 📖 New birth visits, p. 168.

## Marriages

A man and a woman may marry if both are aged 16yrs or over, and single, widowed, or divorced, or in a civil partnership that has been dissolved. Same sex marriage is legal in England and Wales. Those aged 16 and 17 need parental consent. A transsexual person with a full gender recognition certificate can marry someone of the opposite sex. Details of prohibited marriages of relatives are available through the Citizens Advice Bureau (see 📖 Further information, p. 787). It can be a civil or religious ceremony. The legal requirements for a marriage are that it is conducted by, or in the presence of, someone authorized to register it, and it is entered into the marriage register.

## Civil partnerships

A legal relationship that is registered by two people of the same sex who are not related. It can only be ended by death or application for dissolution in a court.

## Deaths

A death must be registered within 5 days, but can be delayed for another 9 days if the registrar knows that a medical certificate of death has been issued. Deaths reported to coroners cannot be registered until investigations are completed. If the death was at home, the registration is in that district. If the death was in hospital or a care home, then registration is in the district of the institution. Death can only be registered by:
• A relative, present at death or last illness, or living in the district where death took place.
• Anyone present at the death.

- The owner/occupier of the building where the death occurred who is aware of the death.
- The person arranging the funeral.

The registrar will require the medical certificate of death and, if possible, certificates of birth and marriage, and an NHS medical card. See also 📖 Bereavement, grief, and coping with loss, p. 528; 📖 Sudden unexpected death of an infant, p. 295.

## Further information

Citizens Advice Bureau. Available at: ℅ www.adviceguide.org.uk

Gov.UK Births, deaths marriages and care. Available at: ℅ www.gov.uk/browse/births-deaths-marriages

# Time off work post-surgery

General guidance on expected recuperation time and time off work for uncomplicated procedures is in Table 14.2.

**Table 14.2** Guidance on time off work for uncomplicated procedures

| Operation | Minimum expected (wks) | Maximum expected if no complications (wks) |
| --- | --- | --- |
| Angiography/angioplasty | <1 | 4 |
| Appendectomy | 1 | 3 |
| Arthroscopy | <1 | <1 |
| Cataract surgery | 2 | 4 |
| Cholecystectomy | 2 | 3 |
| Colposcopy +/– cautery | <1 | <1 |
| CABG or valve surgery | 4 | 8 |
| Cystoscopy | <1 | <1 |
| D&C, ERPC, or TOP | <1 | <1 |
| Femoro-popliteal grafts | 4 | 12 |
| Haemorrhoid banding | <1 | <1 |
| Haemorrhoidectomy | 3 | 7 |
| Hysterectomy | 3 | 7 |
| Inguinal or femoral hernia—unilateral | 1 | 3 |
| Laparoscopy +/– sterilization | <1 | <1 |
| Laparotomy | 6 | 12 |
| Mastectomy | 2 | 6 |
| Pacemaker insertion | <1 | <1 |
| Pilonidal sinus | <1 | <1 |
| Retinal detachment | <1 | Avoid heavy work lifelong |
| Total hip or knee replacement | 12 | 26 |
| TURP | 2 | 5 |
| Vasectomy | <1 | <1 |

Reproduced with permission from Simon C, Everitt H, van Dorp F. (2010). *Oxford Handbook of General Practice*, 3rd edn. Oxford: Oxford University Press.

CABG, coronary artery bypass graft; D&C, dilation and curettage; ERCP, endoscopic retrograde cholangiopancreatography; TOP, termination of pregnancy; TURP, transurethral resection of the prostate

# Benefits and support

## Sources of information on benefits and support

Millions of pounds of state benefits go unclaimed every year in the UK, despite media portrayals of over claiming. Low income is one of the factors affecting health and wellbeing (📖 UK health profile, p. 2). In many places, welfare rights advisors work closely with primary care services to help increase uptake. This is a general guide for practitioners:

- Sources of information and agencies providing help can be found to assist in what is often a complicated eligibility and claim process.
- Agencies and their contact details who provide information and administer schemes of financial or in kind assistance (Table 14.3).
- The types of benefits and help available for:
  - People on low incomes (Table 14.4).
  - For mothers and those responsible for children (Table 14.5).
  - For illness, disability, and carers (Table 14.6).
  - Mobility for disabled people (Table 14.7).
- Types and sources of information about pensions (Table 14.8).

*Benefit fraud*

The DWP provides a freephone number (☎ 0800 854440) and a website. 🕭 https://secure.dwp.gov.uk/benefitfraud to give information about benefit fraud.

## Further information

Age UK. ☎ 0800 169 6565. Available at: 🕭 www.ageuk.org.uk/

Child Poverty Action Group *Annual Welfare Benefits & Tax Credits Handbook*:. Available at: 🕭 www.cpag.org.uk/

Citizens Advice Bureau: local offices. Available at: 🕭 www.adviceguide.org.uk

Department of Work and Pensions (DWP). Available at: 🕭 www.gov.uk/government/organisations/department-for-work-pensions

DWP. A short guide to the benefit system for General Practitioners. Available at: 🕭 www.dwp.gov.uk/docs/gp-benefit-guide.pdf

DWP health and work guidance for health professionals including the Health and Work Handbook (patient care and occupational health). Available at: 🕭 www.dwp.gov.uk/healthcare-professional/guidance/

Government information on benefits. Available at: 🕭 www.gov.uk/browse/benefits

**Table 14.3** Guide to public agencies providing financial or in kind assistance

| Agency | Function | Website: www. + suffix | Telephone |
|---|---|---|---|
| GOV.UK | Information on all UK government services and publicly funded | Benefits information gov.uk/browse/benefits | Benefits enquiry line: 0800 882 200<br>Textphone: 0800 243 355 |
| Job Centre Plus | Helps people of working age to find work and get any benefits they are entitled to | gov.uk/contact-jobcentre-plus | Jobs Centre Plus 0800 055 6688<br>Contact local office (list available on website) |
| Child Support Agency and Child Maintenance Service | Arranges child maintenance when separated parents cannot make own arrangements | gov.uk/child-maintenance | Contact local office (list available on website) |
| Pension service | Provides pensions, benefits (e.g. cold weather payment) and retirement information | gov.uk/contact-pension-service | Contact area office (list available on website) |
| HM Revenue & Customs | Administers tax credits, child benefit | hmrc.gov.uk/ | Tax credit enquiry line: 0345 300 3900<br>Child benefit: 0300 200 3100 |
| Disability and carers service | Delivers a range of benefits to disabled people and their carers | disability.gov.uk | Contact local disability benefits office (list available on gov.uk website) |
| Appeals service | Provides an independent tribunal body for hearing appeals | Appeals-service.gov.uk | N/A |
| Service personnel and veterans agency | Administers Ministry of Defence services including pensions and compensation | veterans-uk.info | 0800 169 22 77 |

❶ 030 numbers are now designated for use only by public bodies and not-for-profit organizations. Calls may be free or at local rates. Callers are advised at the point of the call. 0300 and 0800 numbers usually free.

## Benefits for people with a low income

**Table 14.4** Types of benefits available for those on low incomes

| Type | Detail |
|------|--------|
| Universal Credit | In England only replacing IS, JSA, ESA, CTC, and WTC, housing benefit, and budgeting; loans and crisis loans |
| Income support (IS) | • >18yrs (16yrs in some circumstances) and <state pension age,<br>• Be pregnant, a carer, lone parent with a child <5yrs, or unable to work through sickness or disability<br>• Low income, <£16,000 in savings (2013), not in full-time education |
| Job Seekers Allowance (JSA) | • ≥19yrs and below state pension age,<br>• Not in full time education, unemployed, or working <16hrs/wks<br>• Capable of and available for work<br>• Have Job Seekers agreement that contracts recipient to actively seek work |
| Pension credit | • *Guarantee credit:* >66yrs and low weekly income below a set level, e.g. 2013 £145.40 single person<br>• *Savings credit:* ≥66yrs and evidence of savings towards retirement. |
| Working tax credit (WTC) | Income is below a stated level *and*<br>• Age ≥16yrs, working ≥16h/wk and responsible for a child (<16yrs or 19yrs if in full-time education)<br>• Age ≥16yrs, working ≥16h/wk and has a disability<br>• Age ≥50yrs, working ≥16h/wk and has started work after ≥6mths of receiving 1 of certain benefits or age ≥25yrs and working ≥30h/wk |
| Children's tax credit (CTC) | Age ≥16yrs *and*<br>• Responsible for ≥1 child (<16yrs or 16–19yrs in full-time education)<br>• Family income <£50,000 pa |
| NHS benefits (Free) | *Automatic entitlement:*<br>• Age >60yrs or <16yrs<br>• Claiming IS or income-based JSA<br>• Pregnant or within 1yr of child birth<br>*By application:* low income and savings <£8000<br>*Benefits:* prescriptions, NHS dentistry, NHS eye tests and glasses, NHS wigs, and fabric supports, Travel to hospital, milk and vitamins for pregnant and breastfeeding women, and children <5yrs |
| Housing benefit | • Low income, living in rented housing<br>• *Exclusions:* full-time students without dependents, people in residential care or with savings >£16,000 |

*(continued)*

**Table 14.4** (Continued)

| Type | Detail |
|---|---|
| Council tax benefit | • *Council tax benefit:* low income. Exclusions as for housing benefit<br>• *Second adult rebate:* payable if someone who lives with you is aged >18yrs, does not pay rent or council tax, and has low income<br>• *Council tax reduction:* if single occupier or disabled<br>• *Disregarded occupants:* certain people including students, carers, and children, not counted in calculating number of people living at a property |
| Crisis grants | For those on low income benefits in event of an emergency or disaster. May be available at local authority level in England, through Scottish Welfare Fund and Discretionary Assistance Fund in Wales |

(❶ Subject to change in eligibility, amount, benefit amount caps, always check current information: 📖 Benefits and support, p. 789)

## Benefits for mothers and those responsible for children

**Table 14.5** Types of benefits available for mothers and those responsible for children

| Type | Detail and further information |
|---|---|
| Child benefit | • For those with responsible for the upbringing of a child aged <16yrs or 20yrs if in full-time non-higher education<br>• Tax-free benefit, unless the person claiming or partner has an individual income >£50,000<br>• Claim information available at: ℘ www.hmrc.gov.uk/forms/ch2-online-stubb.htm Child benefit helpline ☏ 0300 200 3100 |
| Child Trust Fund | • Long-term tax free savings account for children, now closed<br>• Born after 1 September 2002 and before 2 January 2011 |
| Child Tax Credit | • Changing to universal credit in England<br>• All families with children <16yrs or <20yrs if in approved education or training<br>• Household income < £20,000 yr (1 child), £30,000 (2 children) and £35,000 (3 children) |
| Healthy Start (milk, vitamins and fruit and vegetables school for those on low income) | • All pregnant ♀ <18yrs<br>• Pregnant (>10wks) and/or children <4yrs<br>• *Plus* receiving IS or JSA or CTC (📖 Benefits for people with a low income)<br>• Application and information at: ℘ www.healthystart.nhs.uk/ |
| NHS Benefits (free) | • *Automatic entitlement:* <16yrs, pregnant or within 1yr of child birth<br>• Prescriptions<br>• NHS dentistry<br>• Available at: ℘ www.nhs.uk/conditions/pregnancy-and-baby/pages/maternity-paternity-leave-benefits.aspx |
| SMP | • Has worked for same employer continuously for 26wks up to 15th week before baby is due<br>• Earning, on average, a stated amount (at least £109 a week in 2013)<br>• Proof of pregnancy should be sent to employer with MATB1 from doctor or midwife<br>• Further information available at: ℘ www.gov.uk/maternity-pay-leave |

*(Continued)*

**Table 14.5** (Continued)

| Type | Detail and further information |
|------|-------------------------------|
| Maternity allowance | • May be available for non-qualifiers for SMP<br>• Employed/self-employed for ≥26wks in the 66wks preceding the baby's due date<br>• Average weekly earnings of ≥£30/wk for at least 13wks of the test period<br>• Information and claim process ℘ www.gov.uk/maternity-allowance/overview |
| Sure Start maternity grant | • A one-off payment of £500 to help towards the cost of a child<br>• To qualify must have no other children (unless expecting multiple birth) and be in receipt of other benefits for low income, e.g. universal credit, IS, pension credit<br>• Information and claim process (within 11wks of EDD and 3mths of birth). Available at: ℘ www.gov.uk/sure-start-maternity-grant/overview |

(❶ Subject to change in eligibility, amount, caps, always check current information: 📖 Table 14.3, p. 790)

## Benefits for illness, disability and carers

**Table 14.6** Types of benefits available for people with illness or disability

| Type and information | Detail |
|---|---|
| Statutory sick pay (SSP). Available at: ℘ www.gov.uk/ statutory-sick-pay/overview | Weekly payment for those too ill to work made by employer for up to 28wks<br>*Eligibility*<br>• Employee age ≥16yrs and <65yrs<br>• Incapable of work due to sickness or disability<br>• Earning ≥National Insurance lower earnings limit (£109/wk in 2013)<br>• Inform employer of sickness within their reporting time |
| Employment and Support Allowance (ESA). Available at: ℘ www.gov.uk/incapacity-benefit | • Financial and work-related support if illness or disability affects ability to work and <state pension age, not receiving SMP, SSP, or JSA<br>• Amount depends on age, length of time ill and national insurance contributions<br>• After 14wks is either placed in a work-related activity group in which weekly meetings with advisor is required (failure to attend results in sanctions) *or*, if severely limited by illness or disability, placed in support-only group, and are not required to go to interviews |
| Disability premiums (income support). Available at: ℘ www.gov.uk/ disability-premiums-income-support/ overview | An extra amount added to income support (🕮 Benefits and support Table 14.4, p. 791) for those <state pension age, and either registered blind or receiving other benefits, such as disabled living allowance |
| Blind Person's Allowance). Available at: ℘ www.gov.uk/ blind-persons-allowance/overview | • Extra amount of income tax-free each year<br>• Eligibility in England and Wales: registered blind with local council<br>• Eligibility in Scotland and Northern Ireland: unable to perform work for which eyesight is essential |
| Disabled facilities grant | For work essential to help a disabled person live an independent life. Information and application via local council. Means tested |

*(Continued)*

**Table 14.6** (Continued)

| Type and information | Detail |
|---|---|
| Disability living Allowance (DLA) being replaced by Personal Independence Payment (PIP)). Available at: ℅ www.gov.uk/dla-disability-living-allowance-benefit/overview? | <ul><li>Disability >3mths or terminally ill (see below)</li><li><65yrs at time of application</li><li>*Mobility component:* help needed to get about outdoors<ul><li>*Higher rate*—unable/virtually unable to walk (age >3yrs)</li><li>*Lower rate*—guidance or supervision outdoors (age >5yrs)</li></ul></li><li>*Care component:* help needed with personal care<ul><li>*Lower rate*—attention/supervision needed for a significant proportion of the day or unable to prepare a cooked meal</li><li>*Middle rate*—attention/supervision throughout day, or repeated prolonged attention, or watching over at night</li><li>*Higher rate*—help or supervision through both day and night, or terminally ill</li></ul></li><li>Special rules for terminally ill (not expected to live >6mths)</li><li>Claim processed faster. Requires DLA claim form with a DS1500 form obtained and completed by doctor, specialist or consultant</li></ul> |
| Attendance allowance (AA). Available at: ℅ www.gov.uk/attendance-allowance | <ul><li>Available to those who need help with personal care, or someone to supervise for their or others safety, as a result of through physical or mental disability and >65yrs. Also not permanently in hospital or accommodation funded by the LA (but can be in sheltered accommodation)<ul><li>*Lower rate payment*—frequent help or constant attention, either during day or night</li><li>*Higher rate payment*—if 24-hr care required or terminal illness</li><li>*Special rules for terminally ill* (not expected to live >6mths)—claim processed faster. Requires AA claim form with a DS1500 form obtained and completed by doctor, specialist, or consultant</li></ul></li></ul> |

*(Continued)*

**Table 14.6** (Continued)

| Type and information | Detail |
|---|---|
| Constant Attendance Allowance (CAA). Available at: ℘ www.gov.uk/constant-attendance-allowance | • Payable to those in receipt of industrial injuries, disablement benefit, or a war disablement pension *and*<br>• 100% disabled as judge by medical examination<br>• In need of daily care and attention |
| Carers allowance. Available at: ℘ www.gov.uk/carers-allowance | • Available to any carer (does not have to be a relative or living with person) who meets eligibility criteria<br>• Has to be ≥16yrs *plus*<br>• Spends ≥35h/wk caring for a person with a disability who is getting AA or CAA, or middle or higher rate care component of DLA<br>• Not available to those earning >£100 a wk. after tax or in full time education |
| Carers Credit. Available at: ℘ www.gov.uk/carers-credit/overview | • This is a National Insurance credit that helps build entitlement to State Pension (💷 Pensions, p. 799)<br>• Eligibility includes >16yrs and <state pension age, and looking after someone in receipt of DLA, AA, or CAA for >20h/wk |

(❶ Subject to change in eligibility, amount, caps, always check current information: 💷 Table 14.3, p. 789)

## Mobility for disabled people

**Table 14.7** Types of support for mobility for people with disabilities

| Type and source of information | Detail |
|---|---|
| Blue badge parking scheme. Available at: ℘ www.gov.uk/apply-blue-badge | • Helps disabled drivers and passengers park close to their destinations<br>• Application through local council and varies by UK country |
| Motability scheme (Helpline 0845 456 4566). Available at: ℘ www.motability.co.uk/ | Run by an independent charity to enable disabled people lease a car at affordable prices |
| Road tax exemption. Available at: ℘ www.gov.uk/vehicle-exempt-from-car-tax | Available on application to disabled people in receipt of mobility component of DLA, or enhanced rate of PIP or war pensions mobility supplement |
| Seatbelt exemption. Available at: ℘ www.gov.uk/seat-belts-law/when-you-dont-need-to-wear-a-seat-belt | GPs issue a certificate of exemption on individual basis |
| Travel concessions for disabled people, e.g. bus pass | • Varies by country and locally<br>• Scotland. Available at: ℘ www.transportscotland.gov.uk<br>• Wales. Available at: ℘ wales.gov.uk/topics/transport/public/concessionary/fares<br>• Northern Ireland. Available at: ℘ www.nidirect.gov.uk/free-bus-travel-and-concessions |

## Related topics

📖 Anti-discriminatory health care, p. 76; 📖 Assistive technology, p. 776.

## Pensions

**Table 14.8** Types of pensions and benefits for pensioners

| Type and source of information | Detail and eligibility |
|---|---|
| State retirement pension. Available at: ℘ www.gov.uk/browse/working/state-pension | Eligibility based on sufficient years of National Insurance contributions paid through working life, currently 30yrs, but planned ↑. ♀ may be at risk of low contributions, but may have home responsibilities protection, or have bought additional voluntary contributions *and* At age of 65, if born after 06/04/1955 (a woman born between 06/04/1950 and 05/04/1955, gets State Pension when reaches State Pension age. This will be between 60 and 65, depending on DOB. |
| Additional State Pension. Available at: ℘ www.gov.uk/additional-state-pension | Automatically paid in addition to basic state pension if eligible If contributed to SERPS or second state pension scheme through employment or as a result of certain benefits |
| Pension Credit. Available at: ℘ www.gov.uk/pension-credit | • An income related benefit for those >65yrs • Guarantee credit tops up weekly income to a fixed amount (£145.40 for 1 person, £222.05 for couple in 2013) • Savings credit is an extra payment to those who have saved towards their retirement, e.g. a pension |
| War Pensions and War Widows Pensions | Information on eligibility and claims at ℘ www.gov.uk/war-widow-pension/overview and ℘ www.veterans-uk.info/ |
| Free TV licence. Available at: ℘ www.tvlicensing.co.uk/check-if-you-need-one/for-your-home/ | All pensioners >75yrs |
| Older persons travel concessions, e.g. bus pass >60yrs | • *England:* free off-peak travel on local buses and other forms of transport in some areas. Available at: ℘ www.gov.uk/apply-for-elderly-person-bus-pass • Scotland: available at: ℘ www.transportscotland.gov.uk/public-transport/concessionary-travel • Wales: available at: ℘ wales.gov.uk/topics/transport/public/concessionary/fares/?lang=en • Northern Ireland: available at: ℘ www.nidirect.gov.uk/free-bus-travel-and-concessions |
| Winter fuel payment. Available at: ℘ www.gov.uk/winter-fuel-payment/overview | • Annual payment to all >60yrs if live in UK, mostly at home (not in e.g. hospital, care home) • Have to apply if not also in receipt of other benefits |
| Cold weather payment. Available at: ℘ www.gov.uk/cold-weather-payment | • Paid when local temperature is either recorded as, or forecast to be, an average of 0°C or below for over 7 consecutive days • Only for those receiving pension credit or IS, JSA, ESA |
| Christmas bonus. Available at: ℘ www.gov.uk/christmas-bonus | One off tax free £10 payment made before Christmas to those receiving state pension and other types of pensions and benefits |

❶ Eligibility and rates may change over time, always check up-to-date information.

# Useful websites

### National Health Service Organizations

NHS England. Available at: ℘ www.england.nhs.uk
Department of Health, England. Available at: ℘ www.gov.uk/government/organisations/department-of-health
NHS Scotland. Available at: ℘ www.scot.nhs.uk
Health & Social Care Directorate, The Scottish Government. Available at: ℘ www.scotland.gov.uk/Topics/Health/About
NHS Wales. Available at: ℘ www.wales.nhs.uk
Health and Social Care Department, Wales. Available at: ℘ wales.gov.uk/topics/health/?lang=en
Department of Health, Social Services and Public Safety, Northern Ireland. Available at: ℘ www.dhsspsni.gov.uk

### Professional and Trade Union Organizations

Nursing and Midwifery Council. Available at: ℘ www.nmc-uk.org
Royal College of Nursing includes country-specific web pages. Available at: ℘ www.rcn.org.uk
Community Practitioner and Health Visitors Association (part of Unite: the Union). Includes country specific websites. Available at: ℘ www.unitetheunion.org/how-we-help/list-of-sectors/healthsector/healthsectoryourprofession/cphva
Queens Nursing Institute (and Scotland). Available at: ℘ www.qni.org.uk
The Queens Nursing Institute (and Scotland). Available at: ℘ www.qni.org.uk Unison (Public Service Trade Union). Available at: ℘ www.unison.org.uk

### Evidence-based health care

NICE Evidence Search Health & Social Care (includes clinical knowledge summaries, journals, and public health). Available at: ℘ www.evidence.nhs.uk
National Institute for Health and Care Excellence includes public health. Available at: ℘ www.nice.org.uk
Scottish Intercollegiate Guidelines Network. Available at: ℘ www.sign.ac.uk

### Evidence-based prescribing

Medicines and prescribing support for NICE. Available at: ℘ www.nice.org.uk/mpc
*British National Formulary*. Available at: ℘ www.bnf.org
*British National Formulary for Children*. Available at: ℘ www.bnfc.nhs.uk/bnfc

### UK Primary and Community Nursing Electronic Network Groups (active in 2013)

Practice nurses discussion group. Available at: ℘ www.practicenursing.co.uk/forum/home.aspx
International Collaboration for Community Health Nursing Research. Available at: ℘ www.icchnr.org

SENATE for health visiting and school nursing. Available at: ℘ health.groups.yahoo.com/group/SENATE-HVSN

## Other sources of information on UK Primary and Community Nursing

The Directory of Community Health Services is published annually by Pavilion Publishing. Available at: ℘ www.pavpub.com/p-636-directory-of-community-health-mental-health-and-learning-disabilities-201314.aspx

## Health Advice and Information Services to the Public

NHS Choices (information). Available at: ℘ www.nhs.uk
NHS Direct England ☎ 111. Available at: ℘ www.nhsdirect.nhs.uk
NHS Direct Wales ☎ 0845 46 47. Available at: ℘ www.nhsdirect.wales.nhs.uk
NHS24 Scotland ☎ 08454 24 24 24. Available at: ℘ www.nhs24.com

## Useful general information sites

Citizens Advice Bureau. Available at: ℘ www.adviceguide.org.uk
UK government information on all public services. Available at: ℘ www.gov.uk
Telephone directories. Available at: ℘
www.thephonebook.bt.com
www.yell.com
Maps. Available at: ℘
www.streetmap.co.uk
www.multimap.com

*Note:* many other websites and sources of information are given at the end of each topic.

# Index